Anatomy&Physiology
for PARAMEDICAL PRACTICE

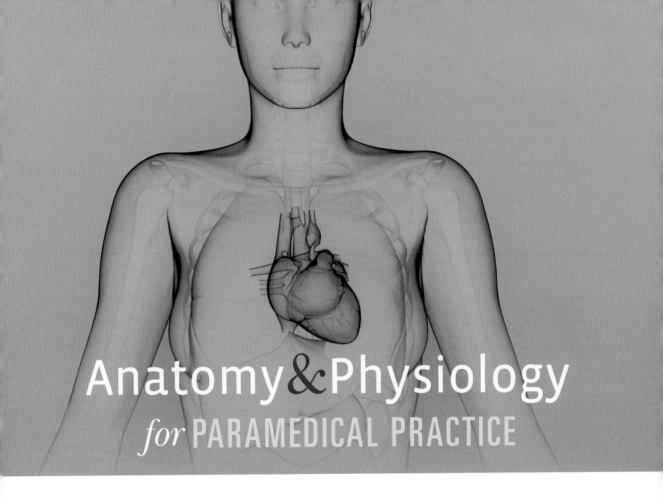

Anatomy & Physiology
for PARAMEDICAL PRACTICE

ROGER W. SOAMES
BSC, PHD

Professor Emeritus
Centre for Anatomy and Human Identification
School of Science and Engineering, University
of Dundee
Dundee, Scotland, UK

ABDUELMENEM ALASHKHAM
MBBS, MSC, PHD

Programme Director for the MSc in Clinical
and Human Anatomy Programmes
Edinburgh Medical School, University of
Edinburgh
Edinburgh, Scotland, UK

ELSEVIER

Notices

ISBN: 978-0-443-11517-2

Content Strategist: Andrae Akeh
Content Project Manager: Shravan Kumar
Design: Brian Salisbury
Illustration Manager: Akshaya Mohan
Marketing Manager: Deborah Watkins

Printed in India

Last digit is the print number: 9   8   7   6   5   4   3   2   1

Working together
to grow libraries in
developing countries

ELSEVIER   Book Aid International

www.elsevier.com • www.bookaid.org

CONTENTS

Preface, ix
Acknowledgements, x
About the authors, xi

Introduction, 1
Organisation of the Book, 1
Aim, 1
Regions and Systems, 1
Terminology, 2
Terms Used to Describe Movement, 3
Physiological Terms, 5

1 Cells, Tissues and Organs, 7
Overview, 8
Cells, 9
Cell Membrane, 9
Cytoplasm, 12
Nucleus, 15
Cell Cycle, 17
Stem Cells, 17
Apoptosis, 19
Tissues 19
Epithelium, 19
Connective Tissues, 25
Muscle, 38
Nervous Tissue, 44
Organs, 53
Skin, 53

2 Thorax (Chest), 65
Overview, 66
Thoracic Cage, 66
Bones and Joints, 68
Muscles, 72
Thoracic Inlet, 79
Thoracic Outlet, 80
Thoracic Cavity, 80
Mediastinum and Contents, 80
Respiratory System, 93
Cardiovascular System, 116
Blood, 164

3 Vertebral Column (Back), 187
Overview, 188
Vertebral Column, 188
Introduction, 188
Bones, 191
Intervertebral Joints, 195
Movements of the Vertebral Column, 200
Stability, 200
Blood and Nerve Supply of the Vertebral Column, 201
Muscles of the Trunk, 202
Spinal Cord, 204
Meninges, 206
Internal Structure and Organisation, 210
Spinal Nerves, 220
Somatic Nervous System, 221
Autonomic Nervous System, 223

4 Head and Neck, 231
Overview, 234
Skull, 234
Growth of the Skull, 235
External Features, 236
Cranial Cavity, 242
Brain, 243
Glial Cells, 247
Adult Morphology, 247
Motor System, 263
Sensory System, 263
Limbic System, 263
Meninges, 264
Arterial Supply, 264
Venous Drainage 269
Cranial Nerves, 270
Olfactory Nerve (I), 272
Optic Nerve (II), 272
Oculomotor Nerve (III), 273
Trochlear Nerve (IV), 273
Trigeminal Nerve (V), 274
Abducens Nerve (VI), 276
Facial Nerve (VII), 276

Vestibulocochlear Nerve (VIII), 277
Glossopharyngeal Nerve (IX), 277
Vagus Nerve (X), 279
Accessory Nerve (XI), 280
Hypoglossal Nerve (XII), 280
Mandible, 282
Growth of the Mandible, 282
Temporomandibular Joint, 283
Infratemporal Fossa, 287
Face, 287
Blood Supply and Innervation, 287
Muscles of the Face, 292
Orbit, 294
External Nose, 304
Nasal Cavity, 304
Oral Cavity, 308
Ear, 314
Neck, 317
Cervical Vertebrae, 317
Regions, 317
Endocrine System, 333
Hormones, 334
Endocrine Glands 334
Pituitary Gland, 335
Thyroid Gland, 340
Parathyroid Glands, 342
Adrenal (Suprarenal) Glands, 343
Islets of Langerhans, 347
Gonads, 351
Pineal Gland 368
Kidneys, 368
Heart, 368
Thymus, 369
Hypothalamus, 369
Local Hormones, 369

5 Upper Limb, 377
Overview, 378
Introduction, 378
Pectoral Region, 379
Clavicle, 379
Sternoclavicular Joint, 381
Scapula, 383
Acromioclavicular Joint, 384
Movements of the Pectoral Girdle, 384
Muscles, 386
Arm, 387
Humerus, 387

Shoulder Joint, 391
Axilla, 398
Compartments of the Arm, 402
Forearm, 404
Radius, 404
Ulna, 406
Elbow Joint, 407
Cubital Fossa, 411
Radioulnar Joints, 412
Compartments of the Forearm, 414
Wrist 418
Carpus, 420
Wrist Joint, 420
Hand, 424
Metacarpals and Phalanges, 425
Carpometacarpal Joints, 426
Metacarpophalangeal Joints, 427
Interphalangeal Joints, 430
Function of the Hand 432
Blood Supply and Lymphatic Drainage, 435
Summary of Nerves and Muscles, 435
Major Nerves of the Upper Limb and the Muscles They Innervate, 435
Muscles Supplied by Each Root of the Brachial Plexus, 441
Movements in Each Region of the Upper Limb, the Muscles Responsible and Their Innervation, 442

6 Abdomen, Pelvis and Perineum, 449
Overview, 450
Abdomen and Pelvis, 450
Anterior and Lateral Abdominal Walls, 453
Pelvic Floor, 458
Abdominal Regions, 459
Digestive System, 461
Digestive Tract, 464
Digestive Physiology, 485
Urinary System, 508
Kidney, 509
Ureter, 523
Bladder, 523
Urethra, 527
Micturition, 528
Reproductive System, 530
Sex Determination, 531
Male Reproductive System, 532
Female Reproductive System, 541

Uterus, 543
Perineum, 550
  Urogenital Triangle, 550
  Anal Triangle, 555
  Neurovascular Supply of the Perineum, 556

7 **Lower Limb, 563**
   Overview, 564
      Introduction, 564
      Pelvic Girdle, 567
        Innominate, 567
        Symphysis Pubis, 569
        Sacrum and Coccyx, 569
        Sacroiliac Joint, 570
        Lumbosacral Joint, 573
        Sacrococcygeal Joint, 573
        Function of the Pelvic Girdle, 574
        Relations, 574
        Gluteal Region/Buttocks, 580
      Thigh, 582
        Femur, 582
        Hip Joint, 584
        Femoral Triangle, 588
        Compartments of the Thigh, 589
      Calf/Leg, 594
        Tibia, 596
        Fibula, 598
        Patella, 598
        Knee Joint, 598
        Popliteal Fossa, 608

Tibiofibular Joints, 611
Compartments of the Calf/Leg, 612
Ankle, 615
  Ankle Joint, 616
Foot, 624
  Tarsus, 625
  Metatarsals and Phalanges, 626
  Joints of the Foot, 626
  Subtalar Joint, 626
  Transverse (Mid) Tarsal Joint, 626
  Tarsometatarsal Joints, 627
  Metatarsophalangeal Joints, 627
  Interphalangeal Joints, 629
  Dorsum of the Foot, 629
  Plantar Aspect (Sole) of the Foot, 634
  Function of the Foot, 636
  Walking, 636
Summary of Nerves and Muscles, 638
  *Major Nerves of the Lower Limb and the
    Muscles They Innervate, 638*
  *Muscles of the Lower Limb Supplied by Each
    Nerve Root, 641*
  *Movements in Each Region of the Lower
    Limb, the Muscles Responsible and Their
    Innervation, 642*

Answers to Self-Test Questions, 649
Index, 655

The processes underlying survival in living organisms occur at many levels, from what happens within individual cells to the complex interaction between cells within different body systems. To appreciate and understand how this happens, how it is controlled and maintained requires a knowledge and understanding of many disciplines, including anatomy, biochemistry, genetics, pathology, pharmacology and physiology among others. A sound knowledge of anatomy (including the relevant embryology and histology) and physiology (including physiological processes) provides the basis for such an understanding. Once this has been achieved, how these disciplines interact can then be appreciated.

Although currently available anatomy and physiology texts present both the anatomy and physiology, it is imperative that physiology and physiological processes are based on a strong anatomical foundation and understanding. In most, if not all, texts the physiology is presented in terms of systems (cardiovascular, reproductive), while in this book the anatomy and physiology are presented regionally with extensive cross referencing to other relevant regions to enable the system to be appreciated and fully understood; this was a conscious decision. When dealing with patients, healthcare professionals are confronted with pathology and/or trauma to a specific body region (chest, abdomen). In addition, most, if not all, texts fail to provide (i) the relevant development required to understand why the body is organised as it is, and (ii) the underlying anatomical structure, in terms of its gross anatomy, histology and/or cell biology, underpinning physiology.

This book brings together anatomy and physiology in a way relevant to those preparing for a career in paramedical and healthcare practice. Anatomy is best taught regionally, that is by considering each region of the body separately, so that the relationships between structures in each region can be emphasised. In contrast, physiology is best taught by systems without recourse to regions, as physiological processes occur in many regions at the same time. This creates a dilemma, should a regional approach be adopted based around anatomy or should a systems approach be adopted based on physiology. In this book a regional approach has been adopted, in which anatomy, including, where appropriate, relevant embryology and histology to aid understanding of adult structure and function, is presented first followed by the systems found within each region.

The underlying tenet of the book is that a sound anatomical knowledge underpins successful understanding of physiology and physiology processes. It is, however, accepted that systems are not entirely contained within any one region. When a system is present in more than one region, which applies to all systems, the reader is directed to other regions. The respiratory system, for example, lies mainly within the thorax (chest), but also in the head and neck. Similarly, the major organ (heart) of the circulatory system also lies within the thorax, but has components (blood vessels) extending into all regions of the body.

In each chapter, the anatomy is covered first, with the physiology of the various structures following. In this way, the reader is logically guided through the structure, intricacies and functioning of the human body. Numerous textboxes are included covering applied anatomy, clinical anatomy, applied physiology and clinical physiology. At the end of each chapter, there are a selection of self-assessment multiple choice questions (MCQs); answers to these MCQs are available at the end of the book. Rather than commission new artwork, existing illustrations from the image collection held by Elsevier have been used (i) to avoid duplication of already excellent artwork, and (ii) to be more environment friendly.

Roger Soames
Abduelmenem Alashkham
2023

ACKNOWLEDGEMENTS

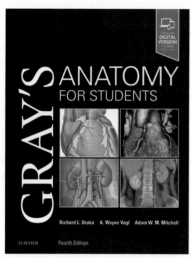

We would like to acknowledge the significant number of figures included in this book from *Gray's Anatomy for Students 4e* (ISBN: 9780323393041) with permission. We extend our sincere thanks to the authors of this leading anatomy text, Richard L Drake, A Wayne Vogel and Adam WM Mitchell.

ABOUT THE AUTHORS

Roger Soames joined the Centre for Anatomy and Human Identification at the University of Dundee in 2007 as Principal Anatomist; he was formerly Associate Professor and Head of Anatomy at James Cook University Queensland Australia. In 2009, he was appointed to a personal chair in Functional and Applied Anatomy and later the same year to the Cox Chair of Anatomy; he is currently Emeritus Professor of Functional and Applied Anatomy. His career has been within the discipline of anatomy, teaching and examining on a wide range of undergraduate and postgraduate degree programmes and courses; he has also developed new programmes of study at both undergraduate and postgraduate levels. He retains research interests in the musculoskeletal system and continues to publish this area.

Abduelmenem Alashkham graduated in medicine from the University of Zawia, Libya. He practiced as an orthopaedic surgeon before coming to the UK. In 2010, he gained an MSc in Human Anatomy (with distinction) and a PhD from the University of Dundee. He is currently Lecturer in Anatomy at the University of Edinburgh and Programme Director of the MSc Human and Clinical Anatomy programmes and teaches anatomy on a number of degree programmes. He has published several manuscripts and abstracts. He is a general reviewer of Grant's Dissector 17th and 18th editions, Grant's Atlas for Anatomy 15th and 16th editions, and Snell Neuroanatomy 9th Edition.

ORGANISATION OF THE BOOK

The processes underlying survival in living organisms occur at many levels, from what happens within individual cells to the complex interaction between cells within different body systems. To appreciate and understand how this happens and how it is controlled and maintained requires a knowledge and understanding of many disciplines, including anatomy, biochemistry, genetics, pathology, pharmacology and physiology, among others. A sound knowledge of anatomy, including the relevant embryology and histology, and physiology, including physiological processes, provides the basis for such an understanding. Once this has been achieved, how these disciplines interact can then be appreciated.

This book brings together anatomy and physiology in a way relevant for those preparing for a career in paramedical practice. Anatomy is best taught regionally, that is, by considering each region of the body separately so that the relationships between structures in each region can be emphasised. In contrast, physiology is best taught by systems without recourse to regions, as physiological processes occur in many regions at the same time. This creates a dilemma: should a regional approach be adopted based around anatomy or should a systems approach be adopted based on physiology? In this book, a regional approach has been adopted, whereby anatomy, including, where appropriate, relevant embryology and histology to aid understanding of adult structure and function, is presented first followed by the systems found within each region.

The underlying tenet of the book is that a sound anatomical knowledge underpins successful understanding of physiology and physiological processes. It is, however, accepted that systems are not entirely contained within any one region. When a system is present in more than one region, which applies to all systems, the reader is directed to other regions. The respiratory system, for example, lies not only mainly within the thorax (chest) but also in the head and neck. Similarly, the major organ (heart) of the circulatory system also lies within the thorax, but it has components (blood vessels) extending into all regions of the body.

AIM

The aim of this book is to provide an integrated and coherent account of anatomy and physiology to underpin a career in paramedical practice.

REGIONS AND SYSTEMS

From an anatomical perspective, the human body is divided into five major regions: head and neck; thorax; abdomen, pelvis and perineum; upper limb and lower limb. However, some structures are found within more than one region: for example, the vertebral column is located in the neck, thorax and abdomen. Nevertheless, each region allows structures to be described and their relationship to one another to be determined. A knowledge of these relationships is important in disease/pathology and/or trauma. The transitional areas between the neck, thorax and upper limb, and between the pelvis and lower limb are extremely important as major structures pass between them. Each region contains parts of several systems, as outlined below.

The *thorax* contains parts of the circulatory, respiratory, digestive, lymphatic, skeletal, muscular, nervous, immune and endocrine systems.

The *abdomen*, *pelvis* and *perineum* contain parts of the digestive, renal, reproductive, endocrine, lymphatic, immune, muscular, skeletal and nervous systems.

The *head* and *neck* contain parts of the skeletal, muscular, nervous, digestive, immune, circulatory, respiratory, endocrine and lymphatic systems.

The *upper limb* contains parts of the skeletal, muscular, nervous, circulatory and lymphatic systems.

Similarly, the *lower limb* also contains parts of the skeletal, muscular, nervous, circulatory and lymphatic systems.

There are a number of systems within the human body; although each is independent structurally and functionally, they are all interdependent. The basic physiological functions include: the provision of oxygen and nutrients; the removal of waste products; the maintenance of blood pressure and body temperature; intellectual functions; and special sensations. In the course of evolutionary development, separate systems have developed for specific functions, these being the circulatory, digestive, endocrine, immune, limbic, lymphatic, muscular, nervous, renal, reproductive, respiratory and skeletal systems. The relationships between them are important in understanding their interaction and the control they have over all body functions.

Parts of the *skeletal, muscular, nervous, circulatory* and *lymphatic* systems are found in all regions of the body.

The *respiratory* system is mainly found in the thorax, but it has components in the head and neck.

The *renal, digestive and reproductive* systems are found in the abdomen, pelvis and perineum.

The effects of the *endocrine* system can be seen in most regions, but its principal components are located in the head and neck, thorax, and abdomen, pelvis and perineum.

The effects of the *immune* system can be seen in all regions; its principal components are located in the head and neck, and abdomen, pelvis and perineum.

The *limbic* system is located entirely within the head and neck.

TERMINOLOGY

To be able to convey information about the position of a structure or a movement, it is important that colleagues in other health professions, as well as those within the same profession, use the same internationally accepted terminology. To facilitate this, the most important descriptive aspect is the adoption of a standard position of the human body to which all terms apply, irrespective of whether the individual is standing, sitting down or lying prone or supine. The standard position (the anatomical position) is shown in Fig. I.1 and is described as: standing erect and facing forwards, the legs together with the feet parallel and toes facing forwards, and the arms hanging loosely by the side, palms facing forwards with the thumbs pointing away from the body.

Mutually perpendicular imaginary reference planes (Fig. I.1) are superimposed on the anatomical position to aid understanding of the relationships between structures, as well as movement between body segments. Passing from front to back through the body dividing it into symmetrical left and right halves is the *sagittal (median) plane*, with any plane parallel to it being a *parasagittal (paramedian) plane*. Passing from top to bottom dividing the body into anterior and posterior parts is the

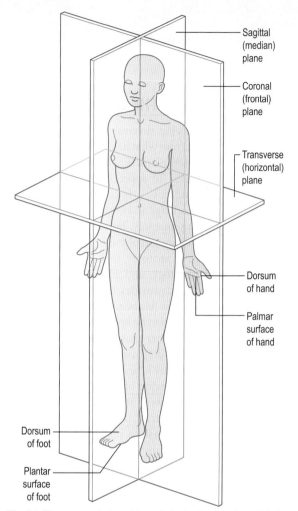

Fig. I.1 The anatomical position of the body, together with the cardinal planes.

coronal (frontal) plane: all planes dividing the body this way are known as coronal planes. Finally, any plane passing through the body horizontally dividing it into upper and lower parts is a *transverse (horizontal) plane*: when discussing or presenting a specific transverse section it is necessary to specify the level at which it is taken, either by referring to the vertebral level or position within a limb.

Anatomy tends to use specific terminology when referring to the position of structures or body parts. These terms are given below and shown in Fig. I.2.

Anterior: in front of or towards the front

Posterior: behind or towards the back

Superior: above (in relation to the trunk and nervous system the term *cephalic* may be used)

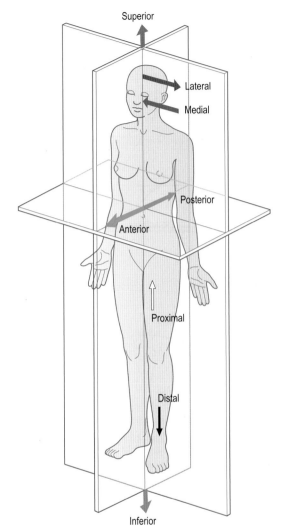

Fig. I.2 Directional terms.

Inferior: below (in relation to the trunk and nervous system the term *caudal* may be used)
Lateral: away from the median sagittal plane (midline)
Medial: towards the median sagittal plane (midline)
Distal: further away from the trunk or root of a limb
Proximal: closer to the trunk or root of a limb
Superficial: closer to the body surface
Deep: further away from the body surface

Terms Used to Describe Movement

In association with a particular joint, a single axis can usually be identified within each plane about which movements occur. In a parasagittal plane, an anteroposterior axis permits *abduction* and *adduction* in a coronal plane. A transverse axis in a coronal plane permits *flexion* and *extension* in a parasagittal plane, while a vertical axis in a coronal plane permits *medial* and *lateral rotation* in a transverse plane.

By arranging the axes to intersect at joint centres, the action of groups of muscles in producing movement at a joint can be understood. However, joint movement rarely occurs about a single axis in a single plane; they invariably occur in two or three planes simultaneously, producing complex patterns of movement. All movements are described with respect to their neutral position, i.e., the anatomical position.

Flexion: bending adjacent body segments in a parasagittal plane so that their anterior surfaces move towards each other, e.g., bending the elbow so that anterior surfaces of the arm and forearm move towards each other (Fig. I.3A). However, due to opposite rotations of the limb buds during development, at the knee joint it is the posterior surfaces of the thigh and calf that move towards each other during flexion.

Extension: bending adjacent body segments in a parasagittal plane so that their posterior surfaces move towards each other, e.g., bending the wrist so that posterior surfaces of the hand and forearm move towards each other (Fig. I.3B). Extension also refers to the moving apart of two opposing surfaces in a parasagittal plane, as in straightening the flexed elbow or knee.

At the ankle and in the foot, flexion and extension are referred to as plantarflexion and dorsiflexion, respectively.

Plantarflexion: moving the top (dorsum) of the foot away from the anterior surface of the calf/leg (Fig. I.3C).

Dorsiflexion: moving the dorsum of the foot towards the anterior surface of the calf/leg (Fig. I.3C).

Abduction: movement in a coronal plane away from the midline of the body or limb, e.g., moving the upper limb away from the trunk (Fig. I.3D).

Adduction: movement in a coronal plane towards the midline of the body or limb, e.g., moving the upper limb towards the trunk (Fig. I.3D).

Lateral flexion (bending): movement of the trunk (vertebral column) to the right or left in the coronal plane (Fig. I.3E).

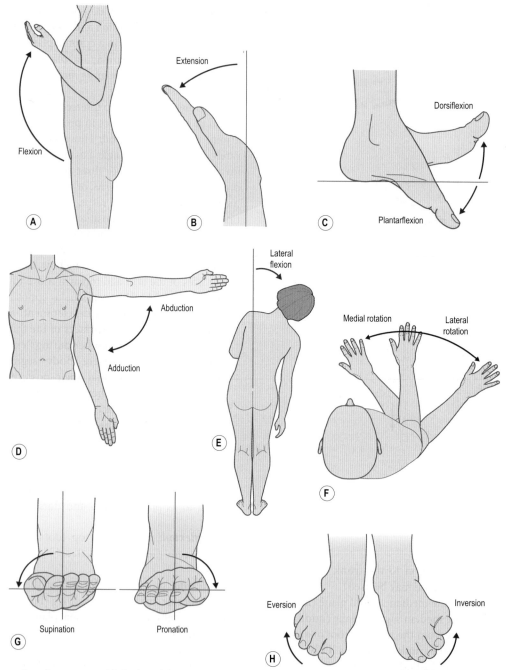

Fig. I.3 Examples of movement: (A) flexion of the elbow; (B) extension of the wrist; (C) plantarflexion and dorsiflexion of the foot at the ankle; (D) abduction and adduction of the upper limb; (E) lateral flexion of the trunk; (F) medial and lateral rotation of the upper limb; (G) supination and pronation of the hand with the wrist flexed; (H) inversion and eversion of the foot.

Medial rotation: rotation of the whole or part of a limb about its longitudinal axis so that its anterior surface faces towards the midline, e.g., moving the flexed forearm and hand towards the midline (Fig. I.3F).

Lateral rotation: rotation of the whole or part of a limb about its longitudinal axis so that its anterior surface faces away from the midline, e.g., moving the flexed forearm and hand away from the midline (Fig. I.3F).

Supination and pronation are used to describe specific movements of the forearm and of the foot.

Supination: in the forearm, supination turns the hand to face forwards, e.g., with the wrist flexed, the palm of the hand faces superiorly (Fig. I.3G). In the foot, supination turns the sole of the forefoot to face medially: it is always accompanied by adduction of the forefoot.

Pronation: in the forearm, pronation turns the hand to face posteriorly, e.g., with the wrist flexed, the palm of the hand faces inferiorly (Fig. I.3G). In the foot, pronation turns the sole of the forefoot to face laterally: it is always accompanied by abduction of the forefoot.

Inversion and eversion are complex composite movements of the foot.

Inversion: movement turning the sole of the foot to face medially (Fig. I.3H); it is a combination of supination and adduction of the forefoot.

Eversion: movement turning the sole of the foot to face laterally (Fig. I.3H); it is a combination of pronation and abduction of the forefoot.

PHYSIOLOGICAL TERMS

Many physiological terms are used within the text; however, most are best considered in context and as such are covered within the relevant chapter and section. Those terms listed below are fundamental to an understanding of the movement of fluid and substances across membranes that they are defined below.

Osmosis: the passage of water and small molecules across a semipermeable membrane so that the concentration on each side becomes the same.

Diffusion (passive transport): the mixing of two substances/gases so that the composition of each becomes the same. It is also used to denote the passage of small molecules of acids and salts through a semipermeable membrane.

Facilitated diffusion: occurs at specific sites in the membrane where substances can cross but can only take place when the concentration of the substance outside the cell is greater than that inside.

Active transport: a process in which substances are accumulated or expelled from cells irrespective of their concentrations on either side of the membrane. For example, the way cells accumulate potassium (K^+) and expel sodium (Na^+) to maintain a high concentration of potassium inside the cell relative to outside. It requires the presence of specific carriers in the membrane, but it differs from facilitated transport as substances can be accumulated irrespective of their concentration on either side of the membrane; it can only do this using energy.

Cells, Tissues and Organs

CONTENTS

Key Concepts, 7
Learning Outcomes, 8
Overview, 8
Cells, 9
Cell Membrane, 9
Transport Across Membranes, 11
Cytoplasm, 12
Endoplasmic Reticulum, 12
Golgi Apparatus/Complex, 12
Lysosomes, 12
Peroxisomes, 13
Proteasomes, 14
Mitochondria, 14
Cytoskeleton, 15
Nucleus, 15
Nuclear Membrane, 16
Chromatin, 17
Nucleolus, 17
Cell Cycle, 17
Mitosis, 17
Stem Cells, 17
Meiosis, 19
Apoptosis, 19
Tissues, 19
Epithelium, 19

Classification, 20
Function, 20
Secretory Epithelia and Glands, 23
Connective Tissues, 25
Cells, 25
Fibres, 26
Ground Substance, 27
Types of Connective Tissue, 27
Blood, 38
Muscle, 38
Smooth Muscle, 38
Cardiac Muscle, 39
Skeletal Muscle, 39
Nervous Tissue, 44
Neuron, 46
Action Potential, 50
Peripheral Nervous System, 50
Nerve Endings, 52
Nerve Injury, 52
Organs, 53
Skin, 53
Functions, 54
Structure, 55
Wound Repair, 57
Appendages of Skin, 58

KEY CONCEPTS

- Cells are the basic living unit of the body.
- Specialised cells have different functions.
- Most cells contain a nucleus surrounded by cytoplasm enclosed by a cell membrane.
- Cell membranes allow communication between the interior and exterior of the cell.
- The movement of substances across cell membranes can be either passive or active.
- The cytoplasm contains several different organelles with specific functions.
- The cytoskeleton determines cell shape and provides structural support for the cell.

- Most cells undergo cycles of growth and division (mitosis); stem cells undergo meiosis.
- There are four basic tissue types: epithelial, connective, muscular and nervous.
- Epithelial cells provide the lining and covering of tissues and organs.
- Connective tissues comprise fat, cartilage, bone and blood.
- Muscular tissue is of three types: smooth, cardiac and skeletal.

- Nervous tissue is present throughout the body enabling it to respond to changes in both the internal and external environments.
- Organs have specific functions determined by the combination of cell types and tissues within them.
- Skin is the largest organ in the body having protective, sensory, thermoregulatory, and metabolic functions.

LEARNING OUTCOMES

At the end of this chapter, you should be able to:
- Understand the difference between cells, tissues and organs.
- Describe the constituent components of cells and understand their function.
- Describe the cell cycle and understand the difference between mitosis and meiosis.
- Describe the classification of epithelium and understand where each type is found and why.
- Describe and understand the way epithelial cells adhere to and communicate with each other.
- Describe the different cell and fibre types present within connective tissue and understand the role of each.
- Describe the different types of connective tissue and their locations.
- Describe the process of ossification, growth and remodelling of bone.
- Describe the structural organisation of bone tissue and the function of different bone cells.
- Describe the types of bone fractures and the process of fracture repair.
- Describe the different types of fibrous, cartilaginous and synovial joints, where they are located and their function.

- Describe the different types of muscle tissue and the role of each type.
- Describe the innervation of muscle, including muscle spindles and Golgi tendon organs.
- Describe the structure and function of a nerve cell and the process of myelination.
- Describe the different types of nerve fibres within the peripheral nervous system.
- Describe the structure of a peripheral nerve and its constituent parts and the ways in which nerve fibres communicate with each other.
- Describe the structure, characteristics and function of skin.
- Describe the location and function of glands associated with skin.
- Describe the variety of nerve endings found within skin and their function.
- Describe the process of wound repair.
- Understand the influence of pathology and/ or trauma on cells, epithelium, and connective, muscular and nervous tissue.

OVERVIEW

This chapter is divided into three parts (cells, tissues, organs). Initially, it considers basic cellular organisation, both histologically (structure) and physiologically (function), followed by the different types of cells in the body and the function of each.

The second part considers how cells are organised to form tissues and includes an account of the function of each tissue type. The third part considers how different types of tissues come together to form organs, of which skin is the largest: the importance of skin, in terms of its structure, organisation and function, is discussed.

CELLS

Cells are the basic living unit of the body, with different cell types adapted to perform a single or limited number of functions (Table 1.1). Although they differ from each other in shape and function, all eukaryotic (animal) cells, except red blood cells (erythrocytes), consist of two major parts (nucleus, cytoplasm): the nucleus is separated from the cytoplasm by the nuclear membrane, while the cytoplasm is separated from the surrounding body fluids by the cell (plasma) membrane (plasmalemma) (Fig. 1.1). Although the cell membrane defines the outer limit of the cell, a continuum exists between the cell interior and extracellular macromolecules. Cells are composed of five basic substances (water, electrolytes, proteins, lipids, carbohydrates) collectively called the protoplasm.

The fluid part of the cytoplasm (cytosol) contains metabolically active structures (intracellular organelles), as well as protein components of the cytoplasmic cytoskeleton, which determine the shape and motility of the cell (Fig. 1.2); there are also numerous other inclusions (deposits of carbohydrates, lipids, pigments) and hundreds of enzymes producing the building blocks for larger molecules or breaking down small molecules to release energy. Oxygen, carbon dioxide, electrolytic ions, low-molecular-weight substrates, metabolites and waste products diffuse freely through the cytosol where they are used or produced or are bound to proteins entering or leaving organelles.

Within cells, oxygen reacts with carbohydrates, fat and protein to release the energy necessary for cell function; cells release the end products of their chemical reactions into the surrounding fluid. In addition, all cells are capable of reproducing cells of their own kind; however, when some cells are destroyed or die, they cannot be replaced, leading to a loss of function of the tissue/organ they are part of.

Cell Membrane

The cell membrane is a thin pliable elastic structure consisting of proteins (55%), phospholipids (25%), cholesterol (13%), other lipids (4%) and carbohydrates (3%). The lipid bilayer (thin double-layered film of lipids) of phospholipid molecules is continuous over the entire surface of the cell, with large globular protein molecules interspersed in the film (Fig. 1.3); the end of the phospholipid molecule in the outer and inner parts of the membrane is soluble in water (hydrophilic), while the middle part of the membrane is soluble only in fats (hydrophobic). The hydrophilic parts of the membrane are in contact with the intracellular and extracellular

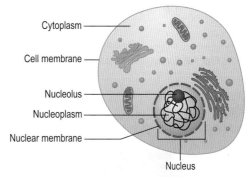

Fig. 1.1 Basic structure of a eukaryotic (animal) cell.

TABLE 1.1 **Different Cell Types and Their Function**	
Cell Type	**Function**
Epithelial cells	The lining/covering of tissues/organs
Fibroblasts, osteoblasts, chondroblasts	Synthesis and secretion of extracellular components
Neurons and sensory cells	Conversion of physical/chemical energy into action potentials
Digestive gland cells	Synthesis and secretion of digestive enzymes
Mucous gland cells	Synthesis and secretion of glycoproteins
Some cells in the adrenal gland, testis and ovary	Synthesis and secretion of steroids
Kidney and salivary gland duct cells	Ion transport
Macrophages and neutrophils	Intracellular digestion
Fat cells	Lipid (fat) storage
Intestinal lining cells	Absorption of metabolites
Muscle and other contractile cells	Movement

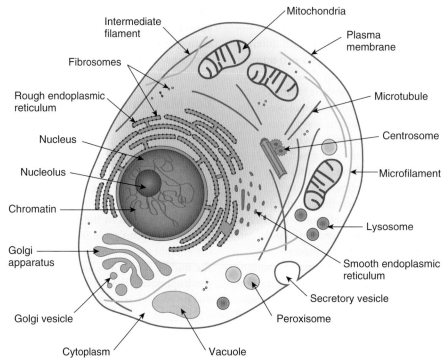

Fig. 1.2 Schematic representation of a typical cell showing the intracellular organelles in the cytoplasm and in the nucleus.

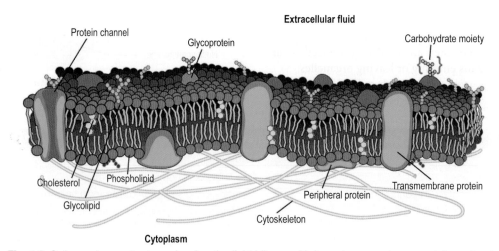

Fig. 1.3 Cell membrane structure showing the lipid bilayer with large transmembrane protein molecules protruding through it.

water on the inside and outside of the cell, respectively, while the middle of the membrane is impermeable to water-soluble substances; however, fat-soluble substances (oxygen, carbon dioxide) can readily penetrate this part.

Integral (transmembrane) proteins extend through the membrane. They provide structural channels through which water molecules and water-soluble substances (ions) can diffuse between the extracellular and intracellular fluids; act as carrier proteins for transporting substances that cannot penetrate the lipid layer; and serve as receptors for water-soluble chemicals (peptide hormones) that cannot easily penetrate the cell membrane. In contrast, peripheral proteins, which are attached to one surface only, function almost entirely as enzymes or controllers of transport of substances through the cell membrane pores; they are often attached to the integral proteins.

The membrane carbohydrates are associated with proteins (glycoproteins) or lipids (glycolipids); 90% of integral proteins are glycoproteins and 10% of membrane lipids are glycolipids.

Transport Across Membranes

The cell membrane is the site where materials are exchanged between the cell and its environment, with many molecules passing through by various mechanisms; small fat-soluble (lipophilic) molecules pass through by simple diffusion; sodium, potassium and calcium ions pass through integral membrane proteins which act as ion channels; and other ions and molecules pass through after binding to carrier (transport) proteins (Fig. 1.4). Simple diffusion is passive; however, ion pumps and carrier proteins involve active transport, using energy from the breakdown of adenosine triphosphate (ATP). Water passively diffuses (osmosis) across selectively permeable membranes through aquaporins, with the direction of movement determined by the relative solute concentrations; it continues until equilibrium is reached.

Passive processes. In addition to simple diffusion and osmosis, facilitated diffusion is also passive and involves the movement of ions and small polar molecules down a concentration gradient; channel-mediated diffusion of ions is movement down a concentration gradient through a protein channel, while carrier-mediated diffusion of small polar molecules is movement down a concentration gradient by a carrier protein.

Active processes. In contrast, active transport (primary, secondary, symport, antiport) of ions and small molecules across a membrane against a concentration gradient by transmembrane protein pumps requires the expenditure of cellular energy. In primary transport, the movement of substances is against its concentration gradient; the calcium ion pump transports calcium out of the cell, while the sodium/potassium ion pump moves sodium out of the cell and potassium into the cell. In secondary transport, the movement of a substance is against its concentration gradient by harnessing the movement of a second substance, such as sodium, down its concentration gradient. In symport transport, a substance moves up its concentration gradient in the same direction as sodium, while in antiport transport a substance moves up its concentration gradient in the opposite direction to sodium.

Similarly, vesicular transport of material released from or brought into a cell requires active transport. Exocytosis is the bulk movement of a substance out of a cell by the fusion of secretory particles with the cell membrane, such as the release of neurotransmitters by nerve cells. Endocytosis (phagocytosis, pinocytosis, receptor-mediated endocytosis) is the bulk movement of substances into a cell by vesicles forming at the cell membrane (Fig. 1.5). Phagocytosis occurs when particles (bacteria) outside the cell are engulfed by pseudopodia,

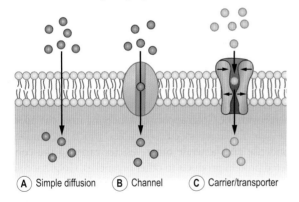

(A) Simple diffusion   (B) Channel   (C) Carrier/transporter

Fig. 1.4 Different types of transport through cell membranes.

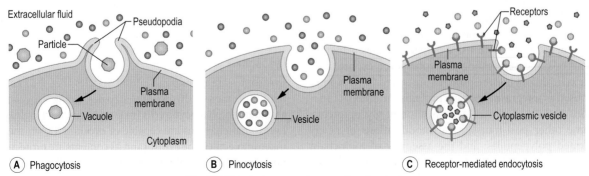

(A) Phagocytosis   (B) Pinocytosis   (C) Receptor-mediated endocytosis

Fig. 1.5 The three general types of endocytosis.

forming vesicles which are then brought into the cell; pinocytosis occurs when the cell membrane forms a pit in which interstitial (extracellular) fluid taken up by the cell; and in receptor-mediated endocytosis receptors on the cell membrane initially bind to specific substances (cholesterol), which are then taken up by the cell.

> **CLINICAL PHYSIOLOGY:** Many diseases are caused by defective receptors on the target cell membrane and cannot, therefore, respond to a substance (hormone).

Cytoplasm

The cytoplasm contains highly organised physical structures (organelles); the clear fluid portion (cytosol) contains small and large dispersed particles (dissolved proteins, electrolytes, glucose). Also within the cytoplasm are neutral fat globules, glycogen granules, ribosomes, secretory vesicles and a number of important organelles (endoplasmic reticulum, Golgi apparatus, lysosomes, peroxisomes, proteasomes, mitochondria); the nucleus is the membrane-bound structure regulating and controlling cell function (Fig. 1.2).

Endoplasmic Reticulum

Endoplasmic reticulum is a convoluted membranous network extending from the surface of the nucleus to the cell membrane (Fig. 1.2), being a major site for the biosynthesis of proteins and lipids; it encloses a series of interconnecting channels and sacs (cisternae) forming a continuous internal cell compartment which collects newly synthesised proteins for modification and delivery to pathways leading to other organelles, as well as for secretion.

Rough endoplasmic reticulum. In rough (granular) endoplasmic reticulum (RER), the cytosol side of the membrane is covered by polyribosomes (segments of ribosomal ribonucleic acid (rRNA) bound to a single messenger ribonucleic acid (mRNA) strand); each mRNA strand specifies the polypeptide sequence to be synthesised. RER is prominent in cells specialising in protein secretion, with its principal activities being the synthesis and segregation of proteins for export from the cell, although some proteins are stored in lysosomes or used as integral membrane proteins. Additional functions include the initial glycosylation of glycoproteins; some other post-translational modifications of newly formed polypeptides; and the assembly of multichain proteins. Defective new proteins are translocated back into the cytosol and then degraded by proteasomes.

> **CLINICAL PHYSIOLOGY:** A number of inherited diseases result from deficient/incomplete degradation of non-functioning proteins; defective procollagen molecules synthesised and secreted by osteoblasts (page 30) produce weak bone tissue (osteogenesis imperfecta).

Smooth endoplasmic reticulum. This lacks the bound polyribosomes present in RER; the smooth (agranular) endoplasmic reticulum (SER) is continuous with RER, but frequently less abundant. SER is specialised for glycogen and lipid metabolism, detoxification reactions and in the sequestering and release of calcium in a controlled way, the latter being part of the rapid response of cells to various stimuli.

> **CLINICAL PHYSIOLOGY:** Underdeveloped SER in liver cells is a frequent cause of jaundice (yellowish discolouration of the skin) in newborn infants; bilirubin and other pigmented compounds in the extracellular fluid are normally metabolised by SER enzymes and converted to a form that can be excreted.

Golgi Apparatus/Complex

The Golgi apparatus consists of smooth membrane saccules (Fig. 1.2) containing enzymes which complete the post-translational modifications of proteins in the RER, packages them up and directs them to their proper destination. It usually has two distinct structural and functional sides; material from the RER moves in transport vesicles to merge with the Golgi apparatus, emerging from the opposite side in larger saccules/vacuoles which accumulate, condense and generate other vesicles carrying the completed protein products to other organelles. Golgi saccules at sequential locations contain different enzymes; they are important for glycosylation (Fig. 1.6), sulfation, phosphorylation and limited proteolysis of proteins. The Golgi apparatus also initiates packing, concentration and storage of secretory products: secretory granules store a product until its release by exocytosis triggered by metabolic, hormonal or neural stimuli (regulated secretion).

Lysosomes

Lysosomes are membrane-bound vesicles (Fig. 1.2) containing numerous hydrolytic enzymes, being especially abundant in phagocytic cells (macrophages, neutrophils). Lysosomal enzymes are capable of breaking down most macromolecules; the cytosol and its contents are protected not only by the membrane but also because the enzymes act optimally at an acidic pH (~5.0) so that any leaked

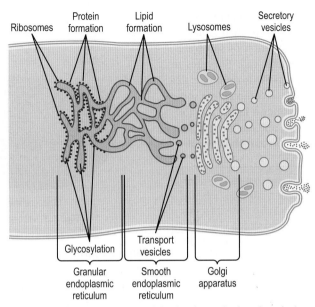

Fig. 1.6 Formation of proteins, lipids and cellular vesicles by the endoplasmic reticulum and Golgi apparatus.

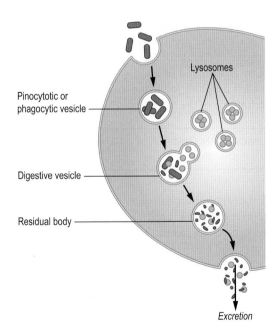

Fig. 1.7 Lysosome enzymes digesting substances in pinocytotic or phagocytic vesicles.

lysosomal enzymes are effectively inactive in the cytosol (pH ~7.2) and are therefore harmless to the cell. When material entering the cell through pinocytosis fuses with a lysosome it is digested; indigestible material is retained within a small vacuole remnant (residual body) (Fig. 1.7). In addition to degrading exogenous macromolecules,

lysosomes also remove excess or non-functioning organelles and other cytoplasmic structures (autophagy); autophagy is enhanced in secretory cells which have accumulated excess secretory granules, as well as in times of nutritional stress (starvation). The digested products of autophagy are reused in the cytoplasm.

> **CLINICAL PHYSIOLOGY:** Some conditions of the cell break the membranes of some lysosomes allowing the release of the digestive enzymes, which split the organic substances they come into contact with into small highly diffusible substances (amino acids, glucose).

> **CLINICAL PHYSIOLOGY:** Lysosomal storage disorders arise from defects in some of the digestive enzymes present in lysosomes; consequently, the lysosomes are unable to function properly and accumulate large secondary lysosomes or residual bodies filled with the indigestible macromolecule. Such accumulations can interfere with normal cell or tissue function leading to symptoms of the disease. Defective lysosomal enzymes can affect the skeletal and nervous system (mucolipidosis II disease (Hurler syndrome)); skeletal muscle (McArdle syndrome); nervous system (Tay-Sachs disease); and the liver and spleen (Gaucher disease).

Peroxisomes

Peroxisomes are small spherical organelles enclosed in a single membrane formed by self-replication or by budding off from the SER; they contain oxidases rather than hydrolases. Peroxidases break down hydrogen peroxide (H_2O_2), formed by the oxidisation of substrates, which is potentially damaging to the cell. Enzymes in peroxisomes also inactivate potentially toxic molecules (including some prescription drugs); complement some functions of the SER and mitochondria in the metabolism of lipids and other molecules; and enable reactions leading to the formation of bile acids and cholesterol.

> **CLINICAL PHYSIOLOGY:** Zellweger spectrum disorders (Zellweger syndrome, Heimler syndrome, infantile Refsum disease, neonatal adrenoleukodystrophy) are rare congenital disorders characterised by the reduction/absence of functional peroxisomes in cells. Zellweger syndrome affects the brain, liver and kidneys, resulting in severe problems with nerves and metabolism – it is usually fatal; Heimler syndrome causes hearing loss and tooth problems in late infancy and early childhood; infantile Refsum disease causes muscle movement problems and delays in development; and neonatal adrenoleukodystrophy causes hearing and vision loss, as well as problems with the brain, spine and muscles. Symptoms include a broad bridge of the nose, epicanthal folds, flattened face, high forehead, underdeveloped eyebrow ridges, wide-set eyes, difficulty feeding, enlarged spleen, gastrointestinal bleeding, hearing and visual problems, jaundice, seizures, and underdeveloped muscles and movement problems.

Proteasomes

Proteasomes are small abundant protein complexes in the cytoplasm not bound by a membrane; they deal mainly with free proteins as individual molecules by degrading denatured or non-functional polypeptides, as well as removing proteins no longer needed by the cell, thereby providing an important mechanism for restricting the activity of a specific protein to within a certain window. Peptides may be further broken down to amino acids or they may have other destinations (antigen-presenting complexes of cells activating an immune response).

> **CLINICAL PHYSIOLOGY:** Failure of proteasomes can allow large aggregates of protein to accumulate in affected cells, which may in turn adsorb other macromolecules to them and damage or kill the cell; aggregates released from dead cells can accumulate in the extracellular matrix of the tissue, which in the brain can interfere directly with cell function leading to neurodegeneration (Alzheimer disease, Huntington disease).

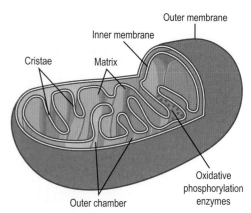

Fig. 1.8 Mitochondrial structure.

Mitochondria

Membrane-enclosed organelles (Fig. 1.2) present throughout the cytoplasm containing arrays of enzymes specialised for aerobic respiration and ATP production, supplying energy for most cellular activities. The number of mitochondria in any given cell depends on its energy requirements; they vary in size and shape, fusing with one another and dividing: they move through the cytoplasm along microtubules. New mitochondria originate by growth and division of existing mitochondria, with each daughter following mitosis receiving half the mitochondria of the parent cell.

> **CLINICAL ANATOMY:** All mitochondria are derived from the mother.

A mitochondrion has outer and inner lipid bilayer-protein membranes creating two compartments, an inner matrix, containing large quantities of dissolved enzymes, and a narrow outer chamber (intermembrane space); the inner membrane forms a series of folds (crests, cristae) projecting into the matrix, greatly increasing its surface area, and on which are oxidative enzymes (Fig. 1.8); the outer membrane contains numerous integral proteins which form channels through which small molecules and other metabolites pass from the cytoplasm to the intermembrane space. The oxidative and matrix enzymes cause oxidation of nutrients forming carbon dioxide and water, at the same time releasing energy, used to synthesise ATP, which is transported out of the mitochondrion to diffuse throughout the cell, releasing its own energy when and where it is needed for cellular functions.

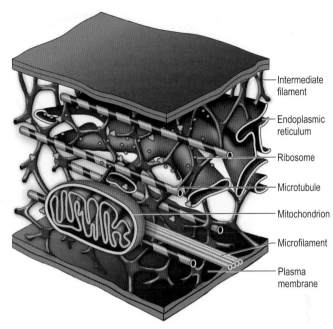

Fig. 1.9 Cytoskeletal components (microtubules, microfilaments, intermediate filaments).

Intermediate filament

Endoplasmic reticulum

Ribosome

Microtubule

Mitochondrion

Microfilament

Plasma membrane

Cytoskeleton

A complex array of microtubules, microfilaments (actin filaments) and intermediate filaments (Fig. 1.9), which determine cell shape, provide structural support to the cell, stabilise junctions between cells, play an important role in cytosol streaming and the movement of organelles and cytoplasmic vesicles, help move chromosomes during cell division, and assist movement of the entire cell.

Microtubules. These form part of the system for intracellular transport of membranous vesicles, macromolecule complexes and organelles; they are also organised into larger arrays (axonemes) in cilia and flagella.

Microfilaments. Composed of actin, microfilaments enable cellular motility and most contractile activity in cells, being thinner, shorter and more flexible than microtubules; they interact with myosin. Microvilli are extensions which increase the surface area of the cell for improved absorption, with other extensions they are used in cell motility. The length of microfilaments and their interaction with other proteins determine the mechanical properties of the local cytoplasm, especially its viscosity. Interactions between F-actin and myosin are the basis of cell movements, including transport of various organelles, vesicles and granules through the cell (cytoplasmic streaming); constriction producing two cells at the end of mitosis (cytokinesis); surface changes underlying phagocytosis and pinocytosis; and rapid shortening/retraction of cellular extensions. Stabilised arrays of actin and myosin filaments allow forceful contraction in specialised cells (muscle) (page 40).

Intermediate filaments. Intermediate in size between microtubules and microfilaments, intermediate filaments are more stable: they have different protein subunits in different cell types (keratins in epithelial cells, vimentin in cells derived from mesenchyme, neurofilaments in neurons, lamins forming a structural framework (nuclear lamina) inside the nuclear envelope).

> **CLINICAL PHYSIOLOGY:** Immunocytochemical methods can reveal specific types of intermediate filaments enabling the cellular origin of tumours in the diagnosis and treatment of cancer.

Nucleus

The nucleus is a large rounded/oval structure near the centre of the cell; it comprises a nuclear envelope (membrane), chromatin (DNA and associated proteins) and

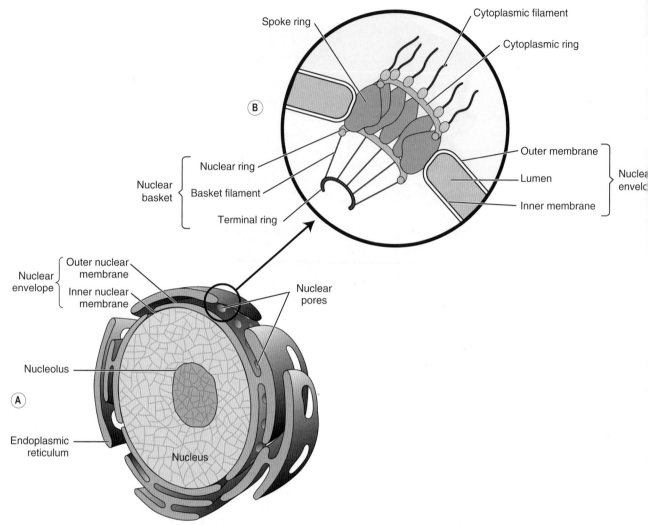

Fig. 1.10 The cell nucleus.

the nucleolus (Figs. 1.2 and 1.10). It is the control centre of the cell containing the code for all the cell's enzymes and proteins; it also contains the molecular machinery to replicate the DNA (genes) and to synthesise and process all types of RNA. During interphase (page 17), pore complexes in the nuclear membrane regulate macromolecular transfer between the nuclear and cytoplasmic compartments; mature RNA molecules pass into the cytoplasm for their role in protein synthesis, and proteins required for nuclear activities are imported from the cytoplasm.

Nuclear Membrane

The nuclear membrane is a selectively permeable barrier comprising two concentric membranes enclosing a narrow perinuclear space; the space and outer membranes are continuous with the cytoplasmic network of the RER. Closely associated with the inner membrane is a network of proteins (nuclear lamina). Bridging the inner and outer membranes are pore complexes enabling ions and small solutes to diffuse through, but control the passage of macromolecules between the nucleus and cytoplasm; pore complexes allow molecular transfer in both directions simultaneously.

Chromatin

Chromatin comprises DNA and its associated proteins; it is of two types, heterochromatin concentrated near the nuclear lamina, and dispersed euchromatin.

Nucleolus

The nucleolus (Fig. 1.2) is an accumulation of large amounts of RNA and proteins found in ribosomes; it is not membrane-bound and becomes enlarged when the cell is actively synthesising proteins. Formation of the nucleolus and ribosomes in the cytoplasm outside the nucleus begins in the nucleus; initially, specific DNA genes in the chromosomes synthesise RNA, some of which is stored in the nucleolus, with most being transported into the cytoplasm through the nuclear pores, where it is used to assemble mature ribosomes important in forming cytoplasmic proteins.

> **CLINICAL PHYSIOLOGY:** Neoplastic proliferation of cells in tissues occurs when cells grow at higher rates and in an uncontrolled way than normal, often following damage to the DNA of proto-oncogenes or failure to eliminate cells. Neoplastic growth can be either benign (slow growing and non-invasive to adjacent organs) or malignant (rapid growth with the capacity to invade other organs); cancer is the result of neoplastic proliferation.

Cell Cycle

Most cells undergo repeated cycles of growth and division (mitosis). The cell cycle has four distinct phases (Fig. 1.11A): mitosis, G_1 (the time between mitosis and DNA replication when cells accumulate the enzymes and nucleotides necessary for DNA replication), S (the period devoted to DNA synthesis) and G_2 (the time between DNA duplication and the next mitosis); when cell cycle activities are suspended (either permanently or temporarily) the cells are referred to as being in G_0. Each phase of the cell cycle has one or more checkpoints where specific cell activities are monitored (Fig. 1.11B).

Mitosis

During mitosis (Fig. 1.11A), a parent cell divides into two daughter cells, each of which receives a set of chromosomes identical to the parent cell.

Prophase. Several changes occur during prophase: the nucleolus disappears; the replicated chromatin condenses into discrete threadlike chromosomes; at the centromere part of each chromosome, the kinetochore (large protein complex) acts as a site for microtubule attachment; the centrosomes separate and migrate to opposite poles of the cell.

Metaphase. There is further condensation of the chromosomes, which attach to the mitotic spindle; the cell becomes more spherical and the chromosomes now become aligned at the equatorial plane.

Anaphase. The chromosomes separate and move towards opposite poles, which move further apart.

Telophase. Each set of chromosomes are at the poles and begin to decondense; a nuclear envelope starts to reassemble around each of the daughter cells; and a contractile ring of actin filaments develops in the peripheral cytoplasm at the cell equator, producing a deep furrow which progresses until the cytoplasm and its organelles become divided into the two daughter cells, each with a single nucleus.

Interphase. The period between mitoses is the interphase.

> **CLINICAL PHYSIOLOGY:** Most tissues (except nerve and cardiac muscle cells) undergo cell turnover; cell turnover is rapid in the epithelial lining of the digestive tract (page 463), uterus (page 543) and epidermis of the skin (page 55).

Stem Cells

Stem cells are small populations of undifferentiated cells which serve to renew the differentiated cells in tissues as and when required; they divide infrequently, with the divisions being asymmetric with one daughter cell remaining as a stem cell and the other (progenitor cell) committed to a path leading to differentiation (Fig. 1.12).

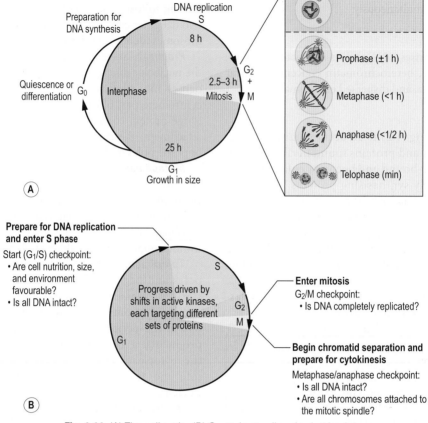

(A)

Quiescence or differentiation

Preparation for DNA synthesis

DNA replication
S

8 h

G_2
+
M

2.5–3 h
Mitosis

G_0 Interphase

25 h

G_1
Growth in size

Prophase (±1 h)

Metaphase (<1 h)

Anaphase (<1/2 h)

Telophase (min)

(B)

Prepare for DNA replication and enter S phase

Start (G_1/S) checkpoint:
• Are cell nutrition, size, and environment favourable?
• Is all DNA intact?

Progress driven by shifts in active kinases, each targeting different sets of proteins

S

G_2
M

G_1

Enter mitosis

G_2/M checkpoint:
• Is DNA completely replicated?

Begin chromatid separation and prepare for cytokinesis

Metaphase/anaphase checkpoint:
• Is all DNA intact?
• Are all chromosomes attached to the mitotic spindle?

Fig. 1.11 (A) The cell cycle. (B) Controls at cell cycle checkpoints.

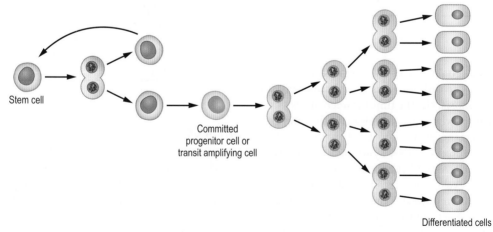

Stem cell

Committed progenitor cell or transit amplifying cell

Differentiated cells

Fig. 1.12 Stem and progenitor cells.

Meiosis

In meiosis, DNA replication is followed by two rounds of cell division producing four daughter cells, each with half the number of chromosomes as the original parent cell; these two divisions are meiosis I and meiosis II. Prior to the start of meiosis, during the S phase of the cell cycle, the DNA of each chromosome is replicated so that it consists of two identical sister chromatids held together through cohesion. Following DNA replication, meiotic cells enter a prolonged G_2-like phase during which homologous chromosomes pair up with each other and undergo genetic recombination; this is a programmed process in which DNA is cut and then repaired enabling the exchange of genetic information. Crossovers, resulting from certain recombination events, create physical links (chiasmata) between homologous chromosomes, helping to segregate them away from each other during meiosis I; the result is two haploid cells each with half the number of chromosomes as the parent cell. During meiosis II, the chromatids are released, with all four products forming gametes (sperm); however, in females, three of the products are eliminated by extrusion into polar bodies, with only one cell producing an ovum.

Diploid human cells contain 23 pairs of chromosomes (including one pair of sex chromosomes), half from the mother and half from the father. Meiosis produces haploid gametes (ova or sperm) containing one set of 23 chromosomes; when an egg and sperm fuse at fertilisation the resulting zygote is again diploid, with the mother and father each contributing 23 chromosomes. Sexual reproduction is alternating cycles of meiosis and fertilisation with successive generations maintaining the same number of chromosomes.

Further details of meiosis during spermatogenesis and oogenesis can be found on pages 351 and 356, respectively.

Apoptosis

Apoptosis is a rapid regulated programmed cellular activity that shrinks and eliminates defective and unneeded cells; it is controlled by cytoplasmic proteins regulating the release of death-promoting factors from mitochondria. Small membrane-enclosed bodies (apoptotic bodies) undergo phagocytosis by neighbouring cells or cells specialised in debris removal. The apoptotic cells do not rupture and release their contents, unlike damaged cells which undergo necrosis; therefore, there is no local inflammatory reaction or migration of leukocytes.

> **CLINICAL PHYSIOLOGY:** Cancer cells deactivate genes controlling the apoptotic process, preventing their elimination and facilitating their progression towards a more malignant state.

TISSUES

Despite its complexity, the human body consists of only four basic tissue types (epithelial, connective, muscular, nervous): each contains cells and molecules of the extracellular matrix and exists in association with one another and in variable proportions and morphologies, to form different organs of the body. Epithelial tissue consists of aggregated cells with a small amount of extracellular matrix: they form the covering/lining of surfaces and body cavities, with some cells being secretory. Connective tissue comprises several types of fixed and wandering cells, with an abundant amount of extracellular matrix; it provides support and protection to tissues and organs. Muscle tissue comprises elongated contractile cells with a moderate amount of extracellular matrix; they produce movement. Nervous tissue comprises elongated cells with fine processes and contains a very small amount of extracellular matrix; they transmit nervous impulses (action potentials). Also of functional importance are the free cells found in body fluids (blood, lymph).

Epithelium

Epithelium is an avascular tissue which covers body surfaces, lines body cavities and surrounds glands, creating a barrier between the external environment and the underlying connective tissue. Epithelial cells have three primary characteristics: they are closely apposed to each other, being held together by specialised cell junctions;

different parts of the cell (apex, base, sides) have different morphological and functional features; and the basal surface is attached to an underlying basement membrane. Epithelial cells are continually replaced by mitotic division of adult stem cells in different sites within the epithelium.

Classification

The classification of epithelium reflects its structure and not its function, being determined by the shape of the surface cells and the number of layers; in this way, the various configurations of epithelia are classified. When the epithelium is one layer thick it is described as being simple, while if there are two or more layers it is stratified; when cell width is greater than height it is squamous; when cell height exceeds width it is columnar; and when cell width, height and depth are similar it is cuboidal (Fig. 1.13). In stratified epithelium the shape of the surface layer cells is used to classify the type of epithelium; sometimes, the apical specialisation of the cell is also used in the classification (in simple columnar ciliated epithelium the apex of the cell possesses cilia).

Pseudostratified epithelium appears stratified, even though some cells do not reach the surface they are all attached to the basement membrane.

Transitional epithelium (urothelium) is stratified and lines the urinary tract between the minor calyces of the kidney and proximal part of the urethra (page 527); the surface cells change from being large, round dome-shaped to squamous depending on the degree of distension.

Endothelium is the lining of blood and lymphatic vessels; it is simple squamous epithelium.

Endocardium is the lining of the heart (ventricles and atria); it is simple squamous epithelium.

Mesothelium lines the walls and covers the contents of the abdominal, pericardial and pleural cavities; it is simple squamous epithelium.

Function

The function of epithelium depends on the activity of the type of cells present in the epithelium: secretion, cells lining the stomach and gastric glands (page 466); absorption, cells in the intestines (pages 468 and 472) and proximal convoluted tubules of the kidney (page

518); transportation of material or cells along the surface of the epithelium by cilia, as in the bronchial tree (page 98) and the transport of material across an epithelium, as in pinocytosis and endocytosis (page 11); mechanical protection, cells of the epidermis of skin (page 55); and reception of external stimuli, cells in the taste buds of the tongue (page 311) and retina (page 299).

Cell apex. The apices of epithelial cells show surface modifications in relation to cell function: microvilli, small finger-like cytoplasmic processes which increase the surface area for absorption; stereocilia, long microvilli present in the male reproductive system (page 532) for absorption and in the sensory epithelium of the inner ear for sensory perception (page 316); motile cilia, extensions of the plasma membrane, which move in a coordinated way; and primary cilia (monocilia), which are non-motile and function as chemoreceptors, osmoreceptors and mechanoreceptors.

CLINICAL ANATOMY: Coeliac disease (gluten-sensitive enteropathy, sprue) involves the loss of the microvillus border of absorptive cells in the small intestine in response to an immune reaction against wheat protein (gluten) during digestion, giving rise to enteritis (inflammation of the intestine). This changes the epithelial cells and leads to malabsorption, as well as pathologic changes in the intestinal wall: the malabsorption and structural changes are usually reversible when gluten is removed from the diet.

Cell-to-cell adhesion. Several membrane-associated structures in the lateral parts of the cell enable them to adhere together, as well as enabling communication between them; epithelial cells are strongly adherent to neighbouring cells, as well as to the basal lamina, especially where they are subject to mechanical forces (friction). The lateral surfaces of epithelial cells have several specialised intercellular junctions (tight [occluding], adherent [anchoring], gap [communicating]) serving different functions (Fig. 1.14); although numerous and prominent in epithelial cells, some of these junctions are present in other tissues.

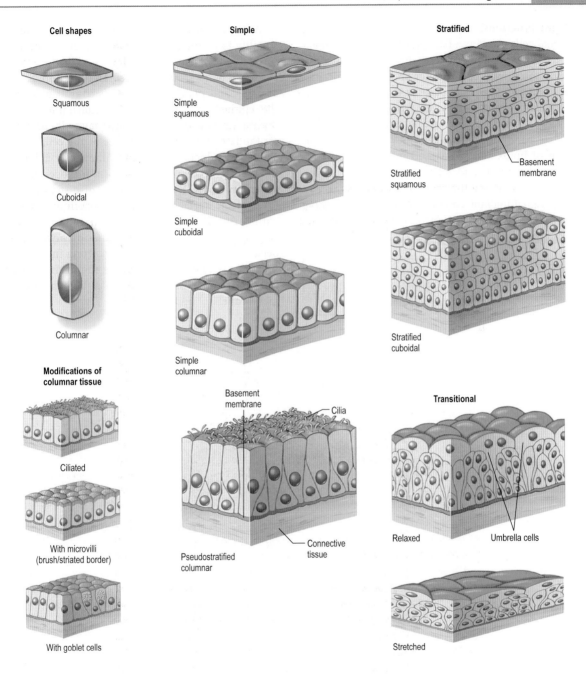

Cell shapes

Squamous

Cuboidal

Columnar

Modifications of columnar tissue

Ciliated

With microvilli (brush/striated border)

With goblet cells

Simple

Simple squamous

Simple cuboidal

Simple columnar

Basement membrane

Cilia

Connective tissue

Pseudostratified columnar

Stratified

Stratified squamous

Basement membrane

Stratified cuboidal

Transitional

Relaxed

Umbrella cells

Stretched

Fig. 1.13 Types of epithelium, their function and location: simple squamous for exchange in the vascular system (endothelium) and kidney (Bowman's capsule) and lubrication in body cavities (mesothelium) and respiratory spaces in the lung; simple cuboidal for absorption and secretion, as well as a conduit, in small ducts of exocrine glands and on the surfaces of the ovary, kidney tubules and thyroid follicles; simple columnar for absorption and secretion in the small intestine and colon, stomach lining and gastric glands and gallbladder; pseudostratified for secretion, absorption and as a conduit in the trachea and bronchial tree, ductus deferens and epididymis; stratified squamous as a barrier and for protection in the epidermis, oral cavity, oesophagus and vagina; stratified cuboidal as a barrier and conduit for sweat gland ducts, large ducts of exocrine glands and the anorectal junction; stratified columnar as a barrier and conduit in the largest ducts of exocrine glands and the anorectal junction and transitional (urothelium) as a distensible barrier in renal calyces, the ureters, bladder and urethra.

Tight junctions. These are impermeable enabling epithelial cells to act as a barrier; they are the primary intercellular diffusion barrier between adjacent cells, limiting the movement of water and other molecules through the intercellular space by maintaining physicochemical separation between tissue compartments. Located towards the apex of the cell and forming a complete band around the cell, they prevent the migration of lipids and specialised membrane proteins between the apical and lateral domains (Fig. 1.14), therefore maintaining their integrity. They also recruit various signalling molecules to the cell surface, linking them to the microfilaments (actin filaments) of the cytoskeleton.

> **CLINICAL PHYSIOLOGY:** Changes to tight junctions (defects in occludins) may compromise the foetal blood-brain barrier, leading to severe neurologic disorders.

Adherent junctions. These provide mechanical stability to epithelial cells by linking the cytoskeleton of one cell to that of the adjacent cell; they form a complete band around the cell and are important in creating and maintaining the structural integrity of the epithelium. Anchoring junctions interact with both actin and intermediate filaments, being found on the lateral and basal surfaces of the cell. By their signal transduction capability, they play important roles in cell-cell recognition, morphogenesis and differentiation. Desmosomes are disc-shaped structures at the surface of one cell, which are matched with identical structures at an adjacent cell surface (Fig. 1.14); they provide firm adhesion between cells because they bind with the very strong intermediate filaments. Hemidesmosomes are found on the basal cell surface attaching it to the basal lamina/basement membrane.

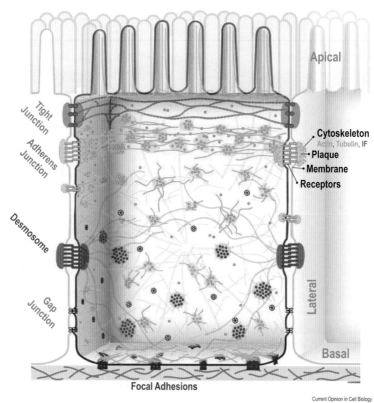

Fig. 1.14 Junctional complexes of epithelial cells. (Source: Sun D, LuValle-Burke I, Pombo-García K, Honigmann A. Biomolecular condensates in epithelial junctions. Curr Opin Cell Biol 2022;77:102089.)

Gap junctions. These enable communication between cells and are abundant in epithelia, although they are functionally important in most tissues; they consist of transmembrane protein complexes forming circular patches in the plasma membrane (Fig. 1.14). Gap junctions permit intercellular exchange of small molecules, some mediating signal transduction by moving rapidly through gap junctions enabling many tissues to act in a coordinated way rather than as independent units; heart and smooth muscle gap junctions promote rhythmic contractions.

Cell base. The cell base is separated from the underlying connective tissue stroma by a basement membrane, being attached to it by focal adhesions and hemidesmosomes and focal adhesions; infoldings of the basal surface increase the cell surface area facilitating interactions between cells and the extracellular matrix proteins.

Secretory Epithelia and Glands

Epithelial cells that mainly function to produce and secrete substances can occur in epithelia with other major functions or comprise specialised organs (glands), with the products produced usually being stored in membrane-bound vesicles (secretory granules) within the cells; the cells may synthesise, store and release proteins (pancreas), lipids (adrenal gland, sebaceous glands), carbohydrate and protein complexes (salivary glands) or water and electrolytes (sweat glands). Unicellular glands (scattered secretory cells) are commonly found in simple cuboidal, simple columnar and pseudostratified epithelia in many organs, especially goblet cells in the lining of the small intestine (page 468) and respiratory tract (page 93). Glands develop from covering epithelium during foetal life by cell proliferation and growth into the underlying connective tissue, followed by further differentiation (Fig. 1.15).

Exocrine and endocrine glands

Exocrine glands. These retain their connection to the surface epithelium via tubular ducts lined with epithelium (Fig. 1.15), with the secreted material leaving the gland by the ducts. Exocrine glands are classified as simple (non-branching ducts) or compound (ducts with branches). The secretory parts can be tubular (short, long, coiled) or acinar (rounded, sac-like), of which either type may be branched, even if the duct is not branched; compound glands can have branching ducts and multiple tubular, acinar or tubuloacinar parts (Fig. 1.16).

In multicellular glands there are three basic mechanisms for releasing their secretory product: merocrine secretion, which involves exocytosis of the protein/glycoprotein from membrane-bound vesicles; holocrine secretion, in which the cell accumulates the secretory product as it matures and then undergoes terminal cell differentiation with complete cell disruption and the release of the product and cell debris into the gland lumen; and apocrine secretion, where the secretion accumulates at the apical end of the cell, parts of which are then extruded to release the product along with some cytoplasm and plasma membrane (Fig. 1.17).

Endocrine glands. In contrast, endocrine glands lose their connection with the surface epithelium and lack ducts; capillaries adjacent to the gland absorb the secretion (hormone) and transport it in the blood to target cells throughout the body (Fig. 1.15).

In both exocrine and endocrine glands, the secretory units are supported by connective tissue, which encloses the gland as a capsule; it also surrounds larger ducts and forms partitions (septa) dividing the glands into separate discrete lobes, which in exocrine glands are connected to the duct system.

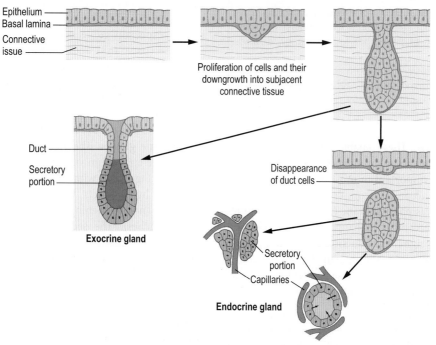

Epithelium
Basal lamina
Connective tissue

Proliferation of cells and their downgrowth into subjacent connective tissue

Duct

Secretory portion

Exocrine gland

Disappearance of duct cells

Secretory portion
Capillaries

Endocrine gland

Fig. 1.15 Formation of glands from surface epithelium.

Compound glands (ducts from several secretory units converge into larger ducts)

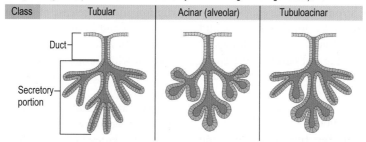

Class	Tubular	Acinar (alveolar)	Tubuloacinar

Duct

Secretory portion

Simple glands (ducts do not branch)

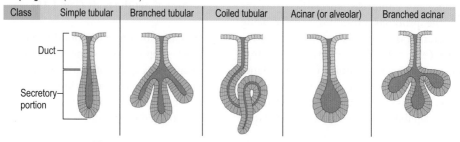

Class	Simple tubular	Branched tubular	Coiled tubular	Acinar (or alveolar)	Branched acinar

Duct

Secretory portion

Fig. 1.16 Simple and compound classes of exocrine glands.

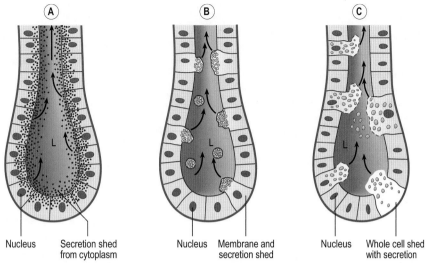

Nucleus Secretion shed
         from cytoplasm

Nucleus Membrane and
         secretion shed

Nucleus Whole cell shed
         with secretion

Fig. 1.17 Modes of secretion of exocrine glands: (A) merocrine, (B) apocrine and (C) holocrine. *L*, Lumen.

CLINICAL ANATOMY: Some epithelial cells undergo abnormal growth (dysplasia), which can progress to pre-cancerous growth (neoplasia); early neoplastic growth may be reversible and does not always progress to cancer. Under some conditions, one type of epithelial tissue may transform into another type in a reversible process (metaplasia). The ciliated pseudostratified epithelium lining the bronchi and trachea can transform into stratified squamous epithelium in heavy smokers, in which case debris/secretions cannot be brought up from the lungs to be swallowed.

CLINICAL ANATOMY: Benign and malignant tumours can arise from almost all types of epithelial cells; malignant tumours of epithelial origin are carcinomas, while those arising from glandular epithelial tissue are adenocarcinomas. Adenocarcinomas are the most common tumours in adults aged over 45.

Connective Tissues

In general, connective tissue consists of cells and an extracellular matrix (Fig. 1.18), which includes protein fibres (collagen, elastic, reticular) and an amorphous component containing specialised molecules (proteoglycans, multiadhesive glycoproteins, glycosaminoglycans), which constitute the ground substance; it originates from embryonic mesenchyme, itself developing mainly from the middle layer (mesoderm) of the embryo. Connective tissue forms a vast continuous compartment throughout the body, bounded by the basal laminae of various epithelia and the basal (external) laminae of muscle cells and nerve-supporting cells. The different types of connective tissue have different functions depending on the organisation of the constituent cells and fibres, as well as the composition of the ground substance in the extracellular matrix.

Cells

Fibroblasts. The most common cells in connective tissue (Fig. 1.18), which produce and maintain most of the extracellular components; they synthesise and secrete collagen and elastin, which form large fibres, as well as glycosaminoglycans, proteoglycans and multiadhesive glycoproteins. Many types of growth factors target fibroblasts influencing cell growth and differentiation.

Adipocytes. Fat cells found in the connective tissue of many organs specialised for cytoplasmic storage of neutral fats, as well as for the production of heat; large deposits of fat in adipose tissue serve to cushion and insulate the skin (page 57) and other organs.

Macrophages. Macrophages are derived from bone marrow precursor cells that divide producing monocytes, which circulate in the blood where they cross the epithelial wall of venules to penetrate connective tissues; here, they further differentiate and mature

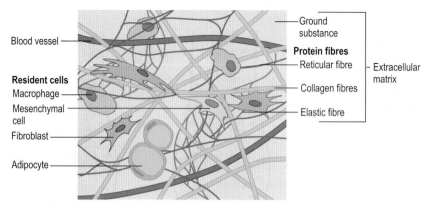

Fig. 1.18 Cells and extracellular components of connective tissue.

becoming macrophages. They play an important role in the early stages of tissue damage, where they accumulate by local proliferation, in addition to monocyte recruitment from the blood. Macrophages specialise in the turnover of protein fibres and the removal of dead cells, tissue debris and other particulate material; they are present in the connective tissue of most organs, where together with other monocyte-derived cells they make up the mononuclear phagocyte system; in the liver, they are known as Kupffer cells (page 480), in the central nervous system as microglial cells (page 247), in the skin as Langerhans cells (page 484) and in bone as osteoclasts (page 30). In addition to the removal of debris, these cells are important for the uptake, processing and presentation of antigens for lymphocyte activation (page 177).

Mast cells. The cytoplasm of these cells contains secretory granules, whose function when released locally has a role in local inflammatory responses, innate immunity and tissue repair; heparin acts locally as an anticoagulant; histamine promotes increased vascular permeability and smooth muscle contraction; chemotactic factors attract leukocytes; cytokines direct the activity of leukocytes and other cells of the immune system (page 176); phospholipid precursors convert prostaglandins and other important lipid mediators in the inflammatory response, while the release of some chemical mediators promote allergic reactions (anaphylactic shock). Mast cells are especially numerous near small blood vessels in skin (page 53), mesenteries (page 452) and in tissue lining the digestive (page 463) and respiratory tracts (page 93).

CLINICAL PHYSIOLOGY: Following exposure to an antigen (allergen) immunoglobulin E (IgE) is produced by plasma cells, which binds to the surface of the mast cell. Subsequent exposures to the antigen results in binding of the antigen to IgE on the mast cell, triggering the release of mast cell granules (histamine, proteoglycans, heparin) initiating an immunologic reaction.

Plasma cells. Large antibody-producing cells derived from β-lymphocytes; at least a few are present in most connective tissues.

Leukocytes. Leukocytes (white blood cells) are a population of wandering cells within connective tissues, which leave blood by migrating between endothelial cells lining venules; the process increases markedly during inflammation, being a vascular and cellular defensive response to injury or foreign substances (pathogenic bacteria, irritating chemical substances). Most leukocytes function for a few days at most in connective tissue and then die; however, some lymphocytes and phagocytic antigen-presenting cells leave the interstitial fluid of the connective tissue, enter blood or lymph and move to selected lymphoid organs.

Fibres

The main types of fibres (collagen, reticular, elastic) are distributed unequally in different connective tissues, with the dominant fibre type giving the tissue its specific properties.

Collagen fibres. Collagen is a key element of all connective tissues, as well as basement epithelial membranes and the external laminae of muscle and nerve cells. It forms a range of extremely strong extracellular structures (fibres (types I, II, III, V, XI); sheets (type IV); networks (types VII, IX, XII, XIV)) resistant to shearing and tearing forces; collagen is a product of fibroblasts. Types I, II, V and XII are found in skin; types I and XII in tendon; types II, IX and XI in cartilage; types I, V and XIV in bone; type III in muscle; type III (often in association with type I) in blood vessels; type V in interstitial and foetal tissues; type IV in basal and external laminae; and type VII in epithelial basement membranes.

Reticular fibres. These consist mainly of type III collagen and form an extensive connective tissue network (reticulum) surrounding many organs; it is the supporting stroma for parenchymal secretory cells and the microvasculature of the liver and endocrine glands. They are also abundant in bone marrow (haematopoietic tissue) and some lymph organs (spleen, lymph nodes), where they support rapidly changing populations of proliferating and phagocytic cells.

Elastic fibres. These form sparse networks interspersed with collagen fibres in many organs, especially those subject to bending or stretching; they have physical properties similar to rubber enabling the tissue to return to its original shape. In large blood vessel walls, especially arteries, elastin occurs as fenestrated sheets (elastic lamellae), being secreted by smooth muscle cells in the vascular wall, as well as by fibroblasts.

Ground Substance

The space between cells and fibres in connective tissue is the ground substance, acting as a lubricant due to its viscosity, as well as a barrier against penetration by invaders. It is highly hydrated and transparent containing a complex mixture of macromolecules (glycosaminoglycans, proteoglycans, multiadhesive glycoproteins); the physical properties of the ground substance influence cellular activity. The largest glycosaminoglycan is hyaluronic acid (hyaluronan), which forms a dense viscous network binding large amounts of water; it has an important role in the diffusion of molecules in connective tissue and in lubricating various organs and joints. Other smaller glycosaminoglycans found in proteoglycans are also highly hydrophilic, and also contribute to ground substance viscosity. Multiadhesive glycoproteins provide binding sites for cell surface receptors and macromolecules within the extracellular matrix.

Types of Connective Tissue

Variations in connective tissue arise from different combinations and densities of cells, fibres and ground substances. Connective tissue proper is classified as loose or dense, depending on the amount of collagen and ground substance present. Loose connective (areolar) tissue contains more ground substance than collagen and is typically found around small blood vessels and in areas adjacent to epithelia. Reticular tissue consists of delicate networks of type III collagen, being most abundant in lymphoid organs where the fibres form attachment sites for lymphocytes and other immune cells. Dense connective tissue is of two types (irregular, regular) and can be further subdivided into white and yellow fibrous tissue; white fibrous tissue is abundant in collagen, while yellow fibrous tissue has a greater amount of elastic fibres. Dense irregular connective tissue contains randomly orientated bundles of type I collagen, with some elastic fibres, and provides resistance to tearing in all directions, as well as some elasticity. Dense white regular connective tissue provides considerable strength without being rigid or elastic; it forms (i) ligaments passing from one bone to another in the region of joints, (ii) tendons for attaching muscles to bone and (iii) protective membranes around muscle (perimysium), bone (periosteum) and many other structures. Dense yellow fibrous tissue is capable of considerable deformation yet returns to its original shape; it is found in the ligamentum flavum (page 199) associated with the vertebral column, as well as in the walls of arteries.

Adipose tissue. Fat (adipose tissue) is a packing and insulating material, with the fat cells (adipocytes) supported by reticular fibres with connective tissue septa dividing the tissue into lobules; adipocytes store lipids from three sources (dietary fats, triglycerides, locally synthesised fatty acids). The presence of dividing septa within the adipose tissue enables it to act as a shock absorber in some circumstances (under the heel, in the buttock, palm of the hand). White adipose tissue is found in many organs and typically accounts for 20% of body weight in adults: fatty acids are released when nutrients are needed and transported throughout the body on plasma proteins (page 165). Brown adipose tissue comprises up to 5% of newborn body weight (smaller amounts in adults); fatty acids released by brown fat adipocytes are used for thermogenesis.

Cartilage. Part of the skeletal system, cartilage is a tough flexible connective tissue able to bear mechanical stresses without permanent deformation, in which the extracellular matrix interacts with collagen and elastic fibres; cartilage cells (chondroblasts: chondrocytes when cell division has ceased) synthesise and maintain the extracellular components, being located in lacunae within the matrix. Cartilage is supplementary to bone wherever strength, rigidity and some elasticity are required; three types of cartilage (hyaline, fibrocartilage, elastic) are present in the body, each having different biomechanical properties. It forms a framework supporting soft tissues and because of its smooth, lubricated surface and resiliency, cartilage provides shock absorption, due to its high water content, and facilitates movement at joints: although a rigid tissue, cartilage is not as hard or strong as bone. It is relatively avascular (being nourished by tissue fluids), aneural and lacks lymphatic vessels; vascular invasion of cartilage results in death of the chondrocytes during the process of ossification of the cartilage and its subsequent replacement by bone. Except for the articular surfaces of synovial joints (page 36), cartilage possesses a fibrous covering (perichondrium); the perichondrium contains blood vessels, nerves and lymphatics.

Hyaline cartilage. The most common form of cartilage. In foetal development, hyaline cartilage provides a temporary tissue later replaced by bone; however, in many places, it persists throughout life as the articular cartilage of synovial joints, in the walls of larger respiratory passages (nose [page 304], larynx [page 328], trachea [page 94], bronchi [page 94]), the anterior ends of ribs [page 70), where they articulate with the sternum, and in epiphyseal growth plates (page 33) enabling bones to grow in length.

At joint surfaces, hyaline cartilage provides a limited degree of elasticity offsetting and absorbing shocks, as well as providing a relatively smooth surface permitting movement. With increasing age, hyaline cartilage tends to become calcified and sometimes ossified.

Fibrocartilage. This is essentially a combination of hyaline cartilage and dense regular fibrous tissue with no distinct perichondrium; it has great tensile strength and elasticity, enabling it to resist considerable pressure. Fibrocartilage is found at many sites in the musculoskeletal system: (i) within the intervertebral disc between adjacent vertebrae (page 196); (ii) in the menisci of the knee joint (page 604); (iii) in the labrum surrounding and deepening the glenoid fossa of the shoulder joint (page 391) and acetabulum of the hip joint (page 584); (iv) in the articular discs of the radiocarpal (wrist) (page 419), sternoclavicular (page 381), acromioclavicular (page 384) and temporomandibular (page 283) joints; and (v) as articular surfaces of bones (clavicle, mandible) which ossify in a membrane (page 31). Fibrocartilage may calcify and ossify.

Elastic cartilage. Contains bundles of elastic fibres with little or no fibrocartilage, being essentially similar to hyaline cartilage; it does not ossify and is not present in the musculoskeletal system. It is found within the auricle of the ear (page 314), walls of the external auditory canal (page 314), auditory (eustachian) tube (page 314), epiglottis and some cartilages of the larynx (page 328).

Bone. Bone, the main component of the adult skeletal system, is essentially an inorganic matrix of fibrous tissue impregnated with mineral salts, giving bone its toughness and elasticity, with the mineral salts providing hardness and rigidity; it is a reservoir for calcium, phosphate and other ions that can be released or stored in a controlled way to maintain constant concentrations in body fluids, with the rate of exchange and overall balance being influenced by several factors, including hormones. It provides support for the body, protects vital organs (brain within the skull, heart and lungs within the thorax), has cavities containing bone marrow, where blood cells are formed, and form a series of levers which magnify the forces generated during skeletal muscle contraction, enabling movement.

> **APPLIED ANATOMY:** The bones of the limbs and their respective girdles (upper limb, pectoral girdle; lower limb, pelvic girdle) comprise the appendicular skeleton, while all remaining bones (skull, vertebrae, sternum, ribs) comprise the axial skeleton.

The external and internal surfaces of each bone are covered in periosteum and endosteum, respectively. The fibrous outer layer of the periosteum contains small blood vessels, collagen bundles and fibroblasts; bundles of collagen fibres (perforating fibres) penetrate the bone matrix attaching the periosteum to bone. The cellular inner layer contains bone lining cells, osteoblasts (bone-forming cells) and stem (osteoprogenitor) cells; osteoprogenitor cells can (and do) proliferate and differentiate into osteoblasts, which have an important role in bone growth and repair. Internally, the thin endosteum covers a system of struts and plates (trabeculae) projecting into the marrow cavity: the endosteum also contains osteoprogenitor cells, osteoblasts and bone lining cells.

The form and structure of bone are adapted to the functions of support and resistance to mechanical stresses; it is continually remodelled to meet these demands, especially during growth. The structure of a bone cannot be satisfactorily considered in isolation; it depends on its relationship to adjacent bones and the type of articulation between them, as well as the attachment of muscles, tendons and ligaments. The internal structure comprises trabeculae (cancellous/spongy bone) running in many directions (Fig. 1.19), especially at the ends of long bones, organised to resist compressive, tensile and shearing stresses; surrounding the trabeculae is a thin layer of condensed (compact) bone. The shaft of long bones has an outer relatively thick ring of compact bone surrounding the marrow cavity containing bone marrow.

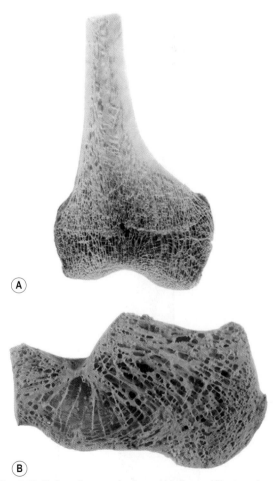

Ⓐ

Ⓑ

Fig. 1.19 Trabecular organisation within bone: (A) coronal section through the distal end of the femur; (B) sagittal section through the calcaneus.

For descriptive purposes, bones can be classified according to their shape: (i) long bones are found within the limbs, with each comprising a shaft (diaphysis) and two expanded ends (epiphyses) (Fig. 1.20); (ii) short bones are those of the wrist (carpus) and part of the foot (tarsus); (iii) flat bones are thin and tend to be curved, they include the bones of the skull vault and ribs, structurally flat bones consist of two layers of compact bone enclosing cancellous bone; and (iv) irregular bones, including the vertebrae and many bones of the skull and face.

APPLIED ANATOMY: The only source of red blood cells and the main source of white cells after birth is red bone marrow; in infants, the cavities of all bones contain red marrow, which is gradually replaced by yellow (fat) marrow. At puberty, red marrow is only present in cavities associated with cancellous bone; with increasing age, most red marrow is replaced by yellow marrow, with red marrow only persisting throughout life in vertebrae, ribs, sternum and the proximal ends of the humerus and femur.

Bone cells:
- **Osteoprogenitor cells:** Derived from mesenchymal stem cells in bone marrow, osteoprogenitor cells have the potential to differentiate into many different cell types (fibroblasts, osteoblasts, adipocytes, chondrocytes, muscle cells) depending on requirements. They are found on the external and internal surface of bones (Fig. 1.21) and resemble periosteal cells in the inner layer of periosteum and endosteal cells lining marrow cavities, osteonal (Haversian) canals and perforating (Volkmann) canals (Fig. 1.22).
- **Osteoblasts:** Bone-forming cells secreting the organic matrix of bone (osteoid) into which mineral salts are deposited forming new bone; mature osteoblasts are located at the surface of the bone matrix (Fig. 1.21).
- **Osteocytes:** As osteoblasts become surrounded, they differentiate into osteocytes, enclosed singly within the regularly spaced lacunae throughout the mineralised matrix; they communicate with each other via dendritic processes which extend from their body and run in canaliculi (Figs. 1.21 and 1.22).

CLINICAL ANATOMY: The dendritic processes detect mechanical stresses on bone, monitoring areas where loading has increased or decreased helping to maintain adequate bone matrix; lack of exercise or weightlessness leads to decreased bone density.

- **Bone lining cells:** Derived from osteoblasts, bone lining cells are essentially inactive osteoblasts; however, they help support the osteocytes embedded in the underlying bone matrix on the external and internal surfaces of bone (Fig. 1.21); they resemble periosteal and endosteal cells, respectively.
- **Osteoclasts:** Large motile cells involved in matrix resorption during bone growth and remodelling (Fig. 1.21).

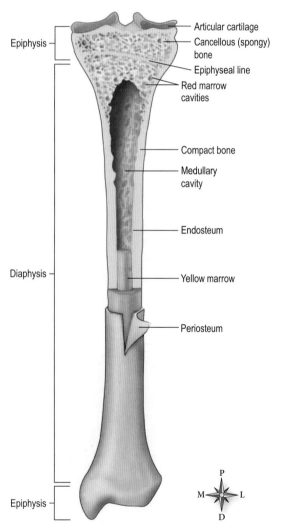

Epiphysis

Articular cartilage
Cancellous (spongy) bone
Epiphyseal line
Red marrow cavities

Compact bone

Medullary cavity

Endosteum

Diaphysis

Yellow marrow

Periosteum

P
M ← → L
D

Epiphysis

Fig. 1.20 Structure of a long bone.

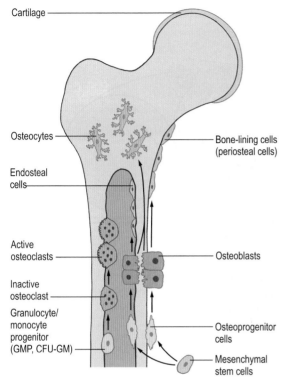

Cartilage

Osteocytes

Bone-lining cells
(periosteal cells)

Endosteal
cells

Active
osteoclasts

Osteoblasts

Inactive
osteoclast

Granulocyte/
monocyte
progenitor
(GMP, CFU-GM)

Osteoprogenitor
cells

Mesenchymal
stem cells

Fig. 1.21 Types of cells associated with bone and their location.

> **APPLIED ANATOMY:** During growth, bone deposition outweighs bone resorption; in adulthood, the two processes are essentially in balance; however, with increasing age bone resorption outweighs bone deposition leading to osteoporosis.

Types of bone. Bone shows two types of organisation (lamellar, woven), of which woven bone is usually more immature than lamellar bone.

- **Lamellar bone:** In adults, most bone, both compact and cancellous, is organised in lamellae, arranged either parallel to each other or concentrically around a central canal forming an osteon (Fig. 1.22); in each lamella, the collagen fibres (type I) are aligned in parallel, but in successive lamellae they are orientated 90 degrees to each other, giving lamellar bone considerable strength. Each osteon (Haversian system) has a central canal containing blood vessels, nerves, loose connective tissue and endosteum; each osteon is long and runs parallel to the long axis of the diaphysis. In compact bone,

remodelling resorbs parts of old osteons and produces new ones (secondary and tertiary osteons).
- **Woven bone:** Type of bone formed in the skeleton of a developing foetus; it does not have a regular appearance, contains relatively more cells, which are randomly arranged, is not heavily mineralised when first formed, and has more ground substance than the matrix of mature bone. Woven bone is present in adults where bone is being remodelled (fracture repair), being present where tendons insert into bones, as well as in alveolar sockets of the jaws.

> **APPLIED ANATOMY:** In healthy adults, 5%–10% of bone is turned over annually.

Bone development. Bone develops either directly in mesoderm by the deposition of mineral salts (intramembranous ossification) or in previously formed cartilage models (endochondral ossification). Intramembranous ossification is the process of calcification followed by ossification without an intervening cartilage model (membrane bone); endochondral ossification is the most common.

- **Intramembranous ossification:** The site of bone formation is initially indicated by a condensation of cells and collagen fibres accompanied by the laying down of organic bone matrix, which becomes impregnated with mineral salts; it occurs in some bones of the skull, the mandible and clavicle.
- **Endochondral ossification:** A cartilage model of the future bone develops from mesodermal cells in the region where the bone is to develop. In long bones, the cartilage model grows mainly at its ends so that the oldest part is near the middle. The cartilage matrix in the older regions becomes calcified following impregnation with mineral salts: the cartilage cells (chondrocytes) are cut off from their nutrient supply and die. The majority of the calcified cartilage is subsequently removed, with bone being formed around its few remaining spicules; the continual process of excavation of calcified cartilage and deposition of bone eventually leads to the complete removal of the calcified cartilage (Fig. 1.23A). The cartilage at the extremities of the bone continues to grow due to cell multiplication, with the deeper layers gradually becoming calcified and replaced by bone.

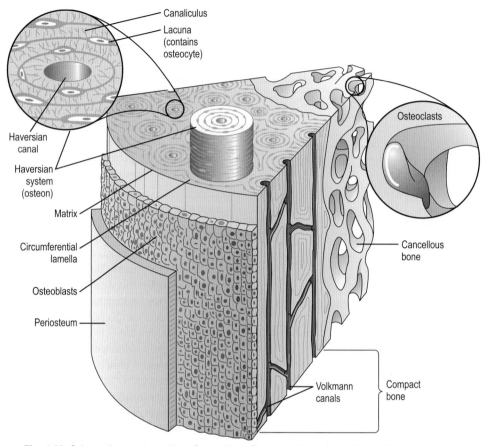

Fig. 1.22 Schematic representation of a section of compact bone from the shaft of a long bone.

APPLIED ANATOMY: The increase in length of a long bone is due to active cartilage at its ends, whereas increases in width are due to deposition of new bone on existing bone.

When first laid down, bone has a cancellous appearance, with no specific organisation (woven bone); in fracture repair, the newly formed bone is also woven in appearance. However, in response to stresses applied to the bone by muscles, tendons and ligaments, in addition to the forces transmitted across joints, the woven bone gradually assumes a specific pattern in response to these stresses.

Growth and remodelling. Growth and remodelling depend on the balanced activity of osteoblasts and osteoclasts facilitating a change in shape. In a growing long bone, new bone is laid down around the circumference

of the shaft increasing its diameter, while at the same time, the deepest layers of bone are removed to maintain a reasonable cortical bone thickness and enlarge the marrow cavity (Fig. 1.23B); failure to match deposition or removal of bone results in either very thick or very thin shafts.

APPLIED ANATOMY: Bone is continually remodelled, mainly under the direct control of hormones to stabilise blood calcium levels, as well as in response to long-term changes in the patterns of stresses applied to it.

Ossification. An ossification centre is a region where bone begins to be laid down; it is from these centres that ossification spreads. The principal (primary) ossification centres appear at different times in different bones but appear in an orderly sequence; they are relatively constant between individuals. The majority of primary ossification

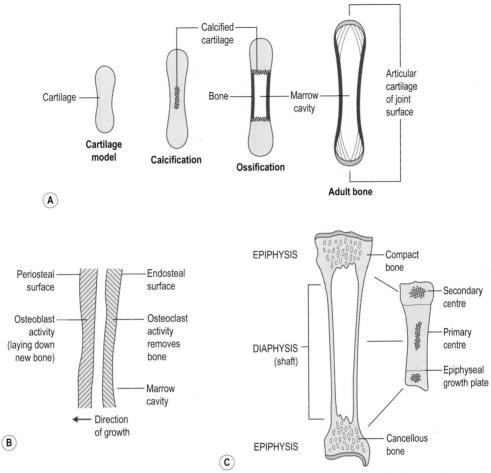

Fig. 1.23 (A) Stages in calcification and ossification of bone from a cartilage model. (B) Schematic representation of osteoblast and osteoclast activity. (C) Sites of ossification centres in long bones and the parts that develop from each.

centres appear between weeks 7 and 12 of intrauterine life, with most being present before birth; in long bones, the primary centre appears in the shaft (Fig. 1.23C). Secondary ossification centres usually appear after birth, appearing in parts of the cartilage model into which ossification from the primary centre has not spread (Fig. 1.23C); the bone formed is almost entirely cancellous.

APPLIED ANATOMY: The part of a long bone ossifying from the primary centre is the diaphysis, and that from a secondary centre is an epiphysis (Fig. 1.23C); the intervening region (epiphyseal growth plate) is where the diaphysis grows in length. When the growth plate disappears and the diaphysis and epiphysis fuse, growth in bone length ceases.

Bone fractures. A fracture is a break in a bone; it can range from a thin crack to a complete break, with most fractures occurring when a bone is impacted by more force than it can support.

- **Open fracture** in which the bone breaks through the skin or there is a deep wound exposing the bone; also referred to as a compound fracture.
- **Closed fracture** where the skin is not broken; also referred to as a simple fracture.
- **Partial fracture** is an incomplete break in the bone.
- **Complete fracture** in which the bone is separated into two or more parts.
- **Stable fracture** in which the two ends of the bone are aligned and not moved out of place.
- **Displaced fracture** in which there is a gap between the broken ends: this type of fracture often requires surgery.

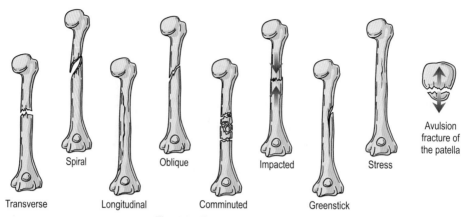

Fig. 1.24 Types of bone fracture.

Types of bone fracture:

- **Transverse fracture:** straight line break across the bone (Fig. 1.24), often caused by falls and traffic accidents.
- **Spiral fractures:** these spiral around the bone (Fig. 1.24), being caused by twisting injuries, often sustained during sports, they occur in long bones of the lower (femur, tibia, fibula) and upper (humerus, radius, ulna) limbs.
- **Greenstick fracture:** a partial fracture in which the bone bends and breaks but does not separate into two separate pieces (Fig. 1.24); it occurs mostly in children as their bones tend to be softer and more flexible.
- **Stress (hairline) fracture:** appears as a crack (Fig. 1.24) which can be difficult to diagnose, they are often caused by repetitive motions (running).
- **Compression fracture:** occurs when bones are crushed, with the broken bone being wider and flatter than before injury, occurring most often in the spine causing vertebrae to collapse; osteoporosis is the most common cause.
- **Oblique fracture:** a diagonal break across the bone occurring most frequently in long bones (Fig. 1.24), often due to a sharp blow at an angle due to a fall or other trauma.
- **Impacted fracture:** a break in which the broken ends of the bone are forced together by the force of the injury causing the fracture (Fig. 1.24).
- **Segmental fracture:** two breaks in the same bone leaving a 'floating' segment between the breaks, often occurring in long bones they can take longer to heal or can cause complications.

- **Comminuted fracture:** three or more breaks in the same bone with bone fragments at the fracture site (Fig. 1.24); they are due to high-impact trauma as in a road traffic accident.
- **Avulsion fracture:** occurs when a fragment is pulled off the bone by a tendon/ligament (Fig. 1.24), being more common in children than adults; in children there can be fracture through the growth plate.

Fracture repair. Repair of fractured bone occurs through four main stages (Fig. 1.25) using mechanisms in place for bone remodelling. At the fracture site, the torn blood vessels release blood that clots producing a large fracture haematoma (stage 1). This is gradually removed by macrophages and replaced by a soft fibrocartilage-like mass of procallus tissue rich in collagen and fibroblasts (stage 2); if disrupted, the periosteum re-establishes continuity over this tissue. The soft procallus is then invaded by ingrowing blood vessels and osteoblasts; over the next few weeks, the fibrocartilage is gradually replaced by woven bone forming a hard callus throughout the original fracture site (stage 3). Finally, the woven bone is remodelled as compact and cancellous bone in continuity with the adjacent non-injured areas, with a fully functional vasculature being established (stage 4).

Joints. The bones of the body come together to form joints; it is by these articulations that movement occurs. The type and extent of movement possible are dependent on the structure and function of the joint; variation in the form and function of joints allows them to be grouped into well-defined classes (fibrous, cartilaginous, synovial), with the degree of mobility gradually increasing from fibrous through to synovial joints.

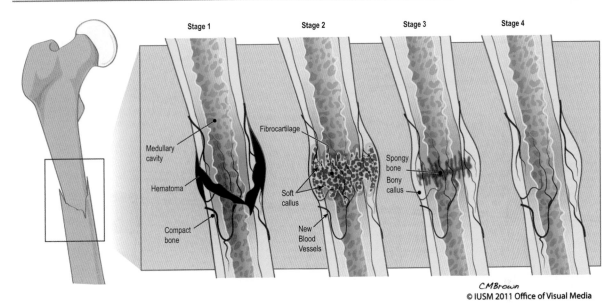

Stage 1   Stage 2   Stage 3   Stage 4

Fibrocartilage

Medullary
cavity

Spongy
bone

Bony
callus

Hematoma

Soft
callus

Compact
bone

New
Blood
Vessels

CMBrown
© IUSM 2011 Office of Visual Media

Fig. 1.25 Stages in the process of fracture repair.

Fibrous joints. There are three types (suture, gomphosis, syndesmosis) of fibrous joint (Fig. 1.26).

- **Sutures:** Between the bones of the skull, they allow no movement as the edges of the articulating bones are usually highly serrated, as well as being united by an intermediate layer of fibrous tissue (Fig. 1.26A). The inner and outer layers of periosteum on either side of the fibrous tissue are continuous, constituting the main bond between them.

> **APPLIED ANATOMY:** Sutures usually become partially obliterated after age 30.

- **Gomphosis:** A type of fibrous joint in which a peg fits into a socket, being held in place by a fibrous band or ligament. The roots of the teeth held within their sockets in the maxilla and mandible are gomphoses (Fig. 1.26B); the fibrous structure is the periodontal ligament/membrane.
- **Syndesmosis:** In these joints, the amount of fibrous tissue between the bones is greater than in sutures, being a ligament or interosseous membrane (Fig. 1.26C); flexibility of the ligament or twisting of the membrane allow limited and controlled movement at the joint. In adults, the inferior tibiofibular joint (page 612) is a syndesmosis, where the two bones

are held together by an interosseous ligament, and between the radius and ulna and the tibia and fibula, which are held together by an interosseous membrane (pages 416 and 612, respectively).

Cartilaginous joints. In cartilaginous joints the two bones are united by a pad of fibrocartilage; there are two types (primary cartilaginous/synchondrosis, secondary cartilaginous/symphysis) of cartilaginous joints (Fig. 1.27).

- **Primary cartilaginous:** The ends of the articulating bones are joined by a continuous layer of hyaline cartilage (Fig. 1.27A); such joints show no movement due to the rigidity of the hyaline cartilage. These joints occur at the epiphyseal growth plates of growing and developing bones but become obliterated with fusion of the diaphysis and epiphysis. There is only one such joint in adults (1st sternocostal joint), in which the hyaline cartilage is relatively long, enabling slight movement between the 1st rib and sternum.
- **Secondary cartilaginous joint:** Slightly more specialised than primary cartilaginous joints having a pad of fibrocartilage between the hyaline cartilage-covered ends of the articulating bones, allowing a small amount of controlled movement to take place. The joints between adjacent vertebrae (Fig. 1.27B) are such joints, where the intervertebral disc (page 196) is the fibrocartilaginous pad: the joint between the body of the pubis of each innominate (page 569) is also a secondary cartilaginous joint.

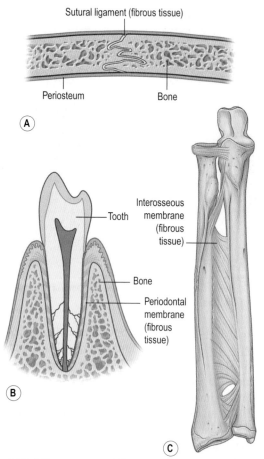

Fig. 1.26 Different types of fibrous joints: (A) suture; (B) gomphosis; (C) syndesmosis.

> **APPLIED ANATOMY:** Secondary cartilaginous joints tend to occur in the midline of the body.

Synovial joints. These are freely mobile joints whose movement is limited by the associated joint capsule, ligaments, muscles and tendons crossing the joint; most joints in the limbs are synovial joints. The articular surfaces are covered in a layer of articular (hyaline) cartilage, which due to its hardness and smoothness enables the bones to move against each other with minimum friction. Surrounding each joint is a fibrous capsule, often strengthened by ligaments and the deep part of muscles crossing the joint; lining the deep surface of the capsule is the synovial membrane covering all non-articular surfaces within the capsule (Fig. 1.28). The synovial membrane secretes synovial fluid into the joint

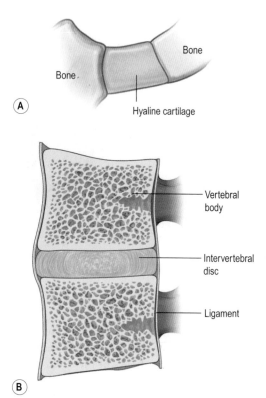

Fig. 1.27 Different types of cartilaginous joints: (A) primary cartilaginous (synchondrosis); (B) secondary cartilaginous (symphysis).

cavity, lubricating and nourishing the articulating surfaces; during movement, the joint surfaces spin, roll or slide past each other (Fig. 1.29). Bursae are often associated with synovial joints, being present where tendons cross the joint: they may or may not communicate directly with the joint cavity.

The tissues surrounding joints (skin, ligaments, fibrous capsule) contain receptors (nerve endings) responsible for detecting stretch, pressure and pain: Ruffini and Paciniform corpuscles (page 52) detect stretch and pressure in joint capsules and/or ligaments, mediating position sense, while free nerve endings (page 52) are thought to be responsible for mediating pain.

> **APPLIED ANATOMY:** In bones ossifying in a membrane (page 31), the articular cartilage has a large fibrous element; in addition, there is a complete or incomplete intra-articular disc within the joint capsule separating the two articular surfaces (Fig. 1.28B).

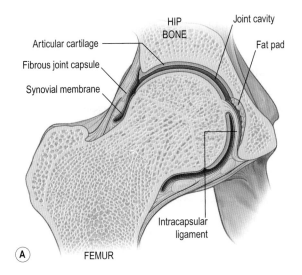

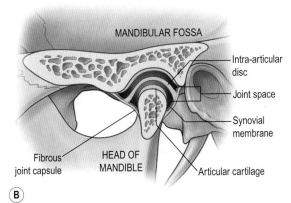

Fig. 1.28 The structure of synovial joints without (A) and with (B) an intra-articular disc.

CLINICAL ANATOMY: Osteoarthritis, the commonest form of arthritis, is a type of degenerative joint disease resulting from the breakdown of articular cartilage and the underlying bone; it is probably caused by mechanical stress on the joint and low-grade inflammatory processes. The most common symptoms are joint pain and stiffness (which usually progress slowly), joint swelling, decreased range of movement and, if the spine is affected, weakness or numbness in the arms and legs. The most commonly affected joints are the small joints of the fingers, the hip and knee joints, and the joints of the neck and lower back; joints on one side of the body can be affected more than on the opposite side. Primary osteoarthritis has no known underlying disease or injury, developing gradually and affecting older individuals; secondary osteoarthritis can often be linked to a previous injury or another medical condition and is more likely to affect younger individuals.

Because of the large number of synovial joints in the body with their differing forms, they are subdivided according to the shape of their articulating surfaces and the movements permitted.

- **Plane joint:** The joint surfaces are flat or relatively flat and of a similar extent and allow limited movements of either gliding or twisting of one bone against the other; the acromioclavicular joint (page 384) is a plane synovial joint.
- **Saddle joint:** The joint surfaces are reciprocally concavoconvex with the principal movements occurring about two mutually perpendicular axes; however, due to the nature of the joint surfaces, there is usually a small amount of movement about a 3rd axis;

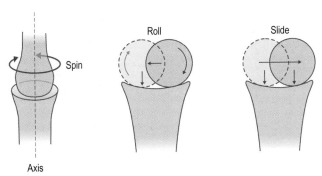

Fig. 1.29 Schematic representation of spin, roll and slide movements between articular surfaces.

the carpometacarpal joint of the thumb (page 426) is such a joint.

- **Hinge joint:** In hinge joints, movement is only permitted about a single axis due to the shape of the articulating surfaces, which fit together very well: the joint is also supported by strong collateral ligaments. The elbow joint (page 407) is a typical hinge joint: however, the knee joint (page 598) is a modified hinge joint as movement is possible about a 2nd axis, due to the poor fit between the articular surfaces.
- **Pivot joint:** Again, movement occurs about a single axis with the articular surfaces arranged so that one bone rotates within a fibro-osseous ring, such as at the atlantoaxial joint (page 194).
- **Ball-and-socket joint:** In this arrangement, movement occurs about three principally mutually perpendicular axes, with the rounded (ball) end of one bone fitting into a cavity (socket) of the other bone: the hip joint (page 598) is an example.
- **Condyloid joint:** A modified form of a ball-and-socket joint allowing active movement about three mutually perpendicular axes; however, passive movement may only be possible about the 3rd axis; condyloid joints are present between the head of the metacarpal and base of the proximal phalanx (metacarpophalangeal joint, page 427) of the fingers.
- **Ellipsoid joint:** Another form of a ball-and-socket joint where the joint surfaces are ellipsoid, with movement being possible about two mutually perpendicular axes; an example of an ellipsoid joint is the radiocarpal joint (page 419) in the wrist.

Blood

Details of blood and its constituents can be found on page 164.

Muscle

Within the body, there are three types of muscle (smooth, cardiac, skeletal), distinguished by morphological and functional characteristics, with the structure of each adapted to its physiological role. Each type has the ability to contract, causing movement within organs, of the blood, and of the body as a whole; contraction is caused by the interaction between thick myosin and thin actin filaments. The cytoplasm of muscle cells is the sarcoplasm, the SER the sarcoplasmic reticulum, and the cell membrane and its external lamina the sarcolemma.

Smooth Muscle

Smooth (involuntary, non-striated) muscle is specialised for slow, steady contraction and is controlled by numerous involuntary mechanisms; on the basis of the arrangement of its fibres and innervation, smooth muscle can be divided into two major types, multi-unit (visceral) and unitary (single unit). Individual fibres are elongated and tapering (Fig. 1.30), each being enclosed by a thin basal lamina and a fine network of reticular fibres (endomysium); in unitary smooth muscle, the connective tissue acts to combine the forces generated by each muscle fibre into a concerted action. The cells are organised with the broadest part of one cell lying adjacent to the narrowest part of another, with cells linked by gap junctions (page 23). In multi-unit smooth muscle, each fibre

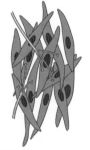
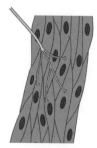

Multi-unit smooth muscle   Unitary smooth muscle

Fig. 1.30 Schematic representation of multi-unit and unitary smooth muscle.

operates independently and is often innervated; while unitary smooth muscle, which is arranged in sheets or bundles with many fibres, is innervated by a single nerve (Fig. 1.30).

Smooth muscle is not under voluntary control, being regulated differently in the viscera, respiratory airways, large and small blood vessels: control can involve the autonomic system (page 223), hormones and similar substances, as well as local physiologic conditions (degree of stretch). Whether smooth muscle fibres contract in small groups or through an entire muscle producing waves of contraction (peristalsis) is largely determined by the degree of autonomic innervation and the density of the gap junctions, both of which vary between organs.

As smooth muscle is most often spontaneously active without nervous stimulation, its nerve supply primarily modifies rather than initiates activity. It receives adrenergic and cholinergic nerve endings, stimulating or depressing its activity, with cholinergic endings activating and adrenergic endings depressing activity in some organs, while in others the reverse occurs. In addition to their contractile properties, smooth muscle cells also supplement fibroblast activity (collagen, elastin and proteoglycan synthesis), having a major impact on the extracellular matrix in tissues where these cells are abundant.

> **CLINICAL ANATOMY:** Benign tumours (leiomyomas) can develop from smooth muscle cells but are seldom problematic; they occur most commonly in the uterus (fibroids).

Cardiac Muscle

Developing heart cells align into chainlike arrays rather than fuse into multinucleated cells, as in developing skeletal muscle fibres, forming complex junctions between interdigitating processes (Fig. 1.31); cells within a fibre often branch and bind to cells in adjacent fibres forming a syncytium. The heart, therefore, comprises tightly knit interwoven bundles of cells exhibiting a cross-striated banding pattern, enabling a characteristic wave of contraction to be propagated. Each cardiac muscle cell is surrounded by a delicate sheath of endomysium containing a rich capillary network and has only one or two nuclei. A unique identifying feature of cardiac muscle

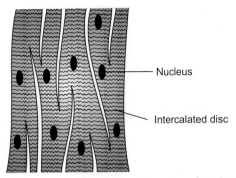

Fig. 1.31 The syncytial interconnecting nature of cardiac muscle fibres.

is the presence of transverse lines crossing the cells at regular intervals where the cells join (intercalated discs) representing the interface between adjacent muscle cells: longitudinal parts of each disc have gap junctions (page 23) providing continuity between cells enabling the cells to contract together.

Cardiac muscle fibre contraction is intrinsic and spontaneous, with impulses for rhythmic contraction (heart beat) being initiated, regulated and coordinated locally by nodes of unique myocardial fibres; the rate of contraction is modified by autonomic innervation of the nodes of conducting cells, with sympathetic activity increasing and parasympathetic activity decreasing the frequency of the impulses.

> **CLINICAL ANATOMY:** Tissue damage (ischaemia), due to lack of oxygen when the coronary arteries and/or their branches are blocked by heart disease, is the most common injury to cardiac muscle; cardiac muscle has little potential to regenerate following injury.

Skeletal Muscle

Skeletal muscle comprises more than one-third of body mass; it consists of non-branching long, cylindrical cells with many peripheral nuclei under the sarcolemma, with a few reserve progenitor cells (muscle satellite cells) associated with most muscle fibres. Each fibre has a delicate connective tissue covering (endomysium) separating it from its neighbours but also connecting them together (Fig. 1.32). Bundles of parallel fibres (fasciculi) are bound together by a thin connective tissue covering (perimysium), with nerves, blood vessels and lymphatics

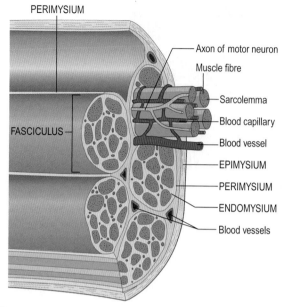

PERIMYSIUM

Axon of motor neuron

Muscle fibre

FASCICULUS

Sarcolemma

Blood capillary

Blood vessel

EPIMYSIUM

PERIMYSIUM

ENDOMYSIUM

Blood vessels

Fig. 1.32 Schematic representation of the organisation of individual muscle fibres into a whole muscle, together with their investing connective tissue coverings.

penetrating the perimysium to supply each fibre: each fascicle is a functional unit in which the fibres work together. Groups of fascicles are bound together to form a whole muscle (Fig. 1.32) enclosed within a fibrous covering (epimysium), which can be thick and strong or thin and relatively weak; septa from the epimysium extend inward carrying larger nerves and blood vessels. The collagen in the connective tissue layers transmits the mechanical forces generated by contracting muscle fibres; the epimysium is continuous with the dense regular connective tissue of a tendon at the myotendinous junction.

Muscle fibre organisation. Skeletal muscle fibres show cross striations of alternating dark (A) and light (I) bands (Fig. 1.33), with each A band having a central H zone (myosin filaments only) bisected by an M line, while each I band is bisected by a dark transverse line (Z disc); I bands contain thin actin filaments, which are attached to the Z disc, and A bands thicker myosin filaments, which are also connected to the Z disc, as well as overlapping portions of thin filaments. The hexagonal arrangement of thin and thick filaments (Fig. 1.33) is responsible for the cross striations seen in skeletal muscle. The functional subunit of the contractile apparatus (sarcomere) extends from Z disc to Z disc (Fig. 1.33);

myofibrils consist of end-to-end repetitive arrangements of sarcomeres. As the degree of overlap between thin and thick filaments increases so each sarcomere, and therefore muscle fibre shortens.

Muscle fibre types. Physiologically, there are three types of skeletal muscle fibre reflecting the muscle's main function: most muscles contain a mixture of all three types. Muscles which are active with slow contractions (postural muscles of the back) tend to have more mitochondria and a higher density of capillaries; these consist of type Ia fibres, which contain iron and store oxygen giving them a red appearance in fresh tissue. Muscles specialised for short-term work and fast contractions (extraocular muscles) consist of large diameter fibres (type IIb) with little myoglobin and appear white in fresh tissue, they depend more on anaerobic (glycolytic) metabolism of glucose, most of which is derived from stored glycogen; glycolysis produces lactate causing rapid muscle fatigue and an oxygen debt (repaid during the recovery period). Intermediate muscles (major muscles of the lower limb) which are active with fast contractions have numerous capillaries and a high myoglobin content; they also appear red in fresh tissue. Differentiation of muscle into red, white and intermediate fibres is partly controlled by the frequency of impulses from its motor innervation; fibres of a single motor unit (all the muscle fibres supplied by a single nerve fibre) are of the same type.

APPLIED ANATOMY: Muscle fibres can change from red to white and vice versa if the frequency of impulses to them changes or the muscle is subject to specific 'training' regimes.

Sensory receptors in muscle. Muscles contain free nerve endings and two types of specialised receptors (Golgi tendon organs, muscle spindles); the free nerve endings are responsible for mediating pain, being sparsely scattered throughout the muscle belly but more densely at the myotendinous junction.

Golgi tendon organs are formed by multiple terminal branches of an axon (page 47) weaving between collagen fibres of the tendon; the region around the branches is surrounded by a fibrous capsule (Fig. 1.34A). When the muscle contracts collagen fibres in the tendon stretch bringing them closer together, compressing the nerve terminals triggering the stimulus: Golgi tendon organs

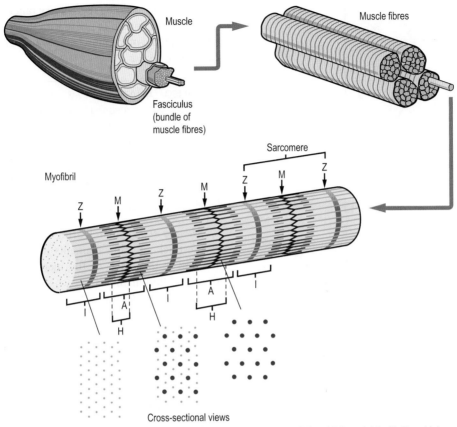

Fig. 1.33 Myofibrils within a muscle fibre showing sarcomeres containing thick and thin fibrils which overlap in some regions; also shown is the hexagonal arrangement of thick and thin filaments.

monitor the extent of muscle contraction, as well as the force exerted by the muscle.

Muscle fibres within a spindle (intrafusal fibres) monitor changes in muscle length; muscle fibres producing movement on contraction are extrafusal fibres. Muscle spindles are highly elaborate structures consisting of two types of modified muscle fibres (nuclear bag and nuclear chain fibres); they are surrounded by a fibrous capsule and occur throughout the muscle belly (Fig. 1.34B). Nuclear bag fibres have nuclei grouped into an expanded region in the middle of the fibre, while nuclear chain fibres have nuclei spread along their length. At their middle, both nuclear bag and nuclear chain fibres are spirally surrounded by branches of a group of Ia sensory neurons (page 51); group II neurons (page 51) form similar spiral endings around nuclear chain fibres and spray-like endings around nuclear bag fibres (Fig. 1.34B).

As a muscle lengthens or shortens, the degree of stretching or relaxation of the intrafusal fibres alters activity in the Ia and II fibres innervating them; this activity is relayed to the central nervous system, where the length of the muscle and its rate of lengthening/ shortening are determined, and indirectly, with other receptors, joint position is determined.

> **APPLIED ANATOMY:** Subgroups of nuclear bag and chain fibres have been identified, which may be responsible for detecting different components of the change in muscle length and its rate of change.

Muscle spindles also receive a motor innervation from δ motor neurons; activity in these neurons causes the ends of the intrafusal fibres to contract, stretching the central region, which changes the sensitivity of the

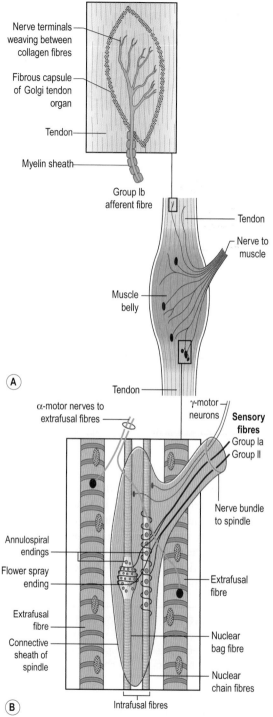

Nerve terminals weaving between collagen fibres

Fibrous capsule of Golgi tendon organ

Tendon

Myelin sheath

Group Ib afferent fibre

γ

Tendon

Nerve to muscle

Muscle belly

(A)

Tendon

α-motor nerves to extrafusal fibres

γ-motor neurons

Sensory fibres
Group Ia
Group II

Nerve bundle to spindle

Annulospiral endings

Flower spray ending

Extrafusal fibre

Extrafusal fibre

Connective sheath of spindle

Nuclear bag fibre

Nuclear chain fibres

(B)

Intrafusal fibres

Fig. 1.34 Location and microscopic appearance of (A) Golgi tendon organs and (B) muscle spindles within a muscle and its tendon.

central region enabling the sensory function of the muscle spindle to remain in phase with the overall lengthening/shortening of the muscle as a whole when it contracts or relaxes.

> **APPLIED ANATOMY:** Without δ activity, muscle spindles would respond to muscle stretch only when it was fully extended; shortening would relieve the stretch with the muscle spindle ceasing to signal muscle length. By contracting, under the control of δ motor neurons, the intrafusal fibres keep the central sensory region taut at all times, enabling it to monitor muscle length throughout the full range of movement.

Muscle contraction. During contraction, the length of the thick and thin filaments does not change; contraction is the result of the increased overlapping of thick and thin filaments in each sarcomere as they slide past each other. Contraction is induced when an action potential arrives at the neuromuscular junction and is transmitted along the T tubules to the sarcoplasmic reticulum triggering the release of calcium. Myelinated motor nerves branch within the perimysium, with each giving rise to several unmyelinated terminal twigs which pass through the endomysium and form synapses with individual extrafusal muscle fibres. Each axonal branch of an α motor neuron forms a dilated termination situated within a trough on the muscle surface: this is the neuromuscular junction or motor endplate (Fig. 1.35).

As the motor neuron approaches its target muscle fibre, it loses its myelin sheath and forms a flattened expansion applied to the surface of the muscle membrane; the expansion is covered by a Schwann cell insulating the neuromuscular junction from the external environment. The apposed muscle fibre surface is also modified, forming a flattened bump on its surface formed by the accumulation of sarcoplasm and organelles within the muscle cell, raising its membrane below the nerve terminal. The part of the nerve cell membrane applied to the muscle cell is the prejunctional membrane, with the corresponding part of the muscle cell membrane being the postjunctional membrane (Fig. 1.35B); the two membranes are separated by a narrow trough (synaptic cleft), with secondary synaptic clefts in the postjunctional membrane increasing the surface area of the receptor muscle membrane (Fig. 1.35B). The terminal end of the motor neuron contains vesicles filled with acetylcholine (neurotransmitter); when an action potential arrives at the nerve terminal, the vesicles release the acetylcholine into the synaptic cleft, where it reacts with receptors on the postjunctional membrane generating an action potential in the muscle membrane. It is this action potential which is propagated into the muscle cell causing contraction of the muscle fibres.

> **CLINICAL ANATOMY:** Denervation of a muscle leads to atrophy and paralysis.

Muscle forms. Muscles have various shapes (forms): some are flat and in sheets, some are short and thick, and others long and slender. The length of a muscle (excluding its tendons) is closely related to the distance

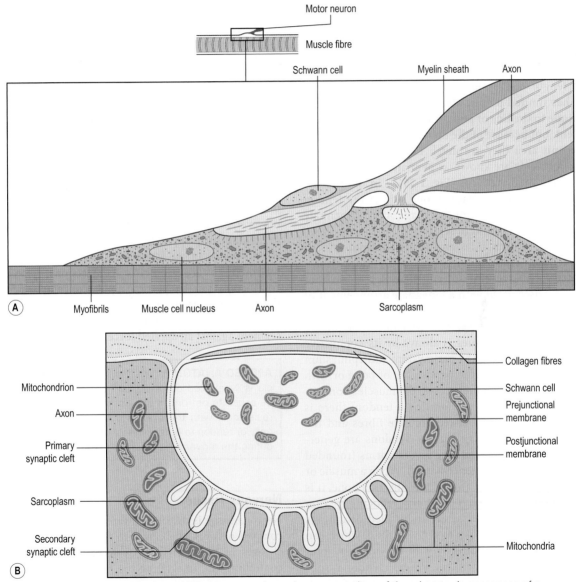

Fig. 1.35 (A) Longitudinal and (B) transverse schematic representations of the microscopic appearance of a neuromuscular junction.

through which it shortens; muscle fibres can shorten to almost half their resting length. The arrangement of fibres within a muscle (parallel or oblique to the direction of pull of the whole muscle) determines how much it can shorten when it contracts; irrespective of muscle fibre arrangement, all movement is brought about by muscle contraction (shortening) with their action across joints changing the relative position of the bones involved.

Muscles with fibres parallel to the line of pull have fibres arranged as discrete bundles forming a fusiform muscle (Fig. 1.36A) or spread out as a broad sheet (Fig. 1.36B); when contraction occurs, it does so through the maximum distance allowed by the length of the muscle fibres; however, the muscle has limited power. Muscles with fibres arranged oblique to the line of pull cannot shorten to the same extent, but because of the increased number of fibres per unit area they are much more powerful; these arrangements are known as pennate, of which there are three main patterns (Fig. 1.36C). In unipennate muscles, the fibres attach to one side of the tendon only (flexor pollicis longus, page 429); bipennate muscles have a central septum with muscle fibres attaching to both sides and to its continuous central tendon (rectus femoris, page 595); multipennate muscles have several intermediate septa, each of which is associated with a bipennate arrangement of fibres (deltoid, page 394).

Muscle attachments. The attachment of muscle to bone or other tissues is always by its connective tissue elements, with the perimysium and epimysium uniting directly with the periosteum of bone or with the joint capsule. In most cases, the muscle's connective tissue elements fuse forming a tendon; there is no direct continuity between muscle fibres and the connective tissue of the tendon. Tendons are generally very strong and can take several forms (rounded cords, thin sheets, flattened bands). When a muscle or tendon passes over or around the edge of a bone, it is usually separated from it by a bursa reducing friction during movement; bursae are fluid-filled dilatations containing a fluid similar to synovial fluid, which can either communicate directly with the adjacent joint cavity or remain independent. Where a tendon is subject to friction a sesamoid bone can develop within it.

CLINICAL ANATOMY: Bursitis is inflammation of a bursa causing a dull aching pain (which is worse when it moves or pressure is applied), swelling, tenderness or warmth in the surrounding skin, and stiffness around a joint; the most commonly affected joints are the shoulders, hips, elbows and knees.

CLINICAL ANATOMY: A tendon is often stronger than the area of bone to which it attaches; brief intense forces generated by the muscle (often in response to potential trauma) can lead to detachment of the tendon from bone taking with it a bone fragment (avulsion fracture).

Muscle action. When a muscle contracts, its two ends are brought closer together changing its length, even though the tension generated may remain more or less constant, these are isotonic contractions; however, if muscle length remains unchanged (due to an externally applied resistance), the tension usually increases in an attempt to overcome the resistance, these are isometric contractions. Isotonic contraction can be of two types: concentric where the muscle shortens or eccentric where the muscle lengthens as in controlling the movement of a body segment against an applied force.

APPLIED ANATOMY: When testing whether a muscle is weakened or paralysed, the individual should be asked to perform the main muscle action against resistance, with the examiner palpating the muscle belly or tendon to determine whether it is contracting during the movement.

Nervous Tissue

Nervous tissue is distributed throughout the body as a complex network enabling it to respond to continuous changes in its internal and external environment by controlling and integrating the functional activities of the organs and organ systems.

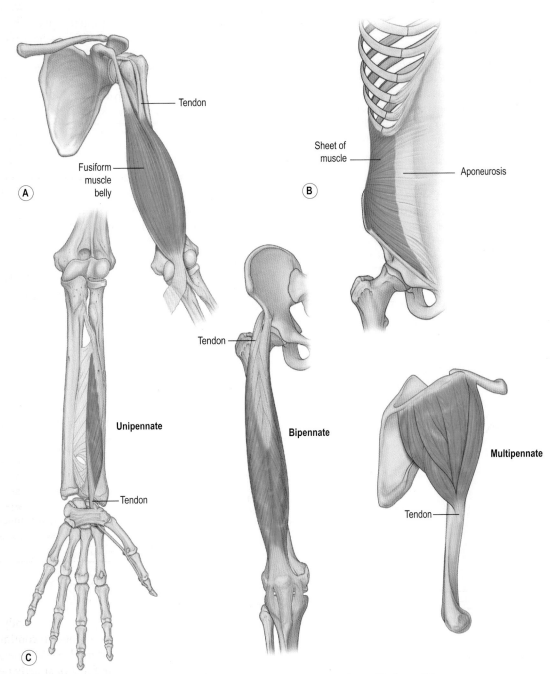

Fig. 1.36 Different arrangements of muscle fibres: (A) fusiform, (B) sheet, (C) pennate.

APPLIED ANATOMY: Anatomically, the nervous system is divided into central nervous system comprising the brain (page 243) and spinal cord (204), and the peripheral nervous system comprising cranial (page 240), spinal (page 220) and peripheral nerves in the limbs and trunk, all of which conduct impulses from (efferent/motor nerves) and to (afferent/sensory nerves) the central nervous system. The autonomic nervous system (page 223) consists of the autonomic parts of both the central and peripheral nervous systems providing efferent involuntary motor innervation to smooth muscle, the conducting system of the heart, and glands, as well as afferent sensory innervation from the viscera (pain and autonomic reflexes); it is subdivided into sympathetic (page 225), parasympathetic (page 225) and enteric (page 464) parts, with the enteric part communicating with the central nervous system via sympathetic and parasympathetic fibres, although it is able to function independently of the other two parts of the autonomic nervous system.

activities (nutrition, defence of cells in the central nervous system).

APPLIED PHYSIOLOGY: By collecting, analysing and integrating information from the body, the nervous system continuously stabilises the intrinsic conditions of the body (blood pressure, oxygen and carbon dioxide content of the blood, hormonal levels) within normal ranges and maintains behavioural patterns (feeding, reproduction, defence against bacteria, viruses and toxins).

Neuron

A number of structural classes of neurons can be identified: multipolar neurons (Fig. 1.37A), including motor neurons and central nervous system interneurons; bipolar neurons (Fig. 1.37B), which include sensory neurons in the retina (page 299), olfactory mucosa and inner ear (page 316); unipolar or pseudounipolar neurons (Fig. 1.37C) which are all other sensory neurons; and anaxonic neurons (Fig. 1.37D) of the central nervous system which lack a true axon and do not produce action potentials, but do regulate local electrical changes in adjacent neurons.

Cell body. The cell body (Fig. 1.37) is the expanded part of the neuron containing the nucleus, with a prominent nucleolus and cytoplasm, containing

The functional unit of the nervous system is the nerve cell (neuron), which is supported by various glial cells (page 247). Neurons have a cell body and many long processes (axon, dendrites), while glial cells have short processes; glial cells support and protect neurons, as well as participating in many neural

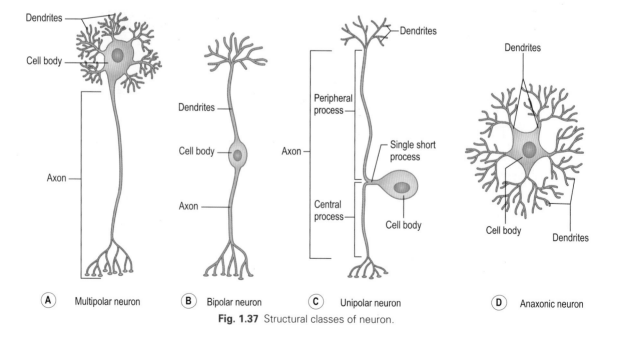

(A) Multipolar neuron   (B) Bipolar neuron   (C) Unipolar neuron   (D) Anaxonic neuron

Fig. 1.37 Structural classes of neuron.

numerous mitochondria, a large perinuclear Golgi apparatus, lysosomes, microtubules, neurofilaments (intermediate filaments, page 15), transport vesicles and other inclusions (Nissl bodies [discrete clumps of RER]); it excludes all processes. The cell body acts as the trophic centre producing cytoplasm for movement into the processes, as well as receiving a large number of nerve endings conveying excitatory or inhibitory stimuli generated in other cells. Nissl bodies and free ribosomes extend into the dendrites, but not the axon; the axon hillock is that part of the cell body connecting to the axon, it lacks large cytoplasmic organelles and has few Nissl bodies, being a distinguishing feature between axons and dendrites.

Dendrites. Short processes emanating from the cell body (Fig. 1.37), with most nerve cells having many dendrites increasing the receptive area of the neuron; they are usually covered with many synapses, being the principal signal reception and processing sites on neurons. The arborisation of dendrites enables a single neuron to receive and integrate a great number of axon terminals from other cells; most synapses impinging on neurons do so on dendritic spines (short blunt structures projecting at points along dendrites).

Axon. Most neurons have a single axon (Fig. 1.37) that can vary in length and diameter depending on their location and function within the nervous system; they are usually very long processes. They originate from a pyramidal-shaped region of the cell body (axon hillock), beyond which is an area (initial segment) where various excitatory and inhibitory stimuli impinging on the neuron are algebraically summated, resulting in the decision whether or not to propagate a nerve impulse. The distal end of an axon forms a terminal arborisation, with the axons of interneurons and some motor neurons having branches (collaterals) that end at synapses influencing the activity of several other neurons; each branch ends as a dilation (terminal bouton) that contacts another neuron or non-nerve cell at a synapse to initiate an impulse in that cell.

> **APPLIED ANATOMY:** The plasma membrane of the axon is frequently called the axolemma and its contents the axoplasm.

> **APPLIED ANATOMY:** Interneurons are situated between sensory and motor neurons, transmitting impulses between them, especially as part of a reflex arc.

Myelination. Myelination is the process by which individual axons are wrapped in a lipid sheath (myelin), which acts as a protective and insulating coating; it enhances the speed of conduction of electrical impulses along it. In the central nervous system, myelination is performed by specialised cells (oligodendrocytes [page 247]), with each oligodendrocyte surrounding several axons (Fig. 1.38); unmyelinated axons are embedded in cytoplasmic extensions/processes of oligodendrocytes.

In the peripheral nervous system, myelination is by Schwann cells which spirally curl an extension of their cell membrane around the axon; as the Schwann cell extension wraps around the axon, its cytoplasm is squeezed out until only a double layer of Schwann cell membrane surrounds the axon (Fig. 1.39A). Outside the myelin sheath, the axon is surrounded by the Schwann cell cytoplasm with the outermost Schwann cell membrane acting as a second membrane to the axon (neurolemma). Along its length, the axon is ensheathed in

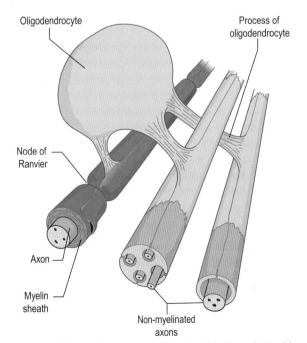

Fig. 1.38 Schematic representation showing the relationship between an oligodendrocyte and several myelinated and unmyelinated axons.

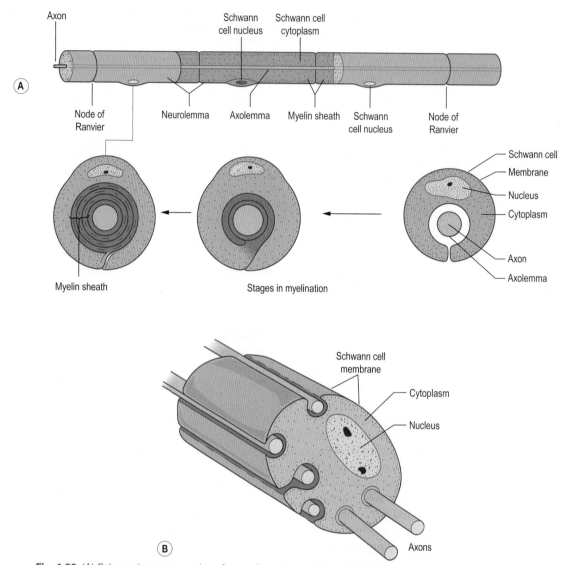

Fig. 1.39 (A) Schematic representation of a myelinated axon in the peripheral nervous system, together with the stages of myelination. (B) The relationship between unmyelinated axons and Schwann cells.

series by a large number of Schwann cells; each Schwann cell is related to a single axon only: junctions between Schwann cells are nodes of Ranvier. An axon, its myelin sheath and the surrounding Schwann cell is a single nerve fibre. Unmyelinated axons run embedded in invaginations of Schwann cell membrane, with a single Schwann cell surrounding several axons (Fig. 1.39B): they have less physical protection; however, the main difference is that unmyelinated axons conduct impulses at much slower velocities.

Neuron communication. A synapse is a site where nerve impulses are transmitted from one neuron to another or to another effector cell; their structure is similar to the neuromuscular junction (page 42), ensuring that transmission is unidirectional. Synapses convert electrical signals (nerve impulses) into a chemical signal that affects the postsynaptic cell, with most synapses acting by releasing neurotransmitters into the synaptic cleft. Neurotransmitters can have either an excitatory or an inhibitory effect depending on the nature of the neurotransmitter and the receptors on the postsynaptic membrane with which it acts; excitatory substances generate an action potential in the postsynaptic neuron, propagating the potential to its other end, while inhibitory substances temporarily alter the electrical potential of the postsynaptic neuron, reducing its capacity to be stimulated by other neurons. The activity of postsynaptic cells is determined by the summation of the interplay between excitatory and inhibitory effects. Different types of synapses occur between neurons (Fig. 1.40). When an axon forms a synapse with a cell body, it is an axosomatic synapse; with a dendrite, an axodendritic synapse; and with another axon, an axoaxonic synapse. Axoaxonic synapses modulate the activity of the other two synaptic types.

Being connected to one another in diverse ways, groups of neurons are organised to subserve different functions within the nervous system; these patterns of connections (circuits) vary in complexity; however, in general, the more sophisticated the function, the more complex the circuitry.

CLINICAL PHYSIOLOGY: A number of factors can affect synaptic transmission. Repetitive stimulation of excitatory synapses at rapid rates leads to a decrease in the number of discharges by the postsynaptic neuron (fatigue), which is an important characteristic of synaptic function because when areas of the nervous system become overexcited, fatigue causes them to lose the excess excitability after a while; most neurons are responsive to changes in pH of the surrounding interstitial fluids, with alkalosis increasing and acidosis depressing neuronal activity. Neuronal excitability is also dependent on an adequate supply of oxygen; a lack of oxygen, if only for a few seconds, can result in complete inexcitability in some neurons. Many drugs (caffeine, theophylline and theobromine present in tea, coffee and cocoa) decrease excitability; in contrast, strychnine increases neuronal excitability by inhibiting the action of inhibitory transmitter substances, leading to severe tonic muscle spasms due to the excitatory transmitters becoming overwhelmed.

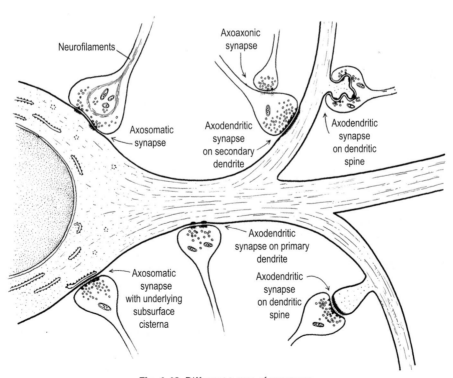

Fig. 1.40 Different types of synapses.

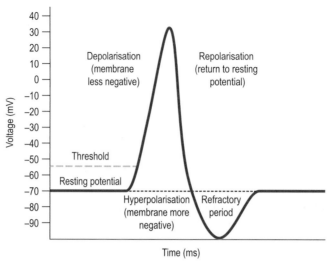

Fig. 1.41 An action potential.

Action Potential

An action potential is an electrochemical process in which a nerve impulse is conducted along an axon; the action potential is effectively a wave of membrane depolarisation initiated at the initial segment of the axon hillock. The membrane (axolemma) contains voltage-gated sodium (Na^+) and potassium (K^+) channels; in response to a stimulus, the Na^+ channels in the initial segment of the membrane open allowing Na^+ ions into the axoplasm, briefly depolarising (reversing) the negative membrane potential of the resting membrane (~70 mV) to positive (+30 mV), following which the Na^+ channels close and the K^+ channels open with K^+ ions rapidly leaving the axon returning the membrane to its resting potential (Fig. 1.41). Depolarisation of one part of the membrane sends an electrical current to neighbouring parts of the unstimulated membrane; the local current stimulates adjacent parts of the membrane causing depolarisation along it. Generation of an action potential is extremely rapid (<1000th of a second); after a very brief (refractory) period, the neuron is able to generate another action potential.

Peripheral Nervous System

Nerves supplying structural tissues (bone, muscle, skin) are somatic nerves, with groups of them innervating specific areas or regions; they are considered in detail in the respective region. Nerves supplying viscera (heart, lungs, digestive tract) are visceral nerves; their functions are largely automatic and subconscious; consequently, the part of the nervous system innervating viscera is the autonomic nervous system (page 223), with components in both the central and peripheral nervous systems.

Structure of peripheral nerves. Peripheral nerves consist of parallel aggregations of myelinated and unmyelinated axons; the greater the number of axons, the larger the nerve. The axons are held together by sheaths of fibrous tissue, providing additional coatings and protecting them from external mechanical and chemical trauma. Individual myelinated axons are surrounded by a tubular sheath of fibrous tissue (endoneurium), with clusters of axons held together by a further fibrous sheath (perineurium); unmyelinated axons are surrounded by endoneurium but run in isolated bundles parallel to myelinated axons, being enclosed with them by the perineurium (Fig. 1.42). Fascicles are bundles of axons within a perineural sheath; axons tend to remain within the same fascicle until their peripheral distribution; however, some axons can leave one fascicle and join another. Fascicles within a peripheral nerve are bound together within an external fibrous sheath (epineurium) forming the external surface of the nerve.

As peripheral nerves pass through body tissues, they give branches consisting of one or more fascicles, which leave them to reach their specific destination; along the course of the nerve, this process is repeated until all fascicles and axons have been distributed to their target tissues.

Constituents of peripheral nerves. Peripheral nerves consist of different types of axons classified according

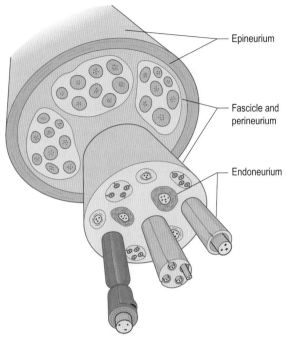

Fig. 1.42 Composition of a peripheral nerve.

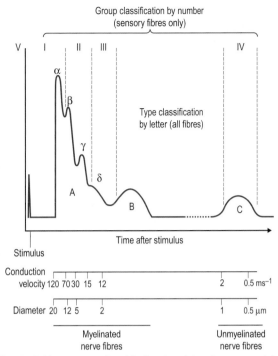

Fig. 1.43 Neurogram of an idealised peripheral nerve: activity in different types of nerve fibres is reflected in depolarisation occurring at different times following stimulation.

to their size, function or physiological characteristics. The broadest classification is into afferent (sensory) and efferent (motor) fibres; afferent fibres conduct information about events in the periphery to the central nervous system, while efferent fibres cause events in the periphery (skeletal or smooth muscle contraction).

Axons can also be classified in relation to their conduction velocities, which are proportional to their size; recording electrical activity in a nerve following its stimulation represents the summation of electrical activity in each axon in waveform, with the size of each component being proportional to the number of axons present with its shape reflecting the type of axons within the nerve. The waveform (neurogram) from a nerve containing all known types of axons has three principal peaks (A, B, C) (Fig. 1.43). The A peak is produced by rapidly conducting axons (A fibres) with velocities between 12 and 120 ms⁻¹; it can be broken down into several secondary peaks (Aα, Aβ, Aγ, Aδ), each being produced by a subgroup of rapidly conducting axons. The B wave is produced by more slowly conducting but still fast fibres (B fibres); the C wave is produced by slow conducting (0.5 to 2 ms⁻¹) fibres (C fibres). Not all peripheral nerves contain every type of fibre; B fibres are not always present. Myelinated axons (A and B fibres) conduct impulses faster than unmyelinated axons (C fibres); in myelinated

axons conduction velocity is directly proportional to the total diameter of the axon and its myelin sheath.

Functionally, Aα and Aγ fibres represent motor fibres innervating skeletal muscle but also contain certain sensory fibres transmitting information from skeletal muscle. Aβ fibres mediate touch, vibration and pressure sensations from skin; Aδ fibres are sensory fibres mediating pressure, pain and temperature from skin, pain and pressure from muscles, and pain, pressure and position information from ligaments and joints. B fibres are preganglionic sympathetic efferent fibres; C fibres are mainly unmyelinated sensory fibres arising in almost all body tissues and transmit pain, temperature and pressure sensations; however, some are postganglionic sympathetic neurons. Aβ fibres are sometimes referred to as large diameter afferent fibres, whereas Aδ and C fibres are collectively referred to as small diameter fibres.

Another axon classification system of sensory fibres uses numbers (I, II, III, IV) based on their conduction velocities (Fig. 1.43); they have the same conduction velocities as Aα, Aβ, Aδ and C fibres, respectively (Fig. 1.43), but do not include the Aα and Aβ motor fibres. Fibres in groups III and IV mainly mediate pain and

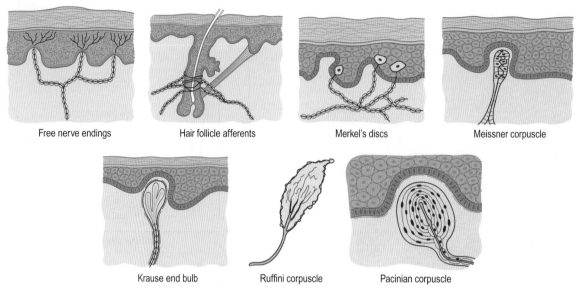

Free nerve endings   Hair follicle afferents   Merkel's discs   Meissner corpuscle

Krause end bulb   Ruffini corpuscle   Pacinian corpuscle

Fig. 1.44 Types of nerve endings (receptors) present in skin.

temperature sensations; group II pressure and touch, as well as fibres from the spray endings in muscle spindles (page 41); and group I, with Ia innervating muscle spindles and Ib innervating Golgi tendon organs.

Nerve Endings

Axon terminals have unique endings depending on their function; motor axon terminals are designed to deliver a stimulus to muscle cells (page 39). Sensory axons have terminals (receptors) designed to detect a specific type of stimulus; Golgi tendon organs (page 40) detect muscle contraction, as well as the force of contraction, and muscle spindles (page 41) detect muscle lengthening and shortening. The types of nerve endings in skin range from simple to complex formations (Fig. 1.44).

Free nerve endings: They are present within the epidermis and dermis (pages 55 and 56): in the epidermis, they run as naked axons between the epidermal cells, branching as they do so, and are usually orientated perpendicular to the skin surface (Fig. 1.44); in contrast, in the dermis, they run parallel to the surface. Free nerve endings detect stimuli generating sensations of pain and temperature; however, many are capable of responding to mechanical stimuli deforming the skin (touch, pressure); they are also present around the roots of hairs (see Fig. 1.46), being stimulated by deformation of the hair, as well as being involved in detecting coarse stimuli causing the hair to bend.

Merkel's discs: Complex endings formed when free nerve endings terminate as an expanded disc-like ending

under a specialised cell in the epidermis (Merkel [tactile] cell) (Fig. 1.44); they are present in hairless skin (especially the fingertips) and mediate touch sensation.

Meissner's corpuscles: Complex encapsulated receptors formed by a spiralling axon surrounded by flattened Schwann cells, in turn, surrounded by fibrous tissue continuous with the endoneurium of the axon (Fig. 1.44); they are probably involved in the sensation of touch.

Krause end bulbs: These consist of an axon that forms a cluster of multiple short branches surrounded by a fibrous capsule (Fig. 1.44); simpler versions occur in which the axon forms a bulbous ending surrounded by a poorly developed capsule, rather than branching. They are present in the dermis and probably respond to mechanical stimulation of the skin.

Ruffini corpuscles: These consist of an axon which forms a flattened tangle of branches embedded in a bundle of collagen fibres (Fig. 1.44); they occur in the dermis and respond to stretching of the collagen fibres when the skin is deformed by pressure.

Pacinian corpuscles: The most complex sensory ending consisting of a single axon surrounded by several concentric lamellae of modified Schwann cells all enclosed in a fibrous capsule (Fig. 1.44); they are found in the dermis and respond to pressure stimuli.

Nerve Injury

Acute injuries are relatively common, being associated with different types of trauma (blunt force, fractures, crush injuries, stretch, penetrating or cutting injuries); nerves of the upper limb tend to be the most commonly affected. The healing process can take from a few weeks to many months, with both the recovery and repair depending on the type of injury and extent of damage.

Neuropraxia: The least severe nerve injury resulting from the complete blocking of nerve transmission despite intact nerve fibres, with neither the axon nor its myelin sheath covering being severed; it can occur after sudden stretching in fractures or dislocations, following a blunt injury or after prolonged pressure on the nerve. Recovery is usually spontaneous over a few hours to a few months.

Axonotmesis: This occurs in traction injuries when the nerve sheath remains intact, but the axon may be divided; it can result in complete loss of muscle function (motor and/or sensory), sensations and autonomic function transmitted by the affected nerve. Recovery can take several months to years.

Neurotmesis: The most severe form of nerve injury in which the axon and its sheath is partially or completely severed; nevertheless, a clean cut has the potential for immediate repair and faster recovery.

CLINICAL ANATOMY: If an axon is severed its peripheral part quickly degenerates. Regeneration in the central nervous system is extremely limited, with functional deficits persisting after spinal cord injury, traumatic brain injury and stroke. However, in the peripheral nervous system, the distal part of the axon undergoes Wallerian degeneration, resulting in fragmentation and disintegration of the axon, with the debris removed by macrophages; regeneration of the proximal part is guided by the presence of important growth factors or neurotropic substances (nerve growth factor), with many other growth factors and cytokines (page 178) also being involved, as well as the intrinsic capacity of the neuron itself. Following degeneration, the nerve begins regeneration, which starts at the proximal site of injury and progresses slowly (1 mm/day) along the distal part of the degenerated nerve; nerve damaged closer to the muscle it innervates recover much earlier than those damaged further away from the muscle. Regenerated nerves may end up with abnormal connections, resulting in abnormal movements or sensations.

ORGANS

An organ is a combination of many different cell types and tissues bound together by intercellular structures, with each organ tending to have a specific function. Details of the major organs of the body can be found elsewhere: heart (page 118), lungs (page 97), brain (page 243), stomach (page 465), small (page 468) and large (page 472) intestine, liver (page 478), pancreas (page 482), spleen (page 162), kidney (page 509) and uterus (page 543), while the largest organ (skin) of the body is considered below.

Organs do not work in isolation, they are arranged into systems, each of which has a specific function or functions; most organ systems interact and cooperate with each other to enable the body to undertake its many and varied tasks. The major systems of the body are the cardiovascular and respiratory systems, both considered in Chapter 2; the nervous system, considered in Chapter 3; the digestive, urinary/renal and reproductive systems, all considered in Chapter 6; the endocrine system, considered mainly in Chapter 2, but also elsewhere in association with particular organs/structures; and the musculoskeletal system, which is considered in Chapters 4 (skull), 3 (vertebral column), 5 (upper limb) and 7 (lower limb).

Skin

Skin is the tough, pliable waterproof covering of the body, blending with the more delicate lining membranes of the body at the mouth, nose, eyelids, urogenital and anal openings; skin (the integument) is the largest organ of the body, accounting for between 15% and 20% of total body weight. In addition to providing a surface covering, it also has a number of specific functions (protective, sensory, thermoregulatory, metabolic, sexual signalling).

APPLIED ANATOMY: In adults, the surface area of the skin is between 1.5 and 2 m², varying with body size, being seven times greater than that at birth; this large surface area is necessary for skin to effectively carry out its metabolic functions. Skin tends to be thicker over posterior and extensor surfaces and thinner over anterior and flexor surfaces, as well as varying with age and from region to region; it is generally between 1 and 2 mm thick. It is thinnest over the eyelids (0.5 mm) and thickest over the back of the neck and upper trunk, palm of the hand and sole of the foot; total skin thickness depends on the thickness of both the epidermis (page 55) and dermis (page 56); on the palm of the hand and sole of the foot, the epidermis is responsible for the thickness, with the dermis being relatively thin.

In young individuals, skin is extremely elastic, rapidly returning to its original shape and position; with increasing age, elasticity is lost so that unless attached to underlying tissues it stretches; stretching tends to occur in one direction due to the orientation of the collagen fibres in the deepest layers running predominantly at right angles to the direction of stretch, parallel to the grooves present on the skin surface. In some places, skin is bound down to the underlying deep fascia, allowing free movement without interference from subcutaneous fat and otherwise highly mobile skin. In adjusting to allow movement, skin follows the body contours through its intrinsic elasticity; nevertheless, it is subject to internal stresses, which vary from region to region.

> **APPLIED ANATOMY:** Skin can be easily displaced as it is loosely applied to underlying tissues; however, in some places, it may be firmly attached to underlying structures (cartilage of the ear, nose, subcutaneous periosteal surface of the tibia, deep fascia around joints). It increases the thickness of its superficial layers in response to continued friction.

> **APPLIED ANATOMY:** Where skin is pulled around a joint it is bound down to the underlying fibrous tissue in loose folds (flexion creases), which are then taken up during flexion.

Functions

Protection. Its protective function is to provide a physical barrier against thermal and mechanical insult and against most potential pathogens and other materials, as well as to alert resident lymphocytes (page 173) and antigen-presenting cells (page 178) to trigger an immune response to microorganisms that penetrate the skin. The dark pigment (melanin) in the epidermis protects cells from ultraviolet light, while skin's waterproofing role provides a selectively permeable barrier against excessive loss or uptake of water. The waterproofing role is essentially concerned with preventing fluid loss from the body rather than keeping fluid out; fatty acid secretions from sebaceous glands help maintain waterproofing.

> **APPLIED PHYSIOLOGY:** The selective permeability of skin allows some lipophilic drugs (some steroid hormones and medications) to be administered via skin patches; it also allows the excretion of certain crystalloids through sweating.

> **CLINICAL PHYSIOLOGY:** A yellowish skin colour (jaundice) results from an accumulation of bilirubin (page 480): it reflects liver dysfunction.

Sensation. The skins' sensory function resides in the numerous nerve endings it contains, enabling it to constantly monitor the environment, as well as help regulate the body's interaction to physical objects (touch, pressure, changes in temperature, painful stimuli).

> **CLINICAL PHYSIOLOGY:** Two-point discrimination tests depend on the density of Meissner corpuscles (page 52) in the skin, with the number decreasing with age; in scleroderma and other connective tissue disorders leading to sclerosis (hardening) of the dermis and tightening of the skin, there is loss or reduction in the number of Meissner corpuscles.

Thermoregulation. An extremely important function of skin as body temperature must be kept within relatively narrow limits in spite of large variations in environmental temperature. Temperature regulation is possibly due to its variable blood supply, as well as the presence of sweat glands, with blood vessels dilating to promote heat loss in warm temperatures and constricting to conserve body heat in cool temperatures.

> **APPLIED PHYSIOLOGY:** Together with the lungs, skin accounts for more than 90% of total body heat loss.

Metabolism. Cells in the skin synthesise vitamin D (page 506), needed in calcium metabolism and bone formation (page 31), through the local action of ultraviolet light on the vitamin's precursor; excess electrolytes can be removed in sweat, while the subcutaneous layer can store a significant amount of energy in the form of fat.

Sexual signalling. Many features of skin (pigmentation, hair) are visual indicators of health involved in sexual attraction; the effects of sex pheromones produced by the apocrine sweat (page 61) and other glands are important contributors to this attraction.

Structure

Skin comprises superficial epithelial (epidermis) and deeper connective tissue (dermal) layers, beneath which lies subcutaneous tissue (hypodermis), a loose connective tissue layer usually containing pads of adipocytes. The subcutaneous tissue binds the skin loosely to the underlying tissues: it corresponds to the superficial fascia. The epidermal-dermal junction is irregular, in which dermal projections interdigitate with invaginating epidermal ridges (Fig. 1.45) to strengthen adhesion between the two layers.

> **CLINICAL PHYSIOLOGY:** Friction blisters are lymph-filled spaces between the epidermis and dermis caused by excessive rubbing (excessive use of hand tools, ill-fitting shoes); it can produce protective thickening and hardening of the outer epithelial layers (corns, calluses).

Epidermis. Epidermis is a layer of stratified squamous keratinised epithelium, as well as less abundant pigment-producing cells (melanocytes), antigen-presenting (Langerhans) cells and tactile (Merkel) cells; it is composed of five layers of cells (Fig. 1.45), from deep to superficial basal (stratum basale), spinous (stratum spinosum), granular (stratum granulosum), translucent (stratum lucidum), corneum (stratum corneum). The basal layer, together with the deep layer of the spinous layer, is where new cells are produced, replacing those lost from the surface; the spinous layer consists of several layers of irregularly shaped cells, which become flattened as they approach the granular layer. In the granular layer, the cells become increasingly flattened and keratinisation begins: the cells are in the process of dying. The translucent layer is relatively thin and transparent, being present only in thick skin, lying below the outer corneum, from which the cells are shed; the corneum is mainly responsible for the thickness of the skin (Fig. 1.45). The epidermis, like all epithelia tissue, is avascular, receiving its nutrients and oxygen by diffusion from the dermis.

> **APPLIED ANATOMY:** The basal and spinous layers are referred to as the germinal zone because of their role in new cell production, with the remaining layers (granular, translucent, corneum) referred to as the horny layer.

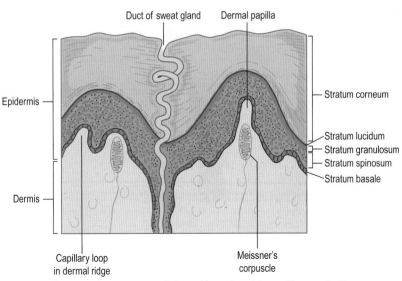

Fig. 1.45 Arrangement of the epidermal and dermal layers of skin.

APPLIED ANATOMY: Epidermal melanocytes responsible for skin pigmentation lie within the deepest epidermal layers.

CLINICAL ANATOMY: One-third of all cancers in adults originate in the skin, most being derived from the basal and spinous layers (basal and squamous cell carcinomas); both types are rarely lethal as they can be readily diagnosed and excised early. Fair-skinned individuals living in regions with high amounts of solar radiation show an increased incidence of skin cancer.

Dermis. Dermis is the deeper interlacing feltwork of collagen and elastin fibres, comprising the greater part of skin thickness; it has superficial finely textured papillary and deeper coarser reticular layers. The papillary layer interdigitates with the epidermis, while the reticular layer gradually blends with the subcutaneous connective tissue. Projecting dermal papillae usually contain capillary networks, bringing blood close to the epidermis (Fig. 1.46); the ability of these networks to open up and close down regulates heat loss through the skin, as well as causing individuals to blush. Some papillae contain tactile receptors, being more numerous in sensitive regions (tips of the fingers, lips) and less so in other regions (back).

APPLIED ANATOMY: On the pads of the fingers and toes, and extending over the palm and sole, are a series of alternating ridges, which have openings of sweat glands (page 60) on them, and depressions; these are due to the specific arrangement of large dermal papillae under the epidermis which improve grip and prevent slippage. These surfaces are devoid of hairs and sebaceous glands.

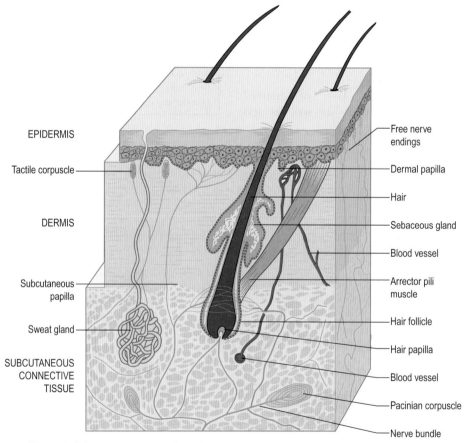

EPIDERMIS

Tactile corpuscle

DERMIS

Subcutaneous papilla

Sweat gland

SUBCUTANEOUS CONNECTIVE TISSUE

Free nerve endings

Dermal papilla

Hair

Sebaceous gland

Blood vessel

Arrector pili muscle

Hair follicle

Hair papilla

Blood vessel

Pacinian corpuscle

Nerve bundle

Fig. 1.46 Schematic representation of the skin and subcutaneous connective tissue layer.

The reticular layer consists of a dense mass of inter-weaving collagen and elastin fibres giving skin its toughness and strength; the fibres run in all directions but are generally tangential to the surface. There is, however, a predominant orientation of fibre bundles with respect to the skin surface which varies from region to region; it is this orientation which gives rise to cleavage (Langer's) lines (Fig. 1.47).

> **CLINICAL ANATOMY:** Skin incisions along cleavage lines heal with a minimum of scarring, whereas incisions or wounds across them usually heal with thicker scars, with the risk of scar contraction because the incision/wound edges are being pulled apart by the skin's internal stresses; cleavage lines do not always correspond with the stress lines of life, rather they reflect the stresses in the skin at rest.

The dermis contains numerous blood vessels and lymphatic channels, nerves and sensory nerve endings, as well as a small amount of fat, hair follicles, sweat and sebaceous glands, and smooth muscle (arrector pili) (Fig. 1.46). Between the papillary and reticular layers is the subpapillary plexus, from which capillary branches extend into the dermal papillae forming a rich, nutritive network just below the epidermis; close to the dermal subcutaneous layer is a deep plexus with larger blood and lymphatic vessels. In addition to its nutritive role, the dermal vasculature also has a thermoregulatory role (page 54), involving numerous arteriovenous anastomoses (shunts) lying between the two plexuses. Lymphatics begin in the dermal papillae converging to form two plexuses alongside the blood vessels. The dermis is also richly innervated with many types of sensory nerve endings (page 52 Fig. 1.44), in addition to autonomic nerves to dermal sweat glands and smooth muscle fibres, in some areas being postganglionic fibres; no parasympathetic fibres are present. The deep layer of dermis is invaginated by projections of subcutaneous connective tissue serving partly for the entrance of blood vessels and nerves into the skin.

Subcutaneous layer. This layer (hypodermis) consists of loosely arranged connective tissue containing fat (adipocytes) and some elastic fibres, binding the skin loosely to the subjacent tissues and organs, enabling it to slide over them. It contains blood and lymphatic vessels,

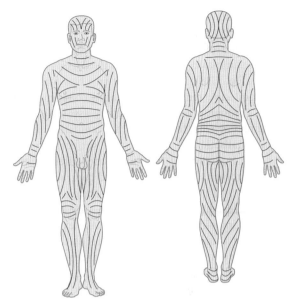

Fig. 1.47 The orientation of cleavage lines in different regions: incisions made along these lines results in minimal scarring.

roots of hair follicles, secretory parts of sweat glands, cutaneous nerves and sensory endings, especially Pacinian (pressure) corpuscles (page 52 Fig. 1.46).

> **APPLIED ANATOMY:** The distribution of fat differs in different body regions, being completely absent in some regions (eyelid, scrotum, penis, nipple, areolar), as well as between men and women, with the amount varying depending on nutritional status; in women, it is a secondary sexual characteristic (breast, rounded contour of the hips).

> **CLINICAL PHYSIOLOGY:** The extensive vascular supply to the subcutaneous layer promotes the uptake of drugs (insulin) injected into it.

Wound Repair

Wound repair is by either primary or secondary union: primary union occurs following surgical incisions (the wound is usually clean and uninfected and has its edges approximated by surgical sutures); secondary union occurs in traumatic wounds with separated edges and more extensive cell and tissue loss. In both cases, repair involves the generation of large amounts of granulation tissue (specialised tissue formed during the repair process).

The repair of an incision or laceration of the skin involves stimulated growth of both the dermis and epidermis (Fig. 1.48). Dermal repair involves formation of a blood clot; removal of damaged collagen fibres, mainly through macrophage activity associated with inflammation; the formation of granulation tissue; re-epithelialisation of the exposed surface; proliferation and migration of fibroblasts and differentiation of myofibroblasts involved in wound contraction; and deposition and remodelling of the extracellular matrix of the underlying connective tissue. The application of sutures in primary union reduces the extent of the repair area through maximal closure of the wound, minimising scar formation. Epidermal repair involves proliferation of the basal layer cells in the surrounding undamaged site, with the wound site quickly being covered by a scab (dehydrated blood clot). The proliferating basal cells migrate (0.5 mm/day) under the scab and across the wound surface; further proliferation and differentiation occur behind the migration front leading to restoration of the multi-layered epidermis. As cells move towards the surface, the overlying scab is freed, with the scab detaching from the periphery inwards. In full-thickness wounds of the epidermis, parts of hair follicles and the follicular bulge containing epidermal stem cells produce cells that migrate over the exposed surface to re-establish a complete epidermal layer.

> **CLINICAL ANATOMY:** When all epithelial structures of the skin have been destroyed (3rd-degree burns, extensive full-thickness abrasions) re-epithelialisation is prevented; such wounds can only be healed by skin (epidermal) grafting to cover the wounded area. Without a graft, the wound would re-epithelialise slowly and imperfectly due to ingrowth of cells from the margins of the wound.

Appendages of Skin

Nails, hairs, sebaceous and sweat glands, and the mammary gland (breast) are all appendages of the skin: they are derived from the epidermis.

Nails. Each nail is an approximately rectangular plate of keratinised horny tissue on the dorsum of the terminal phalanges of the fingers, thumb and toes (Fig. 1.49); it is a special modification of the two superficial layers

(translucent, corneum [page 55]) of the epidermis, mainly the translucent layer. The proximal part of the nail (nail root) is covered by a fold of skin, from which the corneum extends as the cuticle (eponychium); the nail is partly surrounded by a fold of skin (nail wall) firmly attached to the underlying nail bed (basal and spinous layers of the epidermis) with some fibres ending in the periosteum of the distal phalanx. Continuous growth of the nail root pushes the nail forward over the nail bed, becoming free of the nail bed at the epidermal fold (hyponychium).

> **APPLIED ANATOMY:** The transparency of the nail allows the pinkness of the underlying highly vascular nail bed to show through, providing a useful window on the amount of oxygen in the blood of the dermal vessels.

> **APPLIED ANATOMY:** Fingernails grow at 3 mm/month and toenails at 1 mm/month, being greater in summer than winter.

> **APPLIED ANATOMY:** The firm attachment of the nail to the nail bed and proximal phalanx enables it to be used as an instrument for prising open various objects and for scratching.

Hairs. Hairs are widely distributed over most of the body, exceptions being the sides and palmar surfaces of the hands, sides and plantar surfaces of the feet, lips, glans penis (page 540), clitoris (page 552) and labia minor (page 552). Hairs vary in thickness and length, with most being extremely fine giving skin the appearance of hairlessness; there is a marked sexual difference in the distribution of coarse hair, especially on the face and trunk, as well as in its loss from the scalp. Coarse hair tends to become more prominent after puberty, especially in the axilla, over the pubes and on the face in males.

> **APPLIED ANATOMY:** The colour, size, shape and texture of hairs vary according to age, sex, ethnicity and region of the body; they grow discontinuously, with periods of growth (anagen) followed by periods of rest (telogen), with growth not occurring synchronously in all regions of the body or the same area.

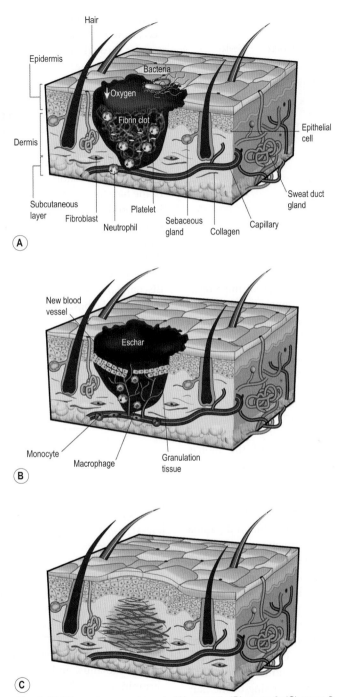

Fig. 1.48 Stages in wound repair: (A) stage 1; (B) stage 2; (C) stage 3.

Hairs emerge obliquely from the skin surface, except for those of the eyelashes, with those in one region doing so in the same direction. The part projecting from the skin surface is the shaft (circular in cross-section) with that under the skin being the root (ensheathed in an epidermal sleeve); the follicle extends into the

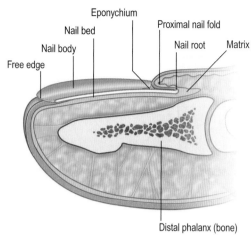

Fig. 1.49 Relationship of nails to the skin.

subcutaneous tissue (Fig. 1.45). Throughout most of its length, hair consists of keratinised remains of cells, with hair colour being due to melanin, a subtle red pigment in hair cells and air in the shaft.

> **APPLIED ANATOMY:** All hairs are intermittently shed: those on the head having a life span of 2–4 years, with those of the eyelashes being 3–5 months.

In growing hair, the deepest part of the follicle expands forming a cap (bulb of the hair), which almost completely surrounds the loose connective tissue (papilla); the follicle cells around the papilla proliferate forming the various layers of the hair. In contrast, in resting hair the follicles around the bulb and papilla shrink. Associated with each hair are one or more sebaceous glands (page 60) in the angle between the slanting hair follicle and skin surface: their ducts open into the upper portion (neck) of the follicle (Fig. 1.46). Bundles of smooth muscle fibres (arrector pili) attach to the hair follicle sheath, deep to the sebaceous gland, passing to the papillary layers of the dermis on the side towards which the hair slopes (Fig. 1.46). Contraction of the muscle fibres causes the hair to stand away from the skin, elevating the skin around the opening of the hair follicle ('goose flesh'); this also compresses the sebaceous glands causing them to empty their secretions onto the skin surface. Elevation of the hairs traps a layer of air against the skin surface producing an insulating layer in an attempt to reduce heat loss, while the sebaceous secretions are important in waterproofing the skin surface, as well as aiding the absorption of fat-soluble substances through the skin.

Glands.

Sebaceous glands. Sebaceous glands are embedded in the dermis over most of the body, except in the thick skin of the palm and sole; they develop as outgrowths (1–4 per hair) of the external root sheath of the hair follicle. They are branched acinar glands with the acini converging on a short duct which empties onto the neck of the hair follicle; the oily substance (sebum) produced is the product of holocrine secretion in which the entire cell produces and becomes filled with the fatty product, while it simultaneously undergoes programmed cell death (apoptosis) as the product fills the cell. (In holocrine secretion the secretory product and cell debris are discharged from the gland, with new cells produced by mitosis of the basal cells at the periphery of the gland.)

> **APPLIED PHYSIOLOGY:** Secretion from sebaceous glands increases greatly at puberty, being stimulated primarily by testosterone in males and by ovarian and adrenal androgens in females; sebum helps maintain the outer layer of the epidermis and hair shafts, as well as having weak antibacterial and antifungal properties.

> **CLINICAL PHYSIOLOGY:** Inflammation and accumulation of secretion within sebaceous glands give rise to acne; permanent plugging of the duct may lead to the formation of a sebaceous cyst, which may require surgical removal if it becomes enlarged.

Sweat glands. Sweat glands develop as long epidermal invaginations embedded in the dermis (Fig. 1.46) and are of two types: eccrine sweat glands are distributed over the entire body surface, except the lips and part of the external genitalia; apocrine sweat glands are limited to the axilla, areola and nipple of the breast, skin around the anus, and external genitalia, as well as the ceruminous glands of the external acoustic meatus. The ducts of sweat glands open onto the summits of the epidermal ridges.

Eccrine sweat glands are not associated with hair follicles, each being a blind-ended, simple coiled structure with two parts, a secretory part deep in the dermis or upper part of the subcutaneous tissue, and a less coiled duct leading to the skin surface: myoepithelial cells on the basal lamina contract to move the watery secretion into the duct. They play a major role in temperature regulation through cooling resulting from evaporation of water from the body surface; they also serve, in part, as an excretory organ as the hypotonic secretion contains sodium chloride, urea, uric acid and ammonia.

> **APPLIED PHYSIOLOGY:** Thermoregulatory sweating occurs first on the forehead and scalp, spreading to the face and rest of the body, with the last areas being on the palms of the hand and soles of the feet; control of thermoregulatory sweating is cholinergic. In contrast, under conditions of emotional stress the palms of the hands, soles of the feet and axillae are the first to sweat; emotional sweating is stimulated by adrenergic parts of the sympathetic nervous system (page 225).

> **CLINICAL PHYSIOLOGY:** Dehydration resulting from excessive sweating involves not only significant water loss but also the loss of electrolytes (sodium, potassium, magnesium); all need to be replaced to return the body to equilibrium.

Apocrine sweat glands development depends on sex hormones and are not functional until after puberty; they show merocrine rather than apocrine secretion. (Merocrine secretion is where the secretion produced within the cell is released through the cell membrane without destroying the cell itself.) The slightly viscous milky secretion is initially odourless, but through bacterial action on the skin surface it may acquire a distinct odour. Apocrine glands respond to emotional and sensory stimuli but not heat.

> **CLINICAL PHYSIOLOGY:** In females, the axillary and areolar apocrine glands undergo morphologic and secretory changes during the menstrual cycle.

> **CLINICAL ANATOMY:** Modified apocrine sweat glands (gland of Moll/ciliary gland) along the distal margin of the eyelid next to the base of the eyelashes secrete sebum onto the adjacent lashes to keep them supple; however, they are prone to infection, with blockage of the duct with sebum and cell debris causing swelling (stye).

Both eccrine and apocrine sweat glands are innervated by the sympathetic part of the autonomic nervous system. Eccrine glands are stimulated by cholinergic neurotransmitters and apocrine glands by adrenergic neurotransmitters.

Breast. The mammary gland (breast) is a modified sweat gland; it is an accessory to reproductive function in females, secreting milk (lactation, page 366) for nourishment of the infant. In children prior to puberty and in adult males, the breast remains rudimentary and functionless. Details of the lymphatic drainage of the breast can be found on page 403.

■ SELF-TEST QUESTIONS

1. Which of the following is NOT a cellular organelle?
   a. Golgi apparatus
   b. Rough endoplasmic reticulum
   c. Nucleolus
   d. Lysosome
   e. Mitochondria

2. Concerning cells, which of the following statements is NOT correct?
   a. The nucleus is separated from the cytoplasm by the nuclear membrane.
   b. The cytoskeleton provides structural support for the cell.
   c. Rough endoplasmic reticulum is associated with ribosomes.
   d. All cells have a nucleus.
   e. Cells undergo a repetitive cycle of growth and division.

3. Which of the following is NOT a characteristic of skin?
   a. Metabolic
   b. Friable
   c. Pliable
   d. Tough
   e. Protective

4. Concerning muscle, which of the following statements is correct?
   a. Cardiac muscle cells are joined together by intercalated discs.
   b. Smooth muscle is under voluntary control.
   c. In fusiform muscles individual muscle fibres attach to an intramuscular tendon.
   d. Skeletal muscle is partly under the control of the autonomic nervous system.
   e. In cardiac muscle, the nucleus lies at the periphery of the cell.

5. Which of the following is NOT a type of connective tissue?
   a. Bone
   b. Areolar tissue
   c. Cartilage
   d. Blood
   e. Epithelium

6. Which of the following is NOT a type of connection between individual cells?
   a. Desmosome
   b. Hemidesmosome
   c. Tight junction
   d. Adherent junction
   e. Gap junction

7. Concerning epithelium, which of the following statements is correct?
   a. In columnar epithelium individual cells are as tall as they are wide.
   b. In simple squamous epithelium the cells are arranged on top of each other.
   c. In pseudostratified epithelium all cells are attached to the basal lamina.
   d. Transitional epithelium is associated with the lining of the digestive system.
   e. Simple epithelium is found in locations where there is a lot of friction.

8. Which of the following is NOT involved in active transport across cell membranes?
   a. Osmosis
   b. Phagocytosis
   c. Endocytosis
   d. Pinocytosis
   e. Exocytosis

9. Concerning mitochondria, which of the following statements is correct?
   a. They are found only in the nucleus of cells.

   b. They have inner and outer lipid monolayer membranes.
   c. The outer membrane is highly folded.
   d. The outer membrane contains integral proteins forming channels.
   e. The number in different cells varies.

10. Concerning cells, which of the following statements is NOT correct?
    a. The nuclear membrane is selectively permeable.
    b. The nucleolus contains large amounts of DNA.
    c. Microfilaments are involved in cell motility.
    d. Lysosomes are membrane-bound vesicles containing hydrolytic enzymes.
    e. Proteasomes are protein complexes found in the nucleus.

11. In which phase of the cell cycle do chromosomes separate and move towards opposite poles?
    a. Prophase
    b. Metaphase
    c. Anaphase
    d. Telophase
    e. Interphase

12. Which of the following is NOT a characteristic of epithelium?
    a. Secretion
    b. Propagation of impulses
    c. Sensory perception
    d. Transportation
    e. Protection

13. In which of the following types of fracture is the skin broken?
    a. Partial
    b. Stable
    c. Closed
    d. Open
    e. Displaced

14. Concerning bone, which of the following statements is correct?
    a. Osteoblasts are bone-forming cells.
    b. Osteocytes are osteoclasts that have become surrounded by bone matrix.
    c. Woven bone is organised into discrete layers.
    d. Intramembranous ossification involves the calcification of a cartilage model of the future bone.
    e. In developing bone the epiphyses are separated from the metaphysis by a layer of cancellous bone.

15. Concerning comminuted fractures, which of the following statements is correct?
    a. It is a diagonal break across the bone.
    b. Two breaks in the same bone leaving a floating fragment.
    c. It is a fragment of bone pulled away by a tendon or ligament.
    d. Three or more breaks in the same bone with fragments at the fracture site.
    e. When broken ends of a bone are forced together.

16. Which of the following is a type of fibrous joint?
    a. Synchondrosis
    b. Syndesmosis
    c. Plane
    d. Symphysis
    e. Pivot

17. Concerning muscle, which of the following statements is NOT correct?
    a. Smooth muscle is specialised for slow steady contraction.
    b. In skeletal muscle groups of fascicles are bound together by epimysium.
    c. Cardiac muscle contraction is spontaneous.
    d. Skeletal muscle with a fusiform arrangement of fibres is stronger than one with a pennate arrangement of fibres.
    e. The connective tissue surrounding skeletal muscle fibres is continuous with that of its tendon.

18. Concerning nervous tissue, which of the following statements is NOT correct?
    a. The enteric nervous system is part of the central nervous system.
    b. The peripheral nervous system comprises the cranial and peripheral nerves of the trunk and limbs.
    c. The autonomic nervous system has sympathetic and parasympathetic parts.
    d. Neurons are the functional units of the nervous system.
    e. Neurons have a cell body, an axon and several dendrites.

19. Concerning nerves, which of the following statements is correct?
    a. An action potential is initiated in the dendrites.
    b. Myelinated fibres conduct impulses faster than non-myelinated fibres.
    c. The resting membrane potential is +70 mV.
    d. Somatic nerves innervate viscera.

    e. The fastest conduction velocities are 200 m/s.

20. Concerning nerve injury, which of the following statements is NOT correct?
    a. Neuropraxia is the complete blocking of nerve transmission even though the nerve fibre is intact.
    b. When severed the distal part of the axon quickly degenerates.
    c. Regenerated nerves always make the same connections as before they were damaged.
    d. Nerve regeneration occurs at 1 mm/day.
    e. Regeneration is facilitated by neurotropic factors.

21. Concerning skin, which of the following statements is NOT correct?
    a. With increasing age skin loses its elasticity.
    b. It is thinnest over posterior and extensor surfaces than over anterior and flexor surfaces.
    c. It accounts for between 15% and 20% of total body weight.
    d. The outer epidermal layer has five distinct regions.
    e. Melanocytes in the deepest epidermal layer are responsible for skin pigmentation.

22. Concerning wound repair, which of the following statements is NOT correct?
    a. The initial response is the formation of a blood clot.
    b. Wound contraction occurs in response to the migration of fibroblasts and differentiation of myofibroblasts.
    c. Proliferating basal cells under the scab migrate at 0.05 mm/day.
    d. The use of sutures can reduce scar formation.
    e. The scab detaches from the periphery inwards.

23. Concerning glands of the skin, which of the following statements is correct?
    a. Sebaceous glands are only found on the palm of the hand and sole of the foot.
    b. Inflammation and accumulation of secretions from sweat glands gives rise to acne.
    c. Apocrine sweat glands only become functional after puberty.
    d. Eccrine sweat glands are associated with hair follicles.
    e. The breast is a modified sebaceous gland.

24. Concerning skin, which of the following statements is NOT correct?

a. Incisions along natural cleavage lines heal with minimal scarring.

b. The hypodermis is the deepest layer.

c. The extensive blood supply to the hypodermis promotes the uptake of drugs injected into it.

d. The epidermal-dermal junction is smooth.

e. The dermis contains numerous sensory nerve endings.

25. Concerning peripheral nerves, which of the following statements is correct?

a. Fascicles within a peripheral nerve are bound together by the epineurium.

b. Axons within peripheral nerves are all of the same size.

c. Afferent fibres cause events in the periphery.

d. Free nerve endings are surrounded by a myelin sheath.

e. Pacinian corpuscles are formed by more than a single axon.

2

Thorax (Chest)

CONTENTS

Key Concepts, 65
Learning Outcomes, 66
Overview, 66
Thoracic Cage, 66
Bones and Joints, 68
Sternum, 68
Ribs, 70
Thoracic Vertebrae, 72
Muscles, 72
Intercostals, 72
Diaphragm, 73
Muscles Attached to the Thoracic Cage, 75
Thoracic Inlet, 79
Thoracic Outlet, 80
Thoracic Cavity, 80
Mediastinum and Contents, 80
Superior Mediastinum, 80
Anterior Mediastinum, 83
Middle Mediastinum, 83

Posterior Mediastinum, 87
Respiratory System, 93
Nose, Pharynx and Larynx, 94
Trachea and Bronchi, 94
Pleurae, 95
Lungs, 97
Respiratory Physiology, 102
Cardiovascular System, 116
Heart, 118
Cardiac Cycle, 127
Cardiac Output, 133
Great Vessels, 136
Circulation, 143
Blood, 164
Plasma, 165
Cells, 165
Immunity, 176

KEY CONCEPTS

- The thorax (chest) is divided into a central area (mediastinum) and right and left pleural cavities.
- The thoracic cage is a musculoskeletal framework surrounding, protecting and supporting the heart and lungs.
- The thoracic contents are continuous with structures in the neck, upper limb and abdomen.
- The respiratory system is restricted to the thorax and neck.
- Expansion of the thoracic cage during inspiration draws air into the lungs, while its recoil during expiration expels air from the lungs.
- External respiration is the exchange of gases in the lungs: internal respiration is the exchange of gases,

nutrients, hormones and enzymes between blood and body tissues.
- The efficiency and effectiveness of respiration is influenced by physiological and pathological changes within the respiratory system.
- The heart serves both the pulmonary and systemic circulations.
- Major cardiovascular vessels lie within the thorax and are continuous with others throughout the body.
- The pattern of blood flow through the foetal and adult heart is different: significant changes occur in some structures at birth.
- The pressure developed during each cardiac cycle forces blood through the pulmonary and systemic circulations.

- Through the circulation nutrients are delivered to body tissues and waste products removed.
- Physiological and pathological changes in the cardiovascular system (heart, blood vessels) and circulation (blood) impact their efficiency and effectiveness.
- Blood consists of plasma and cells, both of which have important roles in maintaining homeostasis.
- Pathological changes to the constituents of blood can have a major impact on life.
- Immunity can be either innate or acquired.

LEARNING OUTCOMES

At the end of this chapter, you should be able to:
- Identify and examine thoracic vertebrae, ribs and the sternum.
- Describe the joints of the thorax.
- Describe and explain the movements of the thorax during respiration.
- Describe the muscles associated with the thorax.
- Describe and locate the surface markings of the pleurae, lungs, their lobes and fissures.
- Describe the organisation of bronchopulmonary segments and their clinical function.
- Describe and understand external and internal respiration.
- Explain and understand the factors influencing lung capacity.
- Understand and appreciate the composition of gases in inspired and expired air.
- Appreciate and understand the changes in PO_2 with altitude and its physiological effects.
- Describe the regulation of air and blood flow in the lungs.
- Describe the neural and chemical control of respiration.
- Understand the effect of physiological changes and pathology on respiratory function.
- Describe the heart, its chambers and valves, their surface markings and where to listen for heart sounds.
- Describe and understand the pattern of blood flow through the heart before and after birth.
- Describe the cardiac cycle and its relationship to the electrocardiogram.
- Describe and understand the influence of electrolyte concentrations on heart function.
- Describe and understand how the heart maintains stroke volume and cardiac output.
- Describe the structure and function of arteries, veins and lymphatics, as well as their inter-relationships.
- Describe and understand how blood pressure, blood volume and blood flow are regulated.
- Describe the microcirculation and its function.
- Understand the effects of physiological changes and pathology on cardiovascular and circulatory function.
- Describe the components of blood and their functions.
- Describe and understand innate and acquired immunity.

OVERVIEW

This chapter considers the anatomy and function of the thorax and the anatomy and physiology of the respiratory and cardiovascular systems, including the circulation and blood. It is organised into six major sections: thoracic cage, thoracic cavity, respiratory system, cardiovascular system, circulation and blood. In the thoracic cage section, the bones, joints and muscles of the thorax, together with its movements during respiration are considered. In the thoracic cavity section, the divisions of the mediastinum are considered, with the relationship between structures in each being presented. The respiratory system considers the anatomy of the airways and lungs, followed by respiratory physiology. In the cardiovascular system, the anatomy of the heart and major vessels is considered, followed by cardiovascular physiology. Finally, the circulation is covered, including the lymphatic system as an important component of the circulation: blood is included in this chapter as it is an integral part of the circulation and cardiovascular system: because of the intimate relationship between white blood cells immunity is also addressed. Throughout this chapter, there are cross-references to other sections within the chapter, as well as to other chapters: the reader is encouraged to follow these to gain a fuller understanding of the topic.

THORACIC CAGE

A conical bony and muscular structure (Fig. 2.1), surrounding, protecting and supporting the heart and

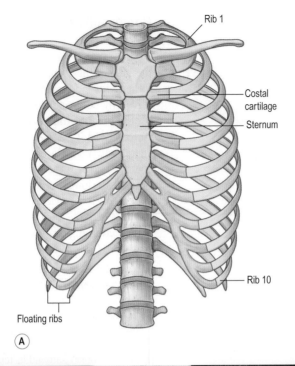

Rib 1

Costal
cartilage

Sternum

Rib 10

Floating ribs

(A)

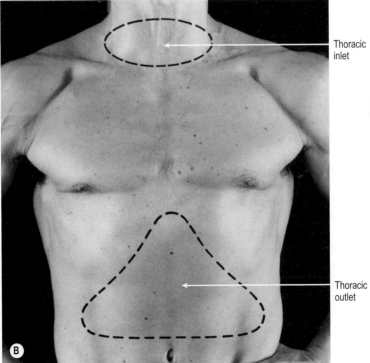

Thoracic
inlet

Thoracic
outlet

(B)

Fig. 2.1 (A) Anterior aspect of the thoracic cage. (B) The positions of the thoracic inlet and outlet.

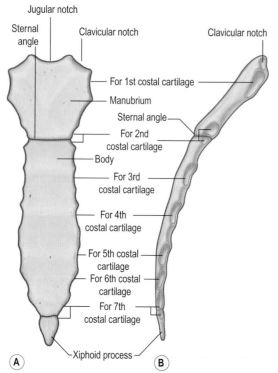

Jugular notch
Sternal angle
Clavicular notch
Clavicular notch
For 1st costal cartilage
Manubrium
Sternal angle
For 2nd costal cartilage
Body
For 3rd costal cartilage
For 4th costal cartilage
For 5th costal cartilage
For 6th costal cartilage
For 7th costal cartilage
Xiphoid process

Fig. 2.2 (A) Anterior and (B) lateral aspects of the sternum.

Bones and Joints
Sternum

Sternum is an elongated flat bone located in the midline of the anterior chest wall extending from the root of the neck to the anterior abdominal wall. It is in three parts: manubrium superiorly, body, and xiphoid process inferiorly (Fig. 2.2).

The **manubrium** lies opposite the 3rd and 4th thoracic vertebrae (T3, T4); it has four borders (upper, lower and two lateral) and two surfaces (anterior and posterior). The upper concave border is the suprasternal (jugular) notch and lies opposite the lower border of the 2nd thoracic vertebra (T2); either side is a clavicular notch for articulation with the medial end of the clavicle; the lower border meets the body at the sternal angle forming a secondary cartilaginous joint (page 35) (Fig. 2.3): it lies at the lower border of T4.

APPLIED ANATOMY: The sternal angle is an important landmark on the anterior chest wall for the 2nd costal cartilage when counting the ribs. A number of structures lie at this level: the beginning and end of the aortic arch; the ligamentum arteriosum with the left recurrent laryngeal nerve hooking around it, together with the superficial cardiac plexus; bifurcation of the trachea and the deep cardiac plexus; end of the pulmonary trunk; the azygous vein joins the superior vena cava; the thoracic duct passes from right to left behind the oesophagus (Fig. 2.4).

lungs; it is narrower towards the neck and wider inferiorly. The upper and lower openings slope obliquely, with the superior opening (thoracic inlet) sloping downwards and forwards some 45 degrees and the lower opening (thoracic outlet) sloping downwards and backwards.

The thoracic cage is bounded anteriorly by the sternum, costal cartilages and anterior parts of the ribs, posteriorly by the 12 thoracic vertebrae and posterior parts of the ribs, and laterally by the ribs.

The ribs pass from the thoracic vertebrae towards the sternum, sloping downwards and forwards so that the anterior end is lower than the posterior part. The intercostal space between adjacent ribs is filled by muscles, between which are blood vessels and nerves. The upper spaces are wider than the lower, which are also narrower posteriorly. The arrangement of the ribs flattens the thorax anteroposteriorly making it wider transversely.

APPLIED ANATOMY: In children the ribs lie more horizontally so that the anteroposterior and transverse diameters of the thorax are similar.

The 1st costal cartilage articulates with the lateral border by a primary cartilaginous joint (page 35), below which the 2nd costal cartilage articulates by a synovial joint (page 36) (Fig. 2.3).

The anterior surface is rough giving attachment to sternomastoid (see Table 4.7) and pectoralis major (see Table 5.2). The posterior surface is smooth giving attachment to sternohyoid and sternothyroid (see Table 4.8), behind which lie the arch of the aorta (lower half), the brachiocephalic, left common carotid and left subclavian arteries (upper half), left brachiocephalic vein (along the upper border of the aortic arch), thymus gland, lymph nodes and connective tissue, and the anterior borders of the lungs and their associated pleura.

The **body** consists of four fused segments (sternebrae): it has four borders (upper, lower and two lateral) and two surfaces (anterior and posterior). The upper border articulates with the manubrium and the lower border with the xiphoid process by a primary cartilaginous joint (Fig. 2.2); the latter lies at the level of the 9th thoracic vertebra (T9) and usually ossifies in old age. On each side, it articulates with the 2nd to 7th costal cartilages by synovial joints (Fig. 2.3).

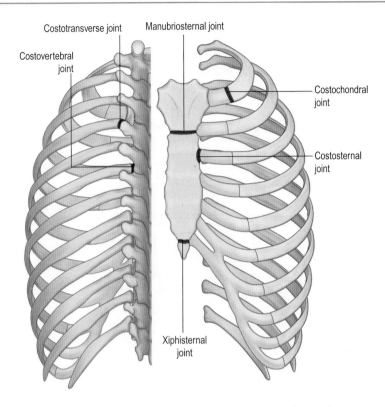

Costotransverse joint   Manubriosternal joint

Costovertebral joint

Costochondral joint

Costosternal joint

Xiphisternal joint

Fig. 2.3 Joints of the thoracic cage viewed anteriorly and posteriorly.

The anterior border is rough giving attachment to pectoralis major (Table 5.2). The posterior border is smooth and gives attachment to the upper and lower sternopericardial ligaments: it is in contact with the pericardium (bare area), thymus and anterior borders of the pleurae and lungs.

The **xiphoid process** has three borders (upper and two lateral) and two surfaces (anterior and posterior). The upper border articulates with the body and the tip gives attachment to the linea alba (page 454). The lateral border articulates with the 7th costal cartilage by a synovial joint at the xiphisternal junction (Fig. 2.3).

The anterior surface gives attachment to the aponeuroses of external oblique and rectus abdominis (see Fig. 6.5, Table 6.1), while the posterior surface gives attachment to two slips of the diaphragm (see Fig. 2.10); it is related to the liver and falciform ligament.

> **APPLIED ANATOMY:** The sternum is shorter in females than in males, with its upper border lying opposite the lower border of T3 rather than the lower border of T2.

Palpation. The inferior margin of the deep hollow at the base of the neck is the jugular notch of the manubrium, either side of which the medial ends of the clavicles can be felt. About 3 cm below the jugular notch a ridge of bone can be felt after which the sternum changes direction; this is the manubriosternal joint (sternal angle). Either side of the joint the costal cartilage of the 2nd rib can be palpated and followed laterally to the 2nd rib, below the 2nd costal cartilage and rib is the 2nd intercostal space. Passing inferiorly from here the 3rd, 4th, 5th, 6th and 7th costal cartilages and ribs can be palpated in succession, together with the intervening intercostal spaces.

At the lower end of the sternum, the tip of the xiphoid process can be palpated, with the costal cartilages of the 7th to 10th ribs passing laterally from it. Where the 9th costal cartilage joins the 8th is a marked change in the direction of the anterior rim of the thorax; this is level with the tip of the 12th rib and spinous process of the 1st lumbar vertebra posteriorly and the pylorus of the stomach (page 465) anteriorly. A transverse plane at this level is referred to as the transpyloric plane. The lateral

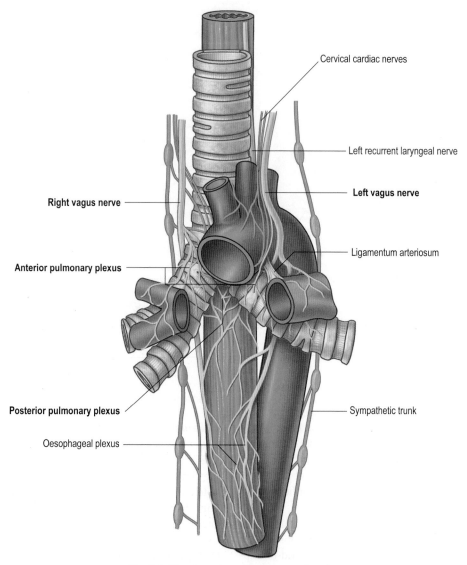

Fig. 2.4 Structures found at the sternal angle.

border of rectus abdominis crosses the costal margin at this level; at this junction on the right the fundus of the gall bladder can be palpated.

Ribs

Long flat bones continuing anteriorly as costal cartilages, which increase in length from above down. The 1st to 7th costal cartilages articulate directly with the body of the sternum (sometimes referred to as true ribs) by synovial joints, the 8th to 10th (sometimes referred to as false ribs) do so via the preceding costal cartilage by synovial joints, while the 11th and 12th ribs (sometimes referred to as floating ribs) end in the anterior abdominal wall (Fig. 2.5).

Typical ribs. The **2nd** to **9th ribs** are typical; the remainder differ in some way. Typical ribs have a large head posteriorly with two flattened facets separated by a crest, a short, flattened neck, and a long curved flattened shaft, which widens anteriorly where it becomes continuous with its costal cartilage. The junction of the neck and shaft is marked by a tubercle with an articular facet. The shaft has smooth convex medial and concave lateral surfaces, and rounded upper and sharp lower borders (Fig. 2.6). The lower border forms the outer margin

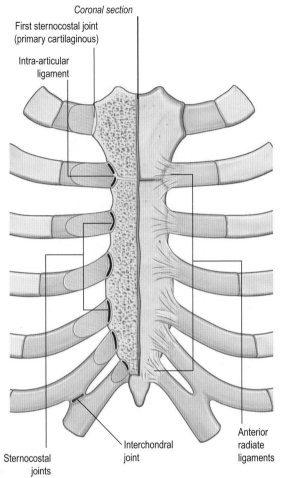

Coronal section

First sternocostal joint
(primary cartilaginous)

Intra-articular
ligament

Sternocostal
joints

Interchondral
joint

Anterior
radiate
ligaments

Fig. 2.5 Ribs 1–7 attaching directly to the sternum, also showing their articulations.

Atypical ribs. The short **1st rib** is C-shaped (Fig. 2.8). Its head has a single articular facet for articulation with T1; the neck and tubercle are similar to typical ribs with the facet on the tubercle articulating with the transverse process of T1. A number of structures pass anterior to the neck; most medial is the sympathetic trunk with the superior thoracic ganglion, often fused with the inferior cervical ganglion forming the stellate ganglion, lateral is the superior intercostal artery and most lateral the 1st thoracic nerve.

The shaft has two surfaces (superior and inferior) and two borders (medial and lateral). The superior surface is crossed obliquely by two grooves separated by a ridge continuous with the scalene tubercle, which gives attachment to scalenus anterior (Table 4.7): the posterior groove transmits the subclavian artery and lower trunk of the brachial plexus, and anterior groove the subclavian vein, with the area in front giving attachment to subclavius (Table 5.1) and the costoclavicular ligament. The inferior surface is covered with parietal pleura. The lateral border is convex and medial border concave, giving attachment to the suprapleural membrane.

The **10th rib** has a single facet on its head for articulation with the body of T10.

The short **11th** and **12th ribs** have a single facet on the head for articulation with the body of T11 and T12, respectively. They have no neck, tubercles or costal groove and end in the anterior abdominal wall. On the medial surface of the 12th rib, the internal intercostal muscle, diaphragm (page 73) and quadratus lumborum (see Table 3.2) are attached, and on its lateral surface latissimus dorsi (see Table 5.2), external oblique (see Table 6.1) and erector spinae (see Table 3.2).

APPLIED ANATOMY: The ribs are held under a certain amount of tension between their articulations with the sternum and thoracic vertebrae; as such they help support the thoracic region of the vertebral column.

CLINICAL ANATOMY: Although extremely painful, fracture of a single rib is not life threatening. Fracture of several ribs in several places, due to trauma, can result in a loose segment of the chest wall (flail chest). During inspiration, the flail part of the chest wall moves in the opposite direction to the chest wall preventing full lung expansion; if a large segment is affected, respiration may be impaired and assistance required until the ribs have healed.

---

of the subcostal groove, with its outer margin giving attachment to the external and internal intercostal muscles and its inner margin the innermost intercostal muscle (see Fig. 2.9). Some 3 cm lateral to the tubercle is the angle of the rib, where the shaft turns downwards and inwards giving it a twisted appearance.

The lower facet on the head articulates with the body of the same numbered vertebra and the upper facet with the body of the vertebra immediately above by synovial costovertebral joints; the facet on the tubercle articulates with the transverse process of the same numbered vertebra by a synovial costotransverse joint (Fig. 2.7). The shape of the costotransverse joint surfaces changes from above downwards, becoming flatter lower down. The change in shape is one of the factors responsible for the different movements of the upper and lower ribs during respiration (page 101).

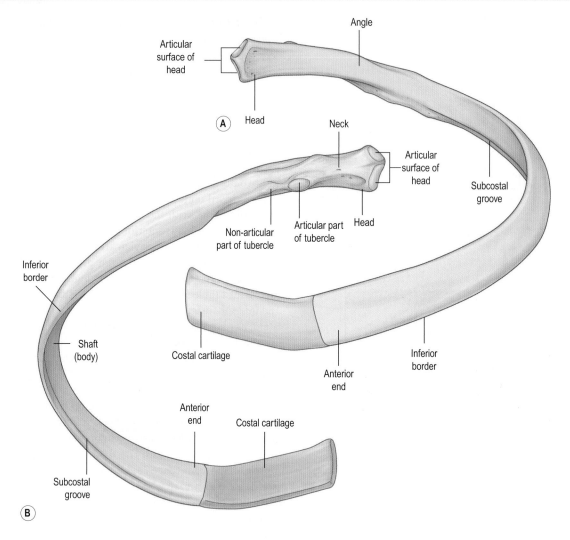

Fig. 2.6 (A) Anterior and (B) posterior aspects of a typical left rib.

Thoracic Vertebrae

Details of the thoracic vertebrae and the joints between them can be found on pages 195 to 199.

Muscles

Intercostals

In each of the upper nine intercostal spaces a group of muscles, arranged in three layers, pass between adjacent ribs (Fig. 2.9). The outer layer is external intercostal, with fibres passing obliquely downwards, forwards and medially; it extends from the rib tubercle posteriorly to the rib-costal cartilage junction anteriorly, where it becomes the anterior intercostal membrane to reach the sternum. The middle layer is internal intercostal, with fibres passing obliquely downwards, backwards and laterally; it extends from the sternum to the angle of the rib, where it is replaced by the posterior intercostal membrane. The deepest layer is the incomplete innermost intercostal, being poorly developed in the upper spaces; its fibres pass in the same direction as the internal intercostal.

As a group, the intercostal muscles help to maintain the interspace between the ribs during respiration by forming, with the ribs, a semi-rigid structure. External intercostal may also raise the lower rib helping to increase thoracic volume during inspiration, while

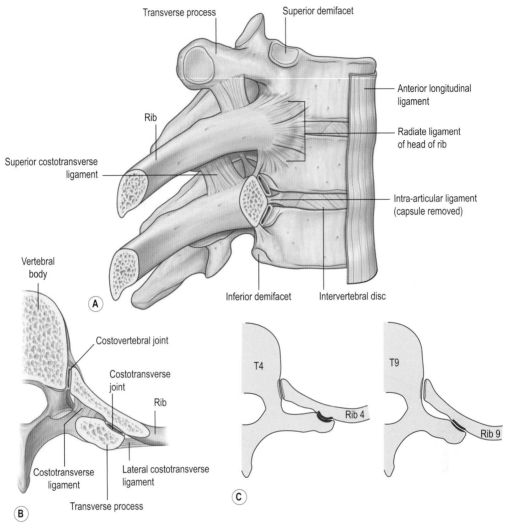

Transverse process   Superior demifacet

Anterior longitudinal ligament

Rib

Radiate ligament of head of rib

Superior costotransverse ligament

Intra-articular ligament (capsule removed)

Vertebral body

(A)

Inferior demifacet   Intervertebral disc

Costovertebral joint

Costotransverse joint

Rib

Costotransverse ligament   Lateral costotransverse ligament

(B)   Transverse process

T4   Rib 4

T9   Rib 9

(C)

Fig. 2.7 (A) Articulation of the ribs with the vertebral column; (B) the costovertebral and costotransverse joints; (C) changes in shape of the costotransverse joint with vertebral level.

internal and innermost intercostal may depress the upper rib helping decrease the thoracic volume during expiration. The intercostals as a group are also active in movements of the trunk, acting to help stabilise the chest wall.

Between the internal and innermost intercostal muscles is the neurovascular plane, in which pass the intercostal vessels and nerve, the arrangement being vein, artery and nerve from superior to inferior (Fig. 2.9).

The intercostal muscles are innervated by the adjacent intercostal (thoracic) nerves. The blood supply is from intercostal vessels in the neurovascular plane.

CLINICAL ANATOMY: Marked caving in and bulging out of the intercostal spaces occurs when the intercostal muscles are paralysed, as in quadriplegia, as well as in flail chest.

Diaphragm

A musculotendinous sheet separating the thoracic and abdominal cavities; muscle fibres, which converge to a central trefoil-shaped tendon, attach to the margins of the thoracic outlet (Fig. 2.10). The lumbar part arises by

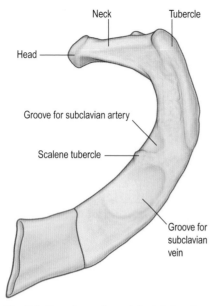

Fig. 2.8 Superior surface of the left 1st rib.

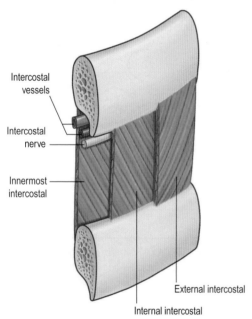

Fig. 2.9 The neurovascular plane showing the relationship between the intercostal vein, artery and nerve.

two crura from the bodies of L1 to L2/L3, and laterally from the medial and lateral arcuate ligaments. Laterally, it arises from the inner surface of the lower costal cartilages and ribs 7–12. Anteriorly it attaches by two slips to the posterior aspect of the xiphoid process. All muscle

fibres arch superomedially towards the central tendon, which is a thin but strong aponeurosis situated slightly anterior to the vault formed by the muscle. The anterior fibres are shorter than those posterior, giving the appearance of an inverted J when viewed from the side. When viewed from the front two small domes (cupolae) on either side of the central tendon are visible, with the right slightly higher than the left; the central tendon lies at the level of the xiphisternal joint.

The superior surface is covered by parietal pleura lining the thoracic cavity, while the inferior surface is lined with parietal peritoneum. The fibrous pericardium is firmly attached to the central tendon. On the right, the inferior surface is related to the right lobe of the liver and right kidney and on the left to the left lobe of the liver, stomach, spleen and left kidney.

Several structures pass between the thorax and abdomen by passing either posterior to or through the diaphragm (Fig. 2.10).

The inferior vena cava and right phrenic nerve pass through the caval opening in the central tendon at the level of T8; the wall of the vena cava is firmly adherent to the margins of the central tendon, ensuring that the vena cava is always held open.

To the left of the midline, the oesophagus, vagus nerves (now the gastric nerves) and oesophageal branches of the left gastric vessels pass through the oesophageal opening at the level of T10, which is surrounded by fibres of the right and left crura. Anterior and to the left of the central tendon passes the left phrenic nerve.

CLINICAL ANATOMY: Hiatus hernia is the most common internal hernia in which the upper part of the stomach, with or without the gastro-oesophageal junction, passes through the oesophageal opening into the posterior mediastinum to lie next to the oesophagus.

In the midline posterior to the arching crura (median arcuate ligament) and anterior to T12 is the aortic opening through which pass the aorta, thoracic duct and azygos vein; the greater and lesser splanchnic nerves pass through the crura.

Behind the medial and lateral arcuate ligaments pass the sympathetic chain and subcostal nerve, respectively.

Anteriorly between the sternal and costal attachments the superior epigastric artery enters the rectus sheath to supply the upper part of rectus abdominis.

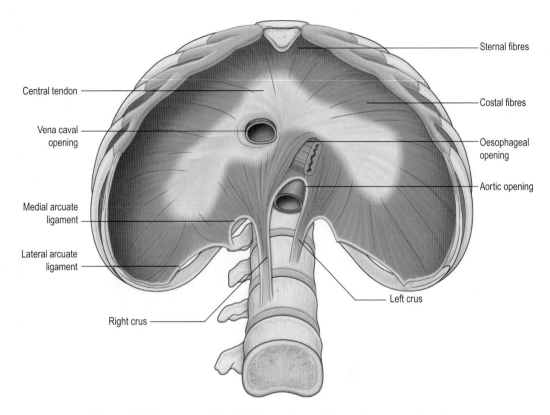

Central tendon

Vena caval opening

Medial arcuate ligament

Lateral arcuate ligament

Right crus

Sternal fibres

Costal fibres

Oesophageal opening

Aortic opening

Left crus

Fig. 2.10 Inferior aspect of the diaphragm showing its attachments and openings.

The diaphragm is innervated by motor and sensory fibres from the right and left phrenic nerves (root value C3, C4, C5), with additional sensory fibres to the periphery from the lower six intercostal nerves.

The diaphragm is the major muscle of inspiration. Downward movement of the diaphragm, elevation of the ribs and forward movement of the sternum increase the dimensions of the thorax causing air to be drawn into the lungs. The diaphragm can also resist upward movement of abdominal contents when the abdominal muscles contract during expulsive acts, such as defaecation, vomiting, micturition and parturition.

Muscles Attached to the Thoracic Cage

Other small muscles also attach between the ribs (subcostalis), between the sternum and ribs (sternocostalis) or between the vertebrae and ribs (levatores costarum, serratus posterior superior, serratus posterior inferior), working to raise or lower the ribs during respiration. They are all supplied by thoracic nerves and receive their blood supply from intercostal vessels.

A number of large powerful muscles also attach to the outer aspect of the thoracic cage, all of which pass to other regions. Anteriorly are pectoralis major (see Fig. 5.20), pectoralis minor (page 389), external oblique (page 457) and rectus abdominis (page 457). Around the sides are serratus anterior (page 389), while posteriorly are trapezius (page 389), latissimus dorsi (page 394) and erector spinae of the vertebral column (page 205). Of these, pectoralis major and minor, serratus anterior, trapezius and latissimus dorsi pass into the upper limb, while external oblique and rectus abdominis form part of the anterior abdominal wall.

Blood and nerve supply

Arterial supply. The intercostal spaces contain posterior and anterior intercostal arteries: there are 11 pairs of posterior arteries, 1 on each side, while the upper 9 spaces have 2 anterior arteries on each side; there are no anterior arteries in the 10th and 11th spaces.

The **1st** and **2nd posterior intercostal arteries** are branches of the superior intercostal artery, a branch of

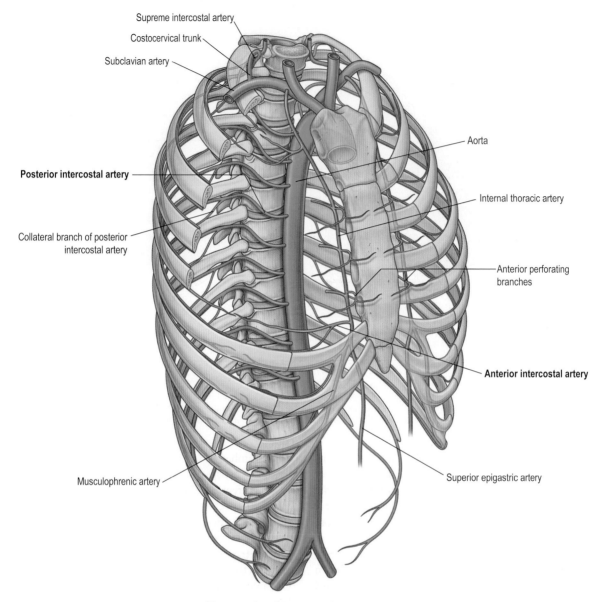

Fig. 2.11 Arterial supply to the chest wall.

the costocervical trunk from the 2nd part of the sub-clavian artery (page 319). The **3rd** to **11th posterior intercostal arteries** arise directly from the descending (thoracic) aorta (Fig. 2.11). Each artery enters the inter-costal space at its posterior end, then passes forwards in the costal groove below the intercostal vein (Fig. 2.9). During its course it gives a collateral branch which runs along the upper border of the rib below. The posterior

artery and its collateral branch anastomose with the anterior arteries.

The upper **1st** to **6th anterior intercostal arteries** are branches of the internal thoracic (mammary) artery (page 77), a branch of the 1st part of the subclavian artery (page 319): each anterior artery almost immedi-ately divides into two branches. The **7th** to **9th anterior intercostal arteries** are branches of the musculophrenic

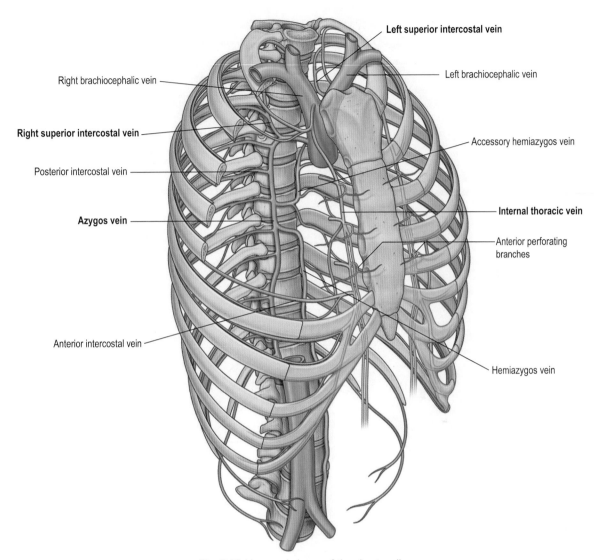

Left superior intercostal vein

Right brachiocephalic vein

Left brachiocephalic vein

Right superior intercostal vein

Accessory hemiazygos vein

Posterior intercostal vein

Azygos vein

Internal thoracic vein

Anterior perforating branches

Anterior intercostal vein

Hemiazygos vein

Fig. 2.12 Venous drainage of the chest wall.

artery, a terminal branch of the internal thoracic artery (Fig. 2.11). There are no anterior intercostal arteries in the 10th and 11th spaces. The anterior arteries run close to the costal cartilages bounding each space, terminating by anastomosing with the posterior intercostal artery and its collateral branch.

The **subcostal artery** arises directly from the descending aorta and passes laterally below the 12th rib to enter the abdomen behind the lateral arcuate ligament of the diaphragm (page 74) with the subcostal nerve to supply the anterior abdominal wall.

Venous drainage. *On the right,* the **1st posterior intercostal vein** drains into the right brachiocephalic vein. The **2nd** and **3rd posterior intercostal veins** join forming the superior intercostal vein, which drains into the arch of the azygos vein. The **4th** to **11th posterior intercostal veins** drain directly into the azygos vein (Figs. 2.12 and 2.13).

On the left, the **1st posterior intercostal vein** drains into the left brachiocephalic vein. The **2nd** and **3rd** (and sometimes **4th**) join forming the left superior intercostal vein which drains into the left brachiocephalic vein. The **4th/5th** to **8th posterior intercostal veins** unite

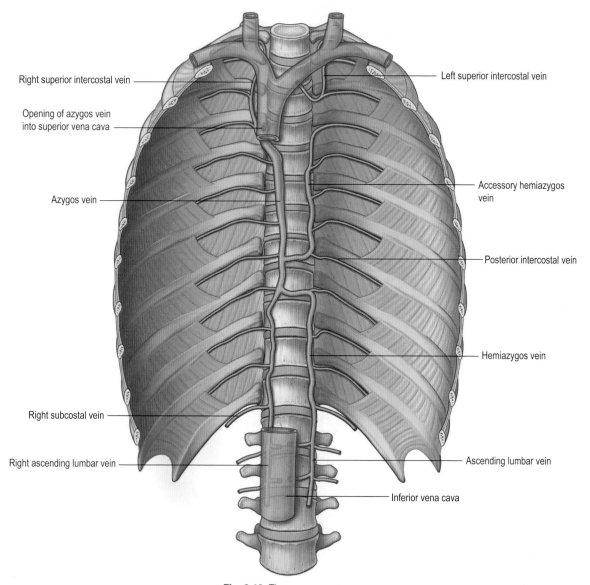

Right superior intercostal vein

Opening of azygos vein
into superior vena cava

Azygos vein

Right subcostal vein

Right ascending lumbar vein

Left superior intercostal vein

Accessory hemiazygos
vein

Posterior intercostal vein

Hemiazygos vein

Ascending lumbar vein

Inferior vena cava

Fig. 2.13 The azygos system.

forming the accessory (superior) hemiazygos vein, while the **9th** to **11th posterior intercostal veins** unite forming the (inferior) hemiazygos vein (Fig. 2.13). The accessory hemiazygos and hemiazygos veins cross the bodies of T7 and T8, respectively, to drain into the azygos vein. Anteriorly, the anterior intercostal veins drain into the internal thoracic veins, which drain into the corresponding brachiocepahlic vein (Fig. 2.12).

Lymphatic drainage. Superficial structures drain into lymph nodes either in the axilla (pectoral and subscapular nodes) or by the sternum (parasternal nodes). Lymph from the anterior chest wall, breast and anterior abdominal wall drains into the pectoral nodes, while that from the posterior chest and back drains into the subscapular nodes. The anteromedial part of the chest wall drains into the parasternal nodes. Details of the lymphatic drainage of the breast can be found on page 403.

Deeper structures drain into either the parasternal, intercostal or diaphragmatic lymph nodes. The upper surface of the liver, anterior and medial parts of the thoracic wall, upper medial part of the abdominal wall as far as the umbilicus drain into four or five parasternal nodes. Intercostal nodes lie in the posterior parts of the intercostal spaces and drain the posterolateral chest wall.

> **APPLIED ANATOMY:** The upper part of the chest wall drains into the deep cervical lymph nodes.

Nerve supply. The intercostal and subcostal nerves are the anterior primary rami of spinal nerves leaving the T1–T12 spinal cord segments (see Fig. 3.34). The upper two intercostal nerves supply the upper limb, T3–T6 supply the thoracic wall, the lower five (T7–T11) supply the thoracic and anterior abdominal walls and the subcostal nerve (T12) supplies skin of the anterior abdominal wall and buttock.

The **1st intercostal nerve** divides into a large branch which ascends to the neck of the 1st rib to join the brachial plexus (page 398): the smaller branch continues as the 1st intercostal nerve, which has no anterior cutaneous branch. The lateral perforating cutaneous branch of the **2nd intercostal nerve** (intercostobrachial nerve) supplies the floor of the axilla.

The **3rd** to **6th intercostal nerves** are considered to be typical (Fig. 2.14). They leave the intervertebral foramen below the vertebrae of the same number and pass laterally between the pleura and posterior intercostal membrane to the costal groove below the posterior intercostal artery and vein (Fig. 2.9). They then pass between the internal and external intercostal muscles, pierce the internal intercostal to lie between it and the innermost intercostal. At the rib-costal cartilage junction, they run between internal intercostal and the parietal pleura. Lateral to the sternum they pierce the internal intercostal, anterior intercostal membrane, pectoralis major and deep fascia becoming the anterior perforating cutaneous nerves, each of which divides into medial and lateral branches.

In the mid-axillary line, the intercostal nerve gives a lateral perforating cutaneous branch, which pierces the intercostal muscles and serratus anterior (see Table 5.1) before dividing into anterior and posterior cutaneous branches (Fig. 2.14).

The **7th** to **11th intercostal** and **subcostal nerves**, having supplied the intercostal muscles, pass into the anterior abdominal wall supplying both muscles and skin.

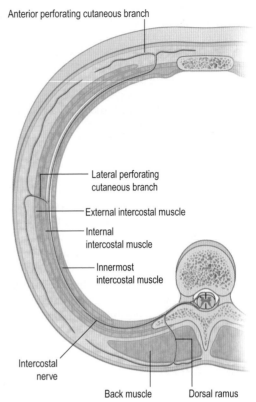

Fig. 2.14 Horizontal showing the course and distribution of a typical intercostal nerve.

Thoracic Inlet

A narrow sloping opening connecting the thoracic cavity with the root of the neck (Fig. 2.1). It is bounded posteriorly by the upper border of the body of T1, laterally by the medial border of the 1st rib and its costal cartilage, and anteriorly by the superior surface of the manubrium.

Through the median part pass small muscles (sternohyoid, sternothyroid, longus cervicis), the trachea and oesophagus, several arteries (brachiocephalic, left common carotid, left subclavian, internal thoracic (mammary) and superior intercostal), veins (brachiocephalic and inferior thyroid), nerves (right and left phrenic, right and left vagus, left recurrent laryngeal, sympathetic trunk (chain) and 1st thoracic), the thoracic duct and right subclavian lymph duct, and remnants of the thymus gland (Figs. 2.15 and 2.16). Each lateral part is occupied by the apex of the lung and cervical pleura covered by the suprapleural membrane.

APPLIED ANATOMY: The suprapleural membrane is a tense triangular layer of fascia attached posteriorly to the transverse process of the 7th cervical vertebra (C7) and anteriorly to the medial border of the 1st rib and costal cartilage. It protects the cervical pleura and apex of the lung, prevents inward suction of structures in the root of the neck during inspiration, and upward bulging of the apex of the lung during expiration.

Thoracic Outlet

The larger thoracic outlet is bounded posteriorly by the body of the 12th thoracic vertebra (T12), laterally by the 11th and 12th ribs and 7th to 10th costal cartilages, and anteriorly by the xiphoid process of the sternum. Most of the outlet is filled by the diaphragm, which has openings to enable the aorta and oesophagus to pass through into the abdomen from the thorax and for the inferior vena cava to pass into the thorax from the abdomen. Other structures also pass between the thorax and abdomen by piercing the diaphragm (page 74).

THORACIC CAVITY

The thoracic cavity is the space within the thoracic cage and is divided into three regions: a central mediastinum, which is further subdivided, and two lateral pleural cavities, each of which contains a lung. It is lined by a loose fibrocellular tissue (endothoracic fascia), which covers the mediastinal structures. Superiorly the fascia is thickened forming the suprapleural membrane, inferiorly it covers the diaphragm, medially it meets in the midline forming the loose connective tissue of the mediastinum, while laterally it binds the parietal pleura to the inner surfaces of the ribs and costal cartilages.

Mediastinum and Contents

The mediastinum is the mass of tissue between the lungs and pleura. Superiorly it extends as far as the thoracic inlet, i.e., from the upper border of the manubrium to the upper border of T1, and inferiorly to the upper surface of the diaphragm from the lower border of the sternum to the lower border of T12. Posteriorly it is bounded by the thoracic region of the vertebral column, anteriorly by the posterior surface of the sternum and laterally by the mediastinal parietal pleura on each side.

Viewed from the right (Fig. 2.15) anteriorly the pericardium and heart (right atrium) form a large bulge continuous with the superior vena cava and right brachiocephalic vein and upper end of the inferior vena cava. The right phrenic nerve runs along the brachiocephalic vein, pericardium and inferior vena cava. Behind the bulge is the root of the right lung, behind which is the azygos vein arching over the lung root to join the superior vena cava. The trachea is posterior to the superior vena cava and superior to the azygos vein, with the right vagus adherent to it. The oesophagus lies posterior to the trachea and lung root. Descending on the neck of the 1st rib and heads of the remaining ribs is the right sympathetic chain.

Viewed from the left (Fig. 2.16) anteriorly the pericardium and heart (left ventricle) form a large bulge, posterior and superior to which is the left lung root. The arch of the aorta, with the left common carotid artery anterior and left subclavian posterior, lies above the lung root. The left phrenic nerve runs along the left common carotid artery, crosses the aortic arch and descends on the pericardium anterior to the root of the lung. The lower part of the oesophagus lies between the pericardium and descending thoracic aorta.

The mediastinum is considered in four parts according to their relationship to the heart and pericardium (Fig. 2.17). The superior mediastinum lies above, the anterior mediastinum in front, the posterior mediastinum behind, while the middle mediastinum contains the heart and pericardium.

APPLIED ANATOMY: The anterior, middle and posterior mediastinum are collectively the inferior mediastinum. The plane between the superior and inferior mediastinum is known as the 'Angle of Louis'. A number of important structures are found here: the concavity of the arch of the aorta; the upper border of the pulmonary trunk bifurcation; bifurcation of the trachea; the azygos vein arches over the right lung root to join the superior vena cava; the thoracic duct passes from right to left behind the oesophagus; the deep and superficial cardiac plexuses; the left recurrent laryngeal nerve (branch of the left vagus) hooks around the ligamentum arteriosum connecting the aortic arch and left pulmonary artery (Fig. 2.18).

Superior Mediastinum

It is bounded superiorly by a line extending between the upper border of the manubrium and the upper border of

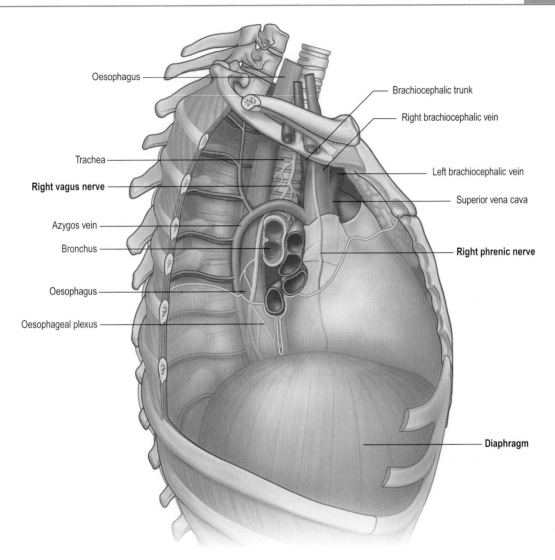

Oesophagus

Brachiocephalic trunk

Right brachiocephalic vein

Trachea

Left brachiocephalic vein

Right vagus nerve

Superior vena cava

Azygos vein

Bronchus

Right phrenic nerve

Oesophagus

Oesophageal plexus

Diaphragm

Fig. 2.15 Right aspect of the mediastinum.

T1, inferiorly by a line extending between the lower borders of the manubrium and T4, posteriorly by thoracic vertebrae T1–T4, anteriorly by the manubrium, and laterally by the mediastinal parietal pleura.

Anterior to the thoracic vertebrae lies the oesophagus (page 87), anterior to which is the trachea (page 94). In front of the trachea and posterior to the lower half of the manubrium is the arch of the aorta (page 83), with the brachiocephalic, left common carotid and left subclavian arteries lying posterior to the upper half of the manubrium. Immediately posterior to the upper half of the manubrium, anterior to the three branches of the aortic

arch, the left brachiocephalic vein passes from left to right to join the right brachiocephalic vein, forming the superior vena cava behind the right border of the lower half of the manubrium; the right brachiocephalic vein lies lateral to the brachiocephalic artery behind the right border of the upper half of the manubrium (Fig. 2.4). The most anterior structure is remnants of the thymus gland.

Also within the superior mediastinum are the right and left vagus nerves, the right descending on the right side of the trachea and the left on the left side of the left common carotid artery; the right and left phrenic nerves, with the right descending on the right side of the right brachiocephalic vein and superior vena cava and the left descending between the left common carotid and subclavian arteries and then crosses anterior to the arch of the aorta (both nerves are accompanied by pericardiophrenic vessels); the left recurrent laryngeal nerve ascends in the gutter between the trachea and oesophagus on the left side; the thoracic duct ascends along the left side of the oesophagus; the arch of the azygos vein lies on the right side of the lower border of the trachea; and the left superior intercostal vein passes anteriorly on the left side of the aortic arch before crossing superficial to the left vagus and phrenic nerves (Figs 2.15 and 2.16).

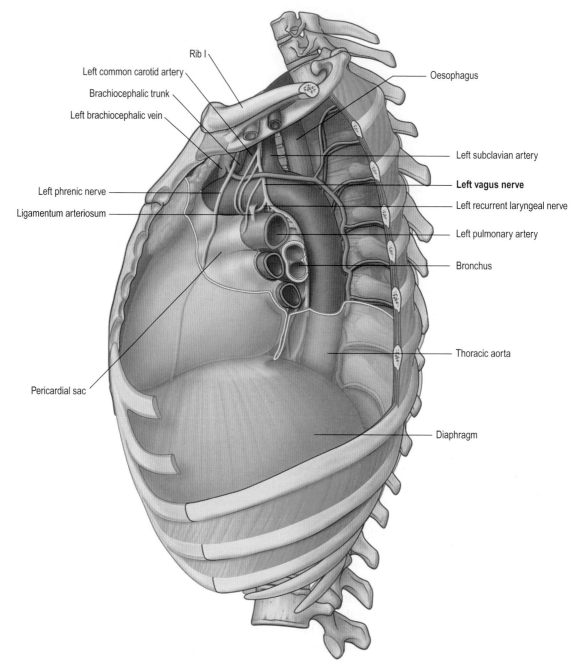

Fig. 2.16 Left aspect of the mediastinum.

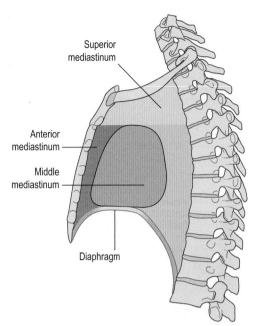

Fig. 2.17 Divisions of the mediastinum.

> **MEDIASTINAL SYNDROME:** Compression of the contents of the superior mediastinum by enlarged lymph nodes or a tumour can give rise to the following: venous congestion in the veins of the head, neck and upper limbs from compression of the veins; ischaemia of the upper limb, head and neck due to arterial compression; dyspnoea due to compression of the trachea; and dysphagia due to compression of the oesophagus.

Arch of the aorta. Continuation of the ascending aorta at the right 2nd sternocostal junction. It then curves from right to left anterior to the trachea and then curves again from anterior to posterior to lie on the left side of the trachea and oesophagus (Fig. 2.4). It is continuous with the descending aorta at the lower border of T4.

The **brachiocephalic artery** arises behind the manubrium terminating behind the right sternoclavicular joint by dividing into the right subclavian and right common carotid arteries. The **left common carotid artery** arises to the left of the brachiocephalic artery and passes superiorly to enter the neck behind the left sternoclavicular joint. The **left subclavian artery** arises to the left of the left common carotid artery and passes superolaterally to enter the neck and then crosses the 1st

rib (Fig. 2.14), with the 1st thoracic nerve, to enter the arm.

Superior vena cava. Formed by the union of the right and left brachiocephalic veins behind the lower border of the 1st right costal cartilage, then descends to drain into the right atrium. During its course, it is joined by the azygos vein prior to entering the fibrous pericardium (Fig. 2.15).

The **right brachiocephalic vein** is formed by the union of the right subclavian and internal jugular veins behind the right sternoclavicular joint: it has a short vertical course. The **left brachiocephalic vein** begins behind the left sternoclavicular joint by the union of the left subclavian and internal jugular veins; it passes immediately above the aortic arch anterior to its three branches (Fig. 2.19). During its course the left brachiocephalic vein receives the left vertebral, left inferior thyroid, left internal thoracic, left 1st posterior intercostal and left superior intercostal veins.

> **SURFACE ANATOMY:** The origin of the brachiocephalic veins is at the sternal end of the clavicle. The origin of the superior vena cava is at the sternal end of the 1st right costal cartilage. The end of the azygos vein is at the end of the 2nd right costal cartilage. The end of the superior vena cava is at the sternal end of the 3rd right costal cartilage.

Anterior Mediastinum

A small space bounded by the body of the sternum anteriorly, the heart and pericardium posteriorly and laterally by the mediastinal parietal pleura. It contains the remnants of the thymus gland, the internal thoracic (mammary) arteries, the superior and inferior sternopericardial ligaments and mediastinal lymph nodes.

Middle Mediastinum

The middle mediastinum contains the heart within the pericardium, the ascending aorta and pulmonary trunk, the lower half of the superior vena cava and the uppermost part of the inferior vena cava, tracheobronchial lymph nodes and the deep cardiac plexus.

Ascending aorta. The ascending aorta arises from the left ventricle at the level of the 3rd left intercostal space. It passes upwards and to the right behind the upper part of the body of the sternum becoming continuous

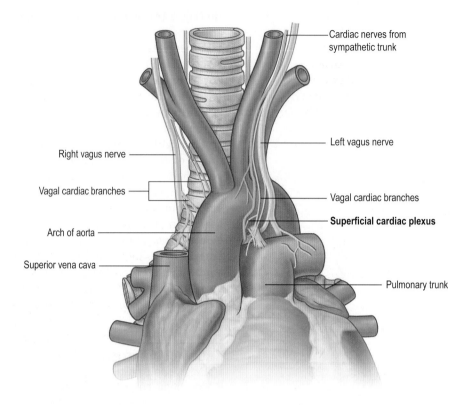

Right vagus nerve

Vagal cardiac branches

Arch of aorta

Superior vena cava

Cardiac nerves from sympathetic trunk

Left vagus nerve

Vagal cardiac branches

Superficial cardiac plexus

Pulmonary trunk

Fig. 2.18 The left recurrent laryngeal nerve hooking around the ligamentum arteriosum.

with the arch of the aorta at the 2nd right sternocostal junction. It is covered by fibrous pericardium and enclosed with the pulmonary trunk in a single sheath of serous pericardium. At its root are three dilations (aortic sinuses) from which the coronary arteries arise: the right coronary artery from the anterior sinus and the left coronary artery from the left posterior sinus.

Details of the heart can be found on pages 118 to 124.

Pericardium. A fibroserous sac surrounding the heart and proximal parts of the ascending aorta, pulmonary trunk, lower half of the superior vena cava, terminal part of the inferior vena cava and the four pulmonary veins. It consists of an outer fibrous layer (fibrous pericardium) with an inner serous lining (serous pericardium).

Fibrous pericardium. Conical in shape with its apex superior and base inferior; it extends anteriorly from the 2nd to 6th ribs and lies in front of the 5th to 8th thoracic vertebrae. The apex fuses with the sheaths of the ascending aorta, pulmonary trunk and superior vena cava, while the base sits on the diaphragm fusing with the central tendon and sheath of the inferior vena cava. Fusion of the fibrous pericardium with the vessel sheaths helps keep them open during cardiac and respiratory movements. Venous return via the inferior vena cava is helped by its attachment to the central tendon of the diaphragm during respiration.

Anterior is the body of the sternum and costal cartilages, from which it is separated by the anterior border of the lungs and pleurae, except for the cardiac notch of the left lung where it lies directly against the sternum (bare area of the pericardium). Posteriorly it lies anterior to the four pulmonary veins with which it fuses, the descending aorta, oesophagus, azygos vein and thoracic duct (Fig. 2.19). Inferiorly it is separated from the liver and fundus of the stomach by the diaphragm, while on each side are the phrenic nerves, pericardiophrenic vessels, mediastinal parietal pleura and lung.

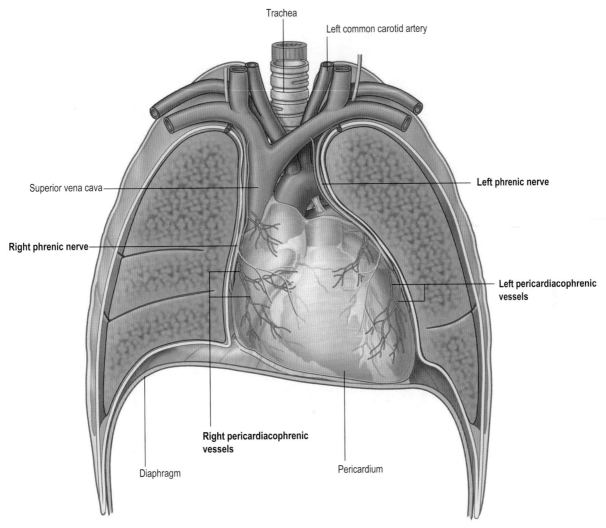

Trachea

Left common carotid artery

Superior vena cava

Right phrenic nerve

Left phrenic nerve

Left pericardiacophrenic vessels

Right pericardiacophrenic vessels

Diaphragm

Pericardium

Fig. 2.19 Pericardium and pericardiophrenic vessels.

APPLIED ANATOMY: The function of the fibrous pericardium is to maintain the central position of the heart within the chest and preventing its over-distension. Several factors help maintain the pericardium and heart in position: the fibrous pericardium is attached to the back of the sternum by superior and inferior sternopericardial ligaments; the lungs provide support laterally, while the diaphragm does so inferiorly. Indirect support is provided by the pretracheal fascia as it blends with the adventitia of the aortic arch, the carotid sheath by its attachment to the base of the skull, the aortic arch as it hooks around the left bronchus, and the subclavian vessels as they cross the apex of the lung and 1st rib.

Serous pericardium. A closed serous sac which is invaginated in foetal life by the developing heart. It has two layers: a visceral layer (epicardium) adherent to the surface of the heart, and a parietal layer which lines the fibrous pericardium. The pericardial cavity is the potential space between the visceral and parietal layers containing a thin film of serous fluid secreted by cells in the serous pericardium. There are two pericardial sinuses, transverse and oblique (Fig. 2.20).

The transverse sinus is a recess of serous pericardium behind the ascending aorta and pulmonary trunk and in

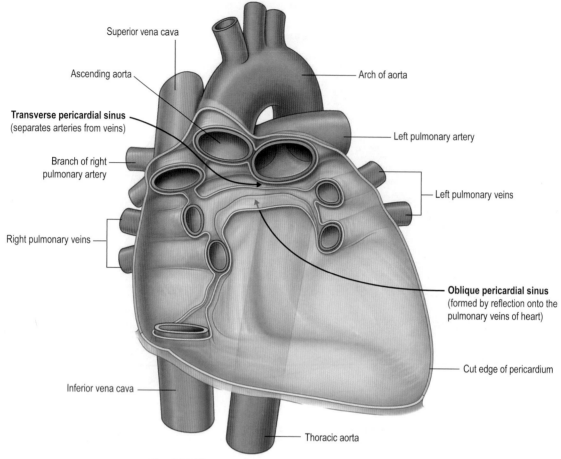

Superior vena cava

Ascending aorta

Transverse pericardial sinus
(separates arteries from veins)

Branch of right
pulmonary artery

Right pulmonary veins

Inferior vena cava

Arch of aorta

Left pulmonary artery

Left pulmonary veins

Oblique pericardial sinus
(formed by reflection onto the
pulmonary veins of heart)

Cut edge of pericardium

Thoracic aorta

Fig. 2.20 The transverse and oblique pericardial sinuses.

front of the superior vena cava and upper parts of both atria; above is the right pulmonary artery and below the two atria, mainly the left.

As the visceral layer of serous pericardium passes upwards on the diaphragmatic surface of the heart over the left atrium, it is reflected downwards onto the fibrous pericardium as the parietal layer forming the oblique sinus separating the left atrium (base of the heart) from the descending aorta and oesophagus. The blind-ending sinus is bounded laterally by the pulmonary veins on each side, with its entrance bounded inferiorly on the right by the inferior vena cava and on the left by the lower left pulmonary vein.

> **APPLIED ANATOMY:** The serous pericardium secretes a small amount of serous fluid sufficient to prevent friction between the heart and fibrous pericardium during movement, as well as preventing adhesion between the heart and surrounding organs.

Blood and nerve supply. The arterial supply to the fibrous pericardium and parietal layer of the serous pericardium is by pericardiophrenic arteries and branches from the internal thoracic artery and descending aorta. Venous drainage is to the internal thoracic and azygos veins, and lymphatic drainage to nodes in the anterior and posterior mediastinum. The innervation is by the phrenic and intercostal nerves; it is therefore sensitive to pain.

The visceral layer of serous pericardium is supplied by branches of the coronary arteries and drained by cardiac veins. Its innervation is by the autonomic nervous system (sympathetic from the sympathetic chain, parasympathetic from the vagus); it is not sensitive to pain.

CLINICAL ANATOMY: The pain of pericarditis originates from the parietal pericardium, while that associated with angina originates from the cardiac muscle or from vessels of the heart.

Posterior Mediastinum

Bounded anteriorly by the pericardium and diaphragm, posteriorly by thoracic vertebrae T5–T12 and laterally by the mediastinal parietal pleura. It contains a number of important structures: the descending thoracic aorta to the left; the oesophagus on the left of the aorta; the azygos vein to the right of the aorta behind the oesophagus; the thoracic duct between the aorta and azygos vein behind the oesophagus; the hemiazygos and accessory hemiazygos veins crossing from left to right behind the oesophagus; the right and left vagi forming the oesophageal plexus; and posterior mediastinal lymph nodes.

Descending aorta. Continuation of the arch of the aorta at the lower border of T4. Initially, it lies on the left side of T5–T7, then anterior to T8–T12, entering the abdomen through the aortic opening of the diaphragm at the lower border of T12 becoming the abdominal aorta. During its course, the descending aorta lies behind (from above down) the left lung root, the fibrous pericardium and oesophagus, and in front of the hemiazygos veins as they pass to the right at the levels of T7 and T8. On its left is the left lung and pleura, which it grooves.

The posterior intercostal and subcostal arteries arise from their posterior surface, as well as pericardial branches. Two left bronchial arteries run on the posterior surface of the left bronchus to enter and supply the left lung: the right bronchial artery is from the 3rd right intercostal or upper left bronchial artery. Oesophageal branches arise from the anterior surface forming a longitudinal chain on the surface of the oesophagus. Phrenic arteries also arise from its anterior surface supplying the upper surface of the diaphragm.

SURFACE ANATOMY: The ascending aorta is represented by a line from the sternal end of the 3rd left costal cartilage to the sternal end of the 2nd right costal cartilage. The arch of the aorta is represented by a curved line from the sternal end of the 2nd right costal cartilage to the sternal end of the 2nd left costal cartilage; its highest point is at the centre of the manubrium. The descending aorta is represented by a line from the sternal end of the left costal cartilage to a point in the sagittal (median) plane 2 cm above the transpyloric plane.

Oesophagus. A flattened, thick, dilatable muscular tube connecting the pharynx and stomach (Fig. 2.21). It begins at the level of the cricoid cartilage (C6) as a continuation of the pharynx and passes downwards through the superior and posterior mediastinum behind the trachea and left atrium, through the diaphragm to the left of the midline at the level of T10 to enter the cardiac region of the stomach; it has cervical, thoracic and abdominal parts. The upper 1/3rd is composed of skeletal muscle, the middle 1/3rd of mixed skeletal and smooth muscle and the lower 1/3rd of smooth muscle. During its course it inclines to the left at T1 and T7 and has four constrictions: at its origin; as it is crossed by the arch of the aorta at T4/T5; as it is crossed by the left bronchus at T4/T5; and as it passes through the diaphragm at T10. Although the last narrowing is not an anatomical sphincter, it is important functionally as it controls the entry of food into the stomach and the reflux of stomach contents (heartburn).

CLINICAL ANATOMY: Oesophageal constrictions are common sites of cancer and strictures. In addition, when introducing instruments through the oesophagus some resistance can be expected in the region of the constrictions.

CLINICAL ANATOMY: Oesophageal atresia is a rare birth defect in which the upper part of the oesophagus is not connected with its lower part; the upper part usually ending in a blind pouch so that food cannot reach the stomach.

In the cervical part, the arterial supply is from the inferior thyroid artery, a branch of the thyrocervical trunk of the subclavian, venous drainage is to the

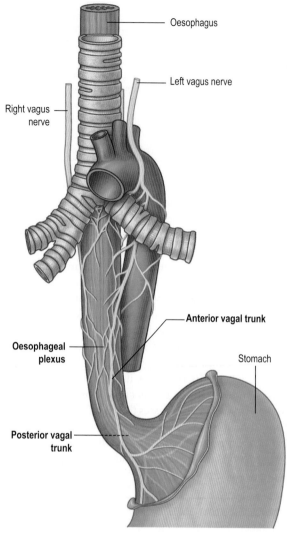

Right vagus nerve

Oesophagus

Left vagus nerve

Anterior vagal trunk

Stomach

Oesophageal plexus

Posterior vagal trunk

Fig. 2.21 The oesophagus.

inferior thyroid vein, and lymphatic drainage is to the deep cervical lymph nodes.

In the thoracic part, the arterial supply is from branches of the descending aorta, with venous drainage into the azygos, accessory hemiazygos and hemiazygos veins; lymphatic drainage is to bronchial and the preaortic group of posterior mediastinal nodes.

In the abdomen, the arterial supply is from the left gastric artery, with venous drainage into the left gastric vein; lymphatic drainage is to the paracardiac group of diaphragmatic nodes.

Throughout its length, parasympathetic innervation is from the vagus; in the neck by the recurrent laryngeal nerve, in the thorax by the oesophageal plexus and in the abdomen by the anterior and posterior gastric nerves. Sympathetic innervation is directly from the sympathetic trunks in the thorax and the greater splanchnic nerves in the abdomen.

Azygos vein. A communicating vein between the superior and inferior venae cavae (Fig. 2.13). It arises in the abdomen from the back of the inferior vena cava at the level of the renal veins (L2); it may also be formed by the union of the ascending lumbar and subcostal veins. It ascends through the aortic opening of the diaphragm on the right side of the aorta and thoracic duct, then runs on the vertebral bodies on the right side of the descending aorta behind the right border of the oesophagus. Passing behind the root of the right lung it curves anteriorly over the right lung root forming the arch of the azygos, which crosses the right side of the oesophagus, trachea and right vagus to drain into the posterior surface of the superior vena cava.

It receives the right ascending lumbar vein; the right subcostal vein; right 4th/5th to 11th posterior intercostal veins; right superior intercostal vein; hemiazygos and accessory hemiazygos veins; bronchial veins of the right lung; and oesophageal and pericardial veins.

> **APPLIED ANATOMY:** All venous blood from the thoracic wall drains into the superior vena cava.

Thoracic duct. The largest lymph duct in the body with a diameter of 5 mm; it is usually beaded in appearance due to its many valves. It drains lymph from the lower limbs, abdomen, pelvis and perineum, left side of the thorax, left upper limb and left side of the head and neck. Its origin is from the cisterna chyli in the abdomen at the lower border of T12 and terminates by draining into the left brachiocephalic vein at the junction of the left internal jugular and subclavian veins (Fig. 2.22).

The thoracic duct passes through the aortic opening behind the diaphragm into the posterior mediastinum behind the right border of the oesophagus. At the level of T4/T5 it crosses obliquely behind the oesophagus to ascend in the superior mediastinum on the left side of the oesophagus. It enters the neck through the thoracic inlet and then arches laterally

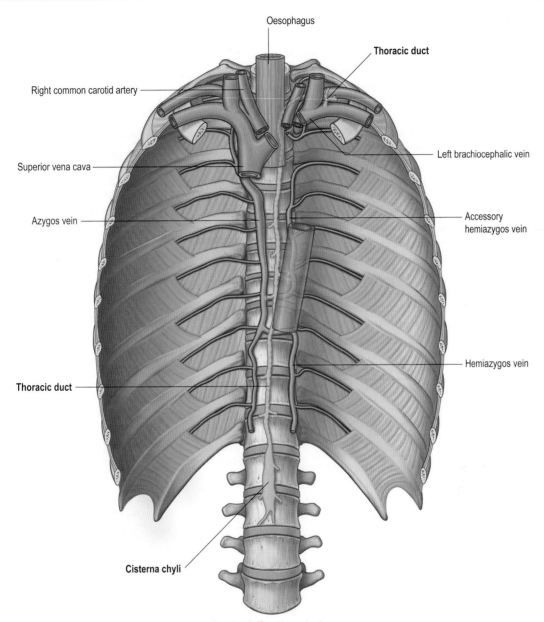

Oesophagus

Thoracic duct

Right common carotid artery

Left brachiocephalic vein

Superior vena cava

Azygos vein

Accessory
hemiazygos vein

Thoracic duct

Hemiazygos vein

Cisterna chyli

Fig. 2.22 The thoracic duct.

over the apex of the left lung behind the carotid sheath (page 325) in front of the left vertebral artery towards its termination.

During its course it receives the left jugular trunk draining the left side of the head and neck, the left subclavian lymph trunk draining the left upper limb, the left bronchomediastinal lymph trunk, and efferents from posterior mediastinal, intercostal, and upper lumbar nodes.

The **cisterna chyli** is a spindle-shaped sac 5 cm long anterior to the upper two lumbar vertebrae (L1 and L2), lying between the abdominal aorta and azygos vein. Its tapered end forms the thoracic duct. It receives lymph from both lower limbs via the right and left lumbar lymph trunks, most of the abdomen and pelvis via the intestinal lymph trunk.

A separate **right lymph trunk** drains lymph from the superior surface of the liver, right half of the thorax via the right bronchomediastinal lymph trunk, right upper limb via the right subclavian lymph trunk and right half of the head and neck. It ascends into the neck to drain into the right brachiocephalic vein.

Sympathetic chain. Running longitudinally along either side of the vertebral column from C1 to the coccyx, crossing the tips of the transverse processes of cervical vertebrae, the heads of the ribs at thoracic levels and the anterolateral aspects of the vertebral bodies at lumbar and sacral levels, are two sets of nerve fibres, the sympathetic chains (trunks) (Fig. 2.23). Each chain consists of preganglionic and postganglionic fibres: at sites along each chain where preganglionic and postganglionic fibres synapse are swellings (sympathetic ganglia). There are usually two (occasionally three) cervical, 11–12 thoracic, 1–6 (usually 4) lumbar, 4 sacral ganglia and a single ganglion impar anterior to the coccyx (Fig. 2.23).

> **CLINICAL ANATOMY:** Sympathetic outflow from the spinal cord is only between the T1 and L2 levels; it is referred to as thoracolumbar outflow.

Cell bodies of the preganglionic neurons are located in the lateral horns of the grey matter of the spinal cord in the T1–L2 segments, the axons of which leave in the ventral roots of the spinal nerves at the same levels to enter the ventral ramus of the spinal nerve just beyond the intervertebral foramen. The fibres then leave the ventral ramus to enter the sympathetic chain conveying preganglionic neurons *to* the sympathetic chain (Fig. 2.24). Because this branch comprises myelinated fibres, it is a *white ramus communicans* (plural: rami communicantes).

On entering the sympathetic chain, the preganglionic neurons usually pass upwards/downwards within it before synapsing in sympathetic ganglia with the cell bodies of postganglionic neurons. At upper thoracic levels, preganglionic neurons tend to pass upwards into the neck before synapsing, while those from lower thoracic and lumbar levels tend to pass downwards into the abdomen and pelvis before synapsing. Those

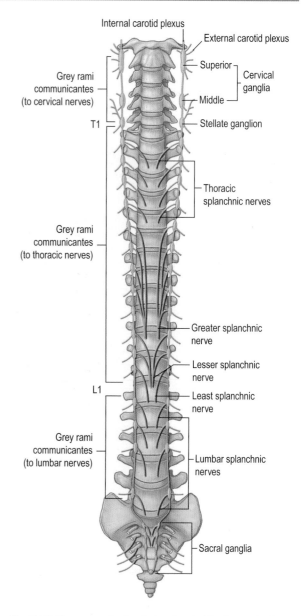

Fig. 2.23 The sympathetic chains (trunks) in the neck, thorax and abdomen.

at midthoracic levels either synapse at their own level or pass up/down a short distance before synapsing. Postganglionic neurons leave the sympathetic chain in one of three ways: by joining a ventral ramus as a *grey ramus communicans*; by following arteries; or by

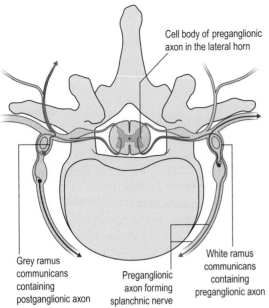

Fig. 2.24 Pre- and post-ganglionic fibres of the sympathetic nervous system.

forming distinct branches passing directly to viscera or plexuses (Fig. 2.24).

> **APPLIED ANATOMY:** All ventral rami of spinal nerves receive a grey ramus communicans, whereas white rami communicantes are only found associated with the ventral rami of spinal nerves T1–L2.

The **thoracic sympathetic chain** is continuous with the cervical part in the neck, where the 1st thoracic ganglion may fuse with the inferior cervical ganglion to form the stellate ganglion at the level of C7/T1 (Fig. 2.23). They leave the thorax behind the medial arcuate ligaments or through the crura to enter the abdomen.

From the upper five thoracic ganglia, small branches pass to the aorta, and its branches, by the aortic plexus. From the 2nd to 4th thoracic ganglia branches pass to the heart by the superficial and deep cardiac plexuses, and lungs by the anterior and posterior pulmonary plexuses. The oesophagus receives branches from the pulmonary and cardiac plexuses.

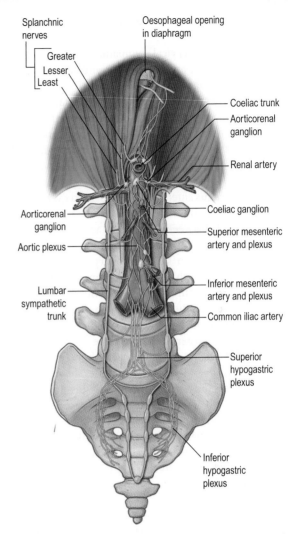

Fig. 2.25 Sympathetic nerves, ganglia and plexuses in the abdomen and pelvis.

The greater splanchnic nerve arises from the 5th to 9th ganglia: it descends on the thoracic bodies, pierces the right crus of the diaphragm and ends in the coeliac ganglion in the abdomen: it gives branches to the oesophagus, aorta and supplies abdominal viscera. The least splanchnic nerve arises from the 10th and 11th ganglia, descending with the greater splanchnic nerve to end in the superior mesenteric and aorticorenal ganglia in the abdomen. The lesser splanchnic nerve arises from the last thoracic ganglion and enters the abdomen with the sympathetic chain to end in the renal plexus (Fig. 2.25).

Details of the cervical sympathetic chain can be found on pages 90, and the lumbar and sacral sympathetic chain on pages 227.

Vagus nerves. Although each vagus contains motor, sensory and parasympathetic fibres, it is mainly a parasympathetic nerve, giving fibres to the respiratory system, the gastrointestinal tract and its associated glands from the oesophagus to the left colic flexure, and to the heart.

The **right vagus** enters the thorax behind the brachiocephalic artery to the right of the trachea, then continues downwards between the trachea and pleura behind the arch of the azygos vein and root of the right lung, where it gives rise to the pulmonary plexus together with branches from the 2nd to 4th sympathetic ganglia (Fig. 2.18). Two or three branches from the pulmonary plexus pass behind the oesophagus to share in the formation of the oesophageal plexus and then pass into the abdomen as the posterior gastric nerve.

The **left vagus** enters the thorax between the left common carotid and subclavian arteries, being crossed by the left phrenic nerve. It then descends downwards crossing the arch of the aorta laterally to pass behind the root of the left lung giving rise to the pulmonary plexus, again with branches from the 2nd to 4th sympathetic ganglia (Fig. 2.18). Two or three branches descend anterior to the oesophagus to share in the formation of the oesophageal plexus and then pass into the abdomen as the anterior gastric nerve.

The left recurrent laryngeal nerve arises as the left vagus crosses the aortic arch (Fig. 2.18). It passes below the arch lateral to the ligamentum arteriosum to pass upwards in the groove between the trachea and oesophagus to reach and supply the larynx (further details of the larynx can be found on pages 328).

Cardiac branches arise from the right vagus and left recurrent laryngeal nerve as they pass alongside the trachea. The oesophageal plexus also gives branches to the posterior aspect of the fibrous pericardium.

> **APPLIED ANATOMY:** Each gastric nerve usually contains fibres from the right and left vagus nerves.

Further details of the vagus nerves and their branches can be found on page 279.

Phrenic nerves. The phrenic nerves are mixed motor and sensory nerves, being motor only to the diaphragm. They arise from the 3rd to 5th cervical nerves (mainly the 4th). Details of their courses in the neck can be found on page 332.

The **right phrenic nerve** descends lateral to the right brachiocephalic vein, superior vena cava, right atrium and inferior vena cava, and medial to the right pleura and lung (Fig. 2.26). It leaves the thorax through the caval opening in the central tendon of the diaphragm with the inferior vena cava.

The **left phrenic nerve** descends between the left common carotid and subclavian arteries lateral to the left vagus, aortic arch, left superior intercostal vein and pericardium over the left ventricle, and medial to the left pleura and lung (Fig. 2.26). It leaves the thorax through an opening in the diaphragm just lateral to the fibrous pericardium.

Both nerves pass anterior to the lung root between the fibrous pericardium and mediastinal parietal pleura accompanied by pericardiophrenic vessels. The nerves ramify over the abdominal surface of the diaphragm supplying it with motor fibres.

During their course through the thorax, the phrenic nerves are sensory to the mediastinal and diaphragmatic pleura, the fibrous and serous pericardium and the diaphragmatic peritoneum under the central tendon. There are sensory communications with the coeliac and hepatic plexuses, while fibres from the right phrenic nerve may reach the gallbladder.

> **CLINICAL ANATOMY:** Inflammation of the gall bladder or diaphragmatic peritoneum may result in referred pain to the right shoulder as both are supplied by the C4 segment of the spinal cord.

An **accessory phrenic nerve** may exist as a separate branch from C5 or as a branch from the nerve to subclavius. When present it lies lateral to the main phrenic nerve, joining it at any level between the 1st rib and lower thorax.

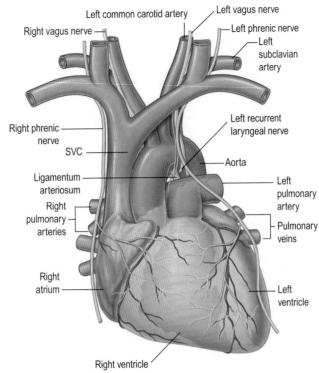

Fig. 2.26 The course of the phrenic nerves in the thorax. *SVC,* Superior vena cava.

CLINICAL ANATOMY: In cases of an accessory phrenic nerve, crushing the main phrenic nerve during surgery (phrenic avulsion) as it passes anterior to scalenus anterior is not sufficient to completely paralyse the diaphragm.

Respiratory System

The respiratory system is concerned with the exchange of gases (oxygen and carbon dioxide) between air in the lungs and blood in the capillaries of the pulmonary circulation; often referred to as external respiration. Internal respiration occurs between blood in the systemic capillaries and cells/tissues of body organs.

DEVELOPMENT: The respiratory system (larynx, trachea, bronchi and lungs) develops as an outgrowth (respiratory diverticulum) from the anterior wall of the primitive pharynx (Fig. 2.27A). A septum forms dividing the foregut into oesophagus and trachea. The distal end of the diverticulum expands forming the lung buds, which grow into the primitive pleural cavities. During the 5th week of development, the right lung bud divides into three main bronchi and the left into two (Fig. 2.27B). The main bronchi continue to divide repeatedly until the end of the 6th month when there have been some 17 divisions; a further 6 divisions occur postnatally. As the vascular supply to the lungs increases the bronchioles continue to divide into smaller and smaller canals until the 7th month. Respiration is not possible until the cells of the respiratory bronchioles become flat and thin (Fig. 2.27C). By the 7th month, an adequate gas exchange is possible potentially enabling premature babies to survive. Considerable growth of the lungs (respiratory bronchioles and alveolar ducts) occurs after birth.

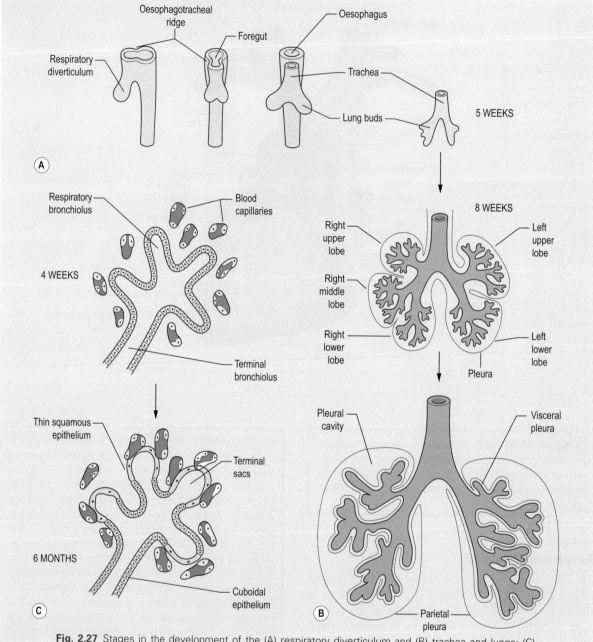

Fig. 2.27 Stages in the development of the (A) respiratory diverticulum and (B) trachea and lungs; (C) histological and functional development of the lungs.

CLINICAL ANATOMY: A connection between the lower part of the oesophagus and trachea may persist giving a tracheo-oesophageal fistula. This can allow air to pass into the oesophagus and stomach, and stomach acid to pass into the lungs. Surgical treatment is required within a few days after birth to prevent life-threatening problems, such as choking and pneumonia.

Nose, Pharynx and Larynx

Details of the nose, pharynx and larynx can be found on pages 304, 326 and 328.

Trachea and Bronchi

The trachea begins at the lower border of the 6th cervical vertebra (C6) and ends at the lower border of

T4 where it divides into right and left principal bronchi (Fig. 2.28). It is a fibromembranous tube reinforced by incomplete cartilage rings, open posteriorly, to keep the lumen open, and completed posteriorly by smooth muscle (trachealis); the lowest tracheal cartilage has a ridge (carina) projecting upwards inside the trachea between the two bronchi.

The wider shorter right bronchus is more in line with the trachea and usually divides into secondary bronchi before entering the lung. The left bronchus is narrower and longer, has a more horizontal course and usually divides into secondary bronchi after entering the lung.

> **CLINICAL ANATOMY:** Foreign bodies entering the trachea usually pass into the right bronchus because it is more vertical and in line with the trachea.

The trachea and larger bronchi are lined by pseudostratified ciliated columnar (respiratory) epithelium (page 20) interspersed with goblet cells. The cilia beat in waves moving mucous and inhaled particles towards the laryngeal inlet and oesophagus, ready for swallowing.

> **CLINICAL ANATOMY:** Prolonged exposure to inhaled organic particles (cigarette smoke) can damage the respiratory epithelium affecting the ability of cilia to beat and therefore effectively remove mucous and inhaled particles.

Blood and nerve supply. The cervical part of the trachea is supplied by the inferior thyroid arteries and drained by the inferior thyroid veins, while the thoracic part is supplied by a single bronchial artery on the right and two bronchial arteries on the left, with venous drainage into the azygos vein on the right and accessory hemiazygos vein on the left. The bronchi are supplied and drained by bronchial vessels.

Lymphatic drainage of the trachea, bronchi and lungs is by tracheobronchial lymph nodes (Fig. 2.28), which are divided into five groups: pulmonary, located in the lung tissue draining it, except for the alveoli where there are no lymphatics; bronchopulmonary, at the hilum of the lung which receives lymph from the pulmonary nodes and also drains superficial tissues of the lung and visceral pleura; inferior tracheobronchial, lying between the principle bronchi receiving lymph from the bronchopulmonary nodes; superior tracheobronchial, around the lower part of the trachea and its bifurcation receiving lymph from the inferior tracheobronchial nodes; and paratracheal, at the sides of the trachea receiving lymph from the superior tracheobronchial nodes.

Innervation of the trachea and bronchi is by autonomic fibres from the right and left vagus and sympathetic chains.

Pleurae

The pleurae are serous membranes consisting of flattened epithelial cells on a basement membrane forming completely closed serous sacs surrounding each lung; each sac is invaginated by the lung from its medial side. **Visceral (pulmonary) pleura** invests the lung and also lines the lung fissures. **Parietal pleura** lines the thoracic wall and covers surrounding structures. The parietal pleura is usually named according to the structures/region it covers: **cervical pleura** projects through the thoracic inlet to the root of the neck covering the apex of the lung and is itself covered by the suprapleural membrane (page 79); **costal pleura** lines the inner surface of the ribs, costal cartilages and intercostal spaces; **mediastinal pleura** covers the sides of the mediastinum and part of the pericardium (pericardial pleura); **diaphragmatic pleura** covers the upper surface of the diaphragm.

The pleurae are continuous around the lung root (Fig. 2.29) forming a fold of pleura known as the pulmonary ligament extending down to the diaphragm. This fold allows free movement of the lung root and distension of the pulmonary veins preventing their collapse during respiration.

The parietal and visceral pleura are separated by a space (pleural cavity) containing serous fluid to lubricate both surfaces allowing the lungs to move freely during respiration. The pleural cavity is enlarged along its anterior margin (costomediastinal recess) and its lower border (costodiaphragmatic recess). During inspiration the anterior and inferior margins of the lung enter these recesses, leaving them during expiration.

> **CLINICAL ANATOMY:** Lack of or loss of serous fluid within the pleural space causes the parietal and visceral pleurae to rub against each other leading to a crackling sound on auscultation and sometimes pain.

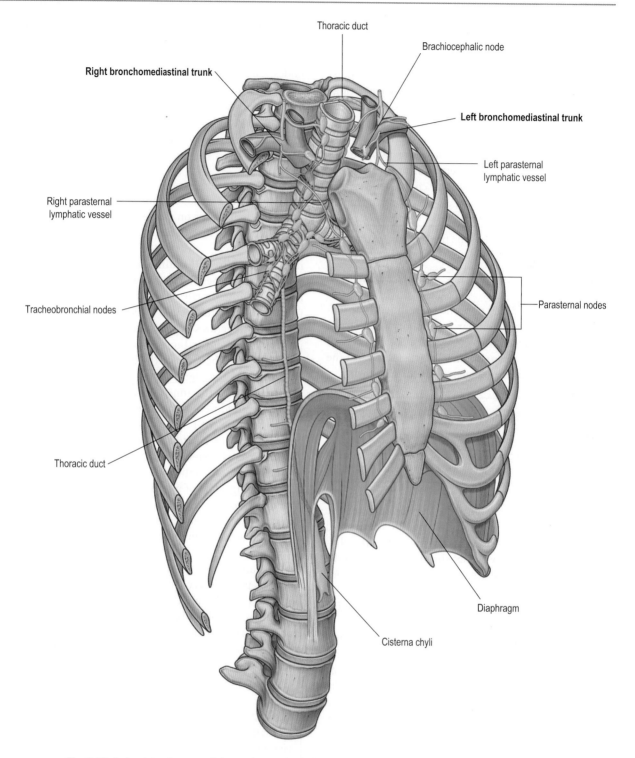

Fig. 2.28 Anterolateral aspect of the trachea and principal bronchi; also shown are the main groups of lymph nodes associated with the lungs.

CLINICAL ANATOMY: The costodiaphragmatic recess is the first to be filled in pleural effusion.

Blood and nerve supply. The arterial supply and venous drainage of the parietal pleura is by vessels from the thoracic wall, being the intercostal, internal thoracic and musculophrenic. Lymph is to intercostal, parasternal, posterior mediastinal and diaphragmatic nodes. The innervation differs depending on its location: the costal and lateral part of the diaphragmatic pleura is by intercostal nerves, and the mediastinal and medial part of the diaphragmatic pleura is by the phrenic nerve.

The blood supply of the visceral pleura is by bronchial vessels supplying the lung tissue; lymphatic drainage is to bronchopulmonary nodes. Innervation is from the vagus and sympathetic nerve plexuses within the lung.

CLINICAL ANATOMY: In inflammation of the parietal pleura, pain is referred to the intercostal spaces or anterior abdominal wall.

CLINICAL ANATOMY: The pleural cavity may fill with air (**pneumothorax**), blood (**haemothorax**) or pus (**empyema**). A **tension pneumothorax** occurs when the heart is pushed to one side severely compromising its function; it requires urgent intervention. To remove fluid from the pleural cavity (**paracentesis**) a chest drain, usually a large needle, is inserted into an intercostal space, usually the 5th in the mid-axillary line. The needle is passed along the upper border of the lower rib to avoid injury to the neurovascular bundle. To avoid injury to the diaphragm and underlying organs the needle should not be inserted below the 7th intercostal space.

Lungs

The lungs occupy most of the space in the thoracic cavity, each lung lying free within its pleural cavity attached by only its root to the mediastinum. The right lung has three lobes (superior, middle, inferior) separated by oblique and horizontal fissures, and the left lung has two lobes (superior (with the lingula), inferior) separated by the oblique fissure (Fig. 2.30). The right lung is larger, shorter and wider than the left.

Each lung has an apex, base, costal and medial surfaces, and anterior, posterior and inferior borders. The costal and medial surfaces are separated by a thin sharp anterior border, extending into the costomediastinal recess anteriorly, and a thick rounded border, lying in the paravertebral gutter posteriorly. An inferior border separates the costal and medial surfaces from the base (Fig. 2.30). On the left the anterior border has a shallow (cardiac) notch below which is the lingula.

Because of the obliquity of the thoracic inlet the rounded apex projects into the root of the neck approximately 1 cm above and behind the medial 1/3rd of the clavicle (Fig. 2.32). It is covered by cervical pleura and the suprapleural membrane and grooved anteriorly by the subclavian artery: posteriorly it is separated from the neck of the 1st rib by the sympathetic chain, superior intercostal vessels and 1st thoracic nerve (T1).

The base is concave upwards, being deeper on the right than the left (Fig. 2.30). The right lung is separated from the right lobe of the liver and the left from the left lobe of the liver, stomach and spleen by the diaphragm.

The costal surface is wide and convex separated from the ribs, costal cartilages and intercostal muscles by costal pleura (Fig. 2.30). The medial surface contains the root (hilum) of the lung and is divided into anterior mediastinal and posterior vertebral parts. The mediastinal part is applied to the side of the mediastinum and has a number of impressions and grooves from adjacent structures; the hilum of the lung lies in its posterior part. The vertebral part lies behind the lung root and is related to the sides of thoracic vertebrae, intervertebral discs, posterior intercostal vessels, sympathetic trunk and roots of the splanchnic nerves.

The **medial surface of the right lung** (Fig. 2.30) has a large impression of the right atrium anterior to the hilum and pulmonary ligament. The inferior vena cava makes a short groove below the hilum, while the superior vena cava makes a vertical groove anterior to the upper part of the hilum, being continuous with that formed by the right brachiocephalic vein; a groove for the arch of the azygos passing over the hilum joins that for the superior vena cava. The ascending aorta is related to the area anterior to the superior vena cava and remains of the thymus gland. The trachea and right vagus are related to an area behind the superior vena cava above the arch of the azygos vein, while the oesophagus lies posterior to the hilum. The right phrenic nerve runs along the grooves of the right

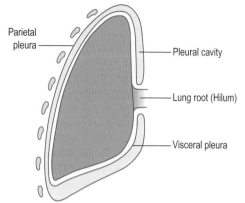

Parietal pleura

Pleural cavity

Lung root (Hilum)

Visceral pleura

Fig. 2.29 Organisation of the parietal and visceral pleurae covering the lungs, as well as formation of the pleural cavity.

brachiocephalic vein, superior vena cava, pericardial impression and inferior vena cava.

The **medial surface of the left lung** (Fig. 2.30) has a large impression of the left ventricle anterior to the hilum and pulmonary ligament. The arch of the aorta, together with the left common carotid and subclavian arteries, form distinct grooves above the hilum, with that for the aortic arch being continuous with the groove for the descending aorta behind the hilum and pulmonary ligament. The oesophagus makes a short groove anterior to the lower end of that for the descending aorta. The left phrenic nerve runs along the grooves of the left common carotid artery, arch of the aorta and pericardial impression.

Root (hilum) of the lung. The part of the medial surface, lying opposite the 5th to 7th thoracic vertebrae, where several structures enter (bronchus, pulmonary artery, bronchial vessels, pulmonary nerve plexuses) or leave (pulmonary vein) the lung; it has no pleural covering (Fig. 2.30). Within the hilum are bronchopulmonary lymph nodes. The bronchial vessels supply the bronchi and their branches, as well as the connective (non-respiratory) tissues of the lung.

In the **right hilum** are two bronchi (superior, middle or inferior lobar) posteriorly, the superior bronchus lying above and behind the pulmonary artery and the middle/inferior below and/or behind (Fig. 2.30). The two pulmonary veins lie inferiorly.

In the **left hilum** the principal bronchus lies posteriorly, with the pulmonary artery above with two pulmonary veins below (Fig. 2.30).

APPLIED ANATOMY: The pulmonary arteries carry de-oxygenated blood from the right ventricle to the lungs, and the pulmonary veins carry oxygenated blood from the lungs to the left atrium for distribution around the body via the systemic circulation.

Bronchopulmonary segments. Each lung consists of several well-defined and distinct bronchopulmonary segments (Fig. 2.31), each of which is functionally independent and can be defined radiologically. Each is pyramidal in shape with the apex directed towards the root of the lung. Their location and relation to the relevant tertiary bronchus are important when drainage of a specific lung segment is required. Within a bronchopulmonary segment, the tertiary bronchus repeatedly subdivides, becoming bronchioles when cartilage is no longer present in their walls. Bronchioles further subdivide, eventually becoming alveoli where respiratory gas exchange occurs.

Each bronchopulmonary segment is surrounded by connective tissue septa forming intersegmental planes. Branches of the pulmonary veins usually run in the intersegmental planes, while those of the pulmonary arteries accompany the bronchi within the segments.

In the **right lung,** the superior lobe bronchus divides into three tertiary segmental bronchi (apical, posterior, anterior), the middle lobe bronchi into two tertiary segmental bronchi (lateral, medial) and the inferior lobe bronchus into five tertiary segmental bronchi (apical basal, medial basal, lateral basal, anterior basal, posterior basal) (Fig. 2.31).

In the **left lung,** the superior lobe bronchus divides into two parts (superior, lingula), with the superior division then dividing into three tertiary segmental bronchi (apical, posterior, anterior) and the lingular division into two tertiary segmental bronchi (superior, inferior). The inferior lobe bronchus divides into five tertiary segmental bronchi (apical basal, medial basal, lateral basal, anterior basal, posterior basal) (Fig. 2.31).

Each tertiary segmental bronchus passes into the same named bronchopulmonary segment supplying it.

APPLIED ANATOMY: There are variations in the pattern of branching of tertiary bronchi giving rise to fewer bronchopulmonary segments in each lung.

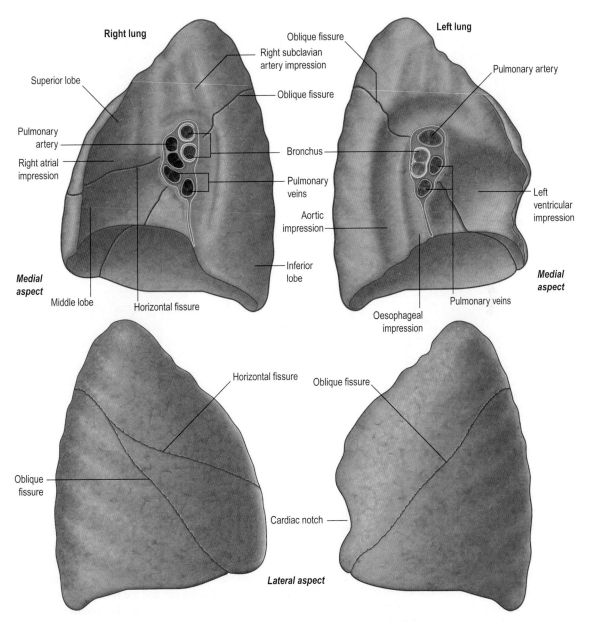

Fig. 2.30 Medial and lateral aspects of the right and left lungs.

CLINICAL ANATOMY: Infection of a bronchopulmonary segment remains restricted to that segment; however, tuberculosis and carcinoma can spread. If a bronchopulmonary segment becomes diseased it can often be surgically removed.

Surface markings of the pleurae and lungs. The surface markings of the parietal pleura and lungs are important in physical examination of the chest: the surface marking of the lungs follows that of the visceral pleura (Fig. 2.32). On both sides, the parietal pleura and lung run down from the apex of the lung 3 cm above the medial 1/3rd of the

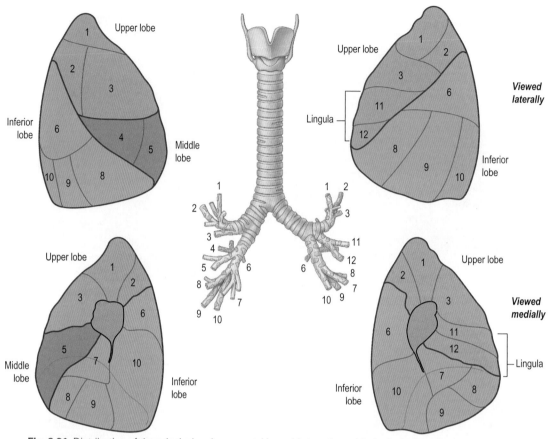

Fig. 2.31 Distribution of the principal and segmental bronchi, together with the bronchopulmonary segments in each lobe of each lung.

clavicle. The anterior border corresponds to an oblique line from the apex to the middle of the manubriosternal joint level with the 2nd costal cartilage. On the right, the anterior borders of both the parietal and visceral pleurae run down to the 6th costal cartilage, where it becomes continuous with the inferior border. On the left, the anterior border of the parietal pleura descends to the 4th costal cartilage and then deviates to the left and continues downwards 1 cm from the sternal margin to the 6th costal cartilage. On the left, at the 4th costal cartilage, the viscera pleura (and lung) deviates to the left 3–4 cm from the margin of the sternum before descending vertically to the 6th costal cartilage (Fig. 2.32).

On both sides a line drawn around the chest wall crossing the 8th rib at the midclavicular line, 10th rib at the mid-axillary line and 12th rib close to the vertebral column represents the position of the parietal pleura; it dips below the costal margin between the vertebral column and lower border of the 12th rib (Fig. 2.32). The posterior border passes vertically 5 cm from the midline parallel to the vertebral column from the posterior end of the inferior border to the apex of the lung (Fig. 2.32).

On both sides, the inferior border of the visceral pleura (and lung) is represented by a line drawn around the chest wall crossing the midclavicular line at the 6th rib, the mid-axillary line at the 8th rib, and the 10th rib close to the vertebral column; the posterior border follows the parietal pleura from the 10th rib to the apex of the lung (Fig. 2.32).

SURFACE ANATOMY: With the arm abducted to 90 degrees the oblique fissure is marked by a line from the spinous process of T3 (level with the spine of the scapula) along the medial border of the scapula as far as the mid-axillary line and then anteriorly along the 6th rib and costal cartilage. The horizontal fissure of the right lung passes laterally along the lower border of the costal cartilage and 4th rib, meeting the oblique fissure at the mid-axillary line (Fig. 2.32).

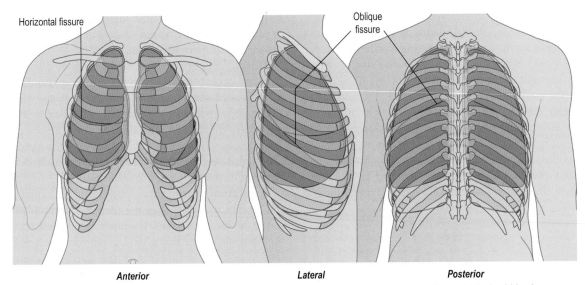

Horizontal fissure

Oblique fissure

Anterior   *Lateral*   *Posterior*

Fig. 2.32 The position of the lung and visceral pleura (dark blue) and parietal pleura (light blue) within the thoracic cavity.

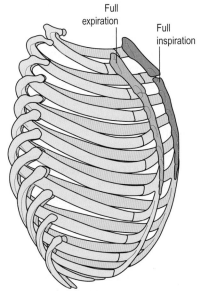

Full expiration

Full inspiration

Fig. 2.33 Lateral aspect of the thoracic cage showing its movement during respiration.

Mechanics of respiration. During respiration the volume of the thorax changes due to movement of the diaphragm, ribs and sternum (Fig. 2.33). The vertical, transverse and anteroposterior diameters increase during inspiration and decrease during expiration. Movements of the ribs and their costal cartilages depend on several factors, including their length, whether they are attached directly to the sternum, and the axis about which movement occurs. Increases in thoracic volume create a negative intrathoracic pressure drawing air into the lungs: the lungs expand passively (inspiration). Elastic recoil of the alveoli and thoracic wall expels air from the lungs (expiration).

Inspiration. Movement of the 2nd to 5th ribs occurs about an axis along their necks, resulting in their anterior ends being raised, lifting the body of the sternum upwards and outwards (Fig. 2.34). Because of restricted movement of the 1st rib, the sternum bends at the manubriosternal joint. These movements of the ribs and sternum increase the anteroposterior diameter of the thorax; there is little lateral movement except during the terminal part of a deep inspiration. The movement is often referred to as the 'pump-handle' movement.

Movement of the 8th to 10th ribs occurs about an axis through the costovertebral and sternocostal/interchondral joints (Fig. 2.34), resulting in an outward and upward movement of their anterior ends widening the infrasternal angle, thereby increasing the transverse diameter of the thorax. This movement is often referred to as the 'bucket-handle' movement.

The 6th and 7th ribs show both pump-handle and bucket-handle types of movement. Ribs 11 and 12 have little or no influence on thoracic diameters, but because they give attachment to the lower fibres of the diaphragm they provide, together with quadratus lumborum, a firm attachment for the diaphragm during its contraction.

In quiet respiration movement of the ribs is essentially brought about by contraction of the diaphragm, with the intercostal muscles maintaining the interspace between the ribs by forming a semi-rigid structure. Contraction of the diaphragm lowers the domes thereby increasing the vertical diameter of the thorax.

As the chest wall moves upwards and outwards, the parietal pleura, which is closely attached to it, moves with it. The visceral pleura follows the parietal pleura

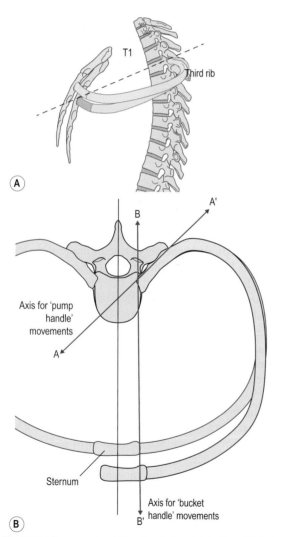

(A)

(B)

Fig. 2.34 Movements of the ribs during respiration. (A) Pump handle movement. (B) Bucket handle movement.

as the volume of the thorax increases. The lungs then expand to fill the increased space and air is drawn into the trachea and bronchial tree.

During deep inspiration, or in cases of respiratory distress, large powerful muscles (sternomastoid, pectoralis major, serratus anterior) attached to the outside of the upper part of the thoracic cage act as accessory muscles of inspiration. By fixing the upper limb, e.g., by holding onto the back of a chair or resting the hands on the thigh/knee, the attachment of these muscles to the ribs and/or sternum helps to raise them.

Expiration. During quiet breathing in expiration, the reverse movements of the ribs and sternum occur as the diaphragm relaxes. The lungs recoil passively and air flows out of the bronchial tree. In forced expiration latissimus dorsi and muscles of the anterior abdominal wall help to compress the thorax.

Respiratory Physiology

Respiration provides oxygen to the tissues and removes carbon dioxide. The first breath occurs after birth and continues throughout life; permanent stoppage occurs at death. Breathing depends on changes in pressure and volume of the thoracic cavity, with increases in volume causing a decrease in pressure, and decreases in volume causing an increase in pressure. Since air flows from areas of high pressure to areas of low pressure, it is the changes in pressure inside the lungs which determine the direction of airflow.

NORMAL RESPIRATORY RATES: Newborn, 30–60 breaths/min; early childhood, 20–40 breaths/min; late childhood, 15–25 breaths/min; adult, 12–16 breaths/min.

Factors influencing breathing

Elasticity is the ability of the lungs to return to their normal shape after each breath. Loss of elasticity of the connective tissues in the lungs, as in emphysema (page 114), leads to increased effort during inspiration and expiration.

Compliance is the stretchiness of the lungs. In healthy lungs, compliance is high requiring little effort to inflate the lungs and alveoli, while low compliance requires increased effort to inflate the lungs (Fig. 2.35). Compliance and elasticity are opposing forces.

Airway resistance determines the effort required to inflate the lungs. Increased airway resistance, as in bronchoconstriction, requires increased respiratory effort.

Lung capacity

Tidal volume (TV) is the volume of air drawn into and expelled from the lungs during normal quiet breathing: it is 500 mL.

Inspiratory reserve volume (IRV) is the additional volume of air that can be inspired forcefully at the end of a normal inspiration, i.e., after inspiring the TV: it is 3300 mL.

Inspiratory capacity (IC) is the maximum volume of air that can be taken in following a normal expiration: it is 3800 mL, being the combined tidal and inspiratory reserve volumes, i.e., IC = TV + IRV (Fig. 2.36).

Expiratory reserve volume (ERV) is the additional volume of air that can be expired after a quiet expiration, i.e., after expiring the TV: it is 1000 mL.

Residual volume (RV) is the volume of air remaining in the lungs after the deepest expiration: it is 1100 mL (Fig. 2.36).

Functional residual capacity (FRC) is the volume of air remaining in the airways and alveoli at the end of quiet expiration. This is an important volume as blood is continuously flowing through the capillaries so that gaseous exchange is not interrupted between breaths preventing changes in blood gas concentrations. Functional RV also prevents the alveoli collapsing during expiration: FRC = ERV + RV.

Vital capacity (VC) is the largest volume of air that can be expelled after a very deep inspiration, i.e., VC = TV + IRV + ERV: it is 4800 mL.

> **APPLIED PHYSIOLOGY:** Vital capacity is less in females, slightly greater in large individuals, greater when standing than lying, greater in athletes, increased in those who play wind instruments, and decreased in those with sedentary jobs.

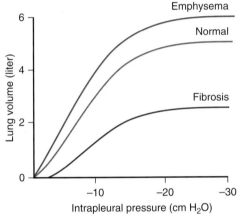

Fig. 2.35 Variations in lung compliance.

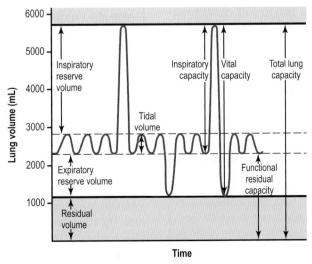

Fig. 2.36 Respiratory excursions during respiration and during maximal inspiration and expiration.

Total lung capacity (TLC) is the maximum volume of air the lungs can hold, i.e., TLC + VC + RV; in healthy adults, it is normally 6000 mL (Fig. 2.36).

Alveolar ventilation is the volume of air moving into and out of the respiratory exchange area (respiratory bronchioles, alveolar ducts, alveolar sacs and alveoli) per minute; it is equal to TV minus the dead space (150 mL) multiplied by respiratory rate. For example, at 14 breaths/min, alveolar ventilation is 4.9 L/min.

> **CLINICAL PHYSIOLOGY:** Dead space is that part of the respiratory tract where gaseous exchange does not take place. Anatomical dead space extends from the nose to non-respiratory bronchioles. Physiological dead space includes two additional volumes: air in non-functioning alveoli and air in alveoli which do not receive an adequate blood supply. Factors affecting dead space are body size, lung volume, age, gender and physical training.

Forced expiratory volume (FEV) is an important measure of dynamic lung function, being the volume of air that can be forcefully expired following a deep inspiration in a given amount of time (usually 1 second: FEV_1): it is normally between 75% and 80% of VC (Fig. 2.37). FEV is reduced in both restrictive and obstructive respiratory diseases (Fig. 2.37).

Peak expiratory flow rate is the maximum rate at which air can be expired after a deep expiration; in normal individuals, it is 400 L/min. In restrictive respiratory diseases, characterised by difficulty in inspiration (poliomyelitis, myasthenia gravis, flail chest, paralysis of the diaphragm, spinal cord diseases, pleural effusion), it is 200 L/min; in obstructive respiratory diseases, characterised by difficulty in expiration (asthma, chronic bronchitis, emphysema, cystic fibrosis), it is only 100 L/min.

> **CLINICAL PHYSIOLOGY:** Even after opening the chest 150 mL of air remains in the lung; this is the minimal air/volume. It is used medicolegally in determining whether a newly born baby died before or after delivery. This is determined by placing the baby's lung in water; if it floats this indicates the presence of minimal air in the lung, i.e., the baby was born alive, breathed, and then died. If the lung sinks this indicates the absence of minimal air in the lung, i.e., the baby was born dead and never breathed.

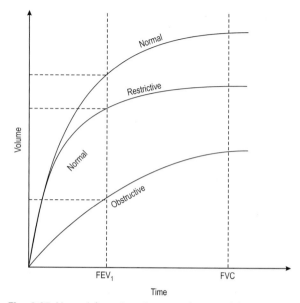

Fig. 2.37 Normal forced expiratory volume and in restrictive and obstructive disease. FEV_1, Forced expiratory volume in 1 second; *FVC*, forced vital capacity.

Gas exchange. Although breathing alternates between inspiration and expiration gas exchange at the respiratory membrane (external respiration) and in the tissues/cells (internal respiration) is a continuous ongoing process. The principle behind both types of respiration is that gases diffuse from regions of higher pressure to those of lower pressure.

> **APPLIED PHYSIOLOGY:** As atmospheric (barometric) pressure reduces, the volume of gases in atmospheric air, as well as in the body, increases; at sea level, atmospheric pressure is 760 mm Hg. With increasing altitude, atmospheric pressure decreases, as does the partial pressure of oxygen in the air, as shown in Table 2.1, together with its effect on the body.

External respiration. Inspired (atmospheric) air consists of 78.6% nitrogen, 20.8% oxygen, 0.04% carbon dioxide and 0.5% water vapour, together with traces of other gases. Each gas exerts a partial pressure (of the total) proportional to its concentration: nitrogen 597 mm Hg (79.6 kPa), oxygen (PO_2) 159 mm Hg (21.2 kPa), carbon dioxide (PCO_2) 0.3 mm Hg (0.04 kPa) and water vapour and traces of other gases 3.7 mm Hg (0.49 kPa), as shown in Table 2.2.

TABLE 2.1 Change in Atmospheric Pressure With the Changes in Altitude

Altitude (feet/m)	Atmospheric Pressure (mm Hg)	Partial Pressure of Oxygen (mm Hg)	Common Effects
50,000/15,250	87	18	Hypoxia becomes more severe even with pure oxygen
30,000/9,150	226	47	Symptoms become severe even when breathing oxygen
25,000/7,600 (Critical level for survival)	250	62	Severe hypoxia: breathing oxygen becomes essential
20,000/6,100 (Highest level of permanent habitation)	349	73	Severe hypoxia, with increased respiratory rate, minute volume, heart rate and cardiac output
15,000/4,600	400	90	Moderate hypoxia
10,000/3,050	523	110	Mild hypoxia
5,000/1,500	600	132	No hypoxia
Sea level	760 (1 atmosphere)	159	-

TABLE 2.2 The Composition and Partial Pressures of Inspired, Alveolar and Expired Air

Gas	INSPIRED AIR		ALVEOLAR AIR		EXPIRED AIR	
	%	P (mm Hg)	%	P (mm Hg)	%	P (mm Hg)
Oxygen	20.8	159	13.3	104	15.7	120
Carbon dioxide	0.04	0.3	5.3	40	3.6	27
Nitrogen	78.6	597	75.3	569	78.6	597
Water vapour + traces of other gases	0.56	3.7	6.1	47	2.1	16
Total	100	760	100	760	100	760

The composition of alveolar air differs from atmospheric air as it is saturated with water vapour. As the total pressure in the alveoli cannot be more than atmospheric pressure (760 mm Hg (101.3 kPa) at sea level) the presence of water vapour reduces the partial pressures of nitrogen from 597 to 569 mm Hg (75.8 kPa) and oxygen from 159 to 104 mm Hg (13.8 kPa), while increasing the partial pressures of carbon dioxide from 0.3 to 40 mm Hg (5.3 kPa) and water vapour from 3.7 to 47 mm Hg (6.3 kPa) as shown in Table 2.2. When the oxygen in alveolar air comes into close contact with blood in the surrounding capillaries, because of the difference in partial pressures (alveolar oxygen is at 104 mm Hg and venous blood oxygen is at 40 mm Hg) oxygen diffuses into the blood until the pressures equalise. At the same time, because the partial pressure of carbon dioxide in venous blood is 46

mm Hg and that in alveolar air is 40 mm Hg, carbon dioxide diffuses from the blood into the alveolar air (Fig. 2.38).

The composition of expired air is 78.6% nitrogen (unchanged), 15.7% oxygen (decreased), 3.6% carbon dioxide (increased) and 2.1% water vapour (increased), together with traces of other gases as shown in Table 2.2.

Oxygen is continually absorbed from the alveoli into the lung capillaries and new oxygen is continually breathed into the alveoli. The oxygen concentration in the alveoli, as well as its partial pressure, is determined by the rate of absorption of oxygen into blood in the lung capillaries and the rate of entry of new oxygen into the lungs. The more rapidly oxygen is absorbed the lower its concentration in the alveolar air becomes; however, the more rapidly new oxygen is breathed into the alveoli the greater its concentration in alveolar air becomes.

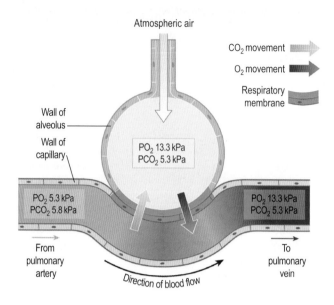

Atmospheric air

CO$_2$ movement

O$_2$ movement

Respiratory membrane

Wall of alveolus

Wall of capillary

PO$_2$ 13.3 kPa
PCO$_2$ 5.3 kPa

PO$_2$ 5.3 kPa
PCO$_2$ 5.8 kPa

PO$_2$ 13.3 kPa
PCO$_2$ 5.3 kPa

From pulmonary artery

To pulmonary vein

Direction of blood flow

Fig. 2.38 External respiration.

> **CLINICAL PHYSIOLOGY:** Lung conditions which increase the distance across which diffusion has to take place decreases the exchange of oxygen and carbon dioxide between the alveolar air and blood in the lung capillaries. Pulmonary oedema (page 114) and pneumonia (page 114) are both associated with reduced gas exchange.

Internal respiration. Oxygen diffused in the blood is carried by oxyhaemoglobin to the cells and tissues where the partial pressure of oxygen is low. Internal respiration is the exchange of gases between blood in the capillaries and that in the body's cells and tissues; it occurs by diffusion. The partial pressure of oxygen (104 mm Hg (13.8 kPa)), being the same as blood leaving the lungs in the capillary bed, is higher than that in the tissues (40 mm Hg (5.3 kPa)), while the partial pressure of carbon dioxide (40 mm Hg (5.3 kPa)) is lower than that in the tissues (46 mm Hg (6.1 kPa)). Oxygen, therefore, diffuses from the bloodstream through the capillary wall into the tissues and carbon dioxide diffuses from the tissues into the extracellular fluid, then into the bloodstream, towards the venous end of the capillary (Fig. 2.39).

Pulmonary circulation. After bifurcation of the pulmonary trunk, the right and left pulmonary arteries enter their respective lung at the hilum, each then divides into branches accompanying the bronchi as they divide; the artery lies dorsolateral to the bronchus. Each branch of

the pulmonary arteries ends in a dense capillary network in the walls of the alveolar sacs and alveoli; the arteries of neighbouring segments are independent. The pulmonary capillaries form plexuses outside the epithelium in the walls and septa of the alveoli and alveolar sacs; the capillaries vary in width but are generally very narrow.

Two pulmonary veins drain the pulmonary capillaries of each lung, their radicles coalescing into larger branches which pass through the lung independent of the arteries and bronchi. The veins communicate freely forming large vessels, which eventually accompany the arteries and bronchi to the hilum of the lung, with the bronchi separating the dorsolateral artery and ventromedial vein. The pulmonary veins from each lung open into the left atrium.

Within a bronchopulmonary segment, the bronchus and its branches are centrally accompanied by the branching arteries, but many tributaries of the pulmonary veins run between segments draining adjacent segments, which drain into more than one vein. A bronchopulmonary segment is, therefore, not a complete vascular unit with an individual bronchus, artery and vein.

> **CLINICAL ANATOMY:** The planes between bronchopulmonary segments are not avascular, being crossed by pulmonary veins and sometimes branches of arteries; therefore, resection of a segment, although undertaken, for example, in lung cancer, has to be done with care.

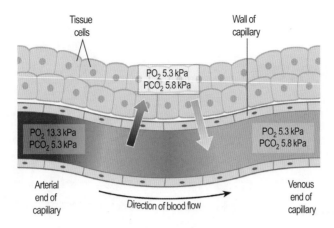

Fig. 2.39 Internal respiration.

Respiratory unit. This comprises a respiratory bronchiole, alveolar ducts, alveolar sacs and alveoli (Fig. 2.40). The lungs contain about 300 million alveoli, each with an average diameter of 0.2 mm. The alveolar walls are extremely thin, between which is a network of interconnecting capillaries. The alveolar epithelium consists of type 1 and type 2 pneumocytes. Type 1 pneumocytes (95% of the cells) are the site of gas exchange between the alveolus and blood. Type 2 (granular) pneumocytes

(5% of the cells) secrete alveolar fluid and surfactant, which helps lubricate the alveoli as they dilate and contract during respiration.

Gas exchange between the alveolar air and blood in the lung capillaries occurs through the membranes of the terminal portions of the lungs, as well as the alveoli. Collectively these membranes are known as the respiratory (pulmonary) membrane (Fig. 2.41); it has an average thickness of 0.6 microns.

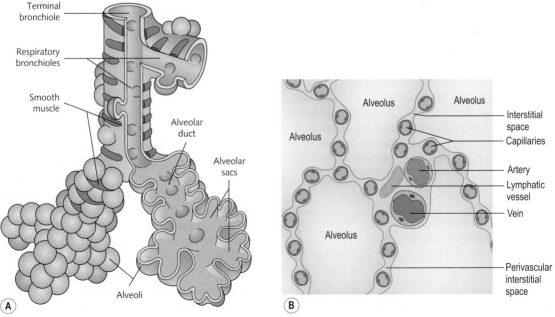

Fig. 2.40 (A) Respiratory unit; (B) cross-section of alveolar walls and their vascular supply.

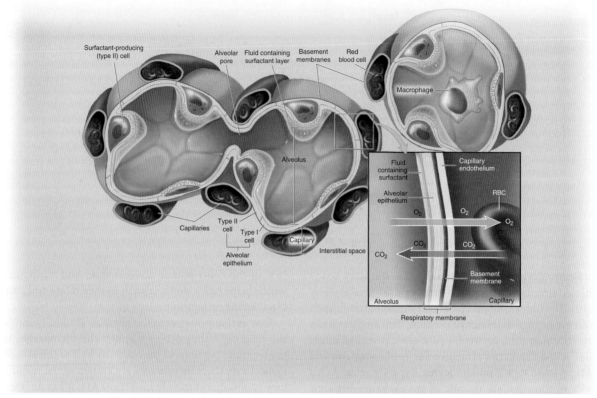

Fig. 2.41 Cross section of the ultrastructure of the alveolar respiratory membrane.

The total surface area of the respiratory membrane is approximately 70 m^2, while the volume of blood in the lung capillaries at any given time is only 60–140 mL. There is, therefore, a rapid exchange of oxygen and carbon dioxide between the alveolar air and capillary blood. The lung capillaries have an average diameter of 5 microns, so that red blood cells (average diameter 7.8 microns) have to squeeze through them. As they do so, the red blood cell membrane touches the capillary wall; oxygen and carbon dioxide do not need to pass through large amounts of plasma as they diffuse between the alveolus and the red blood cell, increasing the rapidity of diffusion.

Oxygen is mainly transported in the blood combined with haemoglobin as oxyhaemoglobin (98.5%), with a small amount in solution in plasma (1.5%). Oxyhaemoglobin is unstable under some conditions (low oxygen levels, low pH, increased temperature) and readily dissociates. In active tissues, there is increased production of carbon dioxide and heat, leading to increased release of oxygen, so that it is available to tissues with the greatest need.

> **APPLIED PHYSIOLOGY:** Oxyhaemoglobin is bright red, and deoxygenated blood has a bluish-purple tinge.

Oxygen-haemoglobin dissociation curve. The ability of haemoglobin to bind with oxygen at the alveolar-capillary barrier and then release it in a physiologically useful way into the tissues of the body is demonstrated by the oxygen-haemoglobin dissociation curve (Fig. 2.42). The curve shows the relationship between the amount of haemoglobin bound to oxygen (its saturation with oxygen) and the amount of oxygen (the partial pressure of oxygen) in the blood; it has a characteristic sigmoid shape. Its shape means that oxygen is readily released into the peripheral tissues from the haemoglobin to enable the tissues to continue to function in response to falling oxygen levels. The curve is sensitive to conditions in the peripheral tissues. It moves to the right, i.e., has a lower affinity for binding oxygen, in response to an increase in temperature, acidity levels (decreased pH), the partial pressure of

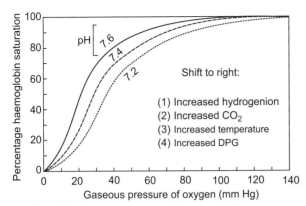

Fig. 2.42 The oxygen-haemoglobin dissociation curve.

carbon dioxide and a decrease in the partial pressure of oxygen, all of which are indicative of increased metabolic activity and a greater demand for oxygen. The curve shifts to the left, i.e., has a greater affinity for binding oxygen, with a decrease in temperature, alkalinity levels (increased pH), the partial pressure of carbon dioxide and the presence of carboxyhaemoglobin or foetal haemoglobin.

P50 of haemoglobin is the partial pressure of oxygen required for the saturation of 50% of haemoglobin with oxygen.

Myoglobin is an iron and oxygen binding protein found in skeletal muscle. It binds with one molecule of oxygen rather than four molecules as is the case of haemoglobin. It takes up oxygen from the haemoglobin in the blood and stores it, then releases it at very low PO_2, e.g., during exercise.

> **CLINICAL PHYSIOLOGY:** The oxygen-haemoglobin dissociation curve is irreversibly shifted to the left in carbon monoxide poisoning (page 113).

> **CLINICAL PHYSIOLOGY:** For foetal blood, the oxygen-haemoglobin curve is shifted to the left as foetal haemoglobin more readily accumulates oxygen than maternal blood, with which it exchanges oxygen and carbon dioxide in the placenta.

Carbon dioxide is a waste product of metabolism, mainly transported to the lungs as bicarbonate ions

(HCO_3^-) in the plasma (70%), as well as loosely combined with haemoglobin as carbaminohaemoglobin (23%) and dissolved in plasma (7%). Carbon dioxide levels must be carefully controlled as either an excess or a deficiency leads to significant disruption of acid-base balance. Sufficient carbon dioxide is essential for the bicarbonate buffering system that protects against a fall in body pH, while excess carbon dioxide reduces blood pH because it dissolves in body water forming carbonic acid.

Regulation of air and blood flow in the lungs. During quiet breathing, only a small fraction of the total alveoli are being ventilated, usually those in the upper lobe. Airways supplying non-functioning alveoli are constricted, directing airflow into functioning alveoli. Pulmonary arterioles bringing blood to ventilated alveoli are dilated to maximise gas exchange, while perfusion past non-functioning alveoli is reduced.

During increased respiration, as in exercise, TV increases with an expansion of additional alveoli accompanied by a redistribution of blood flow to perfuse them. In this way, airflow (ventilation) and blood flow (perfusion) are matched to maximise gas exchange.

Both ventilation and perfusion increase from the apex to the base of the lung due to the effect of gravity. As the specific gravity of blood is more than that of air, the increase is in perfusion rather than in ventilation. This ratio varies from 0.5 for the base of the lung to 3 for the apex of the lung; the average ventilation-perfusion ratio in normal lungs of a resting individual is 0.8.

> **APPLIED PHYSIOLOGY:** The ventilation-perfusion ratio is used to assess the efficiency and adequacy of matching the air reaching the alveoli (ventilation) and blood reaching the alveoli in the capillaries (perfusion). An area with perfusion but no ventilation is termed 'shunt', while an area with ventilation but no perfusion is termed 'dead space'. A low ratio impairs pulmonary gas exchange, while a high ratio can lead to tachypnoea and dyspnoea; the latter being typically associated with emphysema.

Respiratory control. Effective respiratory control enables the body to regulate blood gas levels over a wide range of physiological, pathological and environmental conditions; it is normally involuntary. Voluntary control

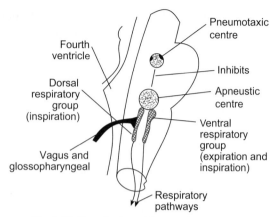

Fig. 2.43 Organisation of the respiratory centre.

is required during speaking and singing but is overridden if blood carbon dioxide levels rise, as in hypercapnia.

The nervous system normally adjusts the rate of alveolar ventilation to meet the body's demands so that the oxygen and carbon dioxide pressures in arterial blood hardly change, even during heavy exercise and most types of respiratory distress.

Respiratory centre. This consists of several groups of neurons located bilaterally in the medulla oblongata (page 247) and pons of the brainstem (Fig. 2.43). It is divided into three major collections of neurons: a dorsal respiratory group mainly responsible for inspiration; a ventral respiratory group mainly responsible for expiration; and the pneumotaxic centre, which mainly controls the rate and depth of breathing.

The **dorsal respiratory group** of neurons play a fundamental role in the control of respiration; most of its neurons are situated within the nucleus of the tractus solitarius in the dorsal part of the medulla (page 247). Other neurons in the adjacent reticular substance of the medulla also play important roles in respiratory control. The nucleus of the tractus solitarius is the sensory termination of the vagus and glossopharyngeal nerves, which transmit sensory signals to the respiratory centre from peripheral chemoreceptors, baroreceptors and receptors in the lungs.

The **pneumotaxic centre** is situated dorsally in the nucleus parabrachialis in the superior part of the pons (page 249). It transmits signals to the dorsal respiratory group (inspiratory area), with its main function being to control the duration of inspiration. A strong pneumotaxic signal may limit inspiration to 0.5 second, thereby limiting the filling of the lungs, whereas a weak signal may allow inspiration to last for 5 seconds, filling the

lung with excess air. A secondary effect of limiting inspiration, and by implication also expiration, is to increase the rate of breathing. A strong signal can increase breathing rates to 30–40 breaths/min, while a weak signal may reduce the rate to 3–5 breaths/min.

The **ventral respiratory group** of neurons situated in the nucleus ambiguus and nucleus retroambiguus in the ventrolateral part of the medulla operates more or less as an overdrive mechanism. Its function differs from that of the dorsal group in several important ways: during quiet respiration, the neurons remain inactive and do not appear to participate in the basic rhythmic oscillations that control respiration; when pulmonary ventilation increases it contributes additional respiratory drive by providing powerful expiratory signals to the abdominal muscles during forced expiration.

There is also an **apneustic centre** located in the reticular centre of the lower pons; it increases the depth of inspiration by acting on the dorsal respiratory group of neurons.

> **APPLIED PHYSIOLOGY:** Apneusis is an abnormal pattern of respiration characterised by prolonged inspiration followed by short inefficient expiration. This can occur as a result of bilateral vagotomy, together with mid-pontine transection.

Hering-Breuer inflation reflex. In addition to the central nervous system control mechanisms, stretch receptors in the muscular walls of the bronchi and bronchioles transmit signals via the vagus nerves to the dorsal respiratory group of neurons when the lungs become overstretched. A feedback response is initiated which 'switches off' inspiration: this is the Hering-Breuer inflation reflex. It also increases the respiratory rate in a similar way as signals from the pneumotaxic centre.

In humans, the reflex is probably not activated until TV is increased to more than 1.5 L / breath. It appears to be mainly a protective mechanism for preventing excess lung inflation rather than an important part of normal respiratory control.

> **CLINICAL PHYSIOLOGY:** If the pneumotaxic centre is destroyed or if the vagal reflex is abolished (e.g., vagotomy), this results in long maintained and powerful inspiratory effort interspersed by short expirations.

Chemical control of respiration. The main aim of respiration is to maintain proper concentrations of oxygen, carbon dioxide and hydrogen ions in the tissues. Respiratory activity is highly responsive to changes in each of these.

Excess carbon dioxide or hydrogen ions in the blood tend to act directly on the respiratory centre, increasing the strength of both inspiratory and expiratory motor signals to the respiratory muscles. However, lack of oxygen has no direct effect on the respiratory centre, tending to act on peripheral chemoreceptors located in the carotid and aortic bodies, which then send appropriate signals to the respiratory centre.

Central chemoreceptors. These are located on the surface of the medulla and are bathed in cerebrospinal fluid. The increase in arterial PCO_2 (hypercapnia) leads to an increase in the concentration of carbon dioxide in the cerebrospinal fluid; this is due to the easy diffusion of carbon dioxide through the blood-brain barrier. When the cerebrospinal fluid carbon dioxide rises these receptors respond by stimulating the respiratory centre, increasing ventilation of the lungs reducing arterial PCO_2. This sensitivity to raised PCO_2 is the most important factor in controlling normal blood gas levels. A small reduction in PO_2 (hypoxaemia) has a similar less pronounced effect, but a substantial reduction depresses breathing.

Peripheral chemoreceptors. Located in the aortic arch and carotid bodies, peripheral chemoreceptors respond to changes in blood carbon dioxide and oxygen levels, but are much more sensitive to carbon dioxide than oxygen. A slight rise in carbon dioxide levels activates them, triggering nerve impulses to the respiratory centre via the glossopharyngeal and vagus nerves, stimulating an immediate rise in the rate and depth of respiration. An increase in blood acidity, either by a decrease in pH or an increase in hydrogen ions, also stimulates the peripheral chemoreceptors, resulting in increased ventilation, increased carbon dioxide excretion and increased blood pH. The peripheral chemoreceptors also help to regulate blood pressure (page 134).

Effect of exercise. Physical exercise increases both the rate and depth of respiration to ensure that the increased oxygen requirements of the muscles are met. Exercising muscles produce more carbon dioxide stimulating both central and peripheral chemoreceptors. The increased respiratory effort persists after the exercise is finished in order to supply sufficient oxygen to repay the 'oxygen debt'; this represents the oxygen needed to get rid of waste products, such as lactic acid. In healthy individuals, alveolar ventilation usually increases in step with the increased level of oxygen metabolism, so that arterial PO_2, PCO_2 and pH remain almost normal. In strenuous exercise, oxygen consumption and carbon dioxide formation can increase up to 20 times.

Breathing can also be modified by the respiratory centre by talking and singing, emotion (crying, laughing, fear), drugs (alcohol, sedatives, recreational), sleep and body temperature. Increased metabolic rate during fever increases respiration, whereas in hypothermia, metabolism and respiration are decreased. Temporary changes in respiration also occur during swallowing, sneezing and coughing (page 116).

Effect of age. With increasing age, the risk of respiratory infections rises due to age-related immune decline and reduced mucous production in the airways, which together with a general loss of elastic tissue in the lungs increases the likelihood that small airways may collapse during expiration, thus decreasing the functional lung volume. The respiratory reflexes that increase respiratory effort in response to rising blood carbon dioxide or falling blood oxygen levels become less efficient. Because of these changes, older individuals may respond less well to adverse changes in blood gases.

Disturbances of respiration

Eupnoea. The normal respiratory pattern.

Tachypnoea. An increase in the rate of respiration.

Bradypnoea. A decrease in the rate of respiration.

Polypnoea. Rapid shallow breathing in which the rate of breathing changes but not the force.

Dyspnoea. Difficulty in breathing. A point is reached (dyspnoea point) when there is increased ventilation with severe breathing discomfort. It occurs (i) in respiratory disorders (pneumonia, pulmonary oedema, pulmonary effusion, pneumothorax, severe asthma) as a result of abnormal respiratory movements and obstruction to the airways; (ii) in left ventricular failure; (iii) in metabolic disorders (diabetic acidosis, uraemia); and (iv) during strenuous and severe exercise.

Orthopnoea. Orthopnoea is the occurrence of dyspnoea in the recumbent position only; it is characteristic of left-side heart failure. Both the TLC and VC are decreased due to pulmonary congestion; lying down leads to a further decrease, due to the excess venous return and visceral pressure on the diaphragm, resulting in dyspnoea.

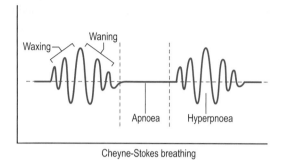

Cheyne-Stokes breathing

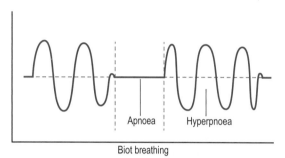

Biot breathing

Fig. 2.44 Types of periodic breathing.

Apnoea. Temporary arrest of breathing; it occurs after hyperventilation. During apnoea, the partial pressure of carbon dioxide in the blood increases stimulating the respiratory centres and respiration restarts.

Periodic breathing. An abnormal or uneven respiratory rhythm; it is of two types.

Cheyne-Stokes breathing: characterised by a rhythmic waxing and waning of the rate and depth of respiration, accompanied by regularly recurring periods of apnoea (Fig. 2.44). It occurs in physiological (during deep sleep, at high altitude, following prolonged voluntary hyperventilation, in the newborn, after severe muscular exercise) and pathological (increased intracranial pressure, advanced cardiac diseases, advanced renal diseases, poisoning by narcotics, premature infants) conditions.

Biot breathing (Biot's respiration): characterised by periods of apnoea and hyperpnoea; waxing and waning do not occur (Fig. 2.44). It only occurs in pathological conditions involving nervous disorders due to lesions/injuries to the brain.

Hyperpnoea. An increase in pulmonary ventilation due to an increase in the rate or force of respiration; it occurs after exercise but may occur during a fever.

Hyperventilation. An abnormal increase in the rate and force of respiration, often leading to dizziness, discomfort and occasionally chest pain. It mostly occurs after exercise when the partial pressure of carbon dioxide in the blood is increased suppressing the respiratory centre, resulting in apnoea. It is followed by Cheyne-Stokes breathing to restore respiration to normal.

Hypoventilation. A decrease in the rate and force of respiration reducing the volume of air moving in and out of the lungs, resulting in hypoxia and hypercapnia. It occurs when the respiratory centre is suppressed or depressed following the administration of some drugs; it also occurs during partial paralysis of the respiratory muscles. There is an increase in the rate and force of respiration leading to dyspnoea; in severe cases, it can lead to lethargy, coma and death.

Hypoxia. Reduced availability of oxygen to the tissues. Acute and severe hypoxia leads to unconsciousness, which, if not treated immediately, can lead to brain death. Chronic hypoxia has various effects on the body, some of which are immediate and others delayed.

The **immediate effects** are wide-ranging and involve the cardiovascular, respiratory, digestive and renal systems. There is an increase in the rate and force of cardiac contraction, cardiac output and blood pressure, followed later by decreases in each of these. Initially, respiratory rate increases, leading to alkalemia, followed later by shallow and periodic breathing. The rate and force of breathing become markedly reduced due to failure of the respiratory centre. There is also a loss of appetite, nausea and vomiting, with the mouth becoming dry and there is a need to drink. In the kidneys there is increased erythropoietin secretion, which increases the production of red blood cells: the urine becomes alkaline.

The effect depends on the length and severity of exposure; individuals become highly irritable, with accompanying nausea, vomiting, depression, weakness and fatigue.

Hypoxic (arterial) hypoxia is due to decreased oxygen content in the blood; it is characterised by reduced oxygen tension in arterial blood.

It can be caused by: (i) low oxygen tension in inspired (atmospheric) air, i.e., insufficient oxygen (high altitude, low partial pressure of oxygen, breathing in closed spaces); (ii) respiratory disorders associated with decreased pulmonary ventilation, i.e., insufficient oxygen intake (asthma, brain tumours affecting the respiratory centre, pneumothorax); (iii) respiratory disorders associated with inadequate oxygenation in the lungs, i.e., insufficient diffusion of oxygen (emphysema, fibrosis, pulmonary oedema/hae-morrhage, pneumonia, bronchiolar obstruction) and (iv) cardiac disorders, i.e., insufficient blood supply to the lungs (congestive heart failure, arteriovenous shunt).

Anaemic hypoxia is the inability of blood to carry sufficient oxygen even though there is enough oxygen available; it is characterised by decreased oxygen-carrying capacity of blood.

It can be caused by: (i) decreased numbers of red blood cells due to bone marrow diseases or haemorrhage; (ii) decreased haemoglobin in the blood due to changes in the structure, shape and size of red blood cells (microcytes, macrocytes, spherocytes, sickle cells, poikilocytes) or a reduced red blood cell count; (iii) the formation of altered haemoglobin due to poisoning (chlorates, nitrates, ferricyanides, carbon monoxide) lowering the quantity of haemoglobin available to combine with oxygen and (iv) the combination of haemoglobin with other gases (carbon monoxide, hydrogen sulphide, nitrous oxide) losing its ability to transport oxygen.

Stagnant (hypokinetic) hypoxia is caused by decreased velocity of blood flow. It can be caused by: (i) congestive heart failure; (ii) haemorrhage; (iii) surgical shock; (iv) vasospasm; (v) thrombosis and (vi) embolism.

Histotoxic hypoxia results from the inability of tissues to utilise oxygen. It occurs due to cyanide or sulphide poisoning, which destroys cellular oxidative enzymes leading to paralysis of the cytochrome oxidase system. Even if sufficient oxygen is available, the tissues are unable to utilise it.

Oxygen toxicity/poisoning. An increase in the oxygen content in tissues beyond a critical level. Excess oxygen is dissolved in the plasma as the haemoglobin has been saturated. Initially, there is tracheobronchial irritation and pulmonary oedema. As the metabolic rate increases in all body tissues, they become burnt out by excess heat, destroying the cytochrome oxidase system and leading to tissue damage. As the brain becomes affected, there is hyperirritability followed by muscle twitching, ringing in the ears and dizziness. The toxicity finally leads to convulsions, coma and death.

> **CLINICAL PHYSIOLOGY:** Retinitis pigmentosa (a critical condition) occurs when premature infants are given pure oxygen; it causes local vasoconstriction of vessels in the retina, leading to the formation of fibrous tissue and blindness.

Hypercapnia. Increased carbon dioxide in the blood resulting from conditions leading to blockage of the respiratory pathways (asphyxia, breathing air containing excess carbon dioxide). The respiratory centre is excessively stimulated leading to dyspnoea; blood becomes acidic. Blood pressure increases accompanied by tachycardia, with flushing of the skin due to peripheral vasodilatation. Individuals complain of headache, depression, and laziness, followed by muscle rigidity, fine tremors and generalised convulsions, and finally giddiness and loss of consciousness.

Hypocapnia. Decreased carbon dioxide in the blood; it is associated with hypoventilation and following prolonged hyperventilation due to the loss of excess carbon dioxide. The respiratory centre is depressed leading to a decrease in the rate and force of respiration. The pH of blood increases (leading to alkalosis) and calcium concentration decreases (leading to tetany). Common features of hypocapnia are dizziness, mental confusion, muscular twitching and loss of consciousness.

Cyanosis. Due to the large amounts of reduced haemoglobin in the blood, characterised by a diffused bluish colouration of the skin and mucous membrane, especially where the skin is thin (lips, cheeks, ear lobes, nose, fingertips at the base of the nail). Occurs in anaemia as haemoglobin content is less.

Carbon monoxide poisoning. Displaces oxygen from haemoglobin as it binds at the same site, thus reducing the capacity of blood to transport oxygen; haemoglobin has a 200 times greater affinity for carbon monoxide than oxygen. Breathing air with 1% carbon monoxide, haemoglobin saturation is 15%–20% leading to headache and nausea. When haemoglobin saturation reaches 30%–40%, it causes convulsions, cardiorespiratory arrest, loss of consciousness and coma; above 50% death occurs.

Airway obstruction

Asphyxia. This results from obstruction of the airways (strangulation, hanging, drowning), being a combination of hypoxia and hypercapnia. There are three stages of asphyxiation: (i) hyperpnoea, lasting about 1 minute, in which breathing becomes deep and rapid due to powerful stimulation of the respiratory centre by excess carbon dioxide, followed by dyspnoea and cyanosis during which the eyes become more prominent; (ii) convulsions, lasting less than 1 minute, with violent expiratory effort, increased heart rate and arterial blood pressure, and loss of consciousness and (iii) collapse, lasting about 3 minutes, with the disappearance of convulsions, pupil dilation, decreased heart rate, loss of all reflexes, respiratory gasping with the duration between gasps gradually increasing, and finally death.

Atelectasis. Partial or complete collapse of the lungs leading to dyspnoea. It can be caused by: (i) deficiency or inactivation of surfactant; (ii) bronchus or bronchiole obstruction and (iii) the presence of air (pneumothorax), fluid (hydrothorax), blood (haemothorax) or pus (pyothorax) in the pleural space.

Bronchitis. Acute bronchitis is a secondary bacterial infection of the bronchi, the spread of which can lead to bronchiolitis and/or bronchopneumonia.

Chronic bronchitis is a progressive inflammatory disease due to prolonged irritation of the bronchial epithelium which may be worsened by cold and/or damp conditions; it can follow episodes of acute bronchitis. Changes in the bronchi include: (i) the size and number of mucous glands increases, with the increased mucous blocking small airways overwhelming the ability of cilia to remove it leading to a persistent cough and infection; (ii) oedema and other inflammatory changes cause swelling of the airway wall obstructing airflow; (iii) replacement of the respiratory epithelium with a non-ciliated epithelium reducing ciliary efficiency, with mucous accumulation and increased risk of infection; (iv) fibrosis and stiffening of the airways reducing airflow and (v) breathlessness, increasing the work of breathing.

These changes lead to hypoxia, pulmonary hypertension and right-side heart failure. With increasing respiratory failure, arterial blood oxygen is reduced (hypoxaemia) while carbon dioxide in the blood increases (hypercapnia): as the condition worsens, the respiratory centre responds to hypoxaemia rather than hypercapnia. In later stages, inflammatory changes affect the smaller bronchioles and the alveoli, leading to emphysema. The condition is referred to as **chronic obstructive pulmonary disease**.

Pneumonia. Inflammation of the lung caused by bacterial/viral infection or inhalation of noxious chemical substances. There is accumulation of blood cells, fibrin and exudate in the alveoli; the affected part of the lung becomes consolidated. It is of two types, lobar pneumonia and lobular pneumonia (bronchopneumonia). It results in fever, chest compression/chest pain, shallow breathing, cyanosis, insomnia and delirium. Delirium is caused by cerebral hypoxia and is manifest by confusion, illusions, hallucination (touch, pain, taste, smell), disorientation, hyperexcitability and memory loss.

Pulmonary oedema. The accumulation of serous fluid in the alveoli and interstitial lung tissue leading to severe dyspnoea, cough with a frothy bloodstained exudate, cyanosis and cold extremities. Alveolar oedema is fatal causing sudden death from suffocation. It can be due to: (i) increased pulmonary pressure due to left ventricular failure or mitral valve disease; (ii) pneumonia or (iii) breathing in harmful chemicals (chlorine or sulphur dioxide).

Pleural effusion. The accumulation of large amounts of fluid in the pleural cavity leading to atelectasis, dyspnoea and other respiratory disorders. It can be caused by: (i) blockage of lymphatic drainage; (ii) excessive transduction of fluid from the pulmonary capillaries due to left ventricular failure and (iii) inflammation of the pleural membrane damaging the capillary membrane allowing fluid and plasma proteins to leak into the pleural cavity.

Emphysema. Develops due to long-term inflammatory conditions or irritation of the airways (smoking, exposure to oxidant gases, untreated bronchitis) leading to progressive destruction of the supporting elastic tissue in the lung, which gradually expand (barrel chest) due to their inability to recoil. This is accompanied by irreversible distension of the respiratory bronchioles, alveolar ducts and alveoli, reducing the surface area for gaseous exchange.

Panacinar emphysema is the breakdown of the walls between adjacent alveoli, with dilation of the alveolar ducts and loss of interstitial tissue elasticity; the lungs become distended and therefore have increased capacity (Fig. 2.45). Although the volume of air in each breath remains unchanged because it constitutes a smaller portion of the total volume of air, its partial pressure is reduced, decreasing the diffusion of oxygen into the blood. Disease progression may lead to hypoxia, pulmonary hypertension and eventually right-side heart failure.

Centrilobular emphysema is irreversible dilation of the respiratory bronchioles supplying lung lobules (Fig. 2.45). When inspired air reaches the dilated area the pressure falls with reduced ventilation and partial pressure of oxygen. Again, disease progression may lead to hypoxia, pulmonary hypertension and eventually right-side heart failure.

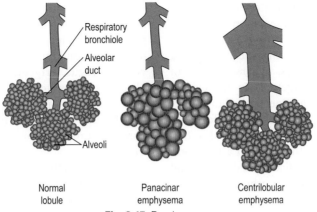

Respiratory
bronchiole

Alveolar
duct

Alveoli

Normal
lobule

Panacinar
emphysema

Centrilobular
emphysema

Fig. 2.45 Emphysema.

Interstitial emphysema is the presence of air in the thoracic interstitial tissues and may be caused by injury from the outside (fractured rib, stab wound) or inside when an alveolus ruptures through the pleura (during an asthma attack, bronchiolitis, whooping cough). The air usually tracks upwards towards the neck where it is gradually absorbed, causing no damage; however, a large quantity in the mediastinum may limit movement of the heart.

Asthma. Asthma is a common inflammatory disease associated with reversible over-activity of the airway smooth muscle in the bronchioles, with thickening of the muscle and mucous membrane and enlargement of the mucous glands. During an attack, the bronchial muscle contracts (bronchospasm) causing further airway narrowing resulting in partial expiration. The lungs become overinflated leading to severe dyspnoea and wheezing. In severe acute attacks, the bronchi may be obstructed leading to acute respiratory failure, hypoxia and possibly death.

There are two clinical categories of asthma which tend to have identical symptoms.

Atopic (extrinsic) asthma occurs in children and young adults who have an allergy to foreign proteins (pollen, dust containing mites, fungi, animal hair or feathers). Inhaled allergens (antigens) are absorbed by the bronchial mucosa stimulating the production of IgE (immunoglobulin E) antibodies that bind to the surface of mast cells and basophils around bronchial blood vessels. When the allergen is encountered again, it triggers the antigen/antibody reaction resulting in the release of histamine and other substances stimulating mucous secretion and muscle contraction narrowing the airways.

Chronic (intrinsic) asthma occurs later in life; it may be associated with chronic inflammation of the upper respiratory tract (chronic bronchitis), exercise or occupational exposure (inhaled paint fumes). Attacks increase in severity over time with possible irreversible lung damage. Impaired lung function leads to hypoxia, pulmonary hypertension and right-side heart failure.

Bronchial asthma. Due to bronchiolar constriction caused by spastic contraction of smooth muscles in the bronchioles, which may be exaggerated by oedema of the mucous membrane and accumulation of mucous in the lumen of the bronchiole; it is characterised by difficulty in breathing with wheezing. It can be caused by inflammation of the airways, hypersensitivity of glossopharyngeal and vagal afferents in the larynx, pulmonary oedema and congestion of the lungs (cardiac asthma). As expiration requires greater effort than inspiration, the lungs are insufficiently deflated so that RV and FRC are increased. There is also a reduction in TV, VC, FEV, alveolar ventilation and the partial pressure of oxygen in the blood. Carbon dioxide accumulates in the blood leading to acidosis, dyspnoea and cyanosis.

Bronchiectasis. A permanent abnormal dilation of bronchi and bronchioles associated with chronic bacterial infection, childhood bronchiolitis or bronchopneumonia, cystic fibrosis or bronchial tumour. The bronchi are blocked by mucous, pus and inflammatory exudate, with the alveoli beyond the blockage collapsing as trapped air is absorbed. Interstitial elastic tissue degenerates and it is replaced by fibrous adhesions attaching the bronchi to the parietal pleura. It usually affects the lower lobe of the lung; suppuration is common. If a blood vessel is eroded, haemoptysis or pyaemia may occur, leading to abscess formation elsewhere (commonly brain). Progressive lung fibrosis leads to hypoxia, pulmonary hypertension and right-side heart failure.

Respiratory protective reflexes. Reflexes which modify respiration to prevent foreign particles from entering the lungs and airways, thereby protecting them. All reflexes are characterised by forced expiration.

Cough reflex. A protective reflex caused by irritation of the respiratory tract. It is mainly caused by irritant agents but can also be produced by cardiac (congestive heart failure) and pulmonary (chronic obstructive pulmonary disease) disorders, and thoracic tumours exerting pressure on the larynx, trachea, bronchi and lungs. It begins with a deep inspiration followed by forced expiration with a closed glottis, increasing intrapleural pressure to more than 100 mm Hg. The glottis then opens suddenly with an explosive outflow of air at a high velocity, resulting in expulsion of the irritant from the respiratory tract.

Receptors initiating the cough are located in the respiratory tract (nose, paranasal sinuses, larynx, pharynx, trachea, bronchi), as well as the pleura, diaphragm and pericardium. Afferent fibres pass via the vagus, trigeminal, glossopharyngeal and phrenic nerves to the medulla oblongata, with efferent fibres arising from the medulla passing through the vagus, phrenic and spinal motor nerves to innervate primary and accessory respiratory muscles.

Sneezing reflex. A protective reflex caused by irritation of the nasal mucous membrane by dust particles, debris, mechanical obstruction and excess fluid accumulation in the nose. It begins with a deep inspiration followed by forceful expiration with an open glottis resulting in expulsion of the irritant.

The reflex is initiated by olfactory receptors and trigeminal nerve endings in the nasal mucosa. Afferent fibres pass via the trigeminal and olfactory nerves to the sneezing centre (diffuse neurons in the nucleus of the trigeminal nerve, nucleus solitarius and reticular formation) in the medulla oblongata. Efferent fibres pass via the trigeminal, facial, glossopharyngeal, vagus and intercostal nerves to innervate pharyngeal, tracheal and respiratory muscles.

Swallowing reflex. A protective reflex preventing food particles entering the larynx, during which respiration is temporarily arrested during the pharyngeal (second) stage of swallowing; it is referred to as swallowing (deglutition) apnoea. Further details of swallowing can be found on page 328.

Cardiovascular System

The cardiovascular system consists of the heart and blood vessels (arteries, veins, capillaries) conveying blood to and from various organs and tissues. Functionally, the heart is a double muscular pump, with the two parts linked via the pulmonary circulation. The right side receives deoxygenated blood via the superior and inferior venae cavae and sends it to the lungs where it is oxygenated, whereas the left side receives reoxygenated blood from the lungs and distributes it throughout the body via the aorta and its branches (systemic circulation).

DEVELOPMENT OF THE HEART: The cardiovascular system starts to develop during the third week; it is the first system to function in the embryo, with the first heartbeat and blood beginning to flow by the end of the third week. As the developing heart and pericardial cavity move to lie in front of the future foregut, a single heart tube is formed (Fig. 2.46A). Between the fourth and seventh weeks the heart tube undergoes considerable changes, with parts be-

coming identifiable (horns of the sinus venosus, pulmonary atrium, atrioventricular canal, pulmonary ventricle, bulbus cordis, truncus arteriosus) foreshadowing the organisation of the adult heart (Fig. 2.46B). The right horn of the sinus venosus becomes incorporated into the right atrium forming its smooth part, while the left horn forms the coronary sinus. The pulmonary atrium gives the rough parts of both atria: the smooth part of the left atrium is due to incorpora-

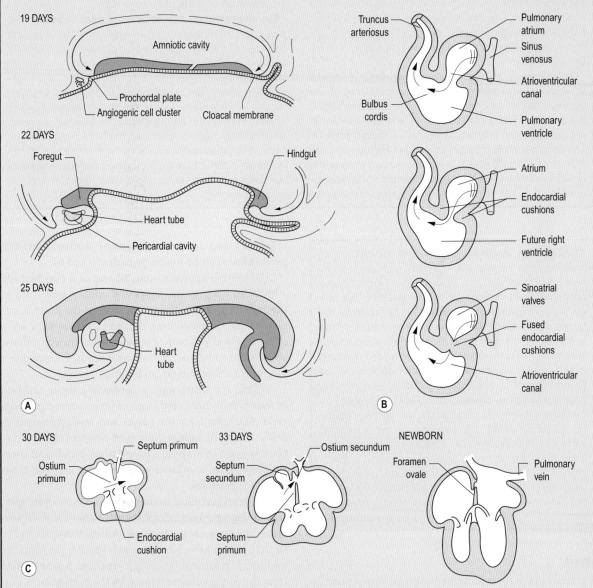

Fig. 2.46 Sagittal sections through (A) the embryo at various stages of development showing formation and migration of the heart; (B) the heart at 4 weeks showing formation of the atrioventricular canal; (C) formation of the interatrial septum.

tion of the pulmonary veins. The atrioventricular canal gives rise to the right (tricuspid) and left (mitral) atrioventricular valves. The pulmonary ventricle forms the adult left ventricle, while the right ventricle arises from the proximal part of the bulbus cordis; its middle part gives the outflow tracts of both ventricles and its distal part the roots of the aorta and pulmonary trunk. The distal part of the bulbus cordis and the truncus arteriosus split longitudinally, separating the aorta from the pulmonary trunk, bringing the aorta into communication with the left ventricle and the pulmonary trunk with the right ventricle; the longitudinal septum becomes continuous with the developing muscular interventricular septum.

Development of the interatrial septum: A sickle-shaped septum primum descends from the roof of the common atrium, just to the left of the sinoatrial orifice, the two ends fusing with the ventral and dorsal endocardial cushions; the foramen formed is the ostium primum. The ostium primum gradually closes, but before complete closure perforations appear in its cephalic part forming the ostium secundum. A sickle-shaped septum secundum appears to the right of the septum primum, which passes caudally towards the atrioventricular cushion covering the ostium secundum; however, the septa do not fuse allowing blood from the inferior vena cava to pass freely from right to left atrium (Fig. 2.46C). The gap formed is the foramen ovale; after birth, it becomes gradually obliterated but may persist in 30% of individuals. In adults, the fossa ovalis is that part of the septum primum enclosed by the ends of the septum secundum: the annulus (limbus fossa) ovalis is the free edge of the septum secundum.

Development of the interventricular septum: The muscular part of the septum develops from the muscle at the apex of the heart and ascends towards the ventricle and endocardial cushions; it is sickle-shaped with its ends binding to the interventricular foramen in the upper part of the septum. The membranous part fills the interventricular foramen with endocardial tissue derived from: (i) an extension of the atrioventricular endocardial cushions (membranous part in adults) (ii) proximal bulbar septum separating the infundibulum of the right ventricle from the vestibule of the left; and (iii) distal bulbar septum dividing the distal part of the bulbus cordis into the aortic and pulmonary openings.

CONGENITAL ANOMALIES OF THE HEART: Heart malformations are relatively common, with the majority being due to genetic and environmental factors. Some congenital malformations cause little disability, but others are incompatible with life; many can be surgically corrected: (1) *dextrocardia*, in which the apex of the heart is directed to the right rather than the left: if associated with transposition of the abdominal viscera the condition is known as situs inversus; (2) *septal defects* can be (i) *atrial* (patent foramen ovale, patent ostium primum, complete absence), (ii) *ventricular* (patent interventricular foramen, a foramen in the muscular part of the septum), (iii) *aorticopulmonary* (transposition of the ascending aorta and pulmonary trunk, aorticopulmonary window (foramen in the septum), complete absence), (iv) *Eisenmenger's complex* (overriding of the aorta, patent interventricular foramen) and (v) *Fallot's tetralogy* (stenosis of the pulmonary trunk, overriding of the aorta, patent interventricular foramen, hypertrophy of the right ventricle).

Heart

The heart lies in the middle mediastinum surrounded by a double fold of serous membrane (serous pericardium), within a dense connective tissue sac (fibrous pericardium) attached to the central tendon of the diaphragm (Figs 2.17 and 2.19). Details of the mediastinum and pericardium can be found on pages 80 and 84.

The heart is approximately the size of a clenched fist, with 2/3rd lying to the left of the midline and 1/3rd to the right (Fig. 2.19). The greater part of the heart is cardiac muscle (myocardium); the serous pericardium and a subserous layer of connective tissue form the epicardium, while the chambers of the heart are lined by endocardium. Details of cardiac muscle can be found on page 39.

Within the heart wall, a connective tissue skeleton of four firmly connected rings of fibrous tissue provides rigid attachment for the valves and myocardium (Fig. 2.47). The myocardium comprises two separate and distinct systems of looping and spiralling bundles of muscle fibres, one associated with the atria and the other with the ventricles.

The heart is conical in shape (Fig. 2.19), with an apex, base and sternocostal, diaphragmatic, right and left surfaces. The **apex** is directed downwards, forwards and to the left, lying in the 5th intercostal space 9 cm from the midline: it is formed by the left ventricle. It is separated from the fundus of the stomach by the pericardium, diaphragm and peritoneum (page 451).

The **base** is directed posteriorly and slightly to the right; it is formed by the two atria (mainly left) and lies

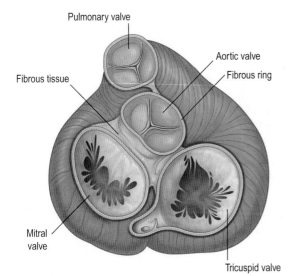

Fig. 2.47 The fibrous framework of the heart supporting the heart valves.

surface of the left lung, left phrenic nerve and left pericardiophrenic vessels (Fig. 2.19). The **right surface** is formed by the right atrium; it is related to the right pleura and mediastinal surface of the right lung, right phrenic nerve and right pericardiophrenic vessels (Fig. 2.19).

> **SURFACE ANATOMY:** Although the position of the heart changes with respiration and posture, its approximate position is as follows. The left border slopes from the left 2nd intercostal space 1 cm to the left of the sternum to the apex of the heart in the left 5th intercostal space 9 cm from the midline; the apex can usually be palpated in the living. The right border extends from the 3rd to 6th intercostal spaces 1 cm to the right of the sternum. The inferior border sits on the central tendon of the diaphragm, indicated by a shallow concavity between the lower points of the right and left borders; joining the upper points of the left and right borders gives the remaining border (Fig. 2.48).

opposite the 5th to 8th thoracic vertebrae. It is separated from the vertebral column by structures in the posterior mediastinum (descending aorta, oesophagus, azygos vein, thoracic duct, oblique sinus of the pericardium), and bounded inferiorly by the atrioventricular (coronary) groove, in which run the coronary sinus and right coronary artery.

The **sternocostal surface** lies behind the body of the sternum from the 3rd to 6th costal cartilages on both sides; it is divided by the atrioventricular groove into two parts. The atrial part lies above and to the right, being formed mainly by the right atrium; the left atrium is masked by the ascending aorta and pulmonary trunk. The ventricular part (majority) lies below and to the left, with the right 2/3rd formed by the right ventricle and the left 1/3rd by the left ventricle. The two ventricles are separated by the anterior interventricular groove, in which run the anterior interventricular artery and great cardiac vein.

The slightly concave **diaphragmatic surface** lies on the diaphragm, being formed by the two ventricles: the left 2/3rd by the left ventricle and right 1/3rd by the right ventricle. The two ventricles are separated by the posterior interventricular groove, in which run the posterior interventricular artery and middle cardiac vein. It is separated from the left lobe of the liver and fundus of the stomach by the pericardium, diaphragm and peritoneum.

The **left surface** is formed by the left ventricle and atrium; it is related to the left pleura and mediastinal

Chambers of the heart. The heart comprises four chambers, right and left atria and right and left ventricles; the upper end of each atrium has a projecting auricle.

The **right atrium** forms the right border and surface of the heart, as well as a small part of the base; the upper part projects to the left as the right auricle. It lies anterior and to the right of the left atrium, from which it is separated by the interatrial septum. The right atrium receives the venous return (deoxygenated blood) from the whole of the body, except the lungs, via the superior and inferior venae cavae and coronary sinus, which open into the smooth posterior part (derived from the right horn of the sinus venosus) (Fig. 2.49). The superior vena cava opening lies opposite the 3rd right sternocostal junction, it has no valve; that of the inferior vena cava lies opposite the 6th right sternocostal junction and is guarded by a small valve. The opening of the coronary sinus lies to the left of the inferior caval opening and is also guarded by a small valve. In the lower anterior part of the atrium lies the right atrioventricular (tricuspid) valve surrounded by a fibrous ring giving attachment to its three cusps (anterior, posterior/inferior, medial/septal), allowing blood to enter the right ventricle. The cusps are attached to papillary muscles via chordae tendineae within the right ventricle (Fig. 2.49).

The rough anterior part (derived from the pulmonary atrium) is separated from the posterior part by the crista terminalis: the rough area is due to a large number of

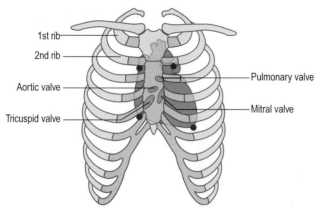

Fig. 2.48 Anterior aspect of the thorax showing the position and surface markings of the heart and heart valves, together with the best sites *(blue dots)* for listening to each valve sound.

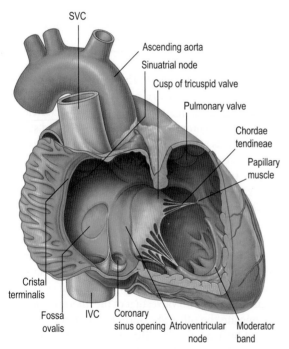

Fig. 2.49 The right atrium and ventricle opened showing the internal features of each chamber. *IVC,* Inferior vena cava; *SVC,* superior vena cava.

muscular ridges (musculi pectinati), which continue into the right auricle (Fig. 2.49). The superior end of the crista terminalis surrounds the sinoatrial node (page 126). On the outside is a vertical groove (sulcus terminalis) corresponding to the crista terminalis on the inside.

On the interatrial septum is an oval-shaped depression (fossa ovalis) above and to the left of the opening of

the inferior vena cava (Fig. 2.49), indicating the site of the foetal foramen ovale, which allowed blood to enter the left atrium bypassing the pulmonary circulation (page 120); the floor of the fossa is the septum primum of the developing interatrial septum. Above and to the sides of the fossa ovalis is a prominent ridge (annulus ovalis), representing the free edge of the septum secundum of the developing interatrial septum.

Small cardiac veins (venae cordae minimae) are found irregularly on the atrial wall, being more numerous on the septum.

The **left atrium** receives venous return (oxygenated blood) from the lungs via four pulmonary veins. It lies behind and to the left of the right atrium and forms the major part of the base of the heart; the left auricle projects forwards and to the right. It lies behind the ascending aorta and pulmonary trunk separated by the transverse sinus, and in front of the descending aorta and oesophagus separated by the oblique sinus. Except for a small rough part (derived from the pulmonary atrium), which extends into the auricle as musculi pectinati, the internal surface is smooth due to the incorporation of the terminal parts of the four pulmonary veins. Two pulmonary veins open into the left atrium on each side; they have no valves. The smaller left atrioventricular (mitral) valve is in the lower part of the left atrium; it is surrounded by a fibrous ring giving attachment to its two cusps (anterior, posterior/inferior), allowing blood to enter the left ventricle. The cusps are attached to papillary muscles via chordae tendineae within the left ventricle. The openings of the mitral and aortic valves are separated by the anterior cusp.

Small cardiac veins (venae cordae minimae) are found irregularly in the atrial walls.

The **right ventricle** lies to the right of the left ventricle; due to the obliquity of the interventricular septum separating the ventricles, it forms the major part of the anterior surface of the heart and its lower border. Its walls are thinner than those of the left ventricle as it pumps blood under lower pressure to the lungs. Because the interventricular septum bulges into its cavity the right ventricle is semilunar in cross section; at its upper end is a funnel-shaped dilation (infundibulum/conus arteriosum) which gives rise to the pulmonary trunk. The inner surface of the infundibulum is smooth, while the remainder of the ventricle is rough due to muscular ridges (trabeculae carneae) and three papillary muscles (anterior, posterior/inferior, medial/septal). Each papillary muscle is attached by its apex to two adjacent cusps by tendinous bands (chordae tendineae). A specialised muscle bundle (moderator band) passes from the interventricular septum to the base of the anterior papillary muscle; it carries the right branch of the atrioventricular bundle. By enabling the wall of the right ventricle to begin contracting slightly before that of the left, it prevents over-distension of the right ventricle during systole (page 127).

The right ventricle has two openings: the right atrioventricular (tricuspid) valve, through which blood from the right atrium flows, and the pulmonary valve, through which blood flows into the pulmonary trunk and then to the lungs.

The **left ventricle** lies posterior and to the left of the right ventricle and forms the apex and most of the diaphragmatic surface of the heart. It has the thickest walls of all chambers due to the extremely high pressures it has to develop to force blood into the systemic circulation. The part below the aortic opening (aortic vestibule) is smooth, while the remainder of the chamber is rough due to muscular ridges (trabeculae carneae) and papillary muscles (anterior, posterior/inferior).

The left ventricle has two openings: the left atrioventricular (mitral) valve, through which blood from the left atrium flows, and the aortic valve, though blood flows into the ascending aorta and then to the rest of the body (except the lungs).

Heart valves. Guarding the chambers of the heart and directing blood flow through the heart are four valves: two atrioventricular (cuspid), one between the right atrium and ventricle (tricuspid valve) and one between

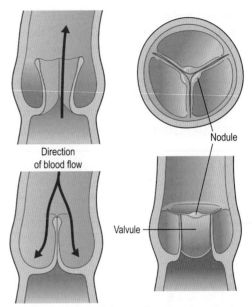

Fig. 2.50 The structure of the semilunar aortic and pulmonary valves, with opening and closing of the valves being dependent on the direction of blood flow.

the left atrium and ventricle (bicuspid/mitral valve), and two semilunar valves, one guarding the entrance to the pulmonary trunk (pulmonary valve) and one guarding the entrance to the ascending aorta (aortic valve) (Fig. 2.47).

The **tricuspid valve** is surrounded by a fibrous ring giving attachment to the three cusps (anterior, posterior/inferior, medial/septal) of the valve. The **mitral (bicuspid) valve** is also surrounded by a fibrous ring giving attachment to the two cusps (anterior, posterior/inferior) of the valve. The atrial surfaces of the cusps are smooth, while their margins and ventricular surfaces are rough. The free margins give attachment to tendinous bands (chordae tendineae), which in turn are attached to the apices of two adjacent papillary muscles (Fig. 2.49). During ventricular systole, the papillary muscles contract pulling on the chordae tendineae, preventing the cusps inverting and allowing blood to flow back into the atrium.

The **pulmonary and aortic valves** are also surrounded by fibrous rings, each giving attachment to three semilunar valvules (Fig. 2.50); the pulmonary valve has two posterior valvules and one anterior valvule, while the aortic has one posterior and two anterior valvules. The free border of each valvule projects upwards into the lumen of its respective vessel. In the middle of each free border is a thickened nodule with a lunule on each side, which assist in approximating the central areas of the edges of the valvule. The concavities formed by the valvules face away from the direction of blood flow so that during systole they lie against the vessel wall. When ventricular pressure falls during diastole there is a tendency for blood to return to the ventricle; the valvules fill approximating their free borders preventing backflow (Fig. 2.50).

> **SURFACE ANATOMY:** All heart valves lie behind the sternum: pulmonary at the 3rd left sternocostal junction; aortic at the 3rd left intercostal space near the midline; tricuspid at the 4th intercostal space near the midline; and mitral at the 4th left sternocostal junction (Fig. 2.48). The heart sounds (i.e., the sound of the valves closing) are best heard downstream in the direction of blood flow: pulmonary valve in the 2nd intercostal space to the left of the sternum; aortic valve in the 2nd intercostal space to the right of the sternum; tricuspid valve 5th intercostal space to the right of the sternum; mitral valve in the 5th intercostal space 9 cm to the left of the midline (Fig. 2.48).

Heart valve disorders. The heart valves prevent backflow of blood into the heart chambers during the cardiac cycle; the mitral and aortic valves are subject to the greatest pressures and so are more susceptible to damage. Damaged valves give rise to abnormal heart sounds (murmurs); severe damage/defects can lead to heart failure. Common causes of valve defects are rheumatic fever; fibrosis following inflammation; and congenital abnormalities.

Stenosis is narrowing of the valve opening, impeding blood flow through the valve; it occurs when inflammation roughens the edges of the cusps so they stick together. With healing, fibrous tissue is formed which tends to shrink with age increasing the stenosis.

Incompetence (regurgitation) is failure of the valve to close completely allowing blood to flow back into the chamber from which it came.

Heart sounds. The characteristic sounds of the heart are the result of vibration of the valves and surrounding fluid following abrupt pressure changes associated with systole. The first heart sound ('lub') is associated with closure of the atrioventricular valves at the start of systole, while the second ('dub') is associated with closure of the semilunar valves at the end of systole; the first heart sound tends to last longer than the second.

In generating the first heart sound, ventricular contraction causes a sudden backflow of blood against the tricuspid and mitral valves, forcing them to close and bulge towards the atria until the chordae tendineae become taut stopping the back bulging. The elastic tautness of the chordae tendineae and valves then causes the back-surging blood to bounce forward again into the ventricles, leading to vibration of the blood, ventricular walls and taut valves causing turbulence in the blood. These vibrations travel through the adjacent tissues to the chest wall, where they can be heard as sound using a stethoscope. The first heart sound is a long, soft low-pitched sound lasting 0.10–0.17 second; it coincides with the peak of the P wave of the electrocardiogram (ECG) (page 127).

The second heart sound is the result of sudden closure of the semilunar valves at the end of systole. When they close they bulge backward towards the ventricles: their elastic stretch recoils the blood back into the arteries causing a short period of reverberation of blood back and forth between the arterial walls and the valves, as well as between the valves and the ventricular walls: the vibrations in the arterial walls are mainly transmitted along the arteries. When the vibrations of the vessels or ventricles come into contact with the chest wall, they create sounds that can be heard. The second heart sound is a short low-pitched sound lasting 0.07–0.10 second: it coincides with the T wave in the ECG, although it may precede it or start after its peak (page 128).

Inaudible third and fourth heart sounds are also present. The third heart sound is produced by the rushing of blood into the ventricles and vibrations in the ventricular wall during the rapid filling period in early diastole; it is a short low-pitched sound lasting 0.07–0.10 second. The third heart sound can be heard in children and athletes, as well as in pathological conditions (aortic regurgitation, cardiac failure, cardiomyopathy with dilated ventricles) when it becomes loud and audible; it occurs between the T and P waves of the ECG (page 127).

The fourth heart sound is produced by contraction of the atrial musculature and its vibrations, as well as ventricular distension during atrial systole; it is a short low-pitched sound lasting 0.02–0.04 second. The fourth heart sound becomes audible when the ventricles become stiff (ventricular hypertrophy, long-standing hypertension, aortic stenosis) and the atria contract forcefully; it coincides with the interval between the P wave and Q of the QRS complex (page 128).

> **CLINICAL PHYSIOLOGY:** A triple heart sound (triple rhythm) is characterised by three clear sounds during each heartbeat; it may be heard in myocardial infarction and severe hypertension. A quadruple heart sound (quadruple rhythm) is characterised by four clear heart sounds during each heartbeat; it is indicative of serious cardiovascular disease (congestive heart failure).

> **CLINICAL ANATOMY:** With increasing age, the cusps of the semilunar valves tend to become stiffer preventing them coming together efficiently and effectively, thus allowing some blood to flow back (regurgitation) into the ventricle. Mitral stenosis is due to stiffness of the cusps causing narrowing of the mitral opening; the usual heart sounds of lub dub are not heard as clearly due to blood flowing back into the left ventricle.

Pattern of blood flow through the heart

Foetal pattern. Oxygenated blood returns from the placenta in the umbilical veins, bypassing the liver via the ductus venosus, flowing directly into the inferior vena cava where it mixes with deoxygenated blood returning from the lower limbs, abdomen, pelvis and perineum (Fig. 2.51A). From the right atrium, blood is directed towards the foramen ovale into the left atrium and then to the left ventricle and aorta to supply the head, neck and upper limbs. Blood also enters the right atrium via the superior vena cava, which passes into the right ventricle and pulmonary trunk. Blood entering the right ventricle from the superior and inferior venae cavae undergo minimal mixing. The high resistance to blood flow in the pulmonary vessels and lungs results in blood bypassing the pulmonary circulation and entering the descending aorta and the systemic circulation via the ductus arteriosus. From the descending aorta, blood

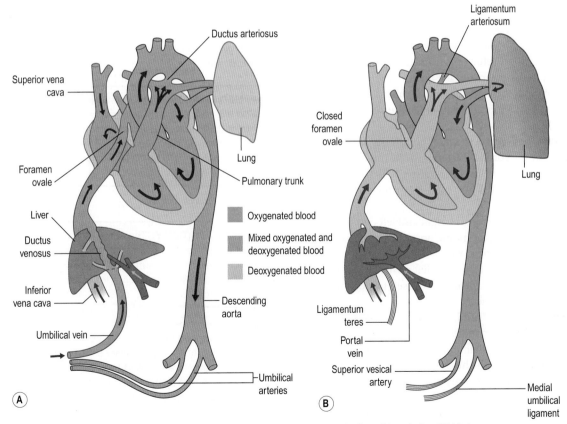

Fig. 2.51 The pattern of blood flow through the heart before (A) and after (B) birth.

flows towards the placenta via two umbilical arteries to be reoxygenated to begin the cycle again.

Changes at birth. At birth, important changes occur due to opening up of the pulmonary circulation and to cessation of blood flow through the placenta. The foramen ovale closes with the first good breath as the septum primum is pushed against the septum secundum; complete fusion of the two septa occurs by the end of the first year. The ductus arteriosus closes with complete anatomical closure by 3 months; the obliterated ductus arteriosus becomes the ligamentum arteriosum (Fig. 2.51B). The umbilical vein and ductus venosus both become obliterated after birth, forming the ligamentum teres in the free edge of the falciform ligament and the ligamentum venosum, respectively. The distal parts of the umbilical arteries close becoming the medial umbilical ligaments.

Adult pattern. In adults, deoxygenated blood enters the right atrium via the superior (from the head, neck, thorax and upper limbs) and inferior (from the abdomen, pelvis, perineum and lower limbs) venae cavae. Blood then passes through the tricuspid valve into the right ventricle and then to the pulmonary trunk and pulmonary circulation via the pulmonary valve. Oxygenated blood returning from the lungs via the pulmonary veins enters the left atrium, then passes to the left ventricle through the mitral valve and then to the aorta and systemic circulation via the aortic valve (Fig. 2.51B).

Blood and nerve supply. The arterial supply to the heart is by the coronary arteries, while the venous drainage is by cardiac veins. Innervation is by the autonomic nervous system; the heart has its own conducting system.

Coronary arteries. The right and left coronary arteries arise from the ascending aorta just above its origin from the left ventricle; the right from the anterior aortic sinus and the left from the left posterior aortic sinus. Both arteries have tortuous courses to accommodate movements of the heart.

The **right coronary artery** passes forward between the pulmonary trunk and right auricle to reach the atrioventricular groove (coronary sulcus) on the anterior of the heart. It continues in the groove around the inferior margin of the heart, giving the right marginal branch before reaching the posterior interventricular groove, where it anastomoses with the circumflex branch of the left coronary artery

(Fig. 2.52A and B). Before anastomosing it gives the posterior interventricular (posterior descending) artery, which runs in the posterior interventricular groove, ending by a poor anastomosis with the terminal part of the anterior interventricular artery near the apex of the heart.

The right coronary artery gives branches supplying both atria and ventricles, as well as providing the major blood supply to the conducting system. The sinoatrial node is supplied by a sinoatrial branch in 60%–70% of individuals; the branch to the atrioventricular node is given off close to the origin of the posterior interventricular artery.

The **left coronary artery** passes anteriorly between the pulmonary trunk and left auricle towards the atrioventricular groove, where it divides into a circumflex branch, which continues around the atrioventricular groove to anastomose with the right coronary artery, and the anterior interventricular (anterior descending) artery, which runs in the anterior interventricular groove (Fig. 2.52A and B), ending by anastomosing with the terminal part of the posterior interventricular artery. The circumflex branch gives the left marginal artery supplying the left ventricle.

APPLIED ANATOMY: When referring to the blood supply to the posterior part of the interventricular septum and the diaphragmatic surface of the left ventricle, the right coronary is dominant in 85% of individuals (right side dominant), with the left coronary artery dominant in the remainder (left side dominant).

CLINICAL ANATOMY: The coronary arteries and their larger branches are functional end-arteries, i.e., the anastomoses are not sufficient to provide an alternative blood supply if the main artery becomes blocked. Sudden blockage of either coronary arteries or one of their larger branches may be fatal; blockage of smaller vessels leads to necrosis of the myocardium (myocardial infarct) supplied by that vessel (heart attack). Narrowing of the lumen of the coronary arteries or their larger branches leads to a reduced blood supply to the myocardium (ischaemia), with the individual complaining of pain behind the sternum, often radiating down the left arm (angina pectoris). The referred pain of ischaemia is carried by sympathetic fibres.

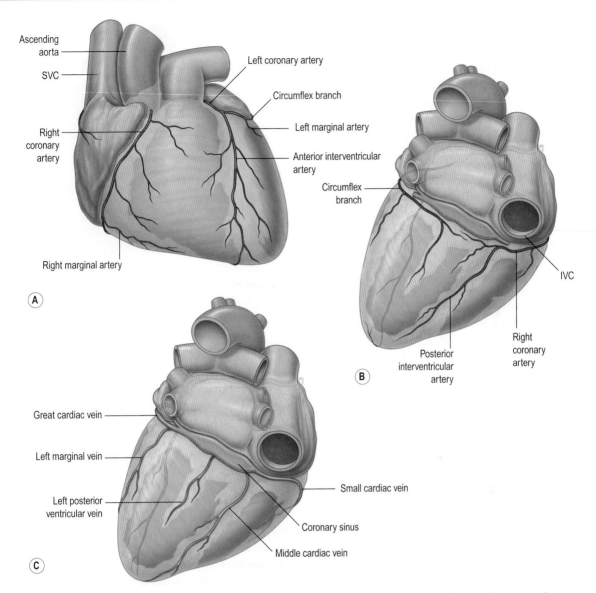

Fig. 2.52 Anterior (A) and posterior (B) aspects of the heart showing its arterial supply; (C) posterior aspect of the heart showing its venous drainage. *IVC,* Inferior vena cava; *SVC,* superior vena cava.

Cardiac veins. The greater part of the venous drainage is by a system of veins draining into the **coronary sinus** lying in the posterior part of the atrioventricular groove (Fig. 2.52C), which opens into the right atrium; it is a continuation of the great cardiac vein and receives the middle and small cardiac veins and the oblique vein of the left atrium.

The **great cardiac vein** begins at the apex of the heart, accompanying the anterior interventricular artery in the anterior interventricular groove, then runs parallel to the circumflex artery in the atrioventricular groove before becoming the coronary sinus (Fig. 2.52C); it receives the left posterior ventricular vein and the left marginal vein. The **middle cardiac vein** accompanies the posterior interventricular artery in the posterior interventricular groove (Fig. 2.52C); it drains into the coronary sinus. The **small cardiac vein** accompanies the right coronary artery in the atrioventricular groove;

it receives the right marginal vein and drains into the coronary sinus. Small **anterior cardiac veins** on the surface of the right ventricle open directly into the right atrium near the opening of the coronary sinus. **Venae cordis minimae** drain the myocardium directly into all chambers of the heart, but mainly into the right atrium.

Lymphatics. Lymph vessels from the myocardium and epicardium (serous visceral pericardium) of the right atrium and diaphragmatic surface of the right ventricle follow the right coronary artery to drain into brachiocephalic lymph nodes. Lymph vessels from the left atrium and both ventricles (except the diaphragmatic surface of the right ventricle) follow the left coronary artery to drain into tracheobronchial lymph nodes.

Innervation. The heart is innervated by both sympathetic and parasympathetic fibres of the autonomic nervous system via deep and superficial cardiac plexuses. The sympathetic fibres arise in six pairs from the right and left superior, middle and inferior cervical ganglia, and the 2nd, 3rd and 4th thoracic ganglia. The parasympathetic fibres arise in three pairs, with the upper two from the right and left superior and inferior cervical branches of the vagus, the lower right from the right vagus and the lower left from the left recurrent laryngeal nerve.

The **superficial cardiac plexus** lies to the right of the ligamentum arteriosum below the arch of the aorta. It receives a superficial cervical cardiac branch from the left sympathetic chain and an inferior cervical cardiac branch from the vagus. It gives branches to the deep cardiac plexus, the right coronary plexus and the left anterior pulmonary plexus.

The **deep cardiac plexus** lies in front of the tracheal bifurcation deep to the aortic arch. It receives cardiac branches from the sympathetic chains (except those to the superficial cardiac plexus) and vagi (except those to the superficial cardiac plexus), as well as from the superficial cardiac plexus. It gives branches to the right and left coronary plexuses, right and left anterior pulmonary plexuses and back to the superficial cardiac plexus.

> **CLINICAL PHYSIOLOGY:** The heart is nerve regulated and not nerve operated; heart rate is a balance between sympathetic and parasympathetic stimulation, with sympathetic stimulation increasing heart rate and parasympathetic stimulation decreasing heart rate.

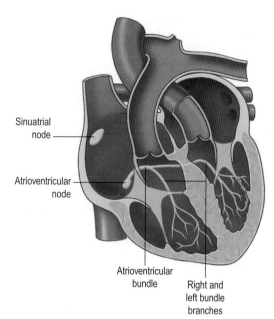

Sinuatrial node

Atrioventricular node

Atrioventricular bundle

Right and left bundle branches

Fig. 2.53 Coronal section through the heart showing the conducting system.

Conducting system. Specialised cardiac muscle fibres arranged in groups of cells (nodes) or bundles of fibres are responsible for the rhythmic initiation and propagation of the impulse associated with the heartbeat and coordinated contraction of the atria and ventricles. Contraction is initiated at the sinoatrial node in the right atrium; the impulse spreads through both atria to the atrioventricular node in the lower part of the interatrial septum on its right side close to the opening of the coronary sinus (Fig. 2.53). From the atrioventricular node, the impulse passes to the atrioventricular bundle and then descends deep to the septal cusp of the tricuspid valve in the interventricular septum. The atrioventricular bundle is the only muscular connection between the atria and ventricles.

At the upper border of the muscular part of the septum, the bundle divides into right and left bundle branches. The right bundle branch descends on the right side of the interventricular septum, then along the moderator band supplying the papillary muscles, to reach the anterior wall of the right ventricle where it divides into fine (Purkinje) fibres supplying the remainder of the right ventricle. The left bundle pierces the interventricular septum and then descends on its left side, where it divides into two or more branches as it passes towards the apex of the heart, dividing into fine fibres supplying the left ventricle.

> **APPLIED ANATOMY:** The blood supply to the conducting system is mainly from the right coronary artery. The sinoatrial node is supplied by both coronary arteries; the atrioventricular node and bundle are supplied by the right coronary artery; the right bundle branch by the right coronary artery; and the left bundle branch by the right and left coronary arteries.

> **CLINICAL ANATOMY:** If the atrioventricular bundle is interrupted (e.g., lack of a blood supply), total heart block results with the ventricles beating slowly and rhythmically at their own rate independent of the atria, which continue to contract at a rate determined by the sinoatrial node.

Cardiac Cycle

The events which occur from the beginning of one heartbeat to the beginning of the next represents the cardiac cycle, each cycle being initiated by the generation of an action potential at the sinoatrial node (electrically unstable specialised cells). The action potential travels rapidly through the atria, causing them to contract, the atrioventricular bundle via the atrioventricular node into the ventricles, causing them to contract. There is a delay of 0.1 second while the impulse travels from the atria to the ventricles, allowing the atria to pump blood into the ventricles before the strong contraction of the ventricles forces blood into the systemic circulation.

> **APPLIED PHYSIOLOGY:** Cardiac muscle starts to contract a few milliseconds after the action potential begins, continuing until a few milliseconds after the action potential ends. The duration of cardiac muscle contraction is effectively a function of the duration of the action potential: 0.2 seconds in atrial muscle and 0.3 seconds in ventricular muscle.

> **APPLIED PHYSIOLOGY:** Instability of the sinoatrial node cells causes them to discharge (depolarise) regularly between 60 and 80 times/min; this is followed by repolarisation and then almost immediately by another depolarisation. Because the sinoatrial node discharges faster than any other part of the heart it sets heart rate, i.e., it is the pacemaker. The atrioventricular node has a secondary pacemaker function if there is a problem with the sinoatrial node or with transmission of impulses from the atria; its intrinsic rhythm is slower (40–60 times/min) than that of the sinoatrial node.

Diastole and systole. The cardiac cycle consists of a period of relaxation (diastole) when the heart fills with blood, followed by a period of contraction (systole). The total duration of the cardiac cycle is the reciprocal of heart rate; if heart rate is 70 beats/min, the duration of the cardiac cycle is approximately 0.86 second/beat. As heart rate increases, the duration of the cardiac cycle decreases, including diastole and systole; at very high heart rates diastole may not be long enough to allow complete filling of the various chambers before the next contraction.

Electrocardiogram. When the cardiac impulse passes through the heart, the electrical activity also spreads to tissues adjacent to the heart, with a small portion reaching the skin surface. Electrodes placed on the skin on opposite sides of the heart can record the electrical potentials generated; this is the electrocardiogram (ECG). A normal ECG shows a P wave, a QRS complex and a T wave (Fig. 2.54); the QRS complex may be present as three separate waves.

The following description of electrical activity originating from the sinoatrial node is the sinus rhythm, which has a rate between 60 and 100 beats/min; bradycardia is a heart rate less than 60 beats/min, tachycardia a heart rate more than 100 beats/min.

P wave. This depolarising wave arises when the impulse from the sinoatrial node sweeps over the atria prior to atrial contraction; its normal duration is 0.10 second and has an amplitude of 0.1–0.12 mV. It is normally positive (upright rounded deflection) in all leads except in aVR. The first and second parts of the wave are due to right and left arterial activation, respectively.

Changes in the P wave can be indicative of several cardiac problems. In right atrial hypertrophy (e.g., tricuspid stenosis), it is tall and usually pointed; in left atrial

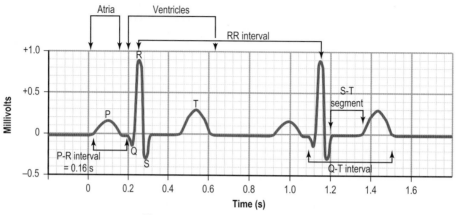

Fig. 2.54 Normal electrocardiogram.

hypertrophy (e.g., mitral stenosis), it is tall and broad or M-shaped; in atrial extrasystole, it is small and shapeless followed by a small compensatory wave; in hyperkalaemia, it is small or absent; in atrial fibrillation and middle atrioventricular nodal rhythm, it is absent; in sinoatrial block, it is absent or inverted; in atrial paroxysmal tachycardia, it is inverted; and in lower atrioventricular nodal block, it appears after the QRS complex.

P-R interval. This corresponds to atrial depolarisation and conduction of the impulse through the atrioventricular node; its normal duration is 0.18 second (range 0.12–0.20 second). In bradycardia, increased vagal tone and 1st-degree heart block, the interval is prolonged, while in tachycardia, A-V nodal rhythm, Wolf-Parkinson-White and Lown-Ganong-Levine syndrome, Duchenne muscular dystrophy and type II glycogen storage disease it is shortened.

QRS complex. This depolarising wave complex represents the rapid spread of the impulse from the atrioventricular node through the atrioventricular bundle and Purkinje fibres to the ventricles prior to ventricular contraction; its normal duration is between 0.08 and 0.10 second and has amplitudes of 0.1–0.2 mV (Q wave), 1 mV (R wave) and 0.4 mV (S wave). The delay between the completion of the P wave and the start of the QRS complex represents conduction of the impulse through the atrioventricular node, which is much slower than conduction elsewhere in the heart; it allows atrial contraction to completely finish before ventricular contraction begins.

Prolongation of the QRS complex occurs in hyperkalaemia, which together with deformation occurs in bundle branch block.

Q-T interval. This is the interval from the onset of the Q wave to the end of the T wave, which corresponds to ventricular depolarisation and repolarisation; its normal duration is 0.4–0.42 second. In long 'Q-T' syndrome, myocardial infarction, myocarditis, hypocalcaemia and hypothyroidism, the interval is prolonged, while in short 'Q-T' syndrome and hypercalcaemia, it is shortened.

T wave. This represents ventricular repolarisation; its normal duration is 0.2 second and has an amplitude of 0.3 mV. Atrial repolarisation occurs during ventricular contraction and is not seen in the ECG because of the large QRS complex.

Changes in the T wave may help in the diagnosis of several cardiac problems. In myocardial infarction it is tall and broad-based with a slight asymmetry (hyperacute T wave); in old age, hyperventilation, anxiety, myocardial infarction, left ventricular hypertrophy and pericarditis, it is small, flat or inverted; in hypokalaemia, it is small, flat or inverted; and in hyperkalaemia, muscular exercise and sympathetic overactivity it is tall and tented.

S-T segment. This is an isoelectric period, with the junction between the QRS complex and S-T segment being the J point; its normal duration is 0.08 second.

Changes in the duration of the S-T segment or a deviation from an isoelectric base can indicate pathology. In anterior or inferior myocardial infarction, left bundle branch block and acute pericarditis, it is elevated (it may also be elevated in athletes); in acute myocardial ischaemia, posterior myocardial infarction, ventricular hypertrophy and hypokalaemia, it is depressed; in

Respiratory Sinus Arrhythmia

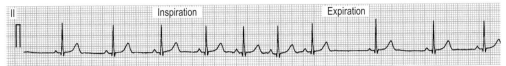

Fig. 2.55 Electrocardiogram showing the R-R interval shortening during inspiration and lengthening during expiration.

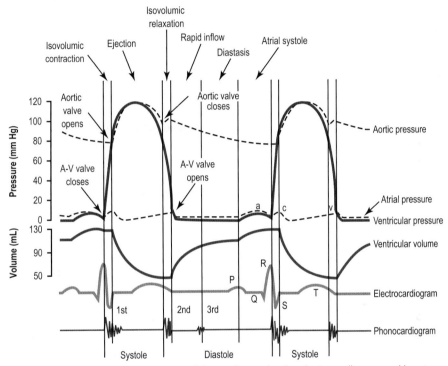

Fig. 2.56 The relationship between events of the cardiac cycle, the electrocardiogram and heart sounds.

hypocalcaemia, it is prolonged; and in hypercalcaemia, it is shortened.

R-R interval. This is the duration (normally 0.86 second) of one cardiac cycle; it is used to calculate heart rate and heart rate variability. Under resting conditions, healthy individuals show some heart rate variability associated with respiration (respiratory sinus rhythm): the interval decreasing during inspiration and increasing during expiration (Fig. 2.55). Heart rate variability decreases in many clinical conditions: cardiovascular dysfunction (hypertension), diabetes mellitus, and psychiatric problems (anxiety, panic).

U wave. This is a small rounded positive wave that follows the T wave representing a slow repolarisation of the papillary muscle. Its normal duration is 0.08 second and has an amplitude of 0.02 mV. It is rarely seen normally but becomes prominent in hypokalaemia.

Relationship between the ECG and the cardiac cycle. The relationship between the ECG, events in the cardiac cycle and heart sounds is shown in Fig. 2.56. Following the P wave, there is atrial contraction resulting in a slight rise in atrial pressure as seen in the minor pressure waves 'a', 'c' and 'v'. The 'a' wave is caused by atrial contraction; right atrial pressure increases from 4 to 6 mm Hg and left atrial pressure from 7 to 8 mm Hg. The 'c' wave occurs at the beginning of ventricular contraction, being caused by slight backflow of blood into the atria but mainly by bulging of the atrioventricular valves towards the atria due to increased pressure in the ventricles. The 'v' wave occurs towards the end of ventricular contraction due to the slow flow of blood into the atria.

During ventricular contraction large volumes of blood accumulate in the atria, because the atrioventricular valves are closed (Fig. 2.56). Once systole is over, ventricular pressure drops (Fig. 2.56), the pressure in the atria opens the atrioventricular valves allowing blood to flow rapidly into the ventricles, producing the third heart sound and causing a rise in ventricular pressure; rapid filling lasts for the first third of diastole. During the middle third of diastole, only a small amount of blood usually flows into the ventricles, being that flowing into the atria from the veins. During the last third of diastole, the atria contract forcing blood into the ventricles; however, this accounts for only 20% of filling during each cardiac cycle. The fourth heart sound is produced in this phase.

Ventricular pressure rises immediately after the start of ventricular contraction causing the atrioventricular valves to close (Fig. 2.56). There is a very short interval (period of isovolumic/isometric contraction lasting 0.02–0.03 second) during which there is no ventricular emptying; the first heart sound is produced in this phase due to closure of the atrioventricular valves. Once left ventricular pressure increases to above 80 mm Hg and right ventricular pressure to above 8 mm Hg, the semilunar valves are pushed open against the pressures in the aorta and pulmonary trunk; this is the period of ejection. The first heart sound continues for a brief period in this phase (Fig. 2.56).

At the end of systole, ventricular relaxation begins causing a rapid decrease in both left and right ventricular pressures (Fig. 2.56). The increased pressures in the distended large arteries, now filled with blood from the ventricles, immediately pushes blood towards the ventricles closing the aortic and pulmonary valves and the second heart sound is produced. The ventricular muscle continues to relax (period of isovolumic/isometric relaxation lasting 0.03–0.06 second) during which time ventricular volume does not change. The atrioventricular valves then open and a new cycle of ventricular pumping begins.

During diastole, normal filling increases the volume of each ventricle to 110–120 mL; the end-diastolic volume (Fig. 2.56). As the ventricles empty during systole, the volume decreases to 70 mL: the stroke volume output. The remaining volume in each ventricle (40–50 mL) is the end-systolic volume. The fraction of the end-diastolic volume that is ejected is the ejection fraction: it is usually 60%.

ECG recording. An ECG can be recorded using either limb leads (standard (I, II, III) or augmented (aVR, aVL, aVF)) or chest leads (V_1, V_2, V_3, V_4, V_5, V_6); the appearance of the ECG differs with each type of recording. It is beyond the scope of this text to discuss each of these leads and their outputs. The reader is referred to a comprehensive textbook of physiology for further details.

Arrhythmias. An arrhythmia is an irregular heart rate or disturbance in the rhythm of the heart; arrhythmias can occur in both physiological and pathological conditions.

Normotopic arrhythmias. These occur when the sinoatrial node is still the pacemaker.

Sinus arrhythmia (respiratory sinus rhythm) is the rhythmical increase and decrease in heart rate related to respiration (Fig. 2.55). It is a normal finding that commonly occurs in children and young adults; it is due to fluctuations in the strength of the vagal tone that affects the rate of sinoatrial node rhythmicity.

Sinus tachycardia occurs when discharges from the sinoatrial node increase; the ECG is normal apart from short R-R intervals (Fig. 2.57). It can occur in physiological (exercise, emotion, high altitude, pregnancy) and pathological (fever, anaemia, hyperthyroidism, hypersecretion of catecholamines, cardiomyopathy, valvular heart disease, haemorrhagic shock) conditions; it is characterised by palpitations, dizziness, fainting, shortness of breath and chest discomfort.

Sinus bradycardia occurs with a reduction in discharges from the sinoatrial node; the ECG shows prolonged waves and prolonged R-R intervals (Fig. 2.58). It occurs during sleep and in athletes in response to the increased force of myocardial contraction. Pathological conditions when it can occur include disease of the sinoatrial node; hypothermia; hypothyroidism; heart attack; congenital heart disease; degenerative processes associated with ageing; obstructive jaundice; increased intracranial pressure; use of some drugs (β-blockers, channel blockers, digitalis); and atherosclerosis, especially of the carotid artery. It is characterised by sick sinus syndrome (dizziness and unconsciousness), fatigue, weakness, shortness of breath, lack of concentration and difficulty in exercising.

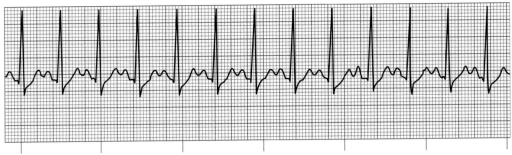

Fig. 2.57 Electrocardiogram in tachycardia: heart rate is greater than 100 beats/min.

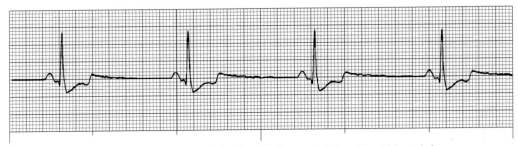

Fig. 2.58 Electrocardiogram in bradycardia: heart rate is less than 60 beats/min.

Ectopic arrhythmias. These occur when another part of the heart (atrial muscle, atrioventricular node, ventricular muscle) becomes the pacemaker: they can be divided into homotopic arrhythmias when the impulses arise from part of the conducting system, and heterotopic arrhythmias when the impulses arise from the heart musculature.

Heart block is blockage of the impulses generated by the sinoatrial node so that they do not reach the cardiac musculature; based on the area affected, it is classified as either sinoatrial (sinus) block or atrioventricular block.

In **sinoatrial block,** the impulses do not reach the atrioventricular node and the heart stops beating; however, the atrioventricular node immediately takes over, with the heart beating at a slower rate (atrioventricular rhythm). Impulses can arise from any part of the atrioventricular node: in upper nodal rhythm the P wave is inverted, but the QRS complex and T waves are normal; in middle nodal rhythm all heart chambers contract at the same time, in which case the P wave is absent as it merges with the QRS complex; in lower nodal rhythm ventricular contraction precedes atrial contraction, in which case the QRS complex appears before the P wave and an R-P interval appears instead of an R-R interval (also known as reverse heart block).

In **atrioventricular block** the impulses are not transmitted to the ventricles due to a defect in the conducting system; it can result in incomplete heart block (1st-degree heart block, 2nd-degree heart block, bundle branch block) or complete heart block (3rd-degree heart block).

In incomplete heart block the transmission of impulses is not completely blocked but slowed down. In *1st-degree heart block,* the transmission of impulses through the atrioventricular node is very slow; the ECG shows prolonged P-R intervals of more than 0.21 second. It is common in young adults and athletes and can also be caused by rheumatic fever and some drugs: it is asymptomatic. In *2nd-degree (partial) heart block,* some impulses from the sinoatrial node do not reach the ventricles, in which case only 1 ventricle may contract for every 2–4 atrial contractions; bradycardia occurs with frequent development of 2nd-degree heart block. The ventricular complex QRST is missing. *Bundle branch block* occurs with dysfunction of the right or left branch of the bundle of His, with the impulse reaching the unaffected ventricle first and then the affected side. The ECG shows a normal ventricular rate but with a prolonged or deformed QRS complex.

In *complete (3rd degree) heart block,* impulses from the sinoatrial node do not reach the ventricles, which beat at their own rhythm independent of the atria (idio-ventricular rhythm): The ECG shows normal P wave and QRS complex, but they are not related (atrioventricular dissociation). This can occur due to disease of the atrioventricular node or a defective conduction system leading from the atrioventricular node. Complete heart block is serious as it decreases the pumping action of the heart, often leading to Stokes-Adams syndrome and heart failure.

CLINICAL PHYSIOLOGY: Some cases with a 2nd-degree heart block exhibit Wenckebach phenomenon, which is manifested by a progressive increase of P-R intervals, in successive complexes till a P wave is not followed by a QRS complex and this process is repeated. It can occur in a variety of pathologic settings, especially inferior myocardial infarction.

CLINICAL PHYSIOLOGY: Stokes-Adams syndrome is a sudden attack of dizziness and unconsciousness caused by heart block; it may be accompanied by convulsions. The ventricles stop beating immediately and restart some 5–30 seconds later once an ectopic pacemaker (atrioventricular node, Purkinje fibres, ventricular muscle) starts functioning. Death may occur if an ectopic discharge does not occur within 30 seconds.

CLINICAL PHYSIOLOGY: Bundle branch block is a serious condition that is commonly due to ischemia and leads to injury of the right or left bundle branches. When one bundle is blocked the excitation wave passes normally through the intact bundle and then passes through the muscle of the ventricle on the blocked side. The ECG shows normal P wave, prolonged slurred QRS complexes, inverted T wave in the leads facing the affected side, and right or left axis deviation (depending on the affected side).

Extrasystole is the premature contraction of the heart before its normal contraction caused by the discharge of an impulse from somewhere other than the sinoatrial node; it is followed by a compensatory pause. Extrasystole can be atrial, nodal or ventricular in origin. When atrial in origin, an additional small shapeless P wave appears immediately after the regular T wave; the R-R interval of this beat is short. When nodal in origin, the P wave merges with the QRS complex and all heart chambers contract together. When ventricular in origin, an extra prolonged QRS complex of high voltage, due to the relatively slow conduction of the impulse through the ventricular muscle, follows the regular T wave, which is inverted.

Extrasystole is associated with organic heart diseases, especially ischaemic areas of the ventricular musculature. Emotion, severe exhaustion, excessive ingestion of coffee or alcohol, excessive smoking, hyperthyroidism and reflexes elicited by abnormal viscera can also initiate extrasystole.

Paroxysmal tachycardia (Bouveret-Hoffmann syndrome) is a sudden increase in heart rate due to an ectopic focus in the atria, atrioventricular node or ventricles; it can last from a few seconds to a few hours, after which it suddenly stops and the heart continues to function normally. Symptoms include palpitations, chest pain, rapid breathing and dizziness. If atrial in origin, the P wave is inverted, but the QRS complex and T wave are normal. If nodal in origin, the P wave is mostly absent with a normal QRS complex and T wave. If ventricular in origin, it can lead to ventricular fibrillation, which is fatal.

Atrial flutter is characterised by rapid ineffective and regular atrial contractions (220–350 beats/min); it is often associated with atrial paroxysmal tachycardia. As the atrioventricular node cannot conduct more than 230 impulses/min, incomplete heart block develops and therefore the ventricles respond once for every two or three atrial beats. In the ECG, each two or three abnormal P waves are followed by one normal QRS complex and T wave. It is common in patients with hypertension and coronary artery disease and initially marked by palpitations, which go unnoticed. Prolonged atrial flutter can lead to atrial fibrillation or heart failure.

Atrial fibrillation is characterised by rapid and irregular contractions (300–400 beats/min); the P wave is absent and replaced by fine oscillations called F waves, the QRS and T waves are normal in shape but irregular in rate. It is common in old people and those with heart diseases but is not life threatening, although it can cause complications (blood clots and blockage of blood flow to vital organs).

Ventricular fibrillation is characterised by rapid and irregular twitching of the ventricles (up to 400–500 beats/min). As the ventricles cannot pump blood around the body, it leads to death. In the ECG, the QRS complexes are quite irregular in shape, rhythm and amplitude, and all waves are not clear and cannot be identified. It is very common during electric shock and ischaemia of the conducting system; it can also occur with coronary occlusion, chloroform and anaesthesia, heart trauma and improper handling of the heart during cardiac surgery.

Cardiac arrest. This results when all electrical signals in the heart have ceased. It can occur during deep anaesthesia when many patients develop severe hypoxia due to inadequate respiration, preventing the muscle and conducting fibres from maintaining normal electrolyte concentration differentials across their membranes, leading to loss of automatic rhythmicity.

In most cases, prolonged cardiopulmonary resuscitation (minutes, hours) is successful in re-establishing a normal heart rhythm. However, severe myocardial disease can cause permanent (or semi-permanent) cardiac arrest, which can lead to death: an implanted electronic cardiac pacemaker can be used to keep patients alive.

Effects of electrolyte concentrations on the heart. The distribution of electrolytes (sodium, potassium and calcium ions) in the extracellular and intracellular fluids is responsible for the electrical activity of tissues, including the myocardium.

Sodium ions. A slight change in the concentration of sodium ions in blood (normal concentration 135–145 mEq/L) does not severely alter the electrical activity of the heart; low concentrations in body fluids reduce the electrical activity of the myocardium, with the ECG showing low voltage waves.

Potassium ions. When potassium ion concentration increases to 6 mEq/L (hyperkalaemia) or drops to 2 mEq/L (hypokalaemia) changes in the ECG appear; the normal concentration is 3.5–5 mEq/L. Hyperkalaemia increases the excitability of the myocardium: at 6–7 mEq/L the T wave is tall and tented, but the QRS complex and R-R interval are normal; at 8 mEq/L the P-R interval and duration of the QRS complex are prolonged, the P wave may be small; above 9 mEq/L the P wave is absent and QRS complex merges with the T wave. This latter situation is fatal as it leads to ventricular fibrillation or the heart stopping in diastole due to the lack of excitability. When potassium ion levels fall to 2 mEq/L, the S-T segment is depressed, the T wave is small, flat or inverted, and a U wave appears sometimes merging with the T wave; because of the U wave the Q-T interval may

be mistaken for being prolonged. With potassium levels below 2 mEq/L the S-T segment is depressed below the isoelectric baseline, the T wave is inverted, a prominent U wave appears, and there is prolongation of the P-R interval.

Calcium ions. The normal concentration of calcium ions in the blood is 4.5–5.5 mEq/L. An elevation in blood calcium levels (hypercalcaemia) increases the excitability and contractility of the myocardium; clinically the effects of hypercalcaemia are rare. There is a shortening of the S-T segment and QT interval, and the appearance of the U wave. Calcium rigour is stoppage of the heart in systole: it is reversible, with the heart functioning normally after the calcium ions have been flushed out. Hypocalcaemia reduces the excitability of the myocardium; there is prolongation of the S-T segment and QT interval, together with the appearance of a prominent U wave.

Cardiac Output

The volume of blood expelled with each contraction of the ventricles is the stroke volume: stroke volume = end of diastolic volume (135 mL) – end of systolic volume (65 mL) = 70 mL. Cardiac output is the amount of blood ejected from each ventricle each minute: cardiac output = stroke volume × heart rate, expressed in L/min. In a healthy heart at rest, stroke volume is approximately 70 mL, which with a heart rate of 70 beats/min gives a cardiac output of 4.9 L/min. This can be increased to 25 L/min during exercise, and up to 35 L/min in elite athletes; the increase during exercise is the cardiac reserve. The means by which the volume pumped by the heart is regulated is by (i) intrinsic cardiac regulation in response to changes in the volume of blood flowing through the heart and (ii) control of heart rate and the strength of ventricular contraction by the autonomic nervous system (Fig. 2.59).

> **APPLIED PHYSIOLOGY:** The intrinsic ability of the heart to adapt to increasing volumes of inflowing blood is the *Frank-Starling mechanism*: the greater the myocardium is stretched during filling the greater the force of contraction and the greater the volume of blood pumped into the aorta.

Stroke volume. This is determined by the volume of blood in the ventricles, i.e., the ventricular

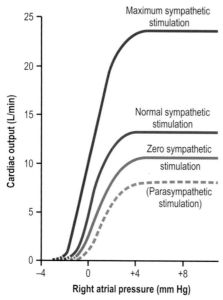

Fig. 2.59 Effect on cardiac output of sympathetic and parasympathetic stimulation.

end-diastolic volume (pre-load), immediately prior to their contraction, which depends on the amount of blood returning to the heart via the superior and inferior venae cavae. Increased pre-load leads to stronger myocardial contraction with more blood being expelled, increasing stroke volume and therefore increasing cardiac output. Within physiological limits the heart always pumps out all of the blood it receives, enabling it to adjust cardiac output to match the body's needs. Factors other than pre-load that increase the force and rate of myocardial contraction include increased sympathetic activity (page 227), and circulating hormones (page 334). However, the ability to increase stroke volume with increasing pre-load is finite; when the limit is reached (e.g., when venous return exceeds cardiac output), cardiac output decreases and the heart begins to fail.

A number of factors influence stroke volume and therefore cardiac output.

Arterial blood pressure. This influences stroke volume as it increases the resistance (afterload) against which the ventricles have to pump; it is determined by the elasticity of the large arteries and the peripheral resistance of the arterioles. An increased afterload could decrease stroke volume if systemic blood pressure is significantly higher than normal.

Blood volume. This is normally kept within strict limits by the kidneys; if blood volume falls, through haemorrhage, this can result in stroke volume, cardiac output and venous return falling. If blood loss is too great for the body's compensatory mechanisms to return blood volume to normal levels the body goes into shock (page 158).

Venous return. The major determinant of cardiac output. Normally, the heart pumps out all of the blood returned to it; however, left ventricular contraction is not by itself sufficient to push blood through the arterial and venous circulation back to the heart: other factors are involved. Firstly, venous return is assisted by posture, with gravity assisting return from the head and neck when standing and sitting, with less resistance to venous return from the lower limbs when lying down. Valves in the veins of the lower limb act to prevent backflow of blood when standing. Secondly, contraction of muscles (skeletal muscle pump) surrounding the deep veins compresses them, pushing blood back towards the heart. Thirdly, expansion of the chest during inspiration creates a negative pressure within the thorax assisting blood flow towards the heart; at the same time, increased intra-abdominal pressure also pushes blood towards the heart.

Heart rate. A major determinant of cardiac output, with a rise in heart rate causing an increase in cardiac output and a fall in heart rate decreasing cardiac output. The most important factor controlling heart rate is the balance between sympathetic and parasympathetic activity reaching the heart via the superficial and deep cardiac plexuses (Fig. 2.59).

Heart rate is regulated by the vasomotor (cardiac) centre situated bilaterally in the reticular formation of the medulla oblongata and lower part of the pons; the centre also regulates blood pressure. It consists of a vasoconstrictor area (cardioaccelerator centre/pressor area), a vasodilator area (cardioinhibitory centre/depressor area) and a sensory area.

The **vasoconstrictor area** increases heart rate and constricts blood vessels via accelerator impulses through sympathetic nerves; it is under the control of the hypothalamus and cerebral cortex.

The **vasodilator area** decreases heart rate and dilates blood vessels via inhibitory impulses through the vagus; it is also under the control of the cerebral cortex and hypothalamus, as well as impulses from baroreceptors (carotid and aortic), chemoreceptors and other sensory inputs.

The **sensory area** receives sensory inputs via the glossopharyngeal and vagus nerves, especially from baroreceptors in the periphery; it controls the vasocon-strictor and vasodilator centres.

Sympathetic stimulation. Increases heart rate from the normal rate of 70 beats/min up to 180–200 beats/min. Stimulation also increases the force of myocardial contraction, in turn increasing cardiac output two- or threefold; however, inhibition of sympathetic activity decreases cardiac output by only 30%.

Parasympathetic stimulation. Decreases both heart rate, to 20–40 beats/min, and the strength of myocardial contraction, by 20%–30%. These changes can result in a decrease in ventricular pumping of 50% or more.

Chemicals circulating in the blood (adrenaline, nor-adrenaline, thyroxine), as well as hypoxia and elevated carbon dioxide levels, have a similar effect on heart rate as sympathetic stimulation. In contrast, electrolyte imbalances (e.g., hyperkalaemia) and some hypertensive drugs (e.g., β-receptor antagonists) can lead to depressed cardiac function and bradycardia.

Other factors can also influence heart rate: **posture** (heart rate is usually higher when standing upright than when lying down); **exercise** (heart rate increases during exercise as active muscles need more blood); **emotion** (excitement, fear and anxiety increases heart rate); **gender** (females have higher heart rates than males); **age** (babies and young children have higher heart rates than older children and adults); **body temperature** (higher temperatures increase heart rate); and the **baroreceptor reflex** (page 149).

CLINICAL PHYSIOLOGY: Baroreceptors regulate heart rate through Marey's reflex, which decreases heart rate when carotid and aortic baroreceptors signal an increase in blood pressure; it is only induced during resting conditions.

CLINICAL PHYSIOLOGY: The Bainbridge (right atrial) reflex increases heart rate when venous return increases.

CLINICAL PHYSIOLOGY: The Bezold-Jarisch reflex (coronary chemoreflex) is characterised by bradycardia and hypotension resulting from stimulation of chemo-receptors in the wall of the left ventricle by substances such as alkaloids. It is a pathological reflex occurring in myocardial infarct, the administration of thrombolytic agents, haemorrhage, aortic stenosis and syncope.

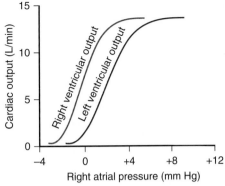

Fig. 2.60 Normal cardiac output curves.

Cardiac function curves. Cardiac output and venous return (systemic vascular function) curves demonstrate the capacity of the ventricles to pump blood and maintain the circulation throughout the body.

Cardiac output curves. These show the relationship between cardiac output and right atrial pressure, which depends on venous return. When pressure in the right atrium is 0 mm Hg right ventricular output is 5 L/min, reaching a maximum of 13–14 L/min when atrial pressure increases to between 2 and 4 mm Hg (Fig. 2.60). When right atrial pressure is 2 mm Hg, left ventricular output is 5 L/min, rising to 13–14 L/min when the pressure increases to between 4 and 8 mm Hg; further increases in right atrial pressure do not increase ventricular output (Fig. 2.60). When atrial pressure rises above 8 mm Hg venous return is decreased; plateauing of the curves shows that the heart can control output by itself. Nevertheless, the curves can be shifted to the left (increased cardiac output) or right (decreased cardiac output) under certain conditions.

A **shift to the left** indicates abnormal functioning of the heart (hypereffective heart) and increased cardiac output. This may be due to hypertrophy of the heart increasing the force of contraction, leading to a cardiac output of 10–19 L/min; combined stimulation of the sympathetic and parasympathetic innervation to the heart leading to an increased rate and force of contraction, with cardiac output increasing to 25 L/min; and excitation of the heart and ventricular hypertrophy increasing cardiac output to more than 35 L/min.

A **shift to the right** indicates a decreased functioning of the heart (hypoeffective heart) and decreased cardiac output. This can occur when there is: increased parasympathetic or decreased sympathetic stimulation;

diphtheria toxins; myocarditis; myocardial infarction; valvular disease; or congenital heart disease.

Changes in **extracardiac pressure** can also lead to changes in cardiac output; intrapleural pressure is the major extracardiac pressure. When intrapleural pressure becomes less negative or becomes positive, venous return decreases leading to decreased cardiac output.

> **CARDIAC TAMPONADE:** An acute compression of the heart caused by increased intrapericardial pressure due to the accumulation of blood or fluid in the pericardial cavity from either rupture of the heart, penetrating trauma or progressive effusion, leads to a decrease in cardiac output.

Venous return curves. These demonstrate the relationship between venous return and right atrial pressure; when right atrial pressure increases, venous return decreases due to back pressure and so does cardiac output (Fig. 2.61).

Cardiac output represents cardiac function while venous return represents vascular function. The relationship between them is shown in Fig. 2.62, where 'A' is the relationship under normal conditions. When venous return increases, cardiac output also increases 'B', together with an increase in right atrial pressure. Factors changing venous return also change cardiac output.

Great Vessels

The heart is connected to the **pulmonary circulation** by the pulmonary trunk taking deoxygenated blood to the lungs and the pulmonary veins returning oxygenated blood to the left atrium, and to the **systemic circulation** by the aorta, thereby distributing oxygenated blood to the tissues of the body. The superior and

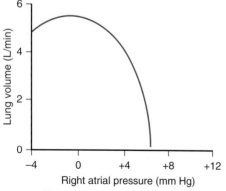

Fig. 2.61 Venous return curve.

inferior venae cavae return deoxygenated blood to the right atrium; the cardiac veins return deoxygenated blood from the heart to the right atrium. Further details of the pulmonary circulation can be found on page 106.

> **DEVELOPMENT OF THE ARTERIES:** The pharyngeal (branchial) arches contribute greatly to the formation of the head and neck. Associated with each pair of pharyngeal arches are a pair of aortic arch arteries, which extend between the aortic sac and the dorsal aortae (Fig. 2.63). The first and second pair disappear except for a small part which forms the maxillary and stapedial arteries on each side; the third pair forms the common carotid arteries and proximal parts of the internal carotid arteries, with the external carotid arteries also coming from the third arches; the fourth pair forms the distal part of the arch of the aorta on the left and the subclavian artery on the right; the fifth pair completely disappears on both sides; the ventral part of the sixth pair gives rise to the pulmonary arteries, while the dorsal part becomes the ductus arteriosus on the left and disappears on the right so that the arch of the aorta becomes continuous with the descending aorta on the left. The aortic sac lies at the upper end of the truncus arteriosus: the left horn gives rise to the proximal part of the aortic arch, while the right horn forms the brachiocephalic artery, which is continuous with the right common carotid artery and stem of the right subclavian artery. The distal part of the arch of the aorta is continuous with the seventh intersegmental artery. Further details of the development of arteries in other regions can be found in the relevant chapter.
>
> **Congenital anomalies:** (i) *Coarctation of the aorta* is narrowing or complete obliteration of the aortic arch distal to the origin of the left subclavian artery; it can be preductal or postductal depending on whether the narrowing is before or after the opening of the ductus arteriosus; (ii) *patent ductus arteriosus* is communication between the arch of the aorta and left pulmonary artery; (iii) *right aortic arch* is directed towards the right due to obliteration of the left aortic arch artery and left dorsal aorta: similar vessels on the right persist; (iv) *abnormal origin of the right subclavian artery* arising from the descending aorta and passes to the right behind the trachea and oesophagus.

The **aorta** arises from the left ventricle, arches to the left and then continues down through the thorax (descending aorta) to the left of the midline to enter the abdomen

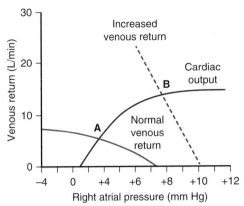

Fig. 2.62 Analysis of cardiac function curves.

by passing behind the diaphragm at the level of T12 to become the abdominal aorta; details of the course and distribution of branches of the abdominal aorta can be found on pages 467, 471, 475 and 513. It ends at the lower border of L4 by dividing into the right and left common iliac arteries; details of the course and distribution of the common iliac arteries can be found on page 578, 579. The ascending aorta gives two branches, right and left coronary arteries, which supply the heart; details of the coronary arteries can be found on page 124. The arch of the aorta gives three branches, the brachiocephalic trunk which divides into the right subclavian and common carotid arteries, the left common carotid artery and the left subclavian artery; details of the course and distribution of these arteries can be found on pages 324, 331.

The **pulmonary trunk** arises from the right ventricle and within the concavity of the aortic arch and divides into right and left pulmonary arteries; the left pulmonary artery is linked to the arch of the aorta by the ligamentum arteriosum, around which the left recurrent laryngeal nerve passes.

DEVELOPMENT OF THE VEINS: The veins of the embryo are identified as vitelline draining the yolk sac, umbilical carrying oxygenated blood from the placenta, and somatic/cardinal (anterior, common, posterior (by the subcardinal and supracardinal)) draining the body. The inferior vena cava develops from the upper part of the right vitelline, subcardinal, supracardinal and posterior cardinal veins. The upper part of the superior vena cava develops from the right anterior cardinal vein, as does the right internal jugular and brachiocephalic veins, while its upper part develops from the right common cardinal vein. The left internal jugular vein develops from the left anterior cardinal vein, while the left brachiocephalic vein develops as an anastomosis between the two anterior cardinal veins.

The **superior** and **inferior venae cavae** convey deoxygenated blood from all body tissues and organs, except the heart, to the right atrium before it is pumped to the lungs for reoxygenation.

Structure of blood vessels. The walls of all blood vessels, except capillaries and venules, consist of three concentric layers: an inner layer (tunica intima), middle layer (tunica media) and outer layer (tunica adventitia). The amount and arrangement of these tissues in vessels are influenced by mechanical (blood pressure) and metabolic (reflecting the local needs of the tissues) factors (Fig. 2.64).

The **tunica intima** has three components: endothelium, a single layer of simple squamous epithelial cells adjacent to the vessel lumen; a basal lamina of the endothelial cells, which is a thin extracellular layer mainly comprising collagen, proteoglycans and glycoproteins; and a subendothelial layer of loose connective tissue (Fig. 2.64). The subendothelial layer in arteries and arterioles contains a sheet-like layer/lamella of fenestrated elastic material (internal elastic membrane), which enables substances to diffuse through it to reach deep cells within the vessel wall.

The endothelium acts as a semipermeable membrane between the blood plasma and interstitial fluid. Together with its basal lamina, it mediates and actively monitors the bidirectional exchange of molecules by simple and active diffusion, receptor-mediated endocytosis, transcytosis and other mechanisms. The endothelium also presents a nonthrombogenic surface on which blood will not clot, actively secretes agents (heparin, tissue plasmogenic activator, von Willebrand factor) that control local clot formation; regulates local vasomotor tone and blood flow by secreting factors that either stimulate (endothelin 1, angiotensin-converting enzyme (ACE)) or cause relaxation (nitric oxide, prostacyclin) of smooth muscle; plays a role in inflammation and local immune responses in venules by inducing specific white blood cells to stop and undergo transepithelial migration at sites of injury or infection; and, under some conditions, secretes growth factors, including proteins promoting specific white blood cell lineage proliferation, as well as cells that make up the vessels wall.

Vascular endothelial growth factor stimulates the formation of the vascular system from embryonic mesoderm (vasculogenesis), helps maintain the vasculature in adults and promotes capillary sprouting and outgrowth from small existing vessels (angiogenesis) during normal growth, tissue repair and regeneration, as well as in tumours and other pathological conditions.

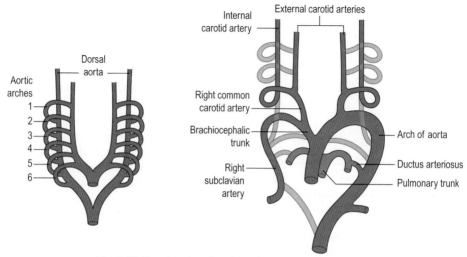

Fig. 2.63 The six pairs of aortic arches and their derivatives.

In both processes, other growth factors (angiopoietins) stimulate endothelial cells to recruit smooth muscle cells and fibroblasts to form other tissues of the vessel's wall.

The **tunica media** mainly consists of circumferentially arranged layers of smooth muscle extending between the internal and external elastic membranes (Fig. 2.64). This layer also contains variable amounts of elastin (fenestrated and arranged in circular concentric lamellae), reticular fibres and proteoglycans between the smooth muscle cells; all extracellular components are produced by the vascular smooth muscle cells.

The **tunica adventitia** consists mainly of longitudinally arranged collagenous tissue, which merges with the loose connective tissue surrounding the vessels, and some elastic fibres (Fig. 2.64). It ranges from being relatively thin in most arteries to fairly thick in the venules and veins, where it is the major part of the vessel wall. In large arteries and veins, there is a system of vessels (vasa vasorum) supplying blood to the vessel walls, as well as a network of autonomic nerves (nervi vasorum/vascularis) which innervate the smooth muscle in the vessel wall.

The various types of arteries and veins can be distinguished from each other by differences in the composition and thickness of the layers (Table 2.3).

Atypical blood vessels. Blood vessels, both arteries and veins, in some locations, have an atypical structure: the **coronary arteries** have large amounts of smooth circular muscle in the tunica media, which progressively thickens with increasing age, together with increasing amounts of fibroelastic tissue; **dural venous sinuses** (page 270) are essentially broad spaces within the dura mater lined with endothelium but devoid of smooth muscle; **long (great) saphenous vein** (page 592) has thick circular smooth muscle in the tunica media and numerous longitudinal smooth muscle bundles in the intima and a well-developed adventitia.

Arteriovenous shunts/anastomoses. These allow blood to bypass capillaries by providing direct routes between arteries and veins (Fig. 2.65); they are commonly found in the skin of the fingertips, nose, lips and the erectile tissue of the penis and clitoris. The tunica media and adventitia of the arteriole are thicker and are richly innervated by the autonomic nervous system, which control the degree of vasoconstriction at the shunts, regulating blood flow through the capillaries.

Portal systems. An alternate pathway in which blood flows through two successive capillary beds separated by a portal vein (Fig. 2.65). In this way, hormones or nutrients picked up by the blood in the first capillary bed network are efficiently delivered to cells around the second network before the blood is returned to the heart for general circulation around the body. Examples are the hepatic portal system of the liver (page 478) and the hypothalamic-hypophyseal portal system (page 335) in the anterior pituitary gland, both of which are of major physiological importance.

Blood vessel pathology

Atheroma. Patchy changes (plaques) develop in the tunica intima of large and medium-sized arteries,

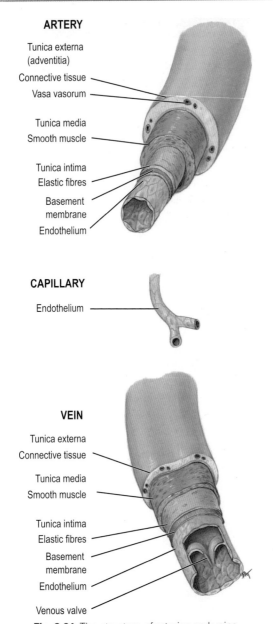

ARTERY

Tunica externa
(adventitia)

Connective tissue

Vasa vasorum

Tunica media

Smooth muscle

Tunica intima

Elastic fibres

Basement
membrane

Endothelium

CAPILLARY

Endothelium

VEIN

Tunica externa

Connective tissue

Tunica media

Smooth muscle

Tunica intima

Elastic fibres

Basement
membrane

Endothelium

Venous valve

Fig. 2.64 The structure of arteries and veins.

Plaques may rupture releasing subintimal material into the blood, which may cause thrombosis and vasospasm compromising blood flow.

The presence of plaques (atherosclerosis) is more common in older people; however, fatty streaks are present in the artery walls of infants but are usually absorbed; incomplete absorption could be responsible for the appearance of plaques in later life. Factors predisposing to atherosclerosis include a family history; obesity; gender (males are more susceptible than females); diet (high in refined carbohydrates and/or saturated fats and cholesterol); increased age; smoking; diabetes mellitus; excessive emotional stress; hypertension; hyperlipidaemia (especially high levels of low-density lipoprotein (LDL)); excessive alcohol consumption; and a sedentary lifestyle.

Atheromatous plaques can cause narrowing or complete obstruction of an artery, which may be further complicated by clot formation. With narrowing, tissues beyond the narrow point become ischaemic, with increases in metabolic rate (increased muscle activity) causing acute ischaemic pain, which disappears when the exertion stops. Cardiac muscle and skeletal muscles of the lower limb are most commonly affected, leading to angina pectoris and intermittent claudication, respectively. With complete blockage, the tissues supplied quickly degenerate (ischaemia), leading to infarction; blockage of a coronary leads to myocardial infarction, while blockage of arteries in the brain leads to cerebral infarction (stroke).

If the fibrous cap of the plaque breaks down, platelets are activated by the damaged cells and an intravascular clot forms (thrombosis) blocking the artery causing ischaemia and infarction. Emboli may detach from the thrombus, travel in the bloodstream and lodge in small arteries distal to the clot causing small infarcts. Plaques can also become calcified making the artery brittle, rigid and prone to aneurysm formation, increasing the risk of rupture and haemorrhage (page 157).

Arteriosclerosis. Arteriosclerosis is the progressive degeneration of arterial walls of mainly large and medium-sized arteries, with the tunica media being infiltrated with fibrous tissue and calcium (Fig. 2.67); it is associated with ageing and hypertension. The vessel becomes dilated, inelastic and often tortuous; the loss of elasticity increases systolic blood pressure and pulse pressure. The involvement of small arteries and arterioles causes narrowing of their lumen by depositions of a hyaline material (Fig. 2.67), reducing their elasticity and increasing blood pressure due to the increased pe-

commonly those of the heart, brain, kidneys, small intestine and lower limbs. They initially appear as fatty streaks in the artery wall, with mature plaques consisting of accumulations of cholesterol and other lipids, excess smooth muscle and fat-filled monocytes (foam cells); the plaque is covered with a rough fibrous cap. As it grows and thickens, the plaque spreads along the artery wall protruding into the lumen (Fig. 2.66).

TABLE 2.3   Characteristic Features of Different Blood Vessels

Vessel	Diameter	Tunica Intima	Tunica Media	Tunica Adventitia	Role in Circulation
Large (elastic) artery	>10 mm	Endothelium; connective tissue with smooth muscle	Smooth muscle; external elastic membrane	Connective tissue (thinner than media) with vasa vasorum; elastic fibres	Conduct blood from heart and with elastic recoil help move blood forward under steady pressure
Medium (muscular) artery	2–10 mm	Endothelium; connective tissue with smooth muscle; prominent internal elastic membrane	Many smooth muscle layers; external elastic membrane	Connective tissue (thinner than media); relatively little elastic tissue; vasa vasorum may be present	Distribute blood to all organs and maintains steady blood pressure and flow with vasodilation and constriction
Small artery	0.1–2 mm	Endothelium; connective tissue; less smooth muscle; internal elastic membrane	3–10 layers of smooth muscle; external elastic membrane; collagen fibres	Connective tissue (thinner than media); some elastic fibres; collagen fibres; no vasa vasorum	Distribute blood to arterioles, adjusting flow with vasodilation and constriction
Arteriole	10–100 μm	Endothelium; no connective tissue or smooth muscle	1–3 layers of smooth muscle	Thin poorly defined connective tissue layer	Resist and control blood flow to capillaries: major determinant of systemic blood pressure
Capillary	4–10 μm	Endothelium	Pericytes	None	Exchange of metabolites by diffusion to and from cells
Post-capillary venule	10–50 μm	Endothelium; pericytes	None	None	Drain capillary bed: site of leukocyte exit from vasculature
Muscular venule	50–100 μm	Endothelium	1–2 layers of smooth muscle	Connective tissue (thicker than media); some elastic fibres	Drain capillary bed: sites of leukocyte exit from vasculature
Small vein	0.1–1 mm	Endothelium; connective tissue; 1–2 layers smooth muscle	2–3 layers of smooth muscle continuous with intima	Connective tissue (thicker than media); some elastic fibres	Collect blood from venules
Medium vein	1–10 mm	Endothelium; connective tissue; smooth muscle; internal elastic membrane; valves	3–5 distinct layers of smooth muscle; collagen fibres	Connective tissue (thicker than media); some elastic fibres; may be some longitudinal smooth muscle	Carry blood to larger veins with no backflow

TABLE 2.3 Characteristic Features of Different Blood Vessels—cont'd

Vessel	Diameter	Tunica Intima	Tunica Media	Tunica Adventitia	Role in Circulation
Large vein	>10 mm	Endothelium; connective tissue with smooth muscle cells; prominent valves	2–15 smooth muscle layers; collagen fibres	Connective tissue (much thicker than media); some elastic fibres; longitudinal smooth muscle: cardiac muscle extensions (myocardial sleeves) into great vessels near heart	Return blood to heart

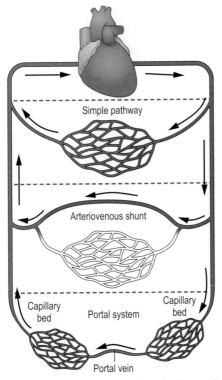

Fig. 2.65 Comparison of simple capillary beds, arteriovenous shunts and portal systems.

ripheral resistance. Damage to small vessels can lead to ischaemia of tissues supplied by the artery; in the limbs, the ischaemia predisposes to gangrene.

Aneurysm. An abnormal local dilation of an artery (Fig. 2.68), which can arise due to atheroma, hyperten-

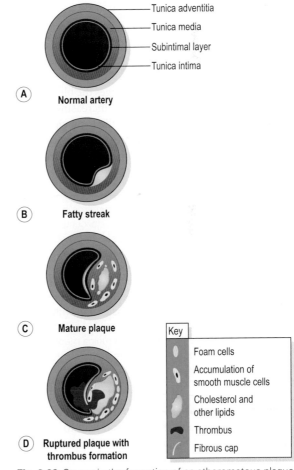

A Normal artery

Tunica adventitia
Tunica media
Subintimal layer
Tunica intima

B Fatty streak

C Mature plaque

D Ruptured plaque with thrombus formation

Key
- Foam cells
- Accumulation of smooth muscle cells
- Cholesterol and other lipids
- Thrombus
- Fibrous cap

Fig. 2.66 Stages in the formation of an atheromatous plaque.

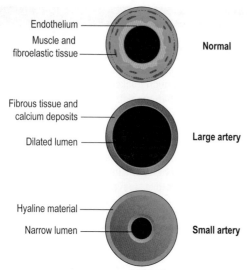

Fig. 2.67 Atherosclerotic arteries.

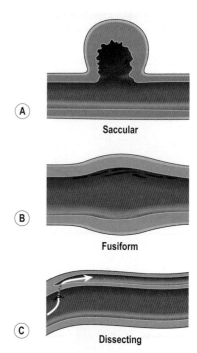

Fig. 2.68 Types of aneurysms.

sion and defective formation of collagen in the arterial wall. Rupture of an aneurysm results in haemorrhage, the consequences of which depend on the site and extent of the bleed. An aneurysm damages the blood vessel endothelium making it rougher and increasing the risk of clot formation, which can block the local circulation or travel as emboli in the bloodstream to other sites. A distended artery can cause pressure on other structures (blood vessels, nerves, organs).

CLINICAL ANATOMY: *Saccular aneurysms* bulge out from one side of the artery and tend to occur in relatively thin-walled arteries (when associated with arteries supplying the brain they are referred to as 'berry' aneurysms); they can be congenital, associated with defective collagen production or atheroma. *Fusiform aneurysms* are spindle-shaped and mainly occur in the abdominal aorta; they are usually associated with atheroma. *Dissecting aneurysms* are caused by infiltration of blood between the endothelium and tunica media starting at the site of endothelial damage; they mainly occur in the arch of the aorta.

Venous thrombosis. A thrombus is a blood clot formed inside a blood vessel and can lead to an interruption of the blood supply to or from the tissue. There is an increased risk of developing a thrombus with slow blood flow, as occurs during periods of immobility (bedrest) or the vessel is compressed by an adjacent structure (tumour) or there is a sustained fall in blood pressure (shock), with damage to the tunica intima or increased blood coagulability as in dehydration, pregnancy and childbirth, blood clotting disorders, the presence of an intravenous cannula and when taking contraceptive pills high in oestrogen.

Superficial thrombophlebitis occurs in superficial veins, with the surrounding tissues becoming inflamed, red and painful; it usually resolves spontaneously.

Deep vein thrombosis (DVT) is usually asymptomatic but may be accompanied by local pain and swelling; it usually affects the lower limb, pelvic and iliac veins, and occasionally upper limb veins. Risk factors include varicose veins; surgery; pregnancy; and immobility. DVT carries a significant risk of death if a clot fragment (embolus) travels to the lungs (pulmonary embolism).

Varicose veins are the result of stretching and damage to the walls of a vein through blood pooling so that it becomes inelastic, dilated and coiled; superficial veins generally become affected as they have little support. Due to distension, the valves are unable to close properly leading to further pooling and engorgement. However, venous return is maintained because the superficial veins are connected to a network of deep veins.

CLINICAL ANATOMY: The superficial veins of the lower limb (great/long and small/short saphenous, anterior tibial) are most commonly affected by varicose veins, causing aching and fatigue of the legs during long periods of standing; when injured they can rupture, with haemorrhage. A varicose ulcer, usually just above the medial side of the ankle, can occur on the skin over the vein due to stasis of blood and poor nourishment. Risk factors include increasing age; obesity; pregnancy; long periods of standing; constrictive clothing; family history and being female.

CLINICAL ANATOMY: Sustained pressure on distended veins at the junction of the rectum and anus leads to increased venous pressure, valve incompetence and haemorrhoids (piles); the most common causes are chronic constipation and increased pressure on the pelvis during the latter stages of pregnancy.

CLINICAL ANATOMY: Increased pressure in the lower oesophageal veins can lead to their rupture (oesophageal varices), with potentially fatal haemorrhage.

CLINICAL ANATOMY: Scrotal varicoceles can develop in men who stand for long periods of time as part of their work; if bilateral the increased temperature due to venous congestion can depress spermatogenesis leading to infertility.

Tumours of blood and lymph vessels. Angiomas are benign tumours of either blood (haemangiomas) or lymph (lymphangiomas) vessels.

Haemangiomas consist of excessive growth of blood vessels in an uncharacteristic way interspersed with collagen in a localised area making a dense network of tissue; each haemangioma is supplied by a single blood vessel. If the vessel thromboses the haemangioma atrophies and disappears.

CLINICAL ANATOMY: Haemangiomas may be present at birth as a purple/red mole (birthmark), where they are usually small; however, they can grow quite fast during the first few months, but after 1–3 years they may begin to atrophy; after 5 years, 80% have disappeared.

Circulation

The function of the circulation is to: (i) transport nutrients to body tissues; (ii) transport waste products away from body tissues; (iii) transport hormones from one part of the body to another; and (iv) maintain an appropriate environment for optimal survival and function.

The rate of blood flow through most tissues is determined in response to their need for nutrients. In some organs, the circulation has additional functions; the kidneys have a high blood flow related to their excretory role. The heart and blood vessels provide the required cardiac output and arterial pressure to facilitate the blood flow requirements of each tissue.

Arteries function to transport blood under high pressure to the tissues; they have strong vascular walls and blood flows at high velocity through them.

Arterioles are the smallest branches of the arterial system through which blood is released into the capillaries. They have strong muscular walls that can close the arteriole completely or relax allowing dilation; they have the ability to control blood flow to the capillaries in each tissue in response to its needs.

Capillaries function to exchange fluid, nutrients, electrolytes, hormones and other substances between the blood and interstitial fluid. They have thin permeable walls (capillary pores) allowing water and small molecular substances to pass through.

Venules collect blood from the capillaries; they gradually coalesce into larger veins.

Veins transport blood from the venules back to the heart. Because venous pressure is very low the walls of veins are thin; however, they are sufficiently muscular to contract or expand and therefore act as controllable reservoirs for extra blood depending on the needs of the circulation.

Details of the histology of arteries, arterioles, capillaries, venules and veins can be found on page 137.

Three principles underlie all functions of the circulation.

The rate of blood flow to each tissue: When tissues are active they need an increased supply of nutrients and a greater blood flow than when at rest: up to 20–30 times resting levels. However, cardiac output can only increase four to seven times. To achieve this microvessels in the tissue constantly monitor its needs (oxygen, nutrients, accumulation of carbon dioxide and other waste products) and then act directly on local blood vessels to control local blood flow to the level required for continued tissue activity.

The central nervous system and hormones also help to control local blood flow.

Cardiac output: This is mainly controlled by the sum of all local tissue flows. Blood flowing through a tissue immediately returns via the veins to the heart, which automatically responds by pumping the blood back into the arteries.

The regulation of arterial pressure: This is generally independent of local blood flow or cardiac output. An extensive system of reflexes controls arterial blood pressure should it fall below normal levels. The nervous signals result in: (i) an increase in the force of myocardial contraction; (ii) contraction of the large venous reservoirs to return more blood to the heart and (iii) generalised constriction of the arterioles so that more blood accumulates in the larger arteries. All of these act to increase arterial pressure. If arterial pressure remains low for prolonged periods of time (hours, days), the kidneys secrete pressure-controlling hormones by regulating blood volume.

Blood volume and blood pressure. The volume of blood in the major components of the circulation is shown in Fig. 2.69, from which it can be seen that 84% of the blood volume is in the systemic circulation, with the remaining 16% in the heart and lungs. Of the 84% in the systemic circulation 64% is in the veins, 13% in the arteries and 7% in the arterioles and capillaries.

Adding together the cross-sectional areas of each type of vessel in the systemic circulation their approximate total cross-sectional areas can be determined (Table 2.4). It is clear that the veins have a much larger cross-sectional area than the arteries, explaining the large storage capacity of the venous system compared with the arterial system. Because the same volume of blood flow (F) must pass through each segment of the circulation each minute, the velocity of blood flow (v) is inversely proportional to vascular cross-sectional area (A), i.e., $v = F/A$.

Under resting conditions, the velocity of blood in the aorta is about 50 cm/second, while in the capillaries it is about 0.05 cm/second (Table 2.4). Because the capillaries are only 0.3–1 mm in length the blood remains there for 1–3 seconds to allow oxygen, nutrients and electrolytes to pass through its walls.

Pressures in different parts of the circulation. The heart continuously pumps blood into the aorta, therefore mean aortic pressure is high (100 mm Hg), alternating between a systolic pressure of 120 mm Hg and a diastolic pressure of 80 mm Hg (Fig. 2.70).

The mean pressure in the capillaries is about 17 mm Hg, low enough that plasma tends not to leak out through pores in the capillary walls but sufficient to allow diffusion of nutrients through the same pores to the surrounding tissues. As blood continues to flow through the systemic circulation its mean pressure continues to fall to almost 0 mm Hg at the termination of the venae cavae as blood enters the right atrium.

Blood flow is also pulsatile in the pulmonary circulation, but the pressures are significantly lower: mean pulmonary artery pressure is 16 mm Hg (mean systolic pressure is 25 mm Hg and mean diastolic pressure 8 mm Hg), and mean pulmonary capillary pressure is 7 mm Hg. Nevertheless, these pressures are sufficient to expose the blood to oxygen and other gases in the alveoli.

Blood flow. In terms of the transport of oxygen and nutrients to tissues and the waste products away

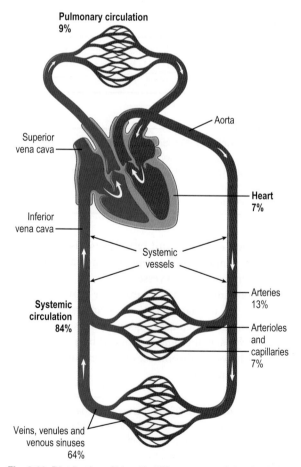

Fig. 2.69 Distribution of blood in different parts of the circulation.

Pulmonary circulation 9%

Aorta

Superior vena cava

Heart 7%

Inferior vena cava

Systemic vessels

Systemic circulation 84%

Arteries 13%

Arterioles and capillaries 7%

Veins, venules and venous sinuses 64%

from the tissues, the mean volume of blood flow (Q) in a given time is of greater physiological importance than linear velocity (v): Q = v/A. Blood flow through vessels is either laminar (streamlined) or turbulent (Fig. 2.71).

In laminar flow, the layer of blood in contact with the vessel wall moves very slowly, with the adjacent layer moving more quickly and so on to the centre of the vessel, where the blood is flowing at its greatest; it occurs only up to a critical velocity. When the velocity is above the critical level the flow becomes turbulent creating sounds. The critical velocity at which blood flow becomes turbulent is determined by the density (P) and viscosity (η) of the blood, the diameter of the vessels (D) through which it is flowing and the velocity (v) of the flow, i.e., the Reynold's number (N_R): $N_R = (PDv)/\eta$. Blood flow is usually not turbulent when N_R is less than 2000. Chances of turbulence are increased when N_R exceeds 2000, and almost always present when N_R is more than 3000.

The volume of blood flowing through a blood vessel is directly proportional to the **pressure gradient** (i.e., the pressure difference between the two ends of the vessel) (Table 2.5).

It is also inversely proportional to the **resistance (friction, tension) against which the blood has to flow**. Although resistance to blood flow is encountered in all blood vessels, with that encountered in the arterioles being of particular significance because they are partially constricted at all times due to sympathetic tone. Peripheral resistance is determined by the diameter of the vessel (the smaller the diameter the greater the resistance), the pressure gradient and the viscosity of the blood.

TABLE 2.4 The Approximate Total Cross-Sectional Area of Different Types of Vessel in the Systemic Circulation, Together With Their Mean Velocity of Blood Flow

Vessel	Cross-Sectional Area (cm²)	Mean Velocity of Blood Flow (cm/second)
Aorta	2.5	50.00
Small arteries	20	5.00
Arterioles	40	0.50
Capillaries	2500	0.05
Venules	250	0.10
Small veins	80	1.00
Venae cavae	8	2.00

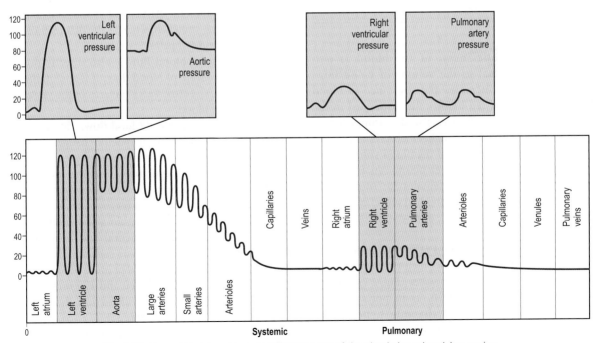

Fig. 2.70 Normal blood pressure in different parts of the circulation when lying supine.

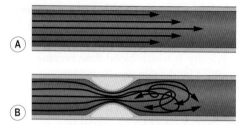

Fig. 2.71 Laminar (A) and turbulent (B) flow in a blood vessel.

TABLE 2.5 **Pressure Gradients in Different Regions of the Vascular Bed**			
Blood Vessels	**Pressure at Proximal End (mm Hg)**	**Pressure at Distal End (mm Hg)**	**Pressure Gradient (mm Hg)**
Aorta to venae cavae	120	0	120
Aorta	120	100	20
Arteries to arterioles	100	30	70
Capillaries	30	15	15
Venules	15	10	5
Veins	10	0	10
Venae cavae	0	−2	−2

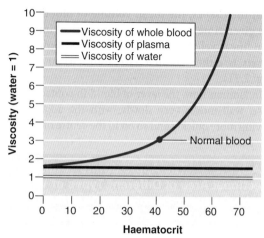

Fig. 2.72 Effect of haematocrit on blood viscosity.

The **viscosity (stickiness) of the blood** is also inversely proportional to the volume of blood flow: increased viscosity increases the resistance to blood flow. The number of red blood cells suspended in the blood determines blood viscosity; the proportion of red blood cells in blood is the haematocrit. A haematocrit of 40 means that 40% of the blood volume consists of cells and the remainder plasma; males have a mean haematocrit of 42 and females 38. These values can vary depending on an individual's level of activity, the altitude at which they live, and whether they have anaemia.

The viscosity of whole blood at normal haematocrit requires three to four times as much pressure to force blood through a vessel as does water (Fig. 2.72). When the haematocrit rises to 60–70, as in polycythaemia (erythrocythaemia/hypercythaemia/hypererycythaemia), blood viscosity can be 10 times that of water, greatly reducing blood flow.

Plasma protein concentration and the types of protein (albumin, globulin) can also affect blood viscosity, but to a much lesser extent than haematocrit; blood plasma has a viscosity about 1.5 times that of water.

The **vessel diameter** is directly proportional to the volume of blood flow; it is not the vessel diameter *per se* but the cross-sectional area through which the blood flows (Table 2.4). Both physiological and pathological conditions can change cross-sectional area; the diameter of the aorta depends upon the elasticity of its wall and ability to recoil after being stretched, whereas the diameter of arterioles depends on sympathetic tone.

The **velocity of blood flow** is also directly proportional to the volume of blood flow; it is maintained by cardiac output, the cross-sectional area of the vessel and the viscosity of blood.

Autoregulation of local blood flow. The regulation of blood flow to an organ in spite of changes in perfusion pressure (arterial–venous pressure) is controlled by the organ itself (autoregulation). Sudden increases or decreases in arterial pressure momentarily increase or decrease blood flow, but local mechanisms bring blood flow back to normal levels within a few minutes. This response is independent of neural and hormonal influences; it is due to the intrinsic capacity of the organ. Blood flow through organs is kept more or less constant between arterial pressures of 60 and 170 mm Hg, after which autoregulation fails and blood flow changes in response to a rise or fall in pressure (Fig. 2.73).

There are two mechanisms by which autoregulation can work. In the first, sudden stretching of blood vessels

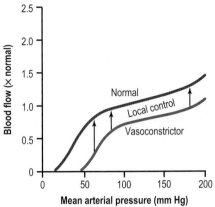

Fig. 2.73 The autoregulation of blood flow in a tissue (e.g., skeletal muscle) with changes in arterial pressure lasting several minutes: blood flow is autoregulated between 60 and 170 mm Hg. The blue line shows the effect of sympathetic stimulation by hormones (e.g., noradrenaline, angiotensin II, vasopressin, endothelin).

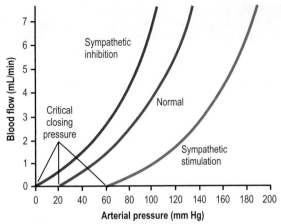

Fig. 2.74 Effect of arterial pressure on blood flow through a vessel with increased and decreased sympathetic stimulation of the vessel.

causes contraction of the smooth muscle in the vessel wall, especially small arteries and arterioles, resulting in vasoconstriction thus controlling blood flow. Stretching of blood vessels due to increased blood pressure increases the influx of calcium ions into the cells from the extracellular fluid, leading to smooth muscle contraction and vasoconstriction. However, when blood pressure falls there is less stretching of the blood vessels leading to vasodilation and an increase in blood flow.

The second mechanism is dependent on the accumulation of metabolites (adenosine, carbon dioxide, lactate, hydrogen) in the blood. With reduced blood flow metabolites cause dilation of the blood vessels restoring blood flow back to normal levels. Similarly, when blood flow increases the metabolites are quickly washed out of the tissues, leading to vasoconstriction returning blood flow back to normal.

The volume of blood flow is regulated by local mechanisms in most tissues of the body; however, it is more effective in some of the vital organs such as the kidney, heart and brain. The mechanism of autoregulation also varies slightly in these organs.

In isolated blood vessels or tissues that do not show autoregulation, changes in arterial pressure can have important effects on blood flow. An increase in arterial pressure not only increases the force pushing blood through the vessel but also distends elastic vessels resulting in a decrease in vascular resistance. Conversely, a decrease in arterial pressure in passive blood vessels increases the resistance as elastic vessels gradually collapse due to a reduced distending pressure. When the pressure falls below a critical level (critical closing pressure) blood flow ceases as the vessel has completely collapsed.

Sympathetic stimulation and other vasoconstrictors can alter the passive pressure-flow relationship, with inhibition of sympathetic activity dilating blood vessels and increasing blood flow and sympathetic stimulation constricting vessels and decreasing blood flow (Fig. 2.74). However, even in tissues that do not effectively autoregulate blood flow during acute changes in arterial pressure, blood flow is still regulated depending on the needs of the tissue when the pressure changes are sustained.

Arterial blood pressure. Arterial blood pressure is the pressure exerted on the walls of arteries when blood flows through them: it can be expressed as systolic pressure, diastolic pressure, pulse pressure and mean arterial pressure.

Systolic pressure is the maximum pressure exerted in the arteries during systole: normal values range between 110 and 140 mm Hg (mean 120 mm Hg).

Diastolic pressure is the minimum pressure exerted in the arteries during diastole: normal values range between 60 and 80 mm Hg (mean 80 mm Hg).

Pulse pressure is the difference between systolic and diastolic pressure: normal value is 40 mm Hg (120–80 mm Hg).

Mean arterial pressure is the average pressure existing in the arteries, being diastolic pressure plus 1/3rd

TABLE 2.6 Changes in Systolic and Diastolic Pressure With Increasing Age		
Age	Systolic Pressure (mm Hg)	Diastolic Pressure (mm Hg)
Newborn	70	40
1 month	85	45
6 months	90	50
1 year	95	55
Puberty	120	80
50 years	140	85
70 years	160	90
80 years	180	95

pulse pressure: normal mean arterial pressure is 80 + (40/3) = 93.3 mm Hg.

Physiological variations in arterial blood pressure. Blood pressure is altered under a number of physiological conditions, with the variation in systolic pressure being over a wider range than that of diastolic pressure.

Age: There is a gradual increase in both systolic and diastolic pressure with increasing age (Table 2.6).

Gender: In females up to menopause arterial pressure is 5 mm Hg less than in males, but afterwards, it is similar to that of males of the same age.

Physique: Arterial pressure is greater in the obese than in leaner individuals.

Diurnal variation: In the morning arterial pressure is lower than at midday, when it is maximum, becoming lower again in the evening.

After meals: Arterial pressure is increased for a few hours after eating due to increased cardiac output.

During sleep: Arterial pressure reduces by 15–20 mm Hg during sleep; however, it increases slightly when dreaming.

Emotion: During excitement or anxiety blood pressure increases due to the release of adrenaline.

Following exercise: After moderate exercise systolic, but not diastolic, pressure increases by 20–30 mm Hg; diastolic pressure depends on peripheral resistance, which is not altered during moderate exercise. After severe muscle exercise, systolic pressure rises by 4–50 mm Hg above basal levels; however, diastolic pressure decreases because peripheral resistance decreases in such exercise.

Pathological variations in arterial blood pressure

Hypertension is a persistent high blood pressure; clinically this is when systolic pressure remains elevated above 140 mm Hg and diastolic pressure remains elevated above 90 mm Hg. An elevation in systolic pressure only is referred to as systolic hypertension, in which pulse pressure is raised.

Primary (essential) hypertension is an elevated blood pressure in the absence of underlying disease; arterial blood pressure is increased because of increased peripheral resistance due to an unknown cause (it can be benign or malignant).

> *Benign hypertension* is when high blood pressure does not cause any problems, having a relatively long and symptomless course. In the early stages, there is an increase in systolic and diastolic pressure to 200 and 100 mm Hg, respectively, which returns to normal when resting or sleeping. Over time there is an increase in blood pressure, which does not return to normal levels when resting; this persistent increase can result in the development of vascular, cardiac and renal diseases.

> *Malignant (accelerated) hypertension* is a severe form quickly leading to progressive cardiac and renal diseases; it develops due to the combined effects of primary and secondary hypertension. Systolic and diastolic blood pressures rise to 250 and 150 mm Hg, respectively. It causes severe damage to the tunica intima of small blood vessels and organs (retina of the eye, heart, brain, kidneys); it is fatal resulting in death within a few years.

Primary hypertension cannot be cured but can be controlled using antihypertensive drugs:

β *adrenoceptor blockers* block the sympathetic nerves to the heart and blood vessels reducing cardiac output and inhibiting vasoconstriction.

α *adrenoceptor blockers* block the effect of sympathetic nerves on blood vessels leading to vasodilation.

Calcium channel blockers block the calcium channels in the myocardium reducing its contractility leading to decreased cardiac output and reduced blood pressure.

Diuretics cause diuresis and a reduction in extracellular fluid.

Angiotensin-converting enzyme (ACE) inhibitors block the formation of angiotensin.

Angiotensin II receptor blockers block the effects of angiotensin (vasoconstriction and aldosterone secretion).

Depressors of the vasomotor centre prevent vasoconstriction.

Vasodilators reduce blood pressure by vasodilation.

Secondary hypertension is an elevation of blood pressure due to an underlying disorder; it can have different forms.

Cardiovascular hypertension is due to cardiovascular disorders, such as hardening of the blood vessels (atherosclerosis) or narrowing (coarctation) of the aorta.

Endocrine hypertension develops due to hyperactivity of some endocrine glands, such as pheochromocytoma (tumour in the adrenal medulla resulting in excess secretion of catecholamines), hyperaldosteronism (excess secretion of aldosterone from the adrenal cortex) and Cushing syndrome (excess secretion of glucocorticoids from the adrenal cortex).

Renal hypertension is due to renal diseases causing hypertension, such as stenosis of the renal arteries, tumour of the juxtaglomerular apparatus leading to excess production of angiotensin II, and glomerulonephritis.

Neurogenic hypertension is due to nervous disorders producing hypertension, such as increased intracranial pressure, lesion in the tractus solitarius, and sectioning of nerve fibres from the carotid sinus.

Hypertension during pregnancy is due to toxaemia during pregnancy. Arterial blood pressure is raised by the low glomerular filtration rate and retention of water and sodium. Hypertension may also be associated with convulsions in eclampsia.

Secondary hypertension can be cured by addressing the diseases causing the hypertension.

CLINICAL PHYSIOLOGY: Goldblatt's hypertension (renovascular hypertension) refers to hypertension due to compression of a renal artery or its branches. It can be of two types: single kidney Goldblatt hypertension occurs when one kidney has already been removed and the renal artery of the other kidney is constricted for any reason; two kidney Goldblatt hypertension occurs when the artery of one kidney is constricted and the other is normal.

Hypotension is when blood arterial blood pressure is below 90 mm Hg.

Primary (essential) hypotension is low blood pressure that develops without any underlying disease or to an unknown cause; it is characterised by frequent fatigue and weakness. Individuals with primary hypotension are not susceptible to heart or renal disorders.

Secondary hypotension is due to an underlying disease, such as myocardial infarction, neurogenic shock, haemorrhagic shock, hypoactivity of the pituitary gland, hypoactivity of the adrenal glands, tuberculosis, and some nervous disorders (myasthenia gravis, tabes dorsalis, syringomyelia, diabetic neuropathy).

Orthostatic (postural) hypotension is a sudden fall in blood pressure while standing for a long time or when rising suddenly from a seated or lying position; it is due to the effects of gravity and some dysfunction of the autonomic nervous system. A common symptom is temporary loss of consciousness (syncope) due to a generalised cerebral ischaemia.

Regulation of arterial blood pressure. Although there is physiological variation in arterial blood pressure, it is soon brought back to within normal levels by a number of mechanisms: nervous (short term), renal (long term), hormonal, and local.

Nervous regulation brings blood pressure back to normal levels within a few minutes; however, it only acts for a short period before adapting to the new pressure. It works through the vasomotor system (vasomotor centre, vasoconstrictor fibres and vasodilator fibres).

The **vasomotor centre** is situated in the medulla oblongata and lower part of the pons and comprises three parts: vasoconstriction area, stimulation of which causes vasoconstriction and an increase in arterial blood pressure (as well as an increase in heart rate); vasodilator area, stimulation of which causes vasodilation by inhibiting vasoconstriction; and the sensory area, which receives sensory impulses from the periphery (particularly the baroreceptors) – it controls the vasoconstrictor and vasodilator areas.

The control of arterial blood pressure through the vasomotor centre is dependent on impulses received from baroreceptors in the carotid sinus and aortic wall, chemoreceptors in the carotid and aortic bodies, higher centres in the brain (cerebral cortex and hypothalamus) and respiratory centres. Baroreceptors and chemoreceptors play a major role in the short-term regulation of blood pressure.

Role of baroreceptors: When arterial blood pressure increases rapidly, they are activated and send impulses via the glossopharyngeal and vagus nerves to the nucleus of the tractus solitarius, which inhibits the vasoconstrictor area and stimulates the vasodilator area. Inhibition of the vasoconstrictor area reduces vasomotor tone with a decrease in peripheral resistance, while stimulation of the vasodilator area increases vagal tone decreasing the rate and force of myocardial contraction leading to a reduction in cardiac output. In this way, arterial blood pressure is brought back to normal levels.

A fall in arterial blood pressure inactivates the baroreceptors, resulting in no inhibition of the vasoconstrictor area or stimulation of the vasodilator area; consequently, blood pressure rises. As the pressure begins to rise both the carotid and aortic baroreceptors respond, with the response depending on the rate of increase in blood pressure. Mean arterial pressure in the range 50–200 mm Hg reaches the vasomotor centre through the carotid baroreceptors, while mean arterial pressure in the range of 100–200 mm Hg goes via the aortic baroreceptors.

Chemoreceptors respond to changes in the chemical composition of blood.

Vasoconstrictor fibres cause the release of noradrenaline, which leads to vasoconstriction; these fibres have a greater role in regulating blood pressure than do vasodilator fibres. The continuous discharge of impulses from the vasomotor centre via vasoconstrictor fibres produces a constant state of constriction of the blood vessels (vasomotor tone/sympathetic vasoconstrictor tone, sympathetic tone); arterial blood pressure is directly proportional to vasomotor tone.

Vasodilator fibres are of three types: parasympathetic vasodilator fibres; sympathetic vasodilator fibres; and antidromic vasodilator fibres. *Parasympathetic vasodilator fibres* cause dilation through the release of acetylcholine. *Sympathetic vasodilator fibres* cause dilation in some areas through the release of acetylcholine; these fibres supply blood vessels in skeletal muscle and are important in increasing blood flow during exercise. *Antidromic vasodilator fibres* cause blood vessels to dilate in response to some cutaneous receptors (e.g., pain receptors).

Renal regulation becomes important when blood pressure changes slowly over time (days/weeks/months), with the kidneys regulating arterial blood pressure by regulating extracellular fluid volume through the renin-angiotensin mechanism.

As blood pressure increases extracellular fluid volume and blood volume decreases as the kidneys secrete large amounts of water (diuresis) and sodium (natriuresis), in the form of salts, in the urine: small increases in blood pressure can double water excretion.

When blood pressure falls the reabsorption of water from the renal tubules is increased, in turn increasing extracellular fluid, blood volume and cardiac output, restoring blood pressure.

As extracellular fluid volume and blood volume decrease the secretion of renin by the kidneys is increased, which converts angiotensinogen into angiotensin, which in turn is converted into angiotensin II by ACE.

Angiotensin II causes arteriolar constriction increasing peripheral resistance and raising blood pressure; it also constricts the afferent arterioles in the kidneys reducing glomerular filtration. There is retention of water and salts leading to an increase in extracellular fluid volume and an increase in blood pressure. At the same time, angiotensin II stimulates the secretion of aldosterone from the adrenal cortex, which increases the reabsorption of sodium from the renal tubules. This in turn increases water reabsorption resulting in an increase in extracellular fluid volume and blood volume, returning blood pressure to normal levels.

Angiotensin II and IV also act to increase blood pressure and stimulate the adrenal cortex to secrete aldosterone.

Hormonal regulation is achieved by a number of hormones, which either act to increase or decrease blood pressure (Table 2.7).

Hormones which increase blood pressure work by different mechanisms.

Adrenaline (secreted by the adrenal medulla) increases systolic pressure by increasing the force of contraction of the myocardium and cardiac output, and decreases diastolic pressure by reducing total peripheral resistance.

Noradrenaline (secreted by the adrenal medulla) increases diastolic pressure by constricting blood vessels leading to an increase in peripheral resistance; there is also a slight increase in systolic pressure due to increasing the force of contraction of the myocardium.

Thyroxine (secreted by the thyroid) increases systolic pressure by increasing cardiac output due to an increase in blood volume and force of contraction of the myocardium. Diastolic pressure decreases due to vasodilation

TABLE 2.7   Hormones Involved in the Regulation of Blood Pressure

Hormones Increasing Blood Pressure	Hormones Decreasing Blood Pressure
Adrenaline	Vasoactive intestinal poly-peptide (VIP)
Noradrenaline	Bradykinin
Thyroxine	Prostaglandin
Aldosterone	Histamine
Vasopressin/antidiuretic hormone (ADH)	Acetylcholine
Angiotensin	Atrial natriuretic peptide
Serotonin	Brain natriuretic peptide
	C-type natriuretic peptide

and a decrease in peripheral resistance. However, mean arterial pressure tends to remain the same, with the change being in pulse pressure.

Aldosterone (secreted by the adrenal cortex) increases extracellular fluid volume and blood volume through the retention of water and sodium, leading to an increase in blood pressure.

Vasopressin/ADH (secreted by the posterior pituitary) causes constriction of all blood vessels, thus increasing blood pressure.

Angiotensins (secreted by the kidneys) cause constriction of systemic arterioles increasing blood pressure.

Serotonin increases blood pressure by vasoconstriction. It is secreted from several sources being synthesised in intestinal chromaffin cells and central and peripheral neurons, and is found in high concentrations in intestinal mucosa, the pineal body and the central nervous system.

Hormones decreasing blood pressure do so by causing vasodilation of blood vessels.

Vasoactive intestinal polypeptide (secreted in the stomach and small intestine) causes dilation of peripheral blood vessels.

Bradykinin is produced in the blood.

Prostaglandins (PGE₂) are secreted by most body tissues.

Histamines are secreted from nerve endings of the hypothalamus, limbic cortex and parts of the cerebral cortex; they are also released from tissues during allergic reactions, inflammation and tissue damage.

Acetylcholine is released from many sources.

Atrial natriuretic peptide is secreted by the myocardium of the atria of the heart.

Brain natriuretic peptide is secreted by the myocardium of the ventricles of the heart.

C-type natriuretic peptide is secreted by several tissues, including the heart and vascular endothelium.

Local regulation is via the action of local vasoconstrictor or vasodilator substances.

Local vasoconstrictors (endothelins) are derived from vascular endothelium when the blood vessel is stretched.

Local vasodilators have either a metabolic (carbon dioxide, lactate, hydrogen ions, adenosine) or an endothelial (nitric oxide) origin. The synthesis of nitric oxide is stimulated by acetylcholine, bradykinin, vasoactive intestinal polypeptide, substance P and the products of platelet breakdown.

Arterial pulse. The arterial pulse is an expression of the pressure changes transmitted through the arterial system following contraction of the heart and ejection of blood into the aorta. This results in a pressure wave produced by the elastic walls of the aorta (central arterial pulse), which is transmitted to the periphery (peripheral arterial pulse). The pulse is not transmitted to capillaries as they do not contain elastic tissue.

The formation and transmission of the pulse wave depend on the elasticity of the blood vessels; when the arterial walls are more distensible the pressure rise is less, as is the transmission of the pulse; when the arterial wall becomes more rigid (loses elasticity) with increasing age the pressure rise is greater, as is the transmission of the pulse. The velocity of pulse wave transmission is 7–9 m/second, which is faster than the maximum velocity of blood (50 cm/second in larger arteries).

A typical peripheral pulse has three main features (Fig. 2.75): the ascending (anacrotic) limb due to the rise in pressure during systole, the descending (catacrotic) limb due to the fall in pressure during diastole, which shows a notch due to the backflow of blood during closure of the semilunar valves at the beginning of diastole producing a slight increase in pressure.

The peripheral pulse can be palpated at several points in the body where major blood vessels are relatively

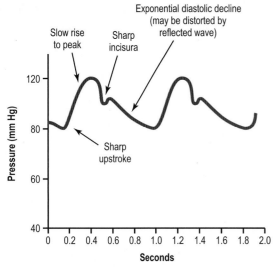

Fig. 2.75 Pressure pulse contour in the ascending aorta.

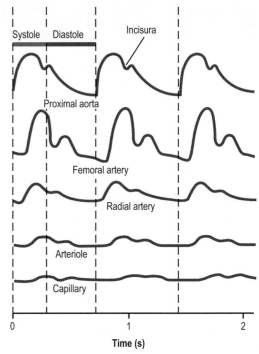

Fig. 2.76 Changes in the pulse pressure contour as the pulse travels towards smaller vessels.

superficial. Details of the temporal, facial and carotid pulse points in the head and neck can be found on pages 286 and 287; of the axillary, brachial, radial and ulnar pulse points in the upper limb on pages 398, 403, 416 and 427; and the femoral, popliteal, dorsalis pedis and tibial pulse points in the lower limb on pages 589, 610, 629 and 635.

As the pressure pulse travels into peripheral vessels, its shape changes due to damping in smaller arteries, arterioles and capillaries (Fig. 2.76); damping is due to the resistance to blood movement in the vessels as well as the compliance of the vessels.

Examining the pulse is a valuable clinical procedure providing important information regarding cardiac function (rate of contraction, rhythmicity) and the characteristics of the blood vessel wall. Pulse (and heart) rate varies with age: in the foetus, it is 150–180/min, at birth 130–140/min, at age 10 90/min and after puberty 72/min.

Pulse (heart) rate increases during exercise, pregnancy, emotional conditions, fever, anaemia, hypersecretion of catecholamines, and hyperthyroidism, and decreases during sleep, hypothermia, hypothyroidism and incomplete heart block.

CLINICAL PHYSIOLOGY: There are a number of abnormal arterial pulses which can be indicative of underlying pathologies. *Pulsus deficit* is when pulse rate is less than heart rate; it occurs in atrial fibrillation and when stroke volume is reduced. *Pulsus alternans* is when every second wave is reduced due to alternate variation in the force of ventricular contraction; it is common in severe myocardial disease, paroxysmal tachycardia and atrial fibrillation. An *anacrotic pulse* is characterised by a slow ascending limb when ejection of blood from the ventricle is slow; it is produced in aortic stenosis. A *thready (weak) pulse* occurs when stroke volume decreases or when there is severe vasoconstriction (severe haemorrhage, severe chills). *Pulsus paradoxus* is when the pulse alternates between being very strong and very weak; it is seen in cardiac tamponade. A *collapsing (water hammer) pulse* is seen in aortic regurgitation, patent ductus arteriosus and atrioventricular fistula (Fig. 2.77). A *Bisferiens pulse* is a combination of an anacrotic and collapsing pulses, both can be felt distinctly, which is seen in combined aortic stenosis (Fig. 2.77) and incompetency.

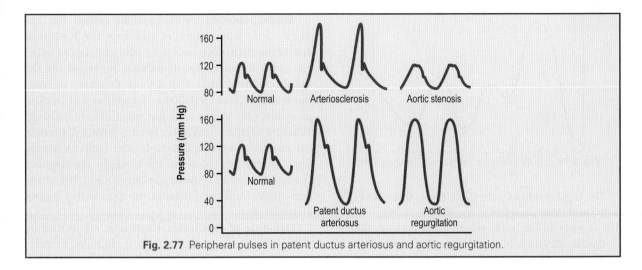

Fig. 2.77 Peripheral pulses in patent ductus arteriosus and aortic regurgitation.

Venous blood pressure. Venous blood pressure is the pressure exerted by the blood contained within the veins: that in the venae cavae and right atrium is central venous pressure and that in peripheral veins is peripheral venous pressure. The pressure is not the same in all veins, varying in different veins (internal jugular, 7 mm Hg; dorsal venous arch, 13 mm Hg) and from central (superior vena cava, 5 mm Hg) to peripheral (antecubital vein, 7 mm Hg) veins; it is less in parts of the body above the heart and more in parts below. Venous pressure is altered in both physiological and pathological conditions.

Physiological variation in venous blood pressure. Venous pressure increases when moving from standing to lying supine; tilting the body; forced expiration (Valsalva manoeuvre); the contraction of abdominal and limb muscles; the effect of gravity during prolonged standing or travelling; and excitement.

Pathological variation in venous blood pressure. Venous pressure increases with low cardiac output; congestive heart failure; venous obstruction; failure of the heart valves; muscle paralysis; immobilisation of a body part; and renal failure. It decreases in severe haemorrhage and surgical shock.

Regulation of venous blood pressure. A number of factors regulate venous blood pressure, these being left ventricular pressure, right atrial pressure, general and peripheral resistance, volume of venous blood, gravity and posture.

Left ventricular pressure forces blood through the systemic system; venous pressure is directly proportional to left ventricular pressure.

Right atrial pressure determines the volume of venous return.

General resistance: Venous pressure is directly proportional to resistance, which can be due to extravascular factors, such as compression of the subclavian vein as it passes over the 1st rib; veins of the neck when standing erect; abdominal veins by increased intra-abdominal pressure; veins passing between or through muscles.

Peripheral resistance: Venous pressure is inversely proportional to peripheral resistance.

Volume of venous blood: Venous pressure is directly proportional to the volume of blood in the venous system.

Gravity and posture: The weight of the column of blood in veins influences venous return. In prolonged standing pooling of blood in the legs leads to increased venous pressure; during movement the pressure decreases as blood is pumped towards the heart by muscle action.

Venous pulse. The venous pulse reflects the transmission of pressure changes from the right atrium to the larger veins (jugular) near the heart. Observations of the venous pulse are an integral part of physical examination as it reflects pressures and haemodynamic events in the right atrium; the venous pulse can be used to determine the rate of right atrial contraction.

CLINICAL PHYSIOLOGY: The inspection of the jugular venous pulse provides valuable information about the cardiac cycle. To observe pulsations of the internal jugular vein, tilt the individual upwards (head up) to 45 degrees; in individuals with increased venous pressure, tilting should be increased. The individual should relax the neck muscles so that the pulsations can be observed directly or when passing a light across the skin over the internal jugular vein.

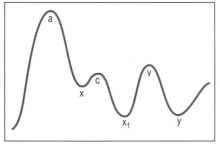

Fig. 2.78 Jugular venous pulse tracing (phlebogram).

The jugular venous pulse wave shows three peaks ('a', 'c', 'v') and three troughs ('x', 'x₁', 'y') (Fig. 2.78).

The *'a' wave* is due to the rise in atrial pressure during systole; elevation of the 'a' wave occurs in tricuspid stenosis and pulmonary hypertension. A giant 'a' wave with an abrupt downward deflection occurs in complete heart block, paroxysmal atrioventricular nodal tachycardia and ventricular tachycardia.

The *'x' wave* is due to the fall in atrial pressure and coincides with atrial diastole and the start of ventricular systole; the 'x' wave appears abnormal in atrial fibrillation, cardiac tamponade and constrictive pericarditis.

The *'c' wave* is due to the rise in atrial pressure during isometric contraction; during this period the tricuspid valve bulges into the right atrium increasing its pressure slightly.

The *'x₁' wave* is due to the fall in atrial pressure during ejection of blood into the right ventricle.

The *'v' wave* is due to the rise in atrial pressure as the right atrium starts to fill during atrial diastole (isometric relaxation); it becomes abnormal in tricuspid incompetence.

The *'y' wave* denotes the fall in atrial pressure due to opening of the tricuspid valve; it appears during rapid and slow filling periods. The wave becomes abnormal in tricuspid regurgitation and constrictive pericarditis.

> **CLINICAL PHYSIOLOGY:** An elevated jugular venous pulse indicates a rise in right ventricular pressure, occurring in bradycardia, pericardial effusion, constrictive pericarditis, tricuspid stenosis and pulmonary hypertension.

> **CLINICAL PHYSIOLOGY:** Kussmaul's sign is distension of the jugular veins during inspiration; it is also present in cardiac tamponade, constrictive pericarditis, restrictive cardiomyopathy, right ventricular infarction and mediastinal tumour.

Microcirculation and the capillary system. The capillaries arise from arterioles and form the functional area of the circulatory system, i.e., the exchange of water, cell nutrients and cell waste between the blood and the tissues. Although narrow and short; they have an enormous surface area (500–700 m²); capillaries lie in close proximity (20–30 μm) to all functional cells of the body. Where a capillary originates from a terminal arteriole (metarteriole) a precapillary sphincter (smooth muscle fibre) controls the blood to the tissue by opening and closing the entrance to the capillary (Fig. 2.79); at the same time, local conditions in the tissues also control arteriolar diameter.

Structure of capillaries. Capillaries are formed by a single layer of endothelial cells surrounded by pericytes (Fig. 2.80), which do not have a muscular coat; however, they can actively alter their diameter in response to nervous, hormonal, chemical and physical stimuli.

Capillary endothelial cells are thin, flattened, nucleated polygonal cells, with adjacent cells surrounded by a thin basement membrane; intercellular clefts (pores) between adjacent cells allow several substances to pass through the cell wall. The clefts are interrupted by short ridges of protein attachments holding the endothelium together but allowing fluid to move freely through it. Also present within endothelial cells are small vesicles (caveolae) thought to play a role in endocytosis and transcytosis of macromolecules across endothelial cells; some caveolae may coalesce forming channels through the cell. The total thickness of the capillary wall is 0.5 μm, with the diameter of the lumen being 4–9 μm, just sufficient for red and other blood cells to squeeze through.

> **APPLIED PHYSIOLOGY:** In some organs, the intercellular clefts/junctions have special characteristics to meet the needs of the organ. In the *brain,* the junctions are mainly tight permitting only very small molecules (water, oxygen, carbon dioxide) into or out of the tissue. In the *liver,* the junctions are wide open allowing almost all dissolved substances of the plasma (including plasma proteins) into the tissues. The junctions of *gastrointestinal capillary membranes* are midway between those in muscle and liver. In the *glomerular capillaries of the kidney,* numerous small oval openings (fenestrae) penetrate all the way through allowing large amounts of small molecules and ionic substances, but not the large plasma proteins, to filter through the glomeruli without passing through the intercellular clefts.

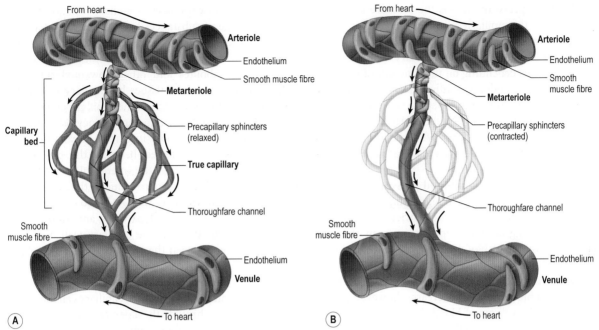

Fig. 2.79 The capillary bed: the precapillary sphincters and metarterioles are open (A) and closed (B) controlling blood flow through the capillary bed.

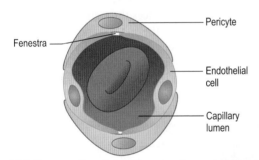

Fig. 2.80 Cross section of a capillary showing endothelial cells, the intercellular cleft and pericytes.

Pericytes (mural cells/Rouget cells) extend long cytoplasmic processes which wrap around the endothelial cells; they are important in remodelling and maintenance of the capillary system. They are contractile and secrete vasoactive substances, growth factors, extracellular matrix and components of the basement membrane; they are also involved in the regulation of blood flow through endothelial junctions in inflammation.

Blood flow in capillaries (vasomotion). Blood flow in capillaries is not continuous but intermittent due to the intermittent contraction of the metarterioles and precapillary sphincters. The most important factor regulating blood flow (opening and closing of the metarterioles and precapillary sphincters) is the concentration of oxygen in the tissues. When tissue oxygen usage is high decreasing tissue oxygen concentrations, the intermittent periods of capillary blood flow occur more frequently, with the duration of each period lasting longer enabling capillary blood to carry increased quantities of oxygen and other nutrients to the tissue.

CLINICAL PHYSIOLOGY: Capillary refill time (CRT) is the time taken for colour to return to an external capillary bed after pressure has been applied to a pink area of skin in an extremity (or the sternum/forehead if the limb is cold) sufficient to cause blanching: the limb should be held above the level of the heart. When the pressure is released, the time taken for blood to return to the area is noted. In the newborn and children, refill time should not exceed 3 seconds. In adults under 65, normal refill times are 2 seconds for males and 3 seconds for females; in the elderly, refill time should not exceed 4 seconds. A prolonged refill time may be a sign of circulatory shock, decreased peripheral perfusion secondary to hypovolaemia, peripheral artery disease or dehydration. The test is influenced by many external factors and should not be relied upon as a universal diagnostic tool.

Capillary pressure. This is the pressure exerted by the blood in the capillaries; it is responsible for the exchange of various substances between the blood and the interstitial fluid through the capillary wall. Capillary pressure varies depending on the function of the organ or region of the body; generally, it is 30–32 mm Hg at the arterial end and 15 mm Hg at the venous end. In the kidneys, capillary pressure is 60 mm Hg, being responsible for glomerular filtration, while in the lungs, it is 7 mm Hg to favour the exchange of gases between the blood and alveoli.

Regulation of capillary blood pressure. The arterioles have an important role in regulating pressure in the capillaries. When the arterioles constrict their resistance increases raising arterial blood pressure; at the same time, the volume of blood flowing into the capillaries decreases causing a fall in capillary pressure.

When the arterioles dilate their resistance decreases and arterial blood pressure decreases; however, it is the increase in the volume of blood flowing into the capillaries which increases capillary pressure.

Capillary oncotic pressure. The capillary membrane is permeable to all substances except plasma proteins, which remain in the capillary and exert pressure (oncotic (colloidal osmotic) pressure); it has an important role in filtration across capillary membranes, especially in renal glomerular capillaries. Normal oncotic pressure is 25 mm Hg, of which albumin exerts 70%.

Function of capillaries. Capillary function involves the exchange of substances between the blood and tissues; oxygen, nutrients and other essential substances enter the tissues from capillary blood, while carbon dioxide, metabolites and other unwanted substances are removed from the tissues by capillary blood. This exchange of materials across the capillary endothelium occurs by diffusion, filtration and pinocytosis.

Diffusion is the most important means by which substances are transferred between the plasma and interstitial fluid through the intercellular clefts in the capillary wall; diffusion occurs due to the pressure gradients across the capillary wall. As blood flows along the capillary lumen dissolved particles and water diffuse back and forth through the capillary wall, with continual mixing between the interstitial fluid and plasma (Fig. 2.81).

Lipid-soluble substances (e.g., oxygen, carbon dioxide) diffuse directly through the capillary cell membrane without going through the intercellular clefts. Water-soluble, non-lipid-soluble substances (e.g., water molecules, sodium ions, chloride ions, glucose, urea) pass through the intercellular clefts.

Filtration of substances through the capillary endothelium depends on the net filtration pressure, being the balance between the hydrostatic pressure in the capillaries, which tends to force fluid and its dissolved substances through the pores into the interstitial space,

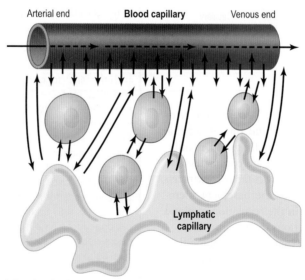

Fig. 2.81 Diffusion of dissolved substances and fluid molecules between the capillary and interstitial fluid spaces.

and (colloid) osmotic pressure caused by the plasma proteins, which tends to cause fluid movement from the interstitial spaces into the capillary blood. Osmotic pressure normally prevents significant loss of fluid volume from the blood into the interstitial spaces.

Also important is the lymphatic system, which returns the small amount of fluid and excess protein that leak from the blood into the interstitial spaces, back to the circulation. Details of the lymphatic system can be found on page 160.

Pinocytosis is the packaging of large molecules as vesicles in the capillary endothelial cells; these are then transported across the endothelial membrane.

Interstitium and interstitial fluid. The spaces between cells of the body are collectively known as the interstitium, with the fluid contained within these spaces being interstitial fluid. The interstitium contains two major types of solid structures: collagen fibre bundles, which extend long distances and provide most of the tensional strength of the tissue, and thin coiled molecules of proteoglycan filaments, which form a mat of fine reticular fibres (Fig. 2.82).

The interstitial fluid is derived by filtration and diffusion from the capillaries; it contains almost the same constituents as plasma, except in lower concentrations. The fluid is mainly trapped in the spaces between the proteoglycan filaments, giving it the characteristics of a gel. Trapped within the gel are small free fluid vesicles and occasionally small rivulets of free fluid; the amount of free fluid in normal tissues is usually less than 1% of the total volume of fluid.

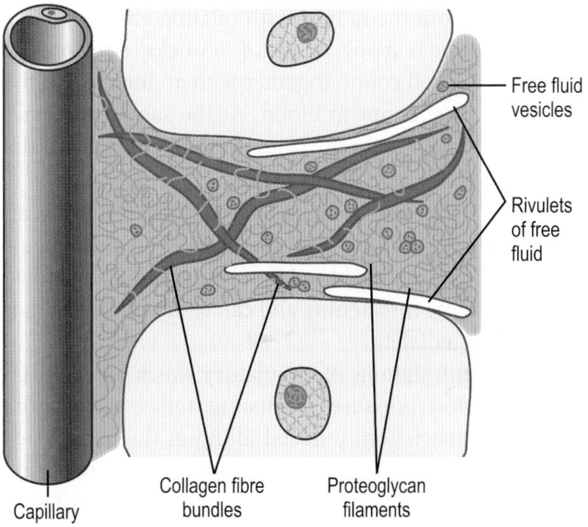

CLINICAL PHYSIOLOGY: In oedema the small pockets and rivulets of free fluid expand until 50% or more of the free fluid becomes freely flowing fluid independent of the proteoglycan filaments; it causes swelling of the tissue. Intracellular oedema is an accumulation of fluid within cells; it can be due to malnutrition, poor metabolism or inflammation of the tissue. Extracellular oedema is the accumulation of fluid in the interstitium due to abnormal leakage of fluid from the capillaries or obstruction of lymphatic vessels preventing fluid returning to the blood. Conditions leading to extracellular oedema are heart failure due to failure to pump blood, low blood pressure and a low blood supply to the kidneys, pulmonary oedema is the accumulation of fluid in the pulmonary interstitium in left heart failure; renal disease due to failure of the kidneys to excrete water and electrolytes (sodium); decreased amounts of plasma protein due to decreased colloidal osmotic pressure, it occurs in malnutrition, liver and renal disease, burns and inflammation; lymphatic obstruction (lymphoedema); and increased endothelial permeability following burns, inflammation, trauma, allergic and immunologic reactions.

Haemorrhage. Haemorrhage is the loss of blood from the circulation. It can be accidental (road and industrial accidents), rupture of capillaries (common in the brain and heart during cardiovascular disease), internal (from rupture of blood vessels supplying viscera) and postpartum (excess bleeding immediately following childbirth).

In **acute haemorrhage,** there is a sudden loss of a large volume of blood, which can lead to hypovolemic shock (page 159). In **chronic haemorrhage,** the blood loss occurs over a long period of time, either from internal or external bleeding, which can lead to anaemia. Following haemorrhage compensatory reactions develop to enable the body to deal with the blood loss, some being immediate and others delayed.

Immediate compensatory effects.

Cardiovascular system: The reduced blood volume decreases venous return, ventricular filling and cardiac output; blood pressure also falls in severe haemorrhage. If blood loss is slow, arterial pressure tends not to be affected, if it is, it is quickly restored.

Fig. 2.82 Proteoglycan filaments fill the spaces between the collagen fibre bundles in the interstitium. Free fluid vesicles and small amounts of free fluid as rivulets occasionally occur.

Free fluid vesicles

Rivulets of free fluid

Capillary

Collagen fibre bundles

Proteoglycan filaments

The loss of 350–500 mL of blood (slow/mild haemorrhage) is accompanied by a slight decrease in blood pressure which soon returns to normal due to: stimulation of the carotid and aortic baroreceptors; an increase in vasomotor tone (except in the heart and brain); vasoconstriction increasing peripheral resistance; reflex constriction of veins; and vasoconstriction in the skin, liver and spleen.

With severe loss of blood (1500–2000 mL) arterial blood pressure drops significantly due to decreased venous return and stroke volume. There is reflex tachycardia increasing the metabolic products in the myocardium, which cause coronary vasodilation.

Skin: Assumes a grey pallor due to the decreased cutaneous blood flow, increased deoxygenation of the blood and large amounts of reduced haemoglobin accumulation; cyanosis may develop in some areas. The skin also feels cold due to the reduced blood flow: sweating is also reduced.

Tissue fluid: Capillary pressure is reduced, due to arteriolar constriction, resulting in tissue fluid entering the capillaries, leading to haemodilution.

Kidneys: Glomerular filtration is reduced due to constriction of both the afferent and efferent arterioles, with a reduction in urine output; urea blood levels increase leading to uraemia. Severe haemorrhage damages the renal tubules resulting in acute renal failure.

Renin secretion: Following blood loss, the kidney increases renin secretion, with the subsequent formation of angiotensin II, which in turn helps to restore blood pressure through generalised vasoconstriction. The release of aldosterone from the adrenal cortex leads to the retention of sodium, which helps increase blood pressure.

Secretion of antidiuretic hormone: This is released following haemorrhage promoting water retention, leading to a restoration of osmolality and the volume of extracellular fluid.

Secretion of catecholamines: Increased sympathetic activity leads to the release of catecholamines, which help restore blood pressure through vasoconstriction.

Respiration: The decrease in venous return, cardiac output and velocity of blood flow causes stagnant hypoxia, which stimulates the chemoreceptors to increase respiratory rate. The released catecholamines also increase respiratory movements.

Nervous system: Increased sympathetic activity causes vasodilation in the brain; blood flow to the brain tends not to be affected due to autoregulation. However, in severe haemorrhage, cardiac output decreases and blood pressure falls, autoregulation fails to cope with the hypotension leading to a reduction in blood flow and fainting. When the blood supply to the brain is severely affected due to hypoxia, cerebral ischaemia of the brain tissues develops within 5 minutes; this can cause irreversible brain damage.

Delayed compensatory effects. If the haemorrhage is not severe, delayed compensatory reactions occur in an attempt to help restore blood volume, blood pressure and blood flow to different regions.

Restoration of plasma volume: During haemorrhage plasma volume increases as tissue fluid enters the blood due to low capillary pressure, resulting in haemodilution and a decrease in the concentration of plasma proteins and haemoglobin; movement of fluid from the tissues continues well after the haemorrhage has finished.

Restoration of plasma protein: Reserve proteins stored in the liver are mobilised within a few hours following haemorrhage; the liver also starts synthesising plasma proteins. The restoration of plasma proteins occurs within 3–4 days, helping to retain fluid transported from the tissues to blood.

Restoration of red blood cell count and haemoglobin content: Hypoxia stimulates the secretion of erythropoietin from the kidneys, stimulating erythropoiesis in red bone marrow; it takes 4–6 weeks to restore the red blood cell count, together with an increase in the reticulocyte count in blood. At the same time, haemoglobin content returns to normal, especially if the diet contains iron and proteins.

Shock. Circulatory shock develops when there is an inadequate blood flow throughout the body, the major cause being decreased blood flow due to reduced cardiac output; it is life threatening and can result in death if not treated immediately.

The manifestations of circulatory shock are reduced arterial blood pressure producing reflex tachycardia and vasoconstriction; reduced filling of the heart leading to decreased stroke volume and systolic pressure, with a reduced pulse pressure (<20 mm Hg) and feeble pulse; hypoxia due to reduced blood flow velocity; pale cold skin, with cyanosis of the ear lobes and fingertips; reduced glomerular filtration rate and urinary output;

increased myocardial metabolism resulting in acidosis, leading to decreased myocardial efficiency and pumping action; and reduced blood flow through organs, which in the brain can result in ischaemia, fainting, irreversible brain damage and death.

Stages of circulatory shock

First (compensatory/non-progressive) stage is when blood loss is less than 10% of total volume and blood pressure decreases only slightly. Regulatory (baroreceptor, renal, antidiuretic) mechanisms, involving negative feedback, successfully restore normal blood pressure and blood flow throughout the body and the individual recovers.

Second (progressive/decompensated) stage occurs when shock is severe, positive feedback develops so that regulatory mechanisms are not adequate to compensate. With immediate and appropriate treatment this stage can be reversed.

During this stage, low blood pressure is not sufficient to maintain blood flow to the myocardium, which starts to deteriorate due to a lack of oxygen and nutrition; toxic substances released by the tissues also suppress the myocardium. The reduced blood flow also causes suppression of the vasomotor and sympathetic systems leading to a further fall in blood pressure with thrombosis occurring in the capillaries, increasing permeability allowing fluid in the blood to pass into the interstitial space. As the tissues begin to deteriorate, severe symptoms appear with shock being irreversible.

Third (irreversible/refractory) stage occurs prior to collapse; there is a dramatic fall in blood pressure, leading to death, irrespective of treatment, due to cerebral ischaemia.

Types and causes of circulatory shock

Hypovolemic (cold) shock is due to decreased blood volume and occurs when there is an acute loss of 10%–15% of total blood volume. There is a decrease in cardiac output, low blood pressure, a thin thready pulse, pale cold skin, increased respiratory rate and lethargy/restlessness. It can occur following haemorrhage (acute and chronic), trauma (crush and reperfusion injuries), surgery, burns and dehydration.

Vasogenic (distributive/low resistance) shock occurs due to an inadequate blood supply to the tissues, with an increase in vascular capacity. It can occur following sudden loss of vasomotor tone (neurogenic shock), anaphylaxis (anaphylactic shock) and sepsis (septic shock).

Cardiogenic shock is due to cardiac disease and can occur in arrhythmia (especially those resulting in reduced cardiac output), depressed myocardial activity due to ischaemia, and congestive cardiac disease.

Obstructive shock can occur when there is an obstruction to blood flow through the circulatory system, due to myocardial tumours, cardiac tamponade and pulmonary embolism.

Treatment for circulatory shock. This is determined by the cause of the shock. In hypovolemic shock, transfusion of whole blood is done, except in burns shock, in which plasma transfusion is useful. Plasma transfusion is also used when there is loss of plasma; plasma substitutes (plasma expanders, concentrated human serum albumin, hypertonic solutions) can be used when plasma is not available.

Sympatheticomimetic drugs (adrenaline, noradrenaline) can be used in neurogenic and anaphylactic shock to restore blood pressure by vasoconstriction; they should not be used for prolonged periods as they can induce severe myocardial activity. Dopamine is used in traumatic and cardiogenic shock. In severe conditions, glucocorticoids and oxygen therapy can be administered.

In neurogenic and haemorrhagic shock, raising the lower limbs/feet increases venous return, cardiac output and cerebral blood flow due to the increased pressure exerted by the abdominal viscera; it should not be used for prolonged periods as it could compromise ventilation.

Heart (cardiac) failure. The inability of the heart to pump sufficient blood to all parts of the body; it can involve the right, left or both ventricles and can be acute or chronic. As both sides of the heart are part of the same overall circuit when one side begins to fail, it often leads to increased strain on, and eventual failure, of the other side. The main clinical manifestations depend on which side of the heart is most affected; left ventricular failure is more common than right, because of the greater workload of the left ventricle.

Compensatory mechanisms. With acute heart failure, there is little time to make compensatory changes, but in chronic heart failure changes ocurr which attempt to maintain cardiac output and tissue perfusion, particularly of the vital organs. In chronic heart failure, there is hypertrophy of cardiac muscle and enlargement of the chambers of the heart, a decreased renal blood flow, which activates the renin-angiotensin-aldosterone system leading to water and salt retention; this increases blood volume and cardiac workload. However, the vaso-constrictor effect of angiotensin II increases peripheral resistance putting additional strain on the heart.

Signs and symptoms of heart failure. Heart failure is accompanied by fatigue and weakness, a rapid and irregular heart rate, shortness of breath, fluid retention and weight gain, loss of appetite, nausea and vomiting, cough and chest pain (caused by myocardial infarction).

Acute heart failure. The sudden and rapid onset of heart failure in which the supply of oxygenated blood to the tissues is abruptly reduced with no time for compensatory mechanisms to occur. If the brain's vital centres are starved of oxygen death may follow; survival of the acute phase may result in myocardial damage leading to chronic heart failure.

Causes include myocardial infarction; pulmonary embolism; life-threatening arrhythmias impairing the pumping action of the heart; rupture of a heart chamber or cusp; and severe malignant hypertension.

Chronic heart failure. The gradual development of heart failure, often without symptoms because of the compensatory changes which ocurr: when further compensation is not possible myocardial function gradually declines. Underlying causes include degenerative heart changes with increasing age and many chronic conditions (anaemia, lung disease, hypertension, cardiac disease).

Right-sided (congestive cardiac) failure occurs when the pressure developed in the right ventricle is insufficient to push blood through the lungs; this may be due to increased vascular resistance in the lungs or weakness of the myocardium. When further compensation is not possible, the right atrium and venae cavae become congested with blood following which there is congestion throughout the whole of the venous system; organs affected first are the liver, spleen and kidneys, followed by oedema of the limbs and excess fluid in the peritoneal cavity (ascites).

Left-sided (left ventricular) failure occurs when the pressure developed in the left ventricle is not sufficient to force blood into the aorta; the ventricle is unable to pump out all of the blood it receives. This leads to dilation of the left atrium and an increase in pulmonary blood pressure, followed by a rise in blood pressure in the right side of the heart and gradual systemic venous congestion. Causes include ischaemic heart disease; hypertension; and mitral and/or

aortic valve disease preventing effective emptying of the chamber.

Lymphatic system. The lymphatic system provides an accessory route through which fluid can flow from the interstitial spaces into the blood. Lymphatics can carry proteins and large particulate matter, which cannot be removed by absorption, from the tissue spaces directly back to the bloodstream; this is an essential function. It also carries bacteria and cell debris from damaged tissues, which can then be filtered out and destroyed by the lymph nodes.

Lymph. A clear yellowish watery fluid similar in composition to plasma, but with only a small amount of plasma proteins (2–5 g/dL), and identical to interstitial fluid. It contains lymphocytes which circulate in the lymphatic system allowing them to patrol all regions of the body. The lymphatic system is a major route for the absorption of nutrients from the gastrointestinal tract, particularly the absorption of nearly all fats. In the small intestine, lacteals absorb fat into the lymphatics giving the lymph a milky appearance (chyle).

Function: Lymph has a number of important roles, including returning proteins from the interstitium to the blood; redistributing fluid within the body; removal of bacteria, toxins and other foreign bodies; maintenance of the structure and functional integrity of the tissues (obstruction to lymph flow affects the myocardium, nephrons and hepatic cells); a route for fat absorption; and the transport of lymphocytes in immunity.

Rate of lymph flow: This is determined by anything that increases interstitial fluid pressure, including elevated capillary hydrostatic pressure, decreased plasma colloid osmotic pressure, increased interstitial fluid colloid osmotic pressure, and increased permeability of the capillary wall. These all change the balance of fluid exchange at the blood-capillary boundary leading to increased interstitial fluid volume, interstitial fluid pressure and thus lymph flow.

When a collecting lymphatic or larger lymph vessel becomes stretched with fluid, the smooth muscle in its wall automatically contracts, with each segment between successive valves acting as a separate pump. In the thoracic duct, the lymphatic pump can generate pressures as high as 50–100 mm Hg, at a rate of 100 mL/h.

Lymph is also moved by intermittent compression of lymph vessels by contraction of surrounding muscles; movement of the body; pulsations of adjacent arteries;

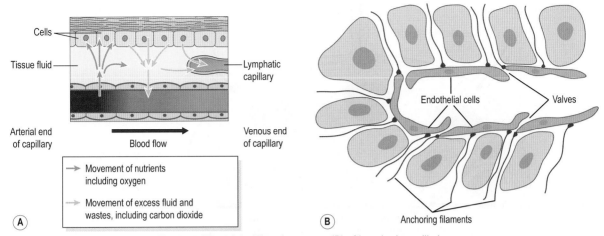

Cells

Tissue fluid

Lymphatic capillary

Arterial end of capillary

Blood flow

Venous end of capillary

→ Movement of nutrients including oxygen

⇢ Movement of excess fluid and wastes, including carbon dioxide

Ⓐ

Endothelial cells

Valves

Anchoring filaments

Ⓑ

Fig. 2.83 The origin (A) and structure (B) of lymphatic capillaries.

and compression of the tissues from objects outside the body. These may become very active during exercise and can increase lymph flow by 10- to 30-fold; during rest, lymph flow is sluggish and may be zero.

Lymph capillaries. Lymph capillaries originate as blind-ending tubes in the interstitial spaces (Fig. 2.83A), with no basal lamina and the endothelial cells attached to the surrounding tissues by anchoring filaments (Fig. 2.83B). At the junctions of adjacent endothelial cells, the edge of one cell overlaps the edge of the adjacent cell with the overlapping edge facing inwards forming a small valve that opens to the interior of the capillary. Interstitial fluid can push the valve open and flow directly into the capillary, backflow is prevented by closure of the flap valve. Although lymphatic capillaries have a similar structure as blood capillaries (single layer of endothelial cells), because of the overlapping of the endothelial cells, their walls are more permeable to all interstitial fluid constituents, including proteins and cell debris.

Almost all tissues have special lymph channels that drain excess fluid directly from the interstitial spaces. Exceptions are superficial skin, central nervous system, endomysium of muscles, bone and cornea of the eye. Nevertheless, these tissues have minute interstitial channels (prelymphatics) through which interstitial fluid can flow, which eventually empties into lymphatic vessels and then back to the blood: in the brain, lymph flows into the cerebrospinal fluid and then back to the blood.

Larger lymph vessels. These usually run with the arteries and veins, with walls of a similar thickness to those of small veins and the same layers (inner endothelium,

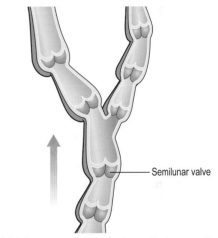

Semilunar valve

Fig. 2.84 Structure of lymphatic capillaries, a collecting lymphatic and lymphatic valves.

middle layer of smooth muscle and elastic tissue, outer fibrous covering); they contain numerous valves to ensure unidirectional lymph flow towards the thorax (Fig. 2.84).

As lymph vessels join together, they become larger and larger, eventually forming two large ducts, the thoracic duct and right lymphatic duct which empty into the left and right brachiocephalic veins, respectively. Details of the thoracic duct and right lymph duct can be found on pages 88 and 90, respectively.

Lymph nodes. These lie, often in groups, along the length of larger lymph vessels; they are oval (bean-shaped) and vary considerably in size. Lymph usually

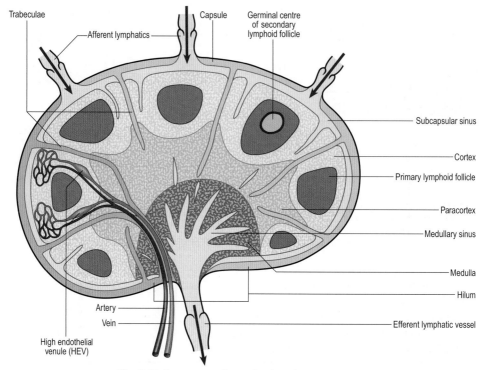

Fig. 2.85 Structure and organisation of a lymph node.

drains through 8–10 lymph nodes before returning to the venous system. The distribution of lymph nodes in the thorax is given on page 95, the head and neck on pages 238 and 290, the upper limb on page 400, the abdomen, pelvis and perineum on page 557, and the lower limb on page 589.

Structure: Lymph nodes have an outer connective tissue capsule which dips down into the substance of the node forming partitions (trabeculae), with the substance consisting of reticular and lymphatic tissue containing lymphocytes and macrophages: the whole being arranged in layers (Fig. 2.85). The paracortex contains T lymphocytes (T cells), as does the medulla together with B lymphocytes (B cells) and macrophages; the cortex consists of primary and secondary lymphoid follicles, also containing B cells and macrophages. When some antigens reach the lymph nodes, cells of the primary follicle proliferate in the germinal centres; after proliferation, the primary follicles become secondary follicles.

Several (1–5) afferent lymph vessels enter a lymph node, dividing into small channels through which lymph passes to reach and circulate through the cortex, paracortex and medulla, before leaving the node via a single efferent vessel (Fig. 2.85).

Function: Lymph is filtered by the reticular and lymphatic tissues as it passes through the node to remove particulate matter (bacteria, dead and live phagocytes containing ingested microbes, malignant tumour cells, worn out and damaged tissue cells, inhaled particles); macrophages and antibodies destroy organic materials. Some inhaled inorganic particles cannot be destroyed by phagocytosis; these remain inside the macrophages either killing them or causing no harm. Material not filtered out and dealt with in one lymph node passes onto successive nodes so that by the time lymph enters the blood it has usually been cleared of foreign matter and cell debris.

Activated T and B cells multiply in lymph nodes, with the antibodies produced by sensitised B cells entering the lymph and blood leaving the node.

CLINICAL ANATOMY: Incomplete phagocytosis of bacteria can stimulate inflammation and enlargement of lymph nodes (lymphadenopathy).

Spleen. Similar in structure to a large lymph node, it lies in the left hypochondriac region (upper left

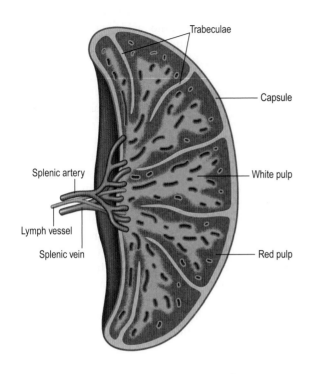

Trabeculae

Capsule

Splenic artery

White pulp

Lymph vessel

Splenic vein

Red pulp

Fig. 2.86 Cross section through the spleen.

quadrant) of the abdomen (page 459). The spleen acts primarily as a blood filter by removing old red blood cells, as well as playing an important role in the immune system. It holds a reservoir of blood, which can be valuable in haemorrhagic shock, and also recycles iron.

Structure: It is slightly oval in shape, with the hilum on the lower medial border; it is enclosed in a fibroelastic capsule, which, as in lymph nodes, dips into the organ forming trabeculae (Fig. 2.86). The cellular material (splenic pulp) consists of lymphocytes and macrophages and lies between the trabeculae; red pulp is suffused with blood, while white pulp consists of areas of lymphatic tissue (sleeves of lymphocytes and macrophages) surrounding blood vessels.

Blood passing through the spleen flows in sinusoids, which have pores between the endothelial cells, allowing it to come into close association with the splenic pulp.

Function: Old and abnormal red blood cells are mainly destroyed in the spleen, with the breakdown products (bilirubin, iron) transported to the liver; leukocytes, platelets and bacteria are phagocytosed.

> **CLINICAL ANATOMY:** The spleen has no afferent lymphatics, so it is not exposed to diseases spread by the lymph.

The spleen contains up to 350 mL of blood; in response to sympathetic stimulation (e.g., haemorrhage), it can rapidly return most of this to the circulation.

T and B cells in the spleen are activated by the presence of antigens.

With the liver, the spleen is an important site of foetal blood cell production; when there is a great need for more blood cells in adults, the spleen fulfils this role.

> **CLINICAL PHYSIOLOGY:** Enlargement of the spleen (splenomegaly) is usually secondary to other conditions: infections, in which the red pulp becomes congested with blood and an accumulation of phagocytes and plasma cells (common primary infections are tuberculosis, typhoid fever, malaria, infectious mononucleosis); circulatory disorders, when blood flow through the liver is impeded, as in cirrhosis due to fibrosis or portal venous congestion due to right-side heart failure; blood diseases (haemolytic and macrocytic anaemia, polycythaemia, chronic myeloid leukaemia); and tumours arising from the infiltration of malignant cells as in chronic leukaemia, Hodgkin disease and Hodgkin lymphoma.

> **CLINICAL PHYSIOLOGY:** Splenomegaly itself may cause some blood disorders, especially in portal hypertension, excessive and premature haemolysis of red cells or phagocytosis of normal white cells and platelets, leading to marked anaemia, leukopenia and thrombocytopenia.

Thymus gland. Lying in the upper part of the mediastinum the thymus consists of two lobes and an intervening isthmus enclosed in a fibrous capsule, which sends septa into the substance dividing it into lobules; each lobule consists of an irregular branching framework of epithelial cells and lymphocytes.

The lymphocytes originate from stem cells in red bone marrow, which on entering the thymus develop into activated T cells. After processing in the thymus mature T cells are produced which can distinguish 'self' tissue from foreign tissue, as well as providing each T cell with the ability to react to a single specific antigen. On leaving the thymus some T cells enter lymphoid tissue, while the remainder circulate in the bloodstream.

T cell production, although most prolific in youth, continues throughout life, probably from a resident population of thymic stem cells. In adolescence, the thymus begins to shrink so that with increasing age the effectiveness of the T cell response to antigens declines.

> **CLINICAL PHYSIOLOGY:** Enlargement of the thymus is associated with some autoimmune diseases (thyrotoxicosis, Addison's disease). Most patients with myasthenia gravis also have either thymic hyperplasia (majority) or thymoma (minority).

Mucosa-associated lymphoid tissue. At strategic locations throughout the body (gastrointestinal, respiratory and genitourinary tracts) are collections of lymphoid tissue where the body is exposed to the external environment. They are not enclosed by a capsule but contain B and T cells, which have migrated from bone marrow and the thymus. Although they have no afferent vessels, do not filter lymph and therefore are not exposed to diseases spread by the lymph, they are important in the early detection of diseases/infections.

The main groups of mucosa-associated lymphoid tissue (MALT) are in the tonsils (page 328) where they will destroy swallowed and inhaled antigens, and in the small intestine (aggregated lymphoid follicles/Peyer patches) (page 469) which intercept swallowed antigens.

Blood

Blood is a fluid connective tissue circulating continuously around the body transporting oxygen from the lungs; carbon dioxide from all tissues to the lungs; nutrients (glucose, amino acids, fatty acids, glycerol, vitamins) from the digestive system to different parts of the body for growth and energy production; waste products (urea, creatinine, uric acid) to the kidneys; hormones from endocrine glands to their target organ/tissue; heat from metabolically active tissues (skeletal muscle, liver) for distribution around the body, contributing to the maintenance of core body temperature; protective substances; and clotting factors (fibrinogen). It is always in motion due to the pumping action of the heart, thereby providing a more or less constant environment for the body's cells. The blood also aids in the regulation of water balance, acid-base balance (plasma proteins and haemoglobin act as buffers) and body temperature, the storage of substances (glucose, sodium, potassium) constantly required by the tissues, and defence (white blood cells).

Blood volume and the concentration of its many constituents are kept within narrow limits by homeostatic mechanisms (Table 2.8).

Blood comprises 7% of body weight in males, slightly less in females and significantly greater in children, which gradually decreases to adult levels. The fluid part of blood is the plasma, in which different types of blood cells are suspended: plasma usually constitutes 55% of blood volume, with the

TABLE 2.8 Normal Values of Some Important Constituents in Blood

Substance	Normal Value
Glucose	100–120 mg/dL
Creatinine	0.5–1.5 mg/dL
Cholesterol	Up to 200 mg/dL
Plasma proteins	6.4–8.3 g/dL
Bilirubin	0.5–1.5 mg/dL
Iron	50–150 µg/dL
Copper	100–200 mg/dL
Calcium	4.5–5.5 mEq/L (9–11 mg/dL)
Sodium	135–145 mEq/L
Potassium	3.5–5.0 mEq/L
Magnesium	1.5–2.0 mEq/L
Chloride	100–110 mEq/L
Bicarbonate	22–26 mEq/L

remaining 45% being the cell fraction. It is slightly alkaline with a pH between 7.35 and 7.45 under normal conditions. The specific gravity of whole blood is 1.052–1.061, with that of plasma being 1.092–1.101 and blood cells 1.022–1.026: it is five times more viscous than water due to the red blood cells and plasma proteins.

> **APPLIED PHYSIOLOGY:** The average volume of blood in a 70 kg adult male is 5 L and in adult females 4.5 L; in the newborn it is 450 mL reaching adult values by puberty.

Plasma

Plasma is the clear straw-coloured fluid portion minus its cellular elements. It constitutes 55% of the blood volume (about 5% of body weight). It is 90%–92% water and 10%–8% dissolved and suspended substances (plasma proteins, electrolytes, nutrients, waste products, hormones and enzymes, gases).

Plasma proteins. These include albumin, globulin, fibrinogen, and prothrombin which comprise some 7% of plasma and are normally retained in the blood. They are mainly responsible for creating the osmotic pressure of blood keeping plasma fluid within the circulation: plasma proteins (except immunoglobulins) are formed in the liver. A fall in plasma protein levels reduces osmotic pressure and fluid moves into the tissues (oedema).

Albumins: The most abundant of the plasma proteins (60% of total), whose main function is to maintain plasma osmotic pressure; they also act as carrier molecules for fatty acids, steroid hormones and some drugs.

Globulins: Their main functions are as antibodies (immunoglobulins) which bind to and neutralise foreign materials (antigens); transportation of some hormones (thyroxine by thyroglobulin) and mineral salts (iron by transferrin); and inhibition of some proteolytic enzymes (trypsin activity by α_2 macroglobulin).

Fibrinogen: Responsible for blood coagulation and plasma viscosity; without the clotting factors plasma is serum.

Prothrombin: Responsible for blood coagulation.

> **CLINICAL PHYSIOLOGY:** The concentration of all plasma proteins increases (hyperproteinaemia) in dehydration, haemolysis, acute infections (acute hepatitis, acute nephritis), respiratory distress syndrome, excess glucocorticoids, leukaemia, rheumatoid arthritis and alcoholism, while they decrease (hypoproteinaemia) in diarrhoea, haemorrhage, burns, pregnancy, malnutrition, prolonged starvation, liver cirrhosis and chronic infections (chronic hepatitis, chronic nephritis). An increase in albumins only (hyperalbuminaemia) occurs in dehydration, excess glucocorticoids and congestive heart failure, while a decrease (hypoalbuminaemia) occurs in malnutrition, liver cirrhosis, burns, hypothyroidism, nephrosis and excessive water intake. An increase in globulins only (hyperglobulinaemia) occurs in liver cirrhosis, chronic infections, nephrosis and rheumatoid arthritis, while a decrease (hypoglobulinaemia) occurs in emphysema, acute haemolytic anaemia, glomerulonephritis and hypogammaglobinaemia. The albumin/globulin ratio increases in hypothyroidism, excess glucocorticoids, hypogammaglobinaemia and a diet high in carbohydrates or protein; in contrast, it decreases in liver dysfunction and nephrosis. The concentration of fibrinogen increases in acute infections, rheumatoid arthritis, glomerulonephritis, myocardial infarction, stroke and trauma, while it decreases in liver dysfunction, and in anabolic steroid and phenobarbital use.

Cells

Blood contains three types of cells: red blood cells (erythrocytes), white blood cells (leukocytes) and platelets (thrombocytes). They are mainly synthesised in red bone marrow; however, some lymphocytes are produced in lymphoid tissue. In the newborn and children, red marrow is present in all bones; however, by age 20 red marrow is replaced by yellow (fat) marrow throughout the skeleton except in flat and irregular bones, and the epiphyses of long bones (page 33), with the main sites of production being the sternum, ribs, pelvis, skull and proximal epiphyses of the humerus and femur. Although the site of production of most blood cells is red bone marrow, 75% of it is involved in the production of leukocytes and 25% in the production of erythrocytes; the life span of leukocytes is between 1 and 10 days, while that of erythrocytes is 120 days, leukocytes, therefore, need to be produced more frequently.

In bone marrow, all blood cells are derived from pluripotent stem cells and go through several stages before entering the blood, with different types of blood cells following different lines of development (haemopoiesis) (Fig. 2.87).

There are significant differences between erythrocytes and leukocytes (Table 2.9).

Erythrocytes. Erythrocytes are the most abundant type of blood cells (99.8% of the total), being biconcave discs (with a size, mean diameter and thickness of 90 μ^3, 7 μm and 2.2 μm, respectively) with no nucleus or intracellular organelles. They have a thin central portion and thicker periphery; their shape increases the surface area for gas exchange, with the thin central part facilitating the fastest exchange of gases, as well as making them flexible enabling them to squeeze through narrow capillaries.

There are some 30 trillion red blood cells, and they constitute approximately 25% of the body's total cell count; about 1% of red blood cells (mainly older cells)

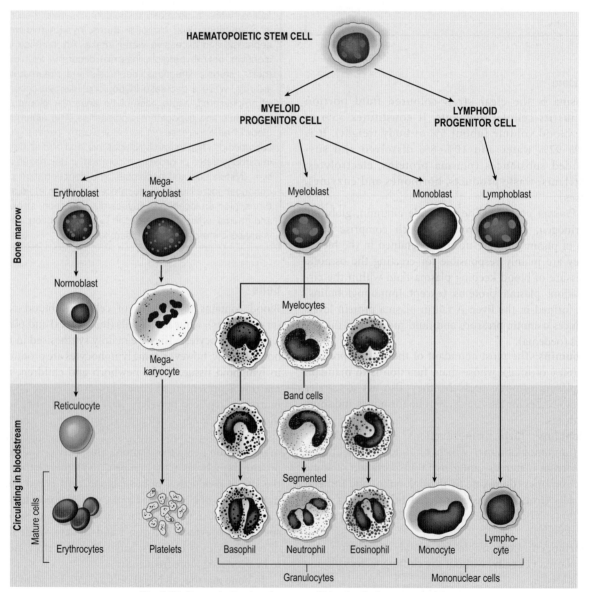

Fig. 2.87 Stages in the development of blood cells (haemopoiesis).

are destroyed each day. The development from stem cells to mature red blood cells (erythropoiesis) takes about 7 days, with reticulocytes released into the bloodstream which then mature into erythrocytes within a couple of days of being in the circulation.

Vitamin B_{12} and folic acid are needed for red blood cell synthesis, both being absorbed in the gastrointestinal tract; vitamin B_{12} must be bound to intrinsic factors for absorption to take place. Also necessary for haemoglobin formation are proteins of high biological value from which are derived amino acids for the synthesis of the protein part of haemoglobin (the haem); iron for the formation of the haem; copper for the absorption of iron from the gastrointestinal tract; cobalt and nickel for the utilisation of iron during haemoglobin formation; and vitamins (vitamin C, riboflavin, nicotinic acid, pyridoxine) for the formation of haemoglobin.

The determination of red cell numbers, volume and haemoglobin content is useful in clinical assessments; normal values are given in Table 2.10.

The main function of erythrocytes is the transportation of gases, mainly oxygen bound to haemoglobin within the cell, but also some carbon dioxide; 97% of oxygen in the blood is transported in the form of oxyhaemoglobin, while 30% of carbon dioxide in the blood is transported in the form of carboxyhaemoglobin.

APPLIED PHYSIOLOGY: Haemoglobin comprises four globin chains and four haem units; each haem unit is associated with one iron atom, which combines with an oxygen molecule forming oxyhaemoglobin. Each red blood cell carries approximately 280 million haemoglobin molecules. Iron is carried in the bloodstream bound to transferrin (its transport protein). Haemoglobin also acts to maintain acid-base balance by regulating hydrogen ion concentration in the blood.

Control of erythropoiesis: Red blood cell numbers are fairly constant as bone marrow produces erythrocytes at a similar rate as they are destroyed due to a negative homeostatic feedback mechanism; red blood cell production is regulated by the hormone erythropoietin, produced mainly in the kidneys.

The main stimulus to increase erythropoiesis is hypoxia resulting from anaemia, low blood volume, poor blood flow, reduced oxygen content of inspired air (such as at high altitude) or lung disease. Erythropoietin stimulates the production of proerythroblasts and the release of reticulocytes into the blood, leading to an increased oxygen carrying capacity of the blood, which reverses the hypoxia; it also increases reticulocyte maturation. Low erythropoietin levels do not lead to increased red blood cell formation even during hypoxia, leading to anaemia.

TABLE 2.9 Differences Between Leukocytes and Erythrocytes

Feature	Leukocytes	Erythrocytes
Colour	Colourless	Red
Number	$4–11 \times 10^3/mm^3$	$4.5–5.5$ million/mm^3
Size	Maximum diameter 18 µm	Maximum diameter 7.4 µm
Shape	Irregular	Biconcave disc
Nucleus	Present	Absent
Granules	Present in some types	Absent
Types	Many	1
Lifespan	0.5–15 days	120 days

TABLE 2.10 Normal Erythrocyte Values

Measure	Normal Value
Erythrocyte count: number of erythrocytes per litre (or cubic millilitre (mm^3)) of blood	Males: $4.5–6.5 \times 10^{12}/L$ ($4.5–6.5$ million/mm^3) Females: $3.8–5.8 \times 10^{12}/L$ ($3.8–5.8$ million/mm^3)
Packed cell volume (PCV, haematocrit): the volume of red cells in 1 L of blood	0.40–0.55 L/L
Haemoglobin: the weight of haemoglobin in whole blood	Males: 13–18 g/100 mL Females: 11.5–16.5 g/100 mL
Mean cell haemoglobin concentration (MCHC): the weight of haemoglobin in 100 mL of red blood cells	30–35 g/100 mL of red blood cells

Destruction of erythrocytes: The breakdown of erythrocytes (haemolysis) is carried out by phagocytic reticuloendothelial cells mainly in the spleen, liver and bone marrow. The iron released is retained in the body, being reused in the bone marrow to form new haemoglobin molecules. Bilirubin, from the haem part of haemoglobin, is transported to the liver bound to plasma globin, where it is transformed from a fat-soluble to a water-soluble form before being excreted as a constituent of bile.

Erythrocyte sediment rate (ESR) is the rate at which erythrocytes settle down when suspended in an anticoagulant and allowed to stand in a graduated vertical tube for 1 hour; the red blood cells settle down due to gravity leaving a supernatant layer of clear plasma. ESR can help in diagnosis as well as prognosis; however, it is non-specific. It is useful in monitoring the progress of patients treated for some chronic inflammatory disorders (pulmonary tuberculosis, rheumatoid arthritis, polymyalgia rheumatic, temporal arteritis).

Physiological variations in ESR occur with age (it is less in children and infants due to the greater number of red blood cells), gender (it is greater in females due to fewer red blood cells), menstruation (due to the loss of blood and red blood cells) and pregnancy (from the third month due to haemodilution).

Pathological variations occur which either increase (tuberculosis, anaemia (except sickle cell anaemia), malignant tumours, rheumatoid arthritis, rheumatic fever, liver disease) or decrease (allergic conditions, sickle cell anaemia, peptone shock, polycythaemia, severe leucocytosis) ESR.

Blood groups. The surfaces of red blood cells carry a range of different proteins (antigens) that can stimulate an immune response when blood is transfused into incompatible individuals; the inherited antigens determine an individual's blood group. Individuals transfused with blood with the same antigens on the red cells will not undergo an immune reaction after the transfusion; however, if the transfused blood has different antigens on the red cells the body generates antibodies to the foreign antigens and destroys the transferred cells.

CLINICAL PHYSIOLOGY: If a particular antigen is present in red blood cells the corresponding antibody is absent in the serum. Conversely, if a specific antigen is absent in red blood cells the corresponding antibody is present in the serum.

TABLE 2.11   Antigen and Antibodies Present in ABO Blood Groups: Group A Has Two Subgroups (A_1, A_2) as Does Group AB (A_1B, A_2B)

Group	Antigen on Red Blood Cells	Antibody in Serum
A	A	Anti-B (β-antibody)
B	B	Anti-A (α-antibody)
AB	A and B	No antibody
O	No antigen	Anti-A (α-antibody) and anti-B (β-antibody)

Although there are more than 20 genetically determined red cell surface antigens, the 2 most important are the ABO and Rhesus systems.

ABO system: Approximately 55% of the population are either blood group A (having A type antigens), B (having B type antigens) or AB (having both A and B type antigens) on the surface of their red blood cells; the remaining 45% (blood group O) have neither A nor B type antigens on the surface of their red blood cells (Table 2.11).

CLINICAL PHYSIOLOGY: Individuals in the AB blood group, which have neither anti-A nor anti-B antibodies on the red cell membranes, can receive either type A or B blood (in small quantities) as it is likely to be safe. Conversely, group O blood, which has neither A nor B antigens on the red cell membranes, can be safely transfused into A, B, AB (in small quantities) or O individuals. Although often referred to as universal recipients and universal donors, respectively, because other antigen systems are associated with the surface of red blood cells, cross-matching of blood prior to transfusion is required to ensure there will be no reaction between the donor and recipient blood.

The inheritance of antigens is shown in Table 2.12.

Rhesus system: The red blood cell membrane also carries the important Rhesus (Rh) D antigen (Rh factor); individuals (85%) with the antigen are Rhesus positive (Rh^+) and do not make anti-Rhesus antibodies, 15% of individuals have no Rhesus antigen and are Rhesus negative (Rh^-). Rh^- individuals can make anti-Rhesus antibodies under certain circumstances (pregnancy) or following an incompatible blood transfusion.

TABLE 2.12   Inheritance of ABO Blood Groups

Gene From Parents	Blood Group of Offspring (Phenotype)	Genotype
A + A A + O	A	AA or AO
B + B B + O	B	BB or BO
A + B O + O	AB O	AB OO

CLINICAL PHYSIOLOGY: Abnormal haemolysis of red blood cells (haemolytic disease) in the foetus and newborn is due to Rh incompatibility (difference between the Rh blood group of mother and baby); it leads to erythroblastosis fetalis characterised by the presence of erythroblasts in foetal blood. When the mother is Rh⁻ and the baby Rh⁺ (the Rh factor is inherited from the father), the first child usually escapes the complications of Rh incompatibility because the Rh antigen cannot cross the placental barrier. During parturition the Rh antigen from foetal blood can leak into maternal blood due to placental detachment; the mother then develops Rh antibodies in her blood. If a subsequent child is Rh⁺, the Rh antibodies cross the placental barrier entering the foetal blood causing agglutination of foetal red blood cells and haemolysis. Severe haemolysis can cause jaundice resulting in the rapid production of red blood cells, with the release of immature cells into the circulation. Due to excessive haemolysis severe complications develop: severe anaemia, hydrops fetalis (oedema, enlargement of the liver and spleen, cardiac failure) which can lead to intrauterine death, and kernicterus (a form of brain damage due to severe jaundice – this happens because the blood-brain barrier is not well developed in infants). Babies born with erythroblastosis fetalis are given a transfusion of Rh⁻ blood to replace their Rh⁺ blood; the new blood replaces the baby's original blood by age 6 months, by which time all the Rh antibodies from the mother have been destroyed.

CLINICAL PHYSIOLOGY: If a mother is Rh⁻ and the foetus is Rh⁺ as a prophylactic measure anti D (antibody against the D antigen) should be given to the mother at 28- and 34-week gestation. However, if an Rh⁻ mother gives birth to an Rh⁺ baby anti D should be given within 48 h of delivery; this develops passive immunity preventing the formation of Rh antibodies in the maternal blood so that haemolytic disease does not occur in subsequent pregnancies.

Anaemia. Anaemia is the inability of the red blood cells to carry sufficient oxygen to meet the body's needs; it is characterised by a reduction in red blood cell count, haemoglobin content and packed cell volume, which can occur due to decreased production or increased destruction of red blood cells and excess loss of blood from the body. These can be caused either by inherited disorders or by environmental influences (nutrition, infection, exposure to drugs and toxins). Anaemia can result in abnormal changes in red blood cell morphology (Table 2.13).

Haemorrhagic anaemia is due to excessive loss of blood; it can be acute (sudden loss of a large amount of blood) or chronic (loss of blood over a long period of time through internal (peptic ulcer, purpura) or external (haemophilia, menorrhagia) bleeding. In acute haemorrhage the plasma portion of blood is replaced within 24 hours, with the replacement of red blood cells taking 4–6 weeks; this leads to haemodilution and hypoxia stimulating the bone marrow to produce more red blood cells. In chronic haemorrhage, the continuous loss of blood leads to iron deficiency, which affects the synthesis of haemoglobin resulting in less haemoglobin in the cells.

Haemolytic anaemia occurs when circulating red blood cells are destroyed or prematurely removed from the blood because the cells are abnormal or the spleen is overactive; it can be classified as being extrinsic (autoimmune) or intrinsic (often inherited). Causes of extrinsic haemolytic anaemia include liver failure; renal disorder; hypersplenism (sometimes accompanied by splenomegaly); burns; infection (hepatitis, malaria, septicaemia); drugs (penicillin, antimalarial drugs; sulphonamides); poisoning by chemicals (lead, coal, tar, arsenic compounds); the

TABLE 2.13   Morphological Classification of Anaemia

Classification of Red Blood Cells	Size of Red Blood Cells	Colour of Red Blood Cells
Normocytic normochromic	Normal	Normal
Normocytic hypochromic	Normal	Pale
Macrocytic hypochromic	Large	Pale
Microcytic hypochromic	Small	Pale

presence of isoagglutinins (anti-Rh); autoimmune diseases (rheumatoid arthritis, ulcerative colitis); and toxins produced by microbes *(Streptococcus pyogenes, Clostridium perfringens)*. In intrinsic haemolytic anaemia (e.g., sickle cell anaemia, thalassaemia), the red blood cells are usually defective and short-lived due to their increased fragility and susceptibility to haemolysis.

Sickle cell anaemia is characterised by the shape of the red blood cells due to sickle cell haemoglobin, in which the α-chains are normal and the β-chains abnormal. The sickle cells do not move smoothly through the circulation obstructing blood flow, leading to intravascular clotting, tissue ischaemia and infarction. Acute episodes (sickle crises) caused by blockage of small vessels cause acute pain, with infarction being common in small bones in the hand and foot resulting in digits of varying length (hand and foot syndrome).

> **CLINICAL PHYSIOLOGY:** Pregnancy, infection and dehydration all predispose to the development of sickle crises due to intravascular clotting and ischaemia leading to severe pain in long bones, the chest and abdomen. Excessive haemolysis results in high bilirubin circulating in the blood; this can lead to the formation of gallstones (cholelithiasis) in the gall bladder (cholecystolithiasis) or common bile duct (choledocholithiasis) and inflammation of the gall bladder (cholecystitis).

Longer-term problems arise from poor perfusion and anaemia include cardiac disease; kidney failure; retinopathy; poor tissue healing; and slow growth in children. Obstruction of blood flow to the brain increases the risk of stroke and seizures. During pregnancy, both mother and child are at significant risk of complications.

> **CLINICAL PHYSIOLOGY:** Some affected individuals have a degree of immunity to malaria, possibly because the sickle cells have a shorter life span than that needed for the malaria parasite to mature within the cells.

Thalassaemia is the result of abnormal haemoglobin production reducing erythropoiesis and stimulating haemolysis; it can range from mild and asymptomatic to severe and life threatening. In moderate to severe forms, symptoms include bone marrow expansion and splenomegaly; in the most severe forms, regular blood transfusions are required, which can lead to iron overload.

Haemolysis in the newborn occurs when the mother's immune system makes antibodies to the baby's red blood cells leading to the destruction of foetal erythrocytes; it is usually the Rhesus antigen system which is involved (page 168).

Nutrition deficiency anaemias are due to a lack of substances (iron, vitamin B_{12}, folic acid) in the diet necessary for erythropoiesis.

Iron deficiency anaemia develops due to a lack of availability of iron for haemoglobin synthesis: it develops over prolonged periods of time, with symptoms (brittle hair and nails, spoon-shaped nails (koilonychias), atrophy of papillae on the tongue, dysphagia) only appearing once the anaemia is established. It can be the result of blood loss (uterine bleeding as in excessive menstruation, repeated miscarriages, postmenopausal bleeding), decreased iron intake (milk-fed infants, anorexia), poor absorption from the intestines (gastrectomy, achlorhydria) and increased demand during growth and pregnancy.

> **CLINICAL PHYSIOLOGY:** The daily iron requirement in men is 1–2 mg, while in women it is 3 mg due to blood loss during menstruation and in pregnancy to meet the needs of the growing foetus; children need more than adults to meet their growth needs.

Protein deficiency anaemia is associated with reduced synthesis of haemoglobin.

Vitamin B_{12} deficiency anaemia impairs erythrocyte maturation leading to large erythrocytes (megaloblasts) in the blood due to a reduction in the rate of DNA and RNA synthesis delaying cell division; the cells are fragile and have a reduced lifespan (40–50 days). *Pernicious anaemia* is the commonest form, especially in women aged over 50; it is an autoimmune disease in which autoantibodies destroy intrinsic factor and parietal cells in the stomach.

Causes of vitamin B_{12} deficiency include gastrectomy; chronic gastritis, malignant disease and ionising radiation (all of which damage the gastric mucosa); and malabsorption when the terminal ileum is removed or inflamed (Crohn's disease). Complications often appear before the signs of anaemia, these being irreversible neurological damage in the spinal cord due to reduced myelin production, and mucosal abnormalities (glossitis), which are usually reversible.

Folic acid deficiency anaemia causes a form of megaloblastic anaemia similar to that seen in vitamin B_{12} deficiency; it is not associated with neurological damage. It may be due to dietary deficiency (a delay in establishing a mixed diet in infants, alcoholism, anorexia, pregnancy), malabsorption from the jejunum (coeliac disease, tropical sprue, anticonvulsive drugs) and interference with folate metabolism caused by cytotoxic and anticonvulsive drugs.

Aplastic anaemia is due to a disorder of the red bone marrow, which is either reduced or replaced by fatty tissue, leading to reduced erythrocytes in the blood; as bone marrow also produces leukocytes and platelets, leukopenia (page 174) and thrombocytopenia (page 174) may also occur. When all three cell types are low (pancytopenia), accompanied by anaemia, there is diminished immunity and a tendency to bruise easily and bleed; the condition may be inherited (15% of cases). Known causes include drugs (cytotoxic therapy and rarely as an adverse reaction to anti-inflammatory and anticonvulsive drugs and some antibiotics); ionising radiation (X-rays, δ-rays); some chemicals (benzene and its derivatives); viral infections (hepatitis, HIV); and tuberculosis.

Chronic disease anaemia is the second most common type, being characterised by a short erythrocyte lifespan due either to disturbances in iron metabolism or to resistance to erythropoietin action; it develops within a few months. Common causes are non-infectious inflammatory diseases (rheumatoid arthritis); chronic infections (tuberculosis, lung abscess); chronic renal failure; and neoplastic disorders (Hodgkin's disease, cancer of the lung and breast).

The characteristic erythrocyte morphology associated with each type of anaemia is given in Table 2.14.

Signs and symptoms of anaemia are related to the inability of the blood to supply the tissues with enough oxygen. The skin and mucous membranes become pale, which is more constant and prominent in buccal and pharyngeal mucous membranes, conjunctiva, lips, ear lobes, palm and nail bed. The skin loses its elasticity and becomes thin and dry; there is also loss and early greying of the hair, with the nails becoming brittle and easily breakable.

There is an increase in heart rate (tachycardia) and cardiac output, with the heart becoming dilated producing cardiac murmurs; the velocity of blood flow also increases. The rate and force of respiration both increase, leading to breathlessness and dyspnoea; the oxygen-haemoglobin dissociation curve is shifted to the right (page 108).

Anorexia, nausea, vomiting, abdominal discomfort and constipation are common. In pernicious anaemia, atrophy of the papillae on the tongue occurs, while in aplastic anaemia, necrotic lesions appear in the mouth and pharynx; in severe anaemia, basal metabolic rate increases.

Renal function is disturbed, with albuminuria being common. In females, the menstrual cycle is disturbed, accompanied by menorrhagia (increased menstrual flow), oligomenorrhea (less frequent menstrual flow) or amenorrhea (no menstrual flow).

TABLE 2.14 Aetiological Classification of Anaemia, Together With Erythrocyte Morphology

Type of Anaemia	Cause	Erythrocyte Morphology
Haemorrhagic	Acute blood loss	Normocytic, normochromic
	Chronic blood loss	Microcytic, hypochromic
Haemolytic	Extrinsic	Normocytic, normochromic
	Intrinsic	Sickle cell: sickle shape
		Thalassaemia: small and irregular
Nutrition deficiency	Iron	Microcytic, normochromic
	Protein	Macrocytic, hypochromic
	Vitamin B_{12}	Macrocytic, normochromic/hypochromic
	Folic acid	Megaloblastic, normochromic
Aplastic	Bone marrow disorder	Normocytic, normochromic
Chronic diseases		Normocytic normochromic, then microcytic hypochromic as the disease progresses

The sensitivity to cold, headache, lack of concentration, restlessness, irritability, dizziness, vertigo (especially when standing) and fainting are all increased. Muscles become weak, with individuals often and easily feeling a lack of energy and fatigued.

Polycythaemia. Polycythaemia is an excess of erythrocytes in the blood, increasing blood viscosity, slowing blood flow and increasing the risk of intravascular clotting, ischaemia and infarction: it can occur when the erythrocyte count is normal, but the volume is reduced through fluid loss (excessive serum from extensive burns). The increase in erythrocyte count can be physiological (prolonged hypoxia as in living at high altitudes, heart or lung disease, heavy smoking) or pathological (some cancers).

Leukocytes. Colourless, nucleated blood cells leukocytes play an important role in defence and immunity by detecting foreign and abnormal material and destroying it through a range of defence mechanisms. There are two main types, granulocytes (neutrophils, eosinophils, basophils) containing granules and agranulocytes (monocytes, lymphocytes) without granules. They are the largest cells in blood, although they comprise less than 1% by volume; differences between leukocytes and erythrocytes are shown in Table 2.9. Increasing numbers of leukocytes in the blood are usually indicative of infection, trauma or malignancy.

> **CLINICAL PHYSIOLOGY:** In infants, the white blood cell count is 20,000/mm³, in children, it is between 10,000 and 15,000/mm³, and in adults, between 4000 and 11,000/mm³. It is also slightly more in females than males; is minimum in the early morning and maximum in the afternoon; increases slightly with exercise and after food intake; decreases during sleep; and increases during menstruation, pregnancy and parturition.

Granulocytes (polymorphonuclear leukocytes): Although they follow a common line of development through myeloblast to myelocyte, they differentiate into three distinct types (neutrophils, eosinophils, basophils), all of which have multilobed nuclei in their cytoplasm (Fig. 2.88); they account for different proportions of white cells and have different sizes and lifespans (Table 2.15).

Neutrophils are active scavengers protecting the body against bacterial invasion, as well as removing dead cells and debris from damaged tissues. They are attracted to infected areas in large number by chemotaxis released

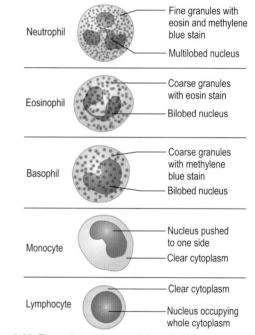

Fig. 2.88 The cellular characteristics of different types of leukocytes present in blood.

TABLE 2.15	The Diameter and Lifespan of Leukocytes, Together With Their Percentage and Absolute Values of the Total Number of Leukocytes			
Leukocyte	Diameter (μm)	Lifespan (Days)	%	Absolute Value/mm³
Neutrophils	10–12	2–5	50–70	3,000–6,000
Eosinophils	10–14	7–12	2–4	150–450
Basophils	8–10	12–15	0–1	0–100
Monocytes	14–18	2–5	2–6	200–600
Lymphocytes	7–12	0.5–1	20–30	1,500–2,700

by damaged cells; pus in an affected area consists of dead tissue cells, dead and live microbes, and phagocytes killed by microbes. Neutrophils are highly mobile, being able to squeeze through the capillary wall (diapedesis) in affected areas where they engulf and kill bacteria by phagocytosis. An increase in the number of neutrophils present (neutrophilia) occurs in acute infections, metabolic disorders, injection of foreign proteins and vaccines, chemical and drug poisoning (lead, mercury, camphor, benzene derivatives), insect venom, and acute haemorrhage. In contrast, a decrease in the number of neutrophils (neutropenia) occurs in bone marrow disorders, tuberculosis, malaria, typhoid, paratyphoid, vitamin deficiencies and autoimmune diseases.

Eosinophils are specialised to eliminate parasites which are too large to be phagocytosed, although they are capable of phagocytosis; when they bind to an infecting organism, they release toxic chemicals stored in the granules. Accumulations of eosinophils occur in allergic reactions (skin allergies) causing tissue inflammation; however, they may also dampen down the inflammatory process through the release of other chemicals (histaminase). An increase in the number of eosinophils (eosinophilia) occurs in asthma and other allergic conditions, blood (malaria, filariasis), intestinal parasitism and scarlet fever. Decreases in eosinophil numbers (eosinopenia) occur in Cushing's syndrome, bacterial infections, stress and the prolonged use of some drugs (steroids, adrenaline, adrenocorticotrophic hormones).

Basophils contain granules packed with heparin (an anticoagulant), histamine (an inflammatory agent) and other inflammation-promoting substances; they are closely associated with allergic reactions. Similar cells (mast cells) are found in tissues (not blood) which rapidly release their granular contents, hence the rapid onset of allergic reactions after exposure (e.g., pollen in hay fever). Increased numbers of basophils (basophilia) occur in influenza, smallpox, chickenpox, chronic myeloid leukaemia and polycythaemia vera, while a decrease in basophil numbers (basopenia) occurs in urticaria, stress and prolonged exposure to chemo or radiotherapy.

Agranulocytes: These comprise between 25% and 35% of the total number of leukocytes present in blood and are of two types (monocytes, lymphocytes); they have a large nucleus and no cytoplasmic granules (Fig. 2.88, Table 2.15).

Monocytes circulate in the blood; some are actively motile and phagocytic, while others migrate into tissues and develop into macrophages (Kupffer cells in the liver, alveolar macrophages in the lungs, macrophages in the spleen). Both monocytes and macrophages produce interleukin-1 which cause an increase in body temperature associated with microbial infection by acting on the hypothalamus, stimulation of the production of some globulins in the liver and enhancement of the production of activated T-lymphocytes; macrophages also play an important role in inflammation and immunity. An increase in the numbers of circulating monocytes (monocytosis) occurs in tuberculosis, syphilis, malaria, subacute bacterial endocarditis, glandular fever and Kala-azar (visceral leishmaniasis), while a decrease (monocytopenia) occurs in prolonged use of prednisone, AIDS and chronic lymphoid leukaemia.

Macrophages have a wide range of protective functions, being more powerful and longer lived than the smaller neutrophils; they synthesise and release many biologically active chemicals (cytokines), have an important role in linking the non-specific and specific (immune) systems of the body's defences, and produce important factors in inflammation and repair. They are capable of isolating indigestible material (resistant bacteria, inhaled organic dust) from surrounding normal tissue.

Lymphocytes develop from pluripotent stem cells in red bone marrow, as well as from precursors in lymphoid tissue; some circulate in the blood, but the majority are found in tissues (lymphatic tissue, lymph nodes, spleen). There are two types of lymphocytes: T cells responsible for developing cellular immunity, and B cells responsible for developing humoral immunity. An increase in the number of lymphocytes (lymphocytosis) occurs in diphtheria, infectious hepatitis, mumps, malnutrition, rickets, syphilis, thyrotoxicosis and tuberculosis. In contrast, a decrease (lymphocytopenia) is seen in AIDS, Hodgkin's disease, malnutrition, radiation therapy and steroid administration.

The role of lymphocytes and other leukocytes in immunity can be found on page 176.

Pathological variation in the total leukocyte count occurs, with the number of neutrophils and lymphocytes tending to vary in opposite direction. An increase in total leukocyte count (leucocytosis) occurs in infections, allergies, the common cold, tuberculosis and glandular fever; leukaemia is an abnormal and uncontrolled increase to more than 1 million/mm³. A decrease in total leukocyte count (leukopenia) occurs in anaphylactic shock, cirrhosis of the liver, disorders of the spleen, pernicious anaemia, typhoid and paratyphoid, and viral infections.

Platelets (thrombocytes). Small (2–4 μm diameter) colourless, non-nucleated cells of varying shape (usually disc-shaped); they are derived from megakaryocyte cytoplasm in red bone marrow (Fig. 2.87). They have a lifespan of 8–11 days, with those not used being destroyed by macrophages, mainly in the spleen. Approximately 2/3rd of platelets are in the circulation, with the remainder in the spleen as an emergency store that can be released when required (excessive bleeding).

> **CLINICAL PHYSIOLOGY:** The normal adult platelet count is between 200,000 and 350,000/mm³ (200 – 350 × 10⁹/L); in infants it is 150,000–200,000/mm³, reaching adult levels 3 months after birth. There is no difference between males and females, although it is reduced in females during menstruation. Platelet count increases after a meal, as well as at high altitudes.

Platelet disorders. These occur due to pathological variations in platelet count, as well as platelet dysfunction. An increase in platelet count (thrombocytosis) occurs in allergic reactions, asphyxia, haemorrhage, fractures, surgical operations, splenectomy, rheumatic fever and trauma; a persistent and abnormal increase (thrombocythaemia) occurs in carcinoma, chronic leukaemia and Hodgkin's disease. A decrease in platelet count (thrombocytopenia), which leads to idiopathic/essential thrombocytopenic purpura, occurs in acute infections, acute leukaemia, aplastic and pernicious anaemia, chickenpox, smallpox, splenomegaly, scarlet fever, typhoid, tuberculosis and purpura. Glanzmann thrombasthenia, which leads to thrombasthenic purpura, is an inherited haemorrhagic disorder due to a structural or functional abnormality of platelets, with a normal platelet count; it is characterised by normal clotting time, normal or prolonged bleeding time, but defective clot retraction.

The cell membrane has extensive invaginations forming an open canalicular system through which platelet granules are extruded. The cell membrane contains lipids (phospholipids, cholesterol, glycolipids), carbohydrates (glycocalyx) and proteins (glycoproteins).

Glycoproteins prevent the adhesion of platelets to normal endothelium but accelerate their adhesion to collagen and damaged endothelium in ruptured blood vessels; they also form receptors for adenosine diphosphate (ADP) and thrombin.

Phospholipids accelerate clotting reactions by forming the precursors of thromboxane A_2 and other prostaglandin-related substances.

Deep to the cell membrane microtubules form a ring around the cytoplasm, providing structural support for the inactivated platelets.

Platelet cytoplasm. Contains proteins (contractile proteins, von Willebrand factor, fibrin-stabilising factor, platelet-derived growth factor, platelet-derived activating factor, vitronectin, thrombospondin), enzymes (adenosine triphosphatase, enzymes for synthesising prostaglandins), hormonal substances (adrenaline, 5-hydroxytryptamine (5-HT, serotonin), histamine) and other chemical substances (glycogen, blood group antigens, calcium, copper, magnesium, iron). Two types of granules (alpha and dense) are found within the cytoplasm; the substances present in each are given in Table 2.16.

Adhesiveness, aggregation and agglutination. These are all properties of platelets. Injury to a blood vessel damages its endothelium exposing the subendothelial collagen; platelets coming into contact with the collagen adhere to it. Adhesion is followed by the activation of greater numbers of platelets, during which the platelets develop long filamentous pseudopodia (filopodia) which help them aggregate together: aggregated platelets then clump together (agglutination).

TABLE 2.16　Substances Found in Alpha and Dense Platelet Granules

Alpha Granules	Dense Granules
Clotting factors: fibrinogen, V and XIII	Nucleotides
Platelet-derived growth factor	Serotonin
Vascular endothelial growth factor (VEGF)	Phospholipid
Basic fibroblast growth factor (FGF)	Calcium
Endostatin	Lysosomes
Thrombospondin	

Platelet function. Platelets only function after they have been activated; they then immediately release many substances to carry out these functions. They play a role in blood clotting, being responsible for the formation of intrinsic prothrombin activator responsible for the onset of clotting; clot retraction, due to the contractile proteins (actin, myosin, thrombosthenin) in their cytoplasm; prevention of blood loss (haemostasis) by causing blood vessel constriction, sealing the damage in the blood vessel wall and forming a temporary plug; repairing ruptured blood vessels via the platelet-derived growth factor; and defence mechanism by encircling and destroying foreign bodies.

Haemostasis. The arrest of bleeding followed by healing via a series of overlapping processes (vasoconstriction, platelet plug formation, coagulation of blood, fibrinolysis), with platelets playing a major role; the greater the damage to the vessel wall, the faster coagulation begins.

Following injury, platelets coming into contact with the damaged surface of the vessel become sticky and adhere to its wall. They then release serotonin, which, with other chemicals released by the damaged vessel wall, causes constriction restricting blood flow through it; the vasoconstriction is local. Adherence of platelets to the exposed collagen is accelerated by the von Willebrand factor, which acts as a bridge between specific proteins on the surface of the platelet and the collagen fibrils.

The adherent platelets aggregate releasing other substances which attract additional platelets to the site of damage creating a positive feedback mechanism to form a temporary seal (platelet plug); plug formation is usually complete within 6 minutes of the original injury.

There then follows a complex process of coagulation involving a positive feedback mechanism, with clotting factors activating each other in a specific order (cascade).

Once the clot has been formed, the process of removing it and healing the damaged blood vessel begins. The first stage is breaking down the clot (fibrinolysis). The plasminogen trapped within the clot as it formed is converted by activators released from the damaged endothelial cells into the enzyme plasmin. Plasmin breaks down fibrin into soluble waste products and removed by phagocytosis; as the clot is removed the integrity of the blood vessel wall is restored.

TABLE 2.17 Blood Clotting Factors	
Factor	
I	Fibrinogen
II[a]	Prothrombin
III	Thromboplastin (tissue factor)
IV	Calcium
V	Labile factor (proaccelerin/accelerator globulin)
VI	*Presence not yet determined*
VII[a]	Stable factor
VIII	Antihaemophilic factor (antihaemophilic globulin)
IX[a]	Christmas factor
X[a]	Stuart-Prower factor
XI	Plasma thromboplastin antecedent
XII	Hageman factor (contact factor)
XIII	Fibrin-stabilising factor (fibrinase)

[a]Vitamin K is essential for the synthesis of these factors.

Coagulation. The process in which blood loses its fluidity; it occurs through a series of cascading reactions due to the activation of clotting factors (Table 2.17).

There are three stages of blood clotting. In stage 1, blood clotting begins with the formation of prothrombin activator which converts prothrombin to thrombin; it is initiated either by platelets within the blood (intrinsic pathway) or by tissue thromboplastin from the damaged tissues (extrinsic pathway). In stage 2, prothrombin is converted to thrombin leading to clot formation. In stage 3, fibrinogen is converted to fibrin by thrombin.

Blood clots are masses of coagulated blood containing red and white cells and platelets within a fibrin mesh, which adheres to the damaged blood vessel preventing further blood loss. Following clot formation, it starts contracting; after 30–45 minutes serum begins to ooze from the clot (clot retraction) due to the action of contractile proteins (actin, myosin, thrombosthenin) in the platelet cytoplasm. The blood clot is removed from the lumen of the vessel by lysis (fibrinolysis); the process requires the presence of plasmin (fibrinolysin).

Intravascular clotting does not normally occur due to physical (continuous circulation of blood, smooth endothelial lining of blood vessels) and chemical (heparin in the blood, thrombomodulin produced by the vessel endothelium, inactivated clotting factors) factors.

Procoagulants accelerate the clotting process. These include thrombin; the venom from some snakes (vipers, cobras, rattlesnakes); thromboplastin extracted from lung and thymic tissue; sodium or calcium alginate substances; and oxidised cellulose activating the Hageman clotting factor.

Anticoagulants prevent or postpone clotting either in (in vivo) or outside (in vitro) the body, the latter being after blood has been collected. *Heparin* can be used *in vivo* and *in vitro* and works by suppressing thrombin activity; it is used to prevent intravascular clotting during surgery, dialysis, cardiac surgery involving a heart-lung machine, and to preserve blood prior to transfusion. *Warfarin* and *dicoumarol* are commonly used as oral anticoagulants and act by inhibiting the action of vitamin K; warfarin is used to prevent myocardial infarction, stroke and thromboses. *Ethylenediaminetetraacetic acid (EDTA)* is a strong anticoagulant and works by removing calcium from the blood; it is administered intravenously in cases of lead poisoning. *Oxalate compounds* also work by removing calcium from the blood; they cannot be used intravenously as they are poisonous. *Citrates* also work by removing calcium from the blood. Other anticoagulants are *peptone*, *C-type lectin* (from viper snake venom) and *hirudin* (from the leach Hirudinaria manillensis).

APPLIED PHYSIOLOGY: Bleeding disorders are characterised by prolonged bleeding or clotting time. *Haemophilia* is characterised by prolonged clotting times but with normal bleeding times; it is due to a deficiency in factor VIII, IX or XI. It usually affects males, with females being carriers; symptoms include spontaneous bleeding; prolonged bleeding following cuts, tooth extraction and surgery; haemorrhage into the gastrointestinal and urinary tracts (blood in the urine); and bleeding into joints with swelling and pain. *Purpura* is characterised by prolonged bleeding time, with normal clotting time; a characteristic feature is spontaneous bleeding under the skin (haemorrhagic/purpuric spots) in many areas of the body, and blood can sometimes collect in large areas under the skin (ecchymoses). It is due to a lack of platelets (thrombocytopenic purpura), reduced platelet count (idiopathic thrombocytopenic purpura) or a structural or functional abnormality of platelets (thrombasthenic purpura). *von Willebrand disease* is characterised by excess bleeding even after a minor injury due to a deficiency in factor VIII, suppressing platelet adhesion.

Thrombosis. Occurs following injury to a blood vessel due to infection or mechanical obstruction; a roughened endothelial lining due to infection or arteriosclerosis; sluggish blood flow causing aggregation of platelets, due to reduced cardiac action, hypotension, low metabolic rate, prolonged bed rest, and immobility of the limbs; erythrocyte agglutination, caused by foreign antigens or toxic substances; toxic thrombosis, due to chemical poisons (arsenic compounds, mercury, poisonous mushrooms, snake venom); and the congenital absence of protein C which inactivates factors V and VIII – its absence in infancy leads to thrombosis and death.

APPLIED PHYSIOLOGY: Thrombi partially or completely occlude the blood vessel lumen resulting in ischaemia, due to hypoxia, of tissues distal to the blockage causing discomfort, pain and tissue death (necrosis). An embolus (detached part of a thrombus) is carried in the bloodstream occluding small vessels causing reduced or no blood flow: common sites of an embolism are in the lungs (pulmonary embolism), brain (cerebral embolism (stroke)) and heart (coronary embolism (heart attack)).

Immunity

Immunity is the capacity of the body to resist the entry of different types of foreign bodies/pathological agents (bacteria, viruses, toxic substances). It can be innate (the inborn capacity of the body to resist pathogens (Table 2.18)) or acquired (resistance developed in the body against bacteria, viruses, toxins, vaccines, transplanted tissue); acquired immunity can be either cellular or humoral, with lymphocytes being necessary for the development of both types.

Lymphocyte processing. Lymphocytes released into the circulation are of two types: T cells responsible for the development of cellular immunity and B cells responsible for the development of humoral immunity.

T lymphocytes. These are processed in the thymus mainly just prior to birth and a few months after birth. Thymosin, secreted by the thymus, accelerates the proliferation and activation of lymphocytes in the thymus, as well as increasing the activity of lymphocytes in lymphoid tissue. During processing T cells are transformed into four cell types: helper T (CD4) cells; cytotoxic T (CD8) cells; suppressor (regulatory) T cells; and

TABLE 2.18   Innate Immunity Mechanisms

Structures and Mediators	Mechanism
Gastrointestinal tract	Secreted enzymes and stomach acidity destroy toxic substances or organisms entering the gastrointestinal tract; lysosomes in saliva destroy bacteria.
Respiratory system	Antimicrobial peptides (defensins, cathelicidins) in epithelial cells of airways; neutrophils, lymphocytes, macrophages and natural killer cells in the lungs act against bacteria and viruses.
Urogenital system	Urine and vaginal fluid acidity destroy bacteria.
Skin	The epidermal keratinised stratum corneum protects the skin against toxic chemicals; β-defensins are antimicrobial peptides; lysozyme secreted in the skin destroys bacteria.
Phagocytic cells	Neutrophils, monocytes and macrophages phagocytose foreign bodies and microorganisms.
Interferons	Inhibit the multiplication of viruses, parasites and cancer cells.
Complement proteins	Accelerate the destruction of microorganisms.

memory T cells. Following transformation, all types of T cells leave the thymus and are stored in lymphoid tissue (lymph nodes, spleen, bone marrow, MALT).

Helper T (CD4) cells activate all other T and B cells; CD4 count in healthy adults is between 500 and 1500/mm^3 of blood. There are two types of helper T cells: Helper-1 (TH1) responsible for cellular immunity; Helper-2 (HT2) cells responsible for humoral immunity. TH1 cells secrete interleukin-2, which activates other T cells, and gamma interferon, which stimulates phagocytic activity of cytotoxin cells, macrophages and natural killer cells. TH2 cells secrete interleukin-4 and interleukin-5, which are concerned with B cell activation, proliferation of plasma cells and production of antibodies by plasma cells.

Cytotoxic T (CD8) cells circulate through blood, lymph and lymphatic tissues destroying invading organism by directly attacking them; they also destroy cancer and transplanted cells. They destroy the body's own tissues which have been infected by viruses trapped in the cell membranes of affected cells. The antigen of the virus attracts cytotoxic T cells, which destroy the affected cells as well as the virus.

Suppressor T cells suppress the activity of cytotoxic (CD8) cells preventing them from destroying the body's own tissues along with the invading organism; they also suppress the activity of helper T cells.

Memory T cells migrate to and remain in lymphoid tissue throughout the body after they have been activated by an antigen. When the body is again exposed to

the same organism memory T cells identify the organism and immediately activate the other T cells, which quickly destroy the invading organism: the response is more powerful the second and subsequent times.

Antigens. Substances which induce specific immune reactions in the body: autoimmune (self) antigens are present on the body's own cells (A and B antigens on erythrocytes) and foreign (non-self) antigens (those which induce the development of immunity or production of antibodies (immunogenicity); those which react with specific antibodies producing an allergic reaction (allergic reactivity)) that enter the body from outside.

Each T cell is activated by one type of antigen only, being capable of developing immunity against that antigen only: it has specificity.

Development of cellular immunity. This involves T cells, macrophages and natural killer cells; it does not involve antibodies. Antigen-presenting cells (macrophages, dendritic cells) release antigenic material from the invading organism and present it to helper T cells. Macrophages digest the invading organism to release the antigen; dendritic cells in the spleen trap antigen in the blood, follicular dendritic cells in lymph nodes trap antigens in the lymph; and Langerhans dendritic cells in the skin trap organisms coming into contact with the body surface.

B cells can also act as antigen-presenting cells as well as antigen-receiving cells; they are the least efficient antigen-presenting cells and need to be activated by helper T cells.

B lymphocytes. These are processed in the liver in the foetus and bone marrow after birth. After processing B cells are transformed into plasma cells and memory B cells, after which they are stored in lymphoid tissue (lymph nodes, spleen, bone marrow, MALT).

Plasma cells destroy foreign organisms by producing antibodies (immunoglobulins), which are released into the lymph and transported to the circulation; the antibodies are produced for the entire lifespan of the plasma cell.

Memory B cells remain inactivate until the body is exposed to an organism for the second time, following which it rapidly produces antibodies which are more potent than those produced during the initial exposure.

Antibodies (immunoglobulins). Proteins produced by B cells in response to the presence of an antigen: five types of antibodies have been identified (immunoglobulin A, IgA; immunoglobulin D, IgD; immunoglobulin E, IgE; immunoglobulin G, IgG; immunoglobulin M, IgM). They comprise 20% of total plasma proteins and enter most tissues of the body. IgA plays a role in localised defence mechanisms; IgD in antigen recognition by B cells; IgE in allergic reactions, while IgG and IgM are responsible for complement fixation.

The complement system consists of a system of 11 inactivated plasma enzymes (C_1 to C_9, with C_1 having three subunits (C_{1q}, C_{1r}, C_{1s})). When C_1 binds with antibodies, it triggers a series of events activating other enzymes in sequence. The enzymes or their by-products lead to activation of neutrophils and macrophages to engulf the bacteria (opsonisation); destruction of the bacteria by rupturing its membrane (lysis); attraction of leukocytes to the site of the antigen-antibody reaction (chemotaxis); clumping of the foreign bodies (agglutination): covering the toxic sites (neutralisation); and activation of mast cells and basophils to release histamine, which dilates blood vessels and increases capillary permeability so the plasma proteins from the blood enter the tissues to inactivate the antigenic products.

The complement system can also be activated by factor I binding with polysaccharides in the cell membrane of invading organisms, which activates C_3 and C_5 stimulating an attack on the invading organisms.

Development of humoral immunity. The immunity mediated by antibodies secreted by B cells. Antigen-presenting cells present the antigenic products bound with human leukocyte antigen (HLA) to B cells, which then activates the B cells through a series of events; HLA is present in class II major histocompatibility complex (MHC) molecules. The B cell recognises the antigen displayed on the antigen-presenting cells (macrophages), initiating a complex interaction between the B cell receptor and antigen, activating the B cells. At the same time, the antigen-presenting cells release interleukin-1 facilitating the activation and proliferation of B cells; the antigen bound to class II MHC molecules activates helper T cells, resulting in the development of cell-mediated immunity.

Natural killer cells. Natural killer cells are large granular cells which are the first line of defence in specific immunity, especially against viruses, and are derived from bone marrow; they are considered a third type of lymphocyte. They kill the invading organism or cells of the body without prior sensitisation. It is not a phagocytic cell; however, its granules contain hydrolytic hormones (perforins, granzymes), which play an important role in the lysis of cells of invading organisms.

They destroy viruses; viral infected and damaged cells which could form tumours; malignant cells preventing the development of cancerous tumours; and secrete cytokines (interleukin-2, interferons, colony stimulating factor (GM-CSF), tumour necrosis factor-α).

Cytokines. Cytokines are small hormone-like proteins acting as intercellular messengers (cell signalling molecules) which bind to specific receptors of target cells. The major function of these non-antibody proteins is to activate and regulate the body's general immune system; they are secreted by leukocytes, as well as some other cell types and classified according to their source and effect (Table 2.19).

Interleukins (IL) act on other leukocytes; 16 types have been identified. IL-1, IL-2, IL-3, IL-4, IL-5, IL-6 and IL-8 are important in the process of immunity: IL-11 and IL-12 (natural killer cell stimulatory factor) are also important cytokines.

Interferons (IFN) (INF-α, INF-β, INF-δ) are glycoprotein molecules considered to be antiviral agents.

Tumour necrosis factors (TNF) are of three types: TNF-α (cachectin), TNF-β (lymphotoxin) and TNF-δ.

Chemokines are cytokines with a chemoattractant action.

Defensins are antimicrobial peptides; α-defensins are secreted by neutrophils, macrophages and Paneth cells in the small intestine; β-defensins are secreted by airway epithelial cells in the respiratory tract, salivary glands and cutaneous cells.

TABLE 2.19 Cytokines, Their Source and Action		
Cytokine	Source	Action
Interleukins	T cells; B cells; eosinophils; basophils; monocytes; mast cells; macrophages; natural killer (NK) cells	Activation of T cells, macrophages and NK cells; promotion of growth of haemopoietic cells; acceleration of inflammatory response by activating eosinophils; chemotaxis of neutrophils, eosinophils, basophils and T cells; destruction of invading organism
Interferons	Leukocytes; NK cells; fibroblasts	Fighting viral infections by suppressing virus replication in target cells; inhibiting replication of parasites and cancer cells
Tumour necrosis factors	T cells; B cells; mast cells; macrophages; NK cells; platelets	Tumour necrosis; activation of general immune system; production of vascular effects; promotion of inflammation
Chemokines	T cells; B cells; monocytes; macrophages	Attraction of leukocytes by chemotaxis
Defensins	Neutrophils; macrophages; Paneth cells in small intestine; salivary glands, cutaneous cells	Role in innate immunity in airways and lungs; destroying phagocytosed bacteria; anti-inflammatory actions; promotion of wound healing; attraction of monocytes and T cells by chemotaxis
Cathelicidins	Neutrophils; macrophages; airway epithelial cells	Antimicrobial activity in airways and lungs
Platelet activating factor	Neutrophils; monocytes	Acceleration of agglutination and aggregation of platelets

Cathelicidins play an important role in a wide range of antimicrobial activity in the airways and lungs: they are antimicrobial peptides.

Platelet-activating factor accelerates agglutination and aggregation of platelets.

Immunisation. The procedure to induce immune resistance of the body to specific diseases; it is of two types (passive and active).

Passive immunisation. Immunity produced without challenging the immune system by administering a serum or gamma globulins from an immunised individual to a non-immune individual.

Passive natural immunisation is acquired from the mother prior to and after birth; before birth maternal antibodies (mainly IgG) pass from the mother to the foetus via the placenta, while after birth antibodies (IgA) are transferred in breast milk. The antibodies do not activate the child's lymphocytes and are soon metabolised; they are short lived.

Passive artificial immunisation is developed by injecting prepared antibodies using serum from individuals affected by the disease; it provides immediate protection against acute infections (tetanus, measles, diphtheria) and poisoning by insects, snakes and venom from other animals. However, this can result in complications and anaphylaxis; there is also a risk of transmitting disease (HIV, hepatitis).

Active immunisation. Immunity acquired by activating the immune system in which the body develops resistance against disease by producing antibodies following exposure to an antigen. Active natural immunisation is achieved in clinical and subclinical infections, while active artificial immunity is achieved by administration of vaccines or toxins.

Immune deficiency diseases. A group of diseases in which some components of the immune system are defective or missing; the deficiency can be either congenital (due to defects in B cells, T cells or both) or acquired through infection (AIDS). Severe combined immune deficiency is due to lymphopenia or the absence of lymphoid tissue, while in Di George syndrome the thymus is absent.

Autoimmune diseases. Diseases in which the body mistakenly attacks its own cells and tissues; it occurs when the body's normal tolerance decreases and the immune system fails to recognise its own tissues as self. They can be organ specific affecting a single organ or non-specific (multisystem) affecting several organs or systems.

The HLA system monitors the immune system; HLA is distributed throughout most tissues. The HLA molecules are recognised by T and B cells and direct antibodies against them. Most autoimmune diseases are HLA linked; common autoimmune diseases are insulin-dependent diabetes mellitus; myasthenia gravis; Hashimoto thyroiditis; Graves' disease; and rheumatoid arthritis.

Insulin-dependent diabetes mellitus is common in childhood; it can be caused by the development of islet cell antibodies against β-cells in the islets of Langerhans in the pancreas; development of an antibody against insulin and glutamic acid decarboxylase; and activation of T cells against islets.

Myasthenia gravis is a neuromuscular disease, due to the development of autoantibodies against acetylcholine receptors in the neuromuscular junction.

Hashimoto thyroiditis occurs when antibodies impair the activity of thyroid follicles and leads to hypothyroidism; it is common in late middle age.

Graves' disease is caused in some cases by autoantibodies activating thyroid stimulating hormone (TSH) receptors leading to hyperthyroidism.

Rheumatoid arthritis is due to chronic inflammation of the synovial lining of joints due to the continuous production of autoantibodies (rheumatoid arthritis factors) leading to swelling around joints and tendons; it is characterised by pain and joint stiffness.

Allergies and immunological hypersensitivity reactions. These may be innate or acquired, being mediated mainly by antibodies, with T cells sometimes being involved. They are characterised by sneezing, itching and skin rashes; symptoms can become severe in some individuals. Common allergic conditions include food allergy, allergic rhinitis, bronchial asthma and urticaria. Allergens are substances that produce an allergic reaction introduced by skin contact (chemicals, metals, animals, plants), inhalation (pollen grains, fungi, dust, smoke, perfumes, disagreeable odours), ingestion (wheat, eggs, milk, chocolate), infectious agents (parasites, bacteria, viruses, fungi), drugs (aspirin, antibiotics) and physical agents (cold, heat, light, pressure, radiation).

Immunological hypersensitive reactions are classified into five types: type I (anaphylactic reactions), type II (cytotoxic reactions), type III (antibody-mediated reactions), type IV (cell-mediated reactions) and type V (stimulator/blocking reactions).

Anaphylactic reactions are mediated mainly by IgE and other factors involved in inflammation; the most serious reactions are a fall in blood pressure due to vasoconstriction, obstruction of the airways and difficulty in breathing due to bronchoconstriction, and shock.

Cytotoxic reactions mainly involve IgG antibodies which bind with antigens on the cell surface, especially blood cells, destroying them; sometimes IgM and IgA antibodies are also involved. Haemolytic diseases in the newborn occur due to Rh incompatibility and autoimmune haemolytic anaemia.

Antibody-mediated reactions are due to excess amounts of IgG and IgM deposited in localised areas such as joints leading to arthritis, the heart leading to myocarditis and the glomeruli of the kidney leading to glomerulonephritis.

Cell-mediated reactions (slow/delayed hypersensitivity) are associated with allergic reactions due to bacteria, viruses and fungi but can also occur in contact dermatitis caused by chemical allergens, and during the rejection of transplanted tissues. The importance of this type of hypersensitivity is the involvement of T cells rather than antibodies.

Stimulatory/Blocking reactions are seen in autoimmune diseases like Graves' disease (stimulatory reaction) and myasthenia gravis (blocking reaction).

SELF-TEST QUESTIONS

1. Which of the following is NOT part of the bony thoracic cage?
   a. 1st rib
   b. Manubrium
   c. 7th thoracic vertebra
   d. Xiphoid process
   e. Clavicle

2. Concerning respiration, which of the following statements is correct?
   a. During inspiration the sternum moves forwards and upwards.
   b. The diaphragm does not contribute to respiration.
   c. Tidal volume is 1500 mL.
   d. The abdominal muscles are important in inspiration.
   e. In quiet respiration, the majority of gas exchange occurs in the lower lobe of the lung.
3. The arrangement of structures in the intercostal space, from above down, is:
   a. Artery, vein, nerve
   b. Vein, artery, nerve
   c. Vein, nerve, artery
   d. Nerve, artery, vein
   e. Artery, vein, nerve
4. The thoracic duct does NOT drain lymph from:
   a. the right side of the head and neck
   b. the right lower limb
   c. the thorax
   d. the abdomen
   e. the left upper limb
5. Concerning the mediastinum, which of the following statements is NOT correct?
   a. The superior mediastinum lies above the level of the sternal angle.
   b. The middle mediastinum contains the heart and roots of the great vessels.
   c. The remnants of the thymus lie in the posterior mediastinum.
   d. The middle mediastinum bulges to the left due to the left ventricle of the heart.
   e. In the posterior mediastinum the descending aorta gives paired posterior intercostal arteries.
6. Concerning the respiratory system, which of the following statements is NOT correct?
   a. The trachea begins at the lower border of C6.
   b. The bronchi are lined with pseudostratified ciliated cuboidal epithelium.
   c. Foreign bodies usually enter the right bronchus.
   d. Lymphatic drainage of the lungs is via tracheo-bronchial lymph nodes.
   e. The bronchi are supplied and drained by bronchial vessels.
7. Concerning the lungs, which of the following statements is correct?
   a. The left lung has transverse and oblique fissures.
   b. The trachea grooves the medial surface of the right lung.
   c. The apex of the lung extends above the middle 1/3rd of the clavicle.
   d. At the hilum, the bronchus is the most posterior structure.
   e. The pulmonary veins carry oxygenated blood to the right atrium.
8. In adults, normal respiratory rate is:
   a. 3–5 breaths/min
   b. 12–16 breaths/min.
   c. 15–25 breaths/min.
   d. 20–40 breaths/min.
   e. 30–60 breaths/min.
9. Concerning lung capacity, which of the following statements is NOT correct?
   a. Elasticity is the ability of the lungs to return to their normal shape after each breath.
   b. Inspiratory reserve volume is 3300 mL.
   c. Vital capacity is the largest volume of air that can be expelled after a very deep inspiration.
   d. In healthy adults, total lung capacity is 6000 mL.
   e. Expiratory reserve volume is the same as vital capacity.
10. Concerning gas exchange, which of the following statements is NOT correct?
    a. Gases diffuse from regions of high pressure to regions of low pressure.
    b. The proportion of oxygen in inspired air is 20.8%.
    c. The proportion of nitrogen in expired air is 78.6%.
    d. In the alveoli oxygen diffuses from blood in the capillaries into the inspired air.
    e. The proportion of carbon dioxide in expired air is 3.6%.
11. Which of the following statements is NOT correct?
    a. Type 1 pneumocytes are the site of gas exchange between the alveolus and blood.
    b. The total surface area of the respiratory membrane is 70 m^2.
    c. In carbon monoxide poisoning the oxygen-haemoglobin dissociation curve is irreversibly shifted to the right.
    d. Carbon dioxide is mainly transported to the lungs in plasma.
    e. A high ventilation-perfusion ratio is typically associated with emphysema.

12. Concerning respiratory control, which of the following statements is NOT correct?
    a. The dorsal respiratory group of cells in the respiratory centre are mainly responsible for expiration.
    b. Apneusis can occur as a result of bilateral vagotomy.
    c. Central chemoreceptors monitor the level of carbon dioxide in cerebrospinal fluid.
    d. An increase in blood acidity increases respiration.
    e. Following exercise, the increased respiratory effort is maintained to repay the 'oxygen debt'.

13. Concerning disturbances of respiration, which of the following is NOT correct?
    a. Tachypnoea is an increase in the rate of respiration.
    b. Polypnoea is slow shallow breathing in which the rate of breathing changes but not the force.
    c. Hyperventilation can lead to dizziness and chest pain.
    d. Apnoea is a temporary cessation of breathing.
    e. Dyspnoea can occur due to left ventricular failure.

14. Which of the following is a partial or complete collapse of the lung?
    a. Asphyxia
    b. Pneumonia
    c. Pulmonary oedema
    d. Atelectasis
    e. Emphysema

15. Which of the following statements is NOT correct?
    a. Atopic asthma occurs in children due to an allergy to foreign proteins.
    b. Bronchial asthma is caused by bronchiolar constriction.
    c. Bronchiectasis is a temporary dilation of the bronchi and bronchioles.
    d. Chronic asthma is associated with possible irreversible lung damage.
    e. Panacinar emphysema is the breakdown of the walls between adjacent alveoli.

16. Concerning the heart, which of the following statements is NOT correct?
    a. The fibrous pericardial covering blends with the central tendon of the diaphragm.
    b. The apex is in right 5th intercostal space 9 cm from the midline.

    c. The coronary sinus drains into the right atrium.
    d. Chordae tendineae attach the papillary muscles to the ventricular myocardium.
    e. The sinoatrial node lies at the superior end of the crista terminalis.

17. Concerning blood flow through the heart, which of the following statements is NOT correct?
    a. In the foetus, blood returning to the heart from the superior vena cava passes directly to the left atrium.
    b. In the foetus, blood destined for the lungs passes through the ductus arteriosus into the systemic circulation.
    c. In adults, an opening may persist in the interatrial septum.
    d. Stenosis of a cuspid valve can give rise to a heart murmur.
    e. Semilunar valves rely on the backflow of blood to cause them to close.

18. Which of the following statements is NOT correct?
    a. The coronary arteries are functional end-arteries.
    b. The right coronary artery supplies blood to the posterior part of the interventricular septum in 85% of individuals.
    c. The heart is innervated by both sympathetic and parasympathetic fibres.
    d. The blood supply to the conducting system of the heart is mainly from the left coronary artery.
    e. In total heart block, the ventricles beat at their own rhythm.

19. Concerning the cardiac cycle, which of the following statements is NOT correct?
    a. Depolarisation of cells in the sinoatrial node sets heart rate.
    b. Heart rate is the reciprocal of the duration of the cardiac cycle.
    c. During diastole the heart fills with blood.
    d. At all heart rates there is complete filing of the heart chambers.
    e. The atrioventricular node can act as a secondary pacemaker.

20. Concerning the electrocardiogram, which of the following statements is NOT correct?
    a. The P-R interval corresponds to atrial depolarisation and conduction of the impulse through the atrioventricular node.
    b. The T wave represents ventricular repolarisation.

c. The QRS complex is a repolarising complex spreading through the atrioventricular node, atrioventricular bundle and Purkinje fibres.

d. The R-R interval represents the duration of a single cardiac cycle.

e. The U wave becomes prominent in hypokalaemia.

21. Concerning arrhythmias, which of the following statements is NOT correct?

a. Sinus arrhythmia is the fluctuation in heart rate associated with respiration.

b. Sinus bradycardia is associated with a reduced R-R interval.

c. Heart block is blockage of impulses generated by the sinoatrial node.

d. Extrasystole is a premature contraction of the heart caused by the discharge of impulses other than at the sinoatrial node.

e. Ventricular fibrillation is a rapid and irregular twitching of the ventricles.

22. Which of the following statements is correct?

a. Low concentrations of sodium ions in blood increases the electrical activity of the myocardium.

b. An increase in calcium ions in the blood reduces the excitability of the myocardium.

c. Small changes in potassium ion concentration in the blood have no effect on the excitability of the myocardium.

d. An increase in calcium ions is associated with a lengthened S-T segment and QT interval.

e. High concentrations of potassium ions in the blood is fatal.

23. Concerning cardiac output, which of the following statements is NOT correct?

a. It is the amount of blood ejected from each ventricle with each heartbeat.

b. It is equivalent to heart rate multiplied by stroke volume.

c. An increased afterload can decrease stroke volume.

d. Stroke volume decreases when venous return exceeds cardiac output.

e. Increased sympathetic activity increases the force and rate of myocardial contraction.

24. Concerning heart rate, which of the following statements is NOT correct?

a. It is a balance between sympathetic and parasympathetic stimulation of the sinoatrial node.

b. The right atrial (Bainbridge) reflex increases heart rate when venous return decreases.

c. It is lower when lying down.

d. It is increased in fear and anxiety.

e. Elevated carbon dioxide levels in the blood lead to bradycardia.

25. Concerning the great vessels, which of the following statements is NOT correct?

a. The mitral valve controls blood flow into the aorta.

b. The pulmonary trunk receives deoxygenated blood from the right ventricle.

c. The adventitia of the inferior vena cava is adherent to the central tendon of the diaphragm.

d. The superior vena cava is formed behind the left sternoclavicular joint.

e. The arch of the aorta gives rise to three branches supplying the head, neck and upper limbs.

26. Concerning blood vessels, which of the following statements is correct?

a. Atheroma develops in the tunica media of large arteries.

b. The tunica adventitia mainly comprises collagenous tissue.

c. The endothelium acts as an impermeable membrane between blood plasma and interstitial fluid.

d. In arteries, the tunica intima contains layers of smooth muscle.

e. Veins do not have valves.

27. Concerning blood vessels, which of the following statement is NOT correct?

a. An aneurysm is a local dilation in an artery.

b. In arteriosclerosis the tunica media is infiltrated with calcium.

c. Deep vein thrombosis is usually asymptomatic.

d. In varicose veins blood flows from the superficial to deep veins.

e. In superficial thrombophlebitis, the surrounding tissues become inflamed and painful.

28. Concerning the circulation, which of the following statements is NOT correct?

a. The rate of blood flow through tissues is determined by their need for nutrients.

b. Cardiac output is determined by the sum of all local tissue blood flows.

c. It functions to transport hormones from one region to another.

d. Arterioles have strong muscular walls which can control blood flow.

e. The regulation of arterial pressure is entirely dependent on local blood flow.

29. What is the pressure gradient between the aorta and right atrium?
   a. 70 mm Hg
   b. 15 mm Hg
   c. 20 mm Hg
   d. 120 mm Hg
   e. 10 mm Hg

30. The volume of blood flow is directly proportional to the:
   a. pressure gradient
   b. resistance
   c. viscosity
   d. vessel compliance
   e. vessel elasticity

31. Concerning arterial blood pressure, which of the following statements is NOT correct?
   a. Mean arterial pressure is diastolic pressure + 1/3rd pulse pressure.
   b. It increases with age.
   c. It is higher in the morning than at midday.
   d. Systolic pressure is the maximum pressure exerted in the arteries.
   e. It is greater in obese individuals.

32. Concerning hypertension, which of the following statements is NOT correct?
   a. Malignant hypertension leads to progressive cardiac and renal disease.
   b. β adrenoreceptor blockers inhibit vasodilation.
   c. Calcium channel blockers decrease cardiac output.
   d. During pregnancy can lead to toxaemia.
   e. In benign hypertension, blood pressure returns to normal when resting or sleeping.

33. Which of the following hormones leads to a decrease in blood pressure?
   a. Thyroxine
   b. Serotonin
   c. Adrenaline
   d. Vasopressin
   e. Histamine

34. Concerning the arterial pulse, which of the following statements is NOT correct?

a. The pulse wave depends on the elasticity of the blood vessels.

b. It is an expression of pressure changes in the systemic circulatory system.

c. At birth pulse (heart) rate is 130–140 beats/min.

d. The anacrotic limb is due to the fall in pressure during systole.

e. It provides important information concerning the rate and rhythmicity of cardiac function.

35. Concerning venous blood pressure, which of the following statements is NOT correct?
   a. It varies in different veins.
   b. It decreases when tilting the body.
   c. It increases with low cardiac output.
   d. It is inversely proportional to peripheral resistance.
   e. It increases with heart failure.

36. Concerning capillaries, which of the following statements is correct?
   a. They comprise several layers of endothelial cells surrounded by pericytes.
   b. Intercellular clefts between cells allow substances to pass through the cell walls.
   c. Blood flow through them is continuous.
   d. A decreased capillary refill time is a sign of circulatory shock.
   e. The capillary membrane is permeable to plasma proteins.

37. Concerning haemorrhage, which of the following statements is NOT correct?
   a. Chronic haemorrhage can lead to anaemia.
   b. The skin has a grey colour.
   c. Capillary pressure increases.
   d. Increased sympathetic activity leads to the release of catecholamines.
   e. Stagnant hypoxia increases respiratory rate.

38. Concerning shock, which of the following statements is NOT correct?
   a. It produces tachycardia and vasoconstriction.
   b. Vasogenic shock is due to an inadequate blood supply to tissues.
   c. In neurogenic shock raising the lower limbs increases venous return.
   d. It can occur in arrhythmia.
   e. In the first stage regulatory mechanisms are unable to successfully restore normal blood pressure and blood flow.

39. Concerning heart failure, which of the following statements is NOT correct?
    a. It is the inability of the heart to supply blood to all parts of the body.
    b. In acute failure there is no time for compensatory mechanisms to occur.
    c. In right-sided congestive cardiac failure blood in the venae cavae continues to flow normally.
    d. Hypertension can be a cause of chronic failure.
    e. There can be nausea and vomiting.

40. Which of the following is NOT a function of lymph?
    a. Transport of lymphocytes.
    b. A route for protein absorption.
    c. Removal of bacteria.
    d. Redistribution of body fluid.
    e. Maintenance of tissue structure.

41. Concerning the lymphatic system, which of the following statements is correct?
    a. Lymph is a yellowish viscous fluid.
    b. Lymphatic capillaries are open-ended tubes.
    c. All lymphatics accompany blood vessels.
    d. Lymph nodes contain lymphocytes and macrophages.
    e. The paracortex of lymph nodes contains T lymphocytes.

42. Which of the following is NOT a function of blood?
    a. It transports carbon dioxide to the lungs.
    b. It aids the regulation of acid-base balance.
    c. It conveys urea to the liver.
    d. It helps maintain core body temperature.
    e. It stores glucose.

43. Concerning blood, which of the following statements is NOT correct?
    a. Plasma is 90% water.
    b. Prothrombin is responsible for blood coagulation.
    c. An increase in plasma proteins occurs in acute infections.
    d. Red bone marrow is the site of most blood cell production.
    e. The lifespan of red blood cells is between 1 and 10 days.

44. Which of the following is NOT a leukocyte?
    a. Neutrophil
    b. Erythrocyte
    c. Basophil
    d. Monocyte
    e. Lymphocyte

45. Concerning anaemia, which of the following statements is NOT correct?

    a. In anaemia there are no changes in red blood cell morphology.
    b. It can be due to excessive blood loss.
    c. Sickle cell haemoglobin changes the shape of red blood cells.
    d. Can be due to a lack of vitamin B_{12} in the diet.
    e. It is associated with a loss of elasticity of the skin.

46. What is the lifespan of lymphocytes?
    a. 120 days
    b. 12–15 days
    c. 7–12 days
    d. 2–5 days
    e. 0.5–1 day

47. Concerning leukocytes, which of the following statements is NOT correct?
    a. Eosinophils cause tissue inflammation.
    b. Monocytes can develop into alveolar macrophages in the lungs.
    c. Neutrophils contain histamine.
    d. A decrease in neutrophils occurs in autoimmune diseases.
    e. Macrophages have a wide range of protective functions.

48. Concerning platelets, which of the following statements is correct?
    a. Platelet count is decreased at high altitude.
    b. Platelet count increases following surgical interventions.
    c. Phospholipids prevent their adhesion to normal endothelium.
    d. Glycoproteins accelerate clotting reactions.
    e. The normal adult platelet count is 100,000–200,000/mm³.

49. Concerning immunity, which of the following statements is NOT correct?
    a. Cytotoxic cells destroy invading organisms.
    b. Memory T cells remain in lymphoid tissue.
    c. Each T cell is activated by a single type of antigen.
    d. B lymphocytes are transformed into plasma cells.
    e. Antibodies comprise 50% of total plasma proteins.

50. Which of the following is NOT an autoimmune disease?
    a. Myasthenia gravis
    b. Graves' disease
    c. Cushing disease
    d. Insulin-dependent diabetes mellitus
    e. Hashimoto thyroiditis

Vertebral Column (Back)

CONTENTS

Key Concepts, 187
Learning Outcomes, 188
Overview, 188
Vertebral Column, 188
  Introduction, 188
    Curvatures, 189
  Bones, 191
    Vertebrae, 191
  Intervertebral Joints, 195
    Between Bodies, 195
    Between Arches, 199
  Movements of the Vertebral Column, 200
  Stability, 200
  Blood and Nerve Supply of the Vertebral
    Column, 201
  Muscles of the Trunk, 202

Spinal Cord, 204
  Meninges, 206
    Epidural Space, 207
    Blood Supply, 207
  Internal Structure and Organisation, 210
    Grey Matter, 211
    White Matter, 212
    Afferent and Efferent Tracts, 212
    Spinal Reflexes, 217
    Spinal Cord Lesions, 219
  Spinal Nerves, 220
    Nerve Root Sheaths, 221
  Somatic Nervous System, 221
  Autonomic Nervous System, 223
    Parasympathetic Nervous System. 225
    Sympathetic Nervous System, 225

KEY CONCEPTS

- The multi-segmented vertebral column is stable.
- Secondary cartilaginous joints between vertebral bodies allow limited movement but, when added together, provide flexibility.
- Synovial joints between vertebral arches control and guide movements.
- Intervertebral discs are viscoelastic.
- The spinal cord is part of the central nervous system: it is bathed in cerebrospinal fluid.
- The rounded spinal cord has an H-shaped central region of grey matter (cells, non-myelinated fibres) surrounded by white matter (myelinated fibres).
- Grey matter is organised into 10 laminae; white matter contains ascending and descending tracts, with short tracts coordinating spinal cord function and long tracts projecting to or originating from higher centres.
- Spinal arteries are reinforced by radicular arteries.
- Vertebral venous plexuses communicate with veins in other regions.
- Thirty-one pairs of spinal nerves arise by dorsal and ventral roots from the spinal cord, with each pair associated with a single spinal cord segment.
- Each spinal nerve divides into dorsal (posterior) and ventral (anterior) rami.
- The autonomic nervous system has two parts: sympathetic part arising between T1 and L2 (thoracolumbar outflow) and parasympathetic from cranial nerves III, VII, IX and X and S2–S4 (craniosacral outflow).

LEARNING OUTCOMES

At the end of this chapter, you should be able to:
- Describe the structure and organisation of the vertebral column and understand its function.
- Describe the movements associated with each region of the vertebral column.
- Describe the structure of the intervertebral disc and understand its function.
- Describe the structure and organisation of the spinal cord.
- Describe the arterial supply and venous drainage of the vertebral column and spinal cord.
- Describe the ascending and descending tracts of the spinal cord and understand the function of each.
- Describe the formation of a spinal nerve and components.
- Describe the components of the autonomic nervous system and their function.
- Understand the effect of pathology and/or trauma on the spinal cord.

OVERVIEW

This chapter considers the structure and function of the vertebral column (back); it is organised into two major sections, the vertebral column and the spinal cord and autonomic nervous system. In the vertebral column section, the features and organisation of the vertebrae in each region are considered, including their ossification, palpation and the articulations between the bodies, including the intervertebral disc, and the vertebral arches: this is followed by a consideration of the major muscle groups and their function. The movements possible in each region of the vertebral column are covered, including those between the base of the skull and cervical spine, as well as the muscles producing movements of the head on the neck. There is also a brief evaluation of the movements of the vertebral column. In the spinal cord and autonomic nervous system section, the major features of each are considered, together with the consequences of trauma and pathology.

VERTEBRAL COLUMN

Introduction

The vertebral column can be considered as a weight-bearing rod held erect by ligaments and muscles. Because of its weight-bearing role, the vertebral bodies increase in size from above downwards (Fig. 3.1A), reflecting the increasing compressive forces lower down the column; the proportions of the vertebral bodies also change from above downwards. To accommodate these increased forces, the sacral vertebrae have fused into a large single bone important in the transmission of weight to the pelvis and lower limbs. Some degree of support is provided by the thorax, its associated ribs and muscles, as well as by the abdominal muscles.

The vertebral column consists of a series of mobile segments held together by ligaments and muscles: each segment is separated from adjacent segments by an intervertebral disc. There are 33 bony segments (vertebrae) of which 24 are usually separate bones: the lower 9 fuse, with 5 forming the sacrum and 4 the coccyx. According to their features, the individual vertebrae are designated cervical, thoracic and lumbar depending on their features and position in the vertebral column: there are 7 cervical, 12 thoracic and 5 lumbar vertebrae (Fig. 3.1A).

Approximately 40% of an individual's height is due to the length of the vertebral column, which is 72–75 cm in length, with a quarter being due to the presence of the intervertebral discs: variations in height are mainly a reflection of an individual's leg length. There are diurnal variations in height (up to 2 cm) due to compression and loss of thickness of intervertebral discs; height loss in the elderly is associated with thinning of the discs, as well as age-related changes.

The vertebral column has a number of important functions: it carries and supports the thoracic cage; gives attachment to muscles of the pectoral and pelvic girdles, which pass into the upper and lower limbs, respectively; provides attachment for many powerful muscles which move the vertebral column, as well as maintaining balance and uprightness of the vertebral column; surrounds and protects the spinal cord against mechanical trauma; acts as a shock absorber by virtue of its inherent curvatures and the intervertebral discs between adjacent vertebral bodies by receiving and distributing the impacts associated with movement; produces and accumulates moments of force, as well as concentrating and transmitting forces received from other parts of the body; and is an important site of haemopoiesis.

Because of the erect posture and independent functioning of the upper limbs increased demands are placed

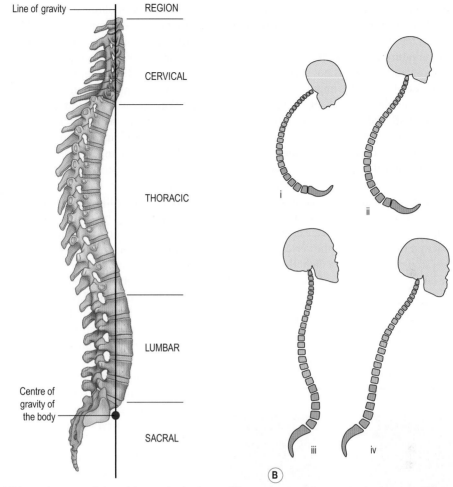

Fig. 3.1 (A) Lateral aspect of the adult vertebral column; (B) curvatures of the vertebral column at different ages, (i) birth, (ii) 6 months, (iii) adulthood, (iv) old age.

on the vertebral column: the adaptations made to meet these demands have not been entirely successful, as seen in the incidence of low back pain and its associated problems in everyday living.

Curvatures

The adult vertebral column has four curvatures, anterior concavities in the thoracic and sacral regions and acquired anterior convexities in the cervical and lumbar regions (Fig. 3.1A): acquired curvatures are not present at birth. Until late in foetal development the vertebral column has a single anterior concave curvature (Fig. 3.1B (i)).

The secondary cervical curvature (Fig. 3.1B (ii)) begins to appear in late foetal life, becoming more accentuated between 6 and 12 weeks after birth; it is relatively shallow extending from the 2nd cervical (C2, axis) to

the 1st thoracic (T1) vertebra and can be reduced by bending the head forwards.

The permanent thoracic curve is due in part to the shape of the vertebral bodies in the thoracic region, which are taller posteriorly than anteriorly; it extends from T1 to the 12th thoracic (T12) vertebra. An increase in the thoracic curvature is known as kyphosis.

The secondary lumbar curve (Fig. 3.1B (iii)) starts to appear as the child begins to sit and stand at about 6 months and develops in response to the need to keep the trunk erect; it is not fully developed until after age 2 following the attainment of a more or less adult pattern of walking. The lumbar curvature starts at T12 and ends at the lumbosacral junction; it is deeper and more prominent in females. During pregnancy, the lumbar curvature becomes more pronounced as the trunk moves backwards to prevent overbalancing. An increase in lumbar curvature is referred to as lordosis, although the normal lumbar curve is also often referred to as a lumbar lordosis.

The sacral curvature is permanent due to its fused parts. The lumbosacral junction is not part of the vertebral curvatures; nevertheless, it is important as the junction between the mobile and immobile regions of the vertebral column, with the associated structures being put under considerable stress.

With increasing age, the vertebral column tends to assume a gentle C-shaped curve (Fig. 3.1B (iv)) due to thinning and degeneration of the intervertebral discs.

The normal curvatures make the vertebral column a flexible support, imparting resilience to axial compressive forces which are absorbed by a concertina action of the curves. Viewed from the front the vertebral column appears almost straight, except for a slight thoracic curve to the right; a large lateral curve (scoliosis) is abnormal.

> **CLINICAL ANATOMY:** Scoliosis is a complex three-dimensional deformity involving lateral flexion and rotation of the vertebrae: in the rotated vertebrae the bodies are rotated towards the convexity and the spinous processes towards the concavity of the curvature (Fig. 3.2).

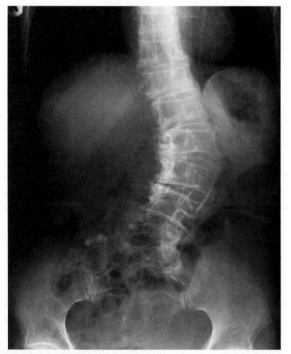

Fig. 3.2 Anteroposterior radiograph of the vertebral column showing thoracolumbar scoliosis.

Scoliosis. Scoliotic curves can be broadly classified into two types: non-structural and structural. Non-structural curves are readily reversed by changing posture or by traction; postural curves are eliminated on forward flexion and show no fixed vertebral rotation. Compensatory curves in the opposite direction develop above and below a single structural curve in an attempt to maintain the alignment of the body; compensatory curves also show no vertebral rotation or structural changes.

In contrast, structural curves demonstrate rib and vertebral rotation to the convexity of the curve in forward flexion. Although scoliotic curves can develop anywhere along the length of the vertebral column, they are most common in the thoracic and lumbar regions; in the thoracic region, there is little resistance to rotation, while in the lumbar region, the existing lordosis may be important in its development.

Scoliosis can be classified according to the age of onset in the individual, particularly important in idiopathic scoliosis, which accounts for 85% of all scolioses. Left thoracic curves present most commonly in infants under age 4 (infantile scoliosis), while right thoracic curves are more common between puberty and skeletal maturity (adolescent scoliosis); infantile scoliosis often regresses naturally. Between age 4 and puberty (juvenile scoliosis) curves occur with equal frequency to the right and left.

While the above age-based classifications are of interest, a more useful classification is in terms of their aetiology and pathogenesis. Three classes of curve can be considered: congenital scoliosis, due to congenital vertebral anomalies, which themselves can be classified; neuromuscular scoliosis, in which there is an obvious neurological or muscular impairment; and idiopathic scoliosis, of which there are four main groups (primary skeletal, neuromuscular, metabolic, genetic), each with an unclear aetiology. Although the aetiology may be reasonably well understood, the mechanisms by which the deformity develops are less clear.

> **CLINICAL ANATOMY:** The incidence of clinically evident scoliosis is 0.1%–0.5% of the population, being more prevalent in white populations than black, and more prevalent in females than males (ratio 5:1). Screening programmes have suggested that 15% of the population show some form of lateral curvature of the vertebral column; most are considered to be non-structural or do not develop to be of any significance.

Bones
Vertebrae

DEVELOPMENT: Typical vertebrae ossify from three primary and five secondary centres: primary centres appear in the body and in each half of the vertebral arch, with secondary centres appearing as annular rings covering the upper and lower surfaces of the bodies and in the tips of the spinous and transverse processes. At birth, the body and vertebral arch are separated by cartilage; this begins to ossify at age 3 in the cervical region extending into other regions by age 7. The laminae begin to unite soon after birth in the lumbar region, spreading to the cervical region by the second year; it is complete in the sacrum between ages 7 and 10. Secondary centres for the upper and lower surfaces of the body appear during the ninth year, forming flat rings of bone around the periphery; those in the tips of the spinous and transverse processes appear between puberty and age 18. Fusion of all secondary epiphyses with the rest of the vertebra begins at age 18 and is complete by age 25.

CLINICAL ANATOMY: A number of congenital conditions associated with the vertebral column are due to incomplete fusion of its constituent parts. Hemivertebrae can cause an abnormal lateral curvature (scoliosis); the laminae may fail to fuse or meet in the midline in any region, but most commonly in the lumbosacral region giving rise to spina bifida; the laminae, spinous and inferior articular processes of L4 and L5 may not fuse with the rest of the vertebra, which under certain loading conditions can lead to forward sliding of the body of L5 on the sacrum (spondylolisthesis).

All vertebrae, except the 1st (C1, atlas) and 2nd (C2, axis) cervical, have a large weight-bearing body anteriorly and a vertebral (neural) arch posteriorly, with a series of projecting processes (Fig. 3.3). Although the shape and size of the body vary, it has flattened upper and lower surfaces with markings for the attachment of the intervertebral disc around the margin, which surrounds a roughened central area. The front and sides are concave from top to bottom with roughened areas at the upper and lower margins; the posterior surface is smooth with a large opening for the basivertebral vein.

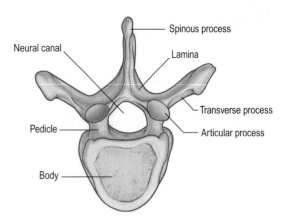

Fig. 3.3 A typical vertebra.

The vertebral arch arises from the posterolateral aspect of the body and, with the body, encloses the vertebral foramen; successive foramen constitute the vertebral canal housing the spinal cord and its coverings. The arch comprises two pedicles and two laminae (Fig. 3.3); the laminae meet in the midline posteriorly where they are continuous with the spinous process. At the junction of the pedicle and lamina, the transverse process projects laterally, as well as the superior and inferior articular processes projecting superiorly and inferiorly, respectively (Fig. 3.3); the articular processes carry articular facets which articulate with adjacent facets by small synovial (zygapophyseal) joints.

With some exceptions, each part of each vertebra is present in all other vertebrae. The major differences between vertebrae in the cervical, thoracic, lumbar and sacral regions are related to the size and fate of their associated costal elements (Fig. 3.4). In the cervical region, the medial end of the costal element fuses with the side of the body anterior to the transverse process; the presence of blood vessels anteriorly leads to the formation of the foramen transversarium (Fig. 3.4). In the thoracic region, the costal element remains separate as the rib (Fig. 3.4), which articulates with the vertebra. In the lumbar and sacral region, the costal element is incorporated into the vertebra (Fig. 3.4).

The number of cervical vertebrae is constant at 7; however, the number of thoracic vertebrae may be increased by the presence of ribs associated with L1, or decreased by the incorporation of L5 into the sacrum; such sacralisation may be partial or complete. The sacrum may also gain or lose segments.

Internal architecture. Within each vertebra are extensive and complex systems of bony plates and struts (trabeculae) which reflect the stresses to which it is exposed (Fig. 3.5A and B). Within each vertebra is a single principle vertical and several oblique and horizontal systems; except for interruption by the intervertebral discs, the vertical system is continuous throughout the length of the vertebral column from C2 to the sacrum. The oblique systems do not reach the anterior margin of the vertebral body, hence the occurrence of vertebral compression fractures (Fig. 3.5C).

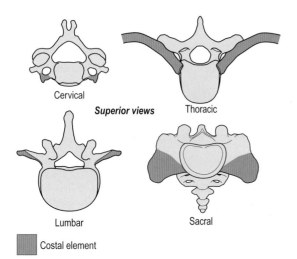

Cervical

Superior views   Thoracic

Lumbar   Sacral

▨ Costal element

Fig. 3.4 Fate of the costal element in each vertebral region.

> **APPLIED ANATOMY:** Mechanically the vertical system sustains body weight and counters the jars and shocks reaching the vertebral column perpendicularly. The oblique systems resist torsion and, together with the vertical system, share in the resistance to bending and shear forces. Systems projecting into the spinous and transverse processes resist tension developed by ligaments during stretching and contraction of muscles. In osteoporosis, the secondary systems are the first to atrophy making the vertical system more prominent on radiographs.

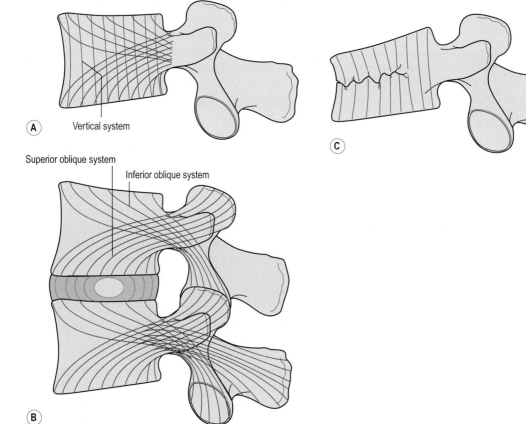

(A) Vertical system

Superior oblique system

Inferior oblique system

(B)

(C)

Fig. 3.5 (A) Vertical and (B) oblique trabecular systems within vertebrae; (C) Compression fracture.

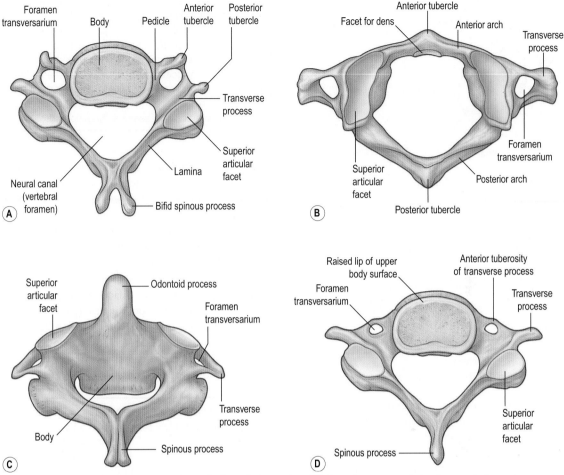

Fig. 3.6 (A) Superior aspect of a typical cervical vertebra. (B) Superior aspect of the 1st cervical vertebra (atlas). (C) Posterosuperior aspect of the 2nd cervical vertebra (axis). (D) Superior aspect of the 7th cervical vertebra.

Cervical vertebrae. All cervical vertebrae are characterised by the presence of a foramen transversarium in each transverse process (Fig. 3.6A). The 3rd to 6th are typical, having a relatively small kidney-shaped body with the superior surface projecting upwards at the sides, while the inferior surface is correspondingly bevelled: these upward projections form small synovial joints between the bodies (uncovertebral joints) which help stabilise movements of the neck (Fig. 3.7). The spinous process is short and bifid. Each superior articular process has a slightly convex articular facet, while the inferior articular process carries a reciprocally concave articular facet; the facets become more vertical in the lower part of the cervical spine.

CLINICAL ANATOMY: Degenerative (arthritic) changes associated with the uncovertebral joints can be painful and lead to restricted movements between adjacent vertebrae and, therefore, of the neck, as well as affecting relevant spinal nerves. In association with hypertrophy of the joints, the degenerative changes can lead to spinal stenosis.

1st cervical vertebra (atlas). A ring of bone with no body or spinous process and slender anterior and posterior arches joined by a large lateral mass carrying superior and inferior articular facets, and a transverse process (Fig. 3.6B); the superior facet articulates with the base of the skull (occipital condyles) and the inferior with C2. The large, wide strong transverse processes may be

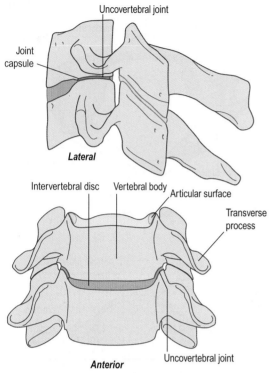

Uncovertebral joint

Joint
capsule

Lateral

Intervertebral disc   Vertebral body
Articular surface

Transverse
process

Anterior   Uncovertebral joint

Fig. 3.7 The uncovertebral joints.

bifid; the foramen transversarium transmits the vertebral vessels and sympathetic nerves. The anterior arch has an articular facet for the odontoid process (dens) of C2.

2nd cervical vertebra (atlas). The strongest of all cervical vertebrae with many features of a typical cervical vertebra but with the addition of an upward projection (odontoid process, dens) from the superior surface of its body (Fig. 3.6C). Large superior articular facets lie at the junction of the body and pedicle and transmit the weight of the head to its body.

7th cervical vertebra (vertebra prominens). Larger than preceding vertebrae it has a long non-bifid spinous process with a large body and pedicles directed posterolaterally (Fig. 3.6D); the inferior articular facets face more anteriorly than inferiorly.

CLINICAL ANATOMY: The costal element of C7 may be longer than its transverse process giving the appearance of a rudimentary rib extending towards the 1st rib, either as a bony or fibrous strip; this can lead to pressure on the C8 nerve root as it passes over the 1st rib to join in the formation of the brachial plexus. Compression of the C8 nerve root leads to neurological signs and symptoms in the area of its distribution.

APPLIED ANATOMY: Approximately 2 cm below the external occipital protuberance (page 239), the spinous process of C2 can be felt; there is a deep hollow between these two landmarks. Some 10 cm further down is the spinous process of C7, immediately below which is the spinous process of T1. Lateral to the muscle mass on either side of the spinous processes the tips of the transverse processes can be palpated.

Thoracic vertebrae. The heart-shaped bodies of thoracic vertebrae have facets on their sides for articulation with the heads of at least one pair of ribs (Fig. 3.8). T1–T9 have an oval facet near their upper borders and smaller demifacets near their lower borders; T10–T12 have a single oval facet at the junction of the body and pedicle. The spinous processes are long and tend to point downwards. The transverse processes project posterolaterally and carry a facet for articulation with the tubercle of the corresponding rib (page 70); those of T11 and T12 have no facets. The articular facets on the superior articular processes tend to face posteriorly and those on the inferior articular processes anteriorly; they lie in an almost vertical plane.

APPLIED ANATOMY: The spinous processes can be felt with the individual sitting with the trunk flexed, especially those of C7 and T1; moving down the column, the remaining processes can be identified. Some 2 cm on either side of the midline the transverse processes can be palpated, just beyond which the rib can be felt passing downwards and laterally around the chest wall; the latter bony points are more readily palpated with the individual lying prone.

Lumbar vertebrae. These are much larger and stronger than either thoracic or cervical vertebrae; they do not possess foramina transversaria or have facets on the body for articulation with the ribs (Fig. 3.9). The large kidney-shaped body has almost parallel upper and lower surfaces, except L5 which is deeper anteriorly than posteriorly; this contributes to the marked change in curvature at the lumbosacral angle. The spinous processes are short and square. The articular facets on the articular processes lie in a vertical parasagittal plane, with the superior facets facing posteromedially and inferior facets facing anterolaterally. The transverse processes are short and thin; L5 may be fused with the lateral part of the sacrum.

APPLIED ANATOMY: Palpation is best when the individual is lying supine with the abdomen supported to raise the lumbar spine; the spinous processes can be palpated in the central midline cleft. On the posterior superior aspect of the buttock is a small dimple 3 cm from the midline, which marks the position of the posterior superior iliac spine (page 567); from these the iliac crest can be traced upwards and forwards. The L5 spinous process can be felt in a deep hollow 2 cm above a line drawn between the iliac spines; from here the gaps between the spinous processes of L4–T12 can be palpated and the individual spinous processes identified. Either side of the midline is a powerful column of muscle running from the posterior of the sacrum up to the thoracic region. Laterally, with deep pressure, the tips of the transverse processes can be felt.

Sacrum and coccyx. The sacrum was originally five separate vertebrae which have fused in adults to form a single curved bone (Fig. 3.10); it is wedged between the posterior parts of the pelvis with which it articulates at the sacroiliac joint (page 570). The coccyx consists of four fused vertebrae forming a single or two pieces of bone (Fig. 3.10A); it is of little significance. Further details of the sacrum and coccyx can be found on page 569.

APPLIED ANATOMY: Between individuals, and sometime between sides, considerable variation exists in the location of bony points. The most obvious surface markings are the posteriorly directed spinous processes; however, their lengths can vary, be angled differently or occasionally be absent. Palpation can also vary due to the lordosis in the cervical and lumbar regions and the kyphosis in the thoracic and sacral regions. The best way to identify vertebral spinous processes is to count upwards or downwards from a known bony landmark and cross-check with other surface markings.

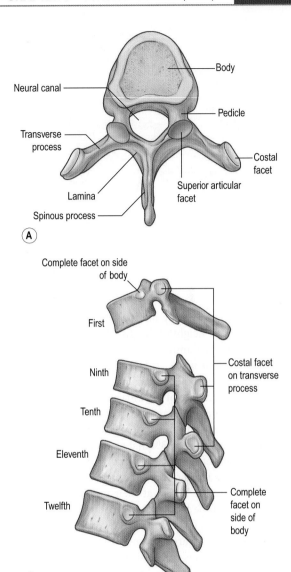

Fig. 3.8 (A) Superior aspect of a typical thoracic vertebra. (B) Lateral aspects of T1 and T9–T12.

Intervertebral Joints

In adults, the vertebrae are arranged in a series of curvatures; nevertheless, the joints between adjacent vertebrae have a common plan, except those between C1 and C2. Anteriorly the bodies are bound together by secondary cartilaginous joints (page 35), while posteriorly the vertebral arches are united by synovial joints (page 36). The vertebral arches are separated by the intervertebral foramen, through which emerge the spinal nerves from the spinal cord; the upper and lower boundaries of the foramen are formed by the pedicles of the arches. Although separate, the joints between bodies and arches function together, giving the vertebral column controlled flexibility and movement.

Between Bodies

Between C2 and S1, the articulations between adjacent vertebral bodies are by a secondary cartilaginous joint,

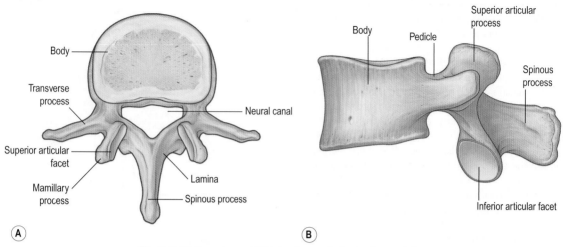

Fig. 3.9 (A) Superior and (B) lateral aspect of a lumbar vertebra.

of which the intervening intervertebral disc is the main component; the height of the disc differs in each region of the vertebral column (Fig. 3.11).

Intervertebral discs. These account for 25% of the length of the vertebral column and are primarily responsible for the presence of the curvatures. On descending the column, the discs increase in thickness (Fig. 3.11), being 40% the height of cervical vertebrae, 25% that of thoracic vertebrae and 33% that of lumbar vertebrae; the relative height of the discs is important in determining the mobility of the vertebral column in each region. The discs are avascular except at their periphery, obtaining the majority of the blood supply from the adjacent vertebral bodies (see Fig. 3.18B).

Individual discs are not uniform in thickness; their shape also conforms to the shape of adjacent vertebral bodies. In the cervical region, the intervertebral discs do not extend the full width of the vertebral body, with small synovial (uncovertebral) joints between the lateral bevelled edges of the bodies (page 193).

CLINICAL ANATOMY: The intervertebral disc forms one of the anterior boundaries of the intervertebral foramen, with the spinal nerves lying directly behind the corresponding disc. It also forms part of the anterior wall of the vertebral canal so that any posterior bulging of the disc may compress the spinal cord, as well as individual spinal nerves.

Each disc comprises three integrated tissues (nucleus pulposus, annulus fibrosis, cartilage end plates) (Fig. 3.12): it is anchored to the vertebral body by fibres of the annulus fibrosis and cartilage end plate.

Nucleus pulposus The soft hydrophilic centre of the disc consisting of a three-dimensional lattice of collagen fibres, enmeshed in which is a proteoglycan gel responsible for its hydrophilic properties. Patchy loss and disappearance of the gel occur with ageing, lowering its water content; in advanced degeneration, the collagen may be devoid of proteoglycan material. In early life, the water content is 80%–88%, but from age 40 it gradually decreases to 70%; the accompanying proteoglycan changes modify the mechanical behaviour of the disc.

There is no clear distinction between the nucleus pulposus and surrounding annulus fibrosis apart from the density of the fibres it contains. The region between the nucleus and annulus is an area of maximum metabolic activity, being sensitive to physical forces and to chemical and hormonal regulation of growth processes; it can be considered to represent the growth plate of the nucleus as it can only increase in size and remodel itself during growth at the expense of the annulus fibrosis. Systemic changes may be the primary cause of pathological change within the disc and possibly of all pathological change within the intervertebral space.

Annulus fibrosis A series of concentric lamellae (bands) surrounding the nucleus pulposus, in which the arrangement of fibres alternates between

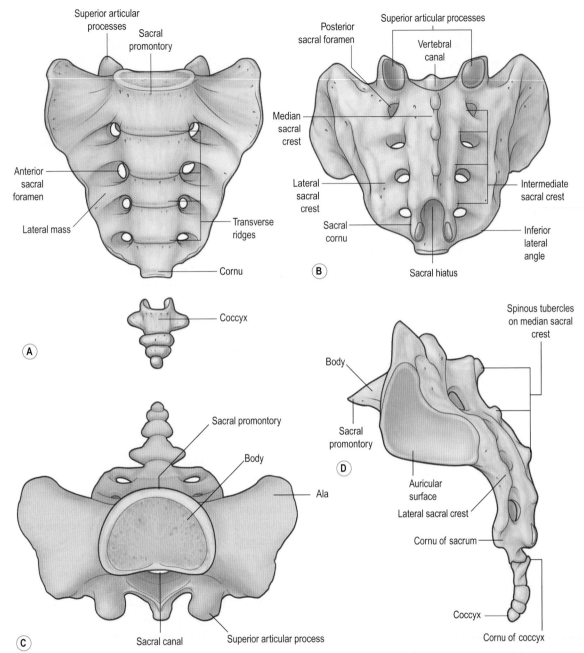

Fig. 3.10 (A) Anterior, (B) posterior, (C) superior and (D) lateral aspects of the sacrum.

adjacent bands; the obliquity of the fibres is greatest in the innermost lamellae. The annulus increases its horizontal diameter by adding new lamellae at the periphery.

The number of lamellae, as well as their size and thickness, vary between vertebral levels and between individuals: the mean number of lamellae is 20, with thicknesses of 200–400 μm. The lamellae are more

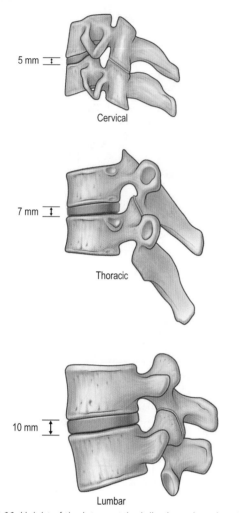

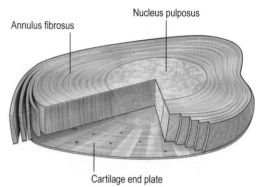

Fig. 3.12 Components of the intervertebral disc. (Adapted from Hendry NG. The hydration of the nucleus pulposus and its relation to intervertebral disc derangement. J Bone Joint Surg 1958;40-B:132–144.)

Fig. 3.11 Height of the intervertebral disc in each region of the vertebral column.

Cartilage end plate Located on each surface of the vertebral body, they represent the anatomical limits of the disc; it is 1 cm in height at the periphery decreasing towards the centre. It has three main functions: protecting the vertebral body from pressure atrophy; confining the annulus fibrosis and nucleus pulposus; and acting as a semipermeable membrane facilitating fluid exchange between the annulus and nucleus and the vertebral body.

Ultrastructurally, the nucleus pulposus, annulus fibrosis and cartilage end plates act as a close-packed system which acts as a shock absorber of forces transmitted to the vertebral column. The ability to absorb shock is due to deformation of the nucleus when compressed, causing it to expand radially against the surrounding annulus, which in turn expands outwards. While the nucleus is important in compressive deformation, the annulus appears to be the primary load-bearing structure, capable of performing this function when part or all of the nucleus has degenerated. However, efficient functioning of the disc depends on the elasticity of the nucleus, which is closely related to its water-binding capacity. Increased pressure in the nucleus through the imbibition of water increases disc height, prestressing the disc, reducing its laxity and increasing vertebral joint stiffness.

Mechanically, the intervertebral disc is a viscoelastic structure capable of maintaining large loads without disintegrating; its mechanical efficiency improves with use, providing a theoretical basis for 'taking the strain' before lifting a heavy load.

densely packed anteriorly and posteriorly than laterally. They do not form complete rings but split or merge with others, with posterolateral regions showing marked irregularities and being less well-ordered; with ageing, the annulus becomes weakest in these regions. The annulus provides limited restriction to movement during compression and tension.

The annulus is attached to the vertebral body by fibres passing over the edges of the cartilage end plate into the compact bone at the margin of the vertebral rim, as well as to the margins of adjacent vertebral bodies and their periosteum.

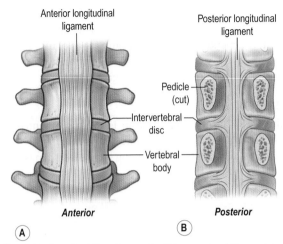

Anterior longitudinal ligament

Posterior longitudinal ligament

Pedicle (cut)

Intervertebral disc

Vertebral body

Anterior

Posterior

(A)

(B)

Fig. 3.13 Anterior (A) and posterior (B) aspects of the vertebral bodies showing the position and attachments of the anterior and posterior longitudinal ligaments.

Ligaments. The vertebral bodies are held together by ligaments (anterior and posterior longitudinal) extending the length of the vertebral column (Fig. 3.13).

The **anterior longitudinal ligament** supports the front of the vertebral column, including the discs, and runs from the anterior tubercle of C1 to the pelvic surface of the upper sacrum; as it descends, it increases in width. It consists of three layers of dense collagen fibres, with the deepest joining adjacent vertebrae and the most superficial extending across several vertebrae. Above the level of the atlas, the anterior longitudinal ligament is continuous with the anterior atlanto-occipital membrane.

The **posterior longitudinal ligament** only attaches to the intervertebral discs and adjacent margins of the vertebral bodies, being denticulate in appearance; it is part of the anterior wall of the vertebral canal. It runs from the back of the body of C2 to the posterior surface of S1; it is broader above than below. Superficial fibres cross several vertebrae, while deeper fibres attach to adjacent vertebrae. Above the level of the atlas, the posterior longitudinal ligament is continuous with the tectorial membrane.

Between Arches

The arches are united by synovial joints between the articular processes (Fig. 3.14), as well as by ligaments passing between the laminae, transverse and spinous processes; the intervertebral foramen lies anterior to the joints.

The shape and orientation of the joints are important in determining the type of movement in each region: those in the cervical region (C2–C7) permit flexion, extension, lateral flexion/bending, and rotation; those in the thoracic region lateral flexion/bending and rotation; and those in the lumbar region flexion, extension and lateral flexion/bending. The movement between C1 and C2 is essentially rotation with limited flexion and extension, while that between C1 and the base of the skull is flexion, extension and lateral flexion/bending. Details of the ranges of movement possible in each region can be found in Table 3.1.

> **CLINICAL ANATOMY:** Arthritic changes in the zygapophyseal joints can give rise to bony projections (osteophytes) which may compress the spinal nerve within the intervertebral foramen.

Ligaments. Accessory ligaments help to stabilise the vertebral arches (Fig. 3.15): these being the ligamentum flavum (C1-sacrum); supraspinous (C7-sacrum), interspinous (cervical–lumbar region) and intertransverse (cervical to lumbar region) ligaments; and ligamentum nuchae (cervical region only).

The ligamentum flavum passes between adjacent laminae between C1/C2 and L4/L5; it forms the posterolateral wall of the vertebral canal. It contains a large amount of elastic tissue, permitting separation of the laminae during flexion and preventing folds from forming when returning to the upright position; folds could become trapped between the laminae or impinge on the dura mater covering the spinal cord.

The ligamentum nuchae is a triangular fibroelastic septum (see Fig. 4.81) replacing the supraspinous ligament between the spinous process of C7 and the external occipital protuberance; it provides muscle attachments without limiting extension of the neck.

> **APPLIED ANATOMY:** Functionally, the vertebral column can be considered as an anterior supporting column comprising the vertebral bodies and intervertebral discs, which has a static role, and a posterior pillar comprising the vertebral arches and ligaments, which has a dynamic role. Alternatively, the vertebrae can be considered to form a passive segment and the intervertebral disc, ligaments and articular processes an active segment; it is the mobility of the active segment which underlies movement of the vertebral column.

CLINICAL ANATOMY: Vertebral fractures can occur anywhere along the vertebral column; less severe fractures tend to heal with appropriate rest and support, although some may require fixation. At the time of injury, it is not the fracture itself which determines the severity of the individual's condition, but the related damage caused to the contents of the vertebral canal and surrounding tissues. Trauma to the craniocervical junction disrupts craniocervical stability, with a significant chance of spinal cord injury resulting in quadriplegia, compromised respiratory function (due to the involvement of the phrenic nerves), and severe hypotension (due to disruption of the sympathetic nervous system). Mid and lower cervical disruption can result in a range of complex neurological problems involving the upper and lower limbs; if the trauma is below C5, respiration is unlikely to be affected. Vertebral injuries can also involve the surrounding soft tissues and supporting structures.

Movements of the Vertebral Column

Movement is due to the slightly flexible intervertebral discs, with the type of movement in each region determined by the shape and orientation of the articular processes; where discs are thick in relation to the vertebral body (cervical and lumbar regions) the range of movement between adjacent vertebrae is increased. However, the amount of movement between adjacent vertebrae is small, being limited by the arrangement of fibres in the annulus fibrosis; when added together over the whole of the vertebral column, the total range of movement becomes considerable.

The basic movements are flexion (forward bending) and extension (backward bending) about a coronal (transverse) axis, lateral flexion/bending about an anteroposterior (sagittal) axis and rotation to the right and left about a vertical axis (Fig. 3.16); lateral flexion and rotation are associated movements and cannot occur independently. The maximum range of movement in each region is shown in Table 3.1; the range of movement decreases with increasing age.

Stability

Although the vertebral column is multi-segmented, it remains stable. Following a long illness many individuals can sit up with little effort long before they can stand;

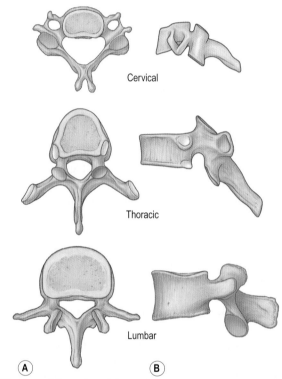

Cervical

Thoracic

Lumbar

A   B

Fig. 3.14 Orientation of the zygapophyseal joints in each region of the vertebral column, viewed from above (A) and laterally (B).

TABLE 3.1	**The Maximum Range of Movement (in degrees) Possible in Each Region of the Vertebral Column**			
Region	**Flexion**	**Extension**	**Lateral Flexion**	**Rotation**
Suboccipital	10	10	10	15
Lower cervical (C2–C7)	25	85	40	50
Thoracic	20–30	30–40	20–25	35
Lumbar	55	30	20–30	–
TOTAL	*110–120*	*155–165*	*90–105*	*100*

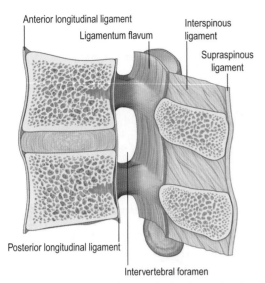

Fig. 3.15 Lateral aspect of the vertebral column showing the anterior and posterior longitudinal, interspinous and supraspinous ligaments and the ligamentum flavum.

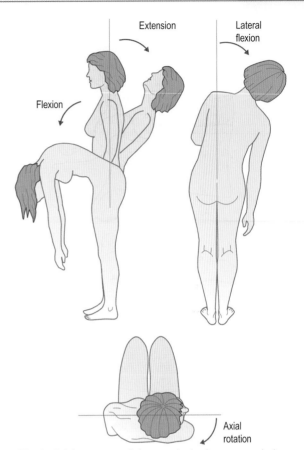

Fig. 3.16 Movements of the vertebral column as a whole.

the vertebral column has an inherent stability requiring little muscle activity to maintain its position. This is achieved due to the interaction between the intervertebral disc and adjacent vertebral bodies producing a self-stabilising unit; tension developed in the annulus fibrosis fibres tend to keep the vertebrae aligned (Fig. 3.17A). In addition, the longitudinal ligaments, as well as the ligamenta flava, interspinous and supraspinous ligaments, are also important in contributing to this inherent stability (Fig. 3.17B). As long as the arches are united with the bodies, they are spread apart putting the ligaments under tension; separation of the arches from the body results in shrinkage of the vertebral column.

The thoracic cage and its articulations posteriorly confer a degree of stability to the thoracic region of the vertebral column; the ribs are under considerable tension between the vertebral column and sternum. The heads of the ribs are held between the vertebral bodies, contributing to its intrinsic stability; this increases the elastic resistance of the thorax, some of which is used in respiration. The intrinsic stability of the vertebral column is important practically and clinically; less muscle activity is needed to maintain an erect posture. The large postvertebral muscles (page 202) play an important role in supporting the ligaments; they are just as important in providing extrinsic stability during dynamic movements.

Blood and Nerve Supply of the Vertebral Column

Arterial Supply. This is segmentally organised from branches of adjacent vessels: vertebral and ascending cervical arteries in the cervical region; posterior intercostal arteries in the thoracic region; lumbar and iliolumbar arteries in the lumbar region; and lateral sacral arteries in the sacral region. There are extensive vertical and horizontal anastomoses between the segmental vessels (Fig. 3.18A); the branches also anastomose with and reinforce the anterior and posterior spinal arteries supplying the spinal cord (page 207).

Venous Drainage. The veins form a complex of freely communicating plexuses extending the whole length of the vertebral column, both inside and out (Fig. 3.19); the plexuses join and drain into the vertebral veins in the neck, the posterior intercostal veins in the chest,

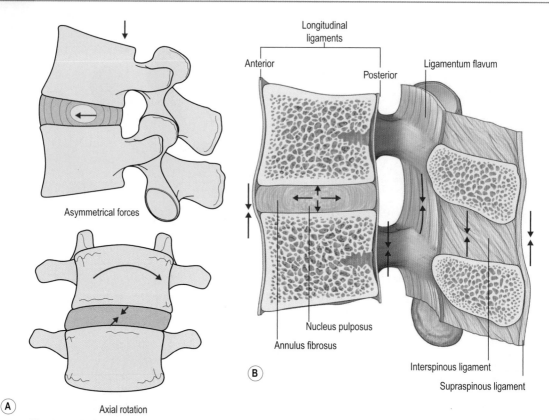

Fig. 3.17 (A) Reaction of the intervertebral disc to asymmetrically applied forces and axial rotation. (B) Interaction of the intervertebral disc and vertebral ligaments providing inherent stability of the vertebral column.

lumbar veins in the lower back and lateral sacral veins in the pelvis.

The internal vertebral venous plexuses form a continuous network between the walls of the vertebral canal and the spinal dura; they communicate above with the basilar and occipital sinuses and with the sigmoid sinus within the skull (page 270).

CLINICAL ANATOMY: The valve-less vertebral venous plexuses form a system of great blood-carrying capacity extending from the pelvis to inside the skull; at all levels, it communicates with the major venous systems of the abdomen, chest, neck and head. It is almost certainly involved in the spread of metastatic cancer cells to widely separated parts of the body under the influence of differences in venous pressure; secondary metastases associated with the prostate or breast invariably involve the vertebrae.

Innervation. The innervation of the periphery of the intervertebral disc and the presence of nervous tissue within related structures (ligaments) is clinically important. That of the anterior longitudinal ligament and lateral aspect of the intervertebral disc appears to be extensive and complex, especially in the lumbar region.

CLINICAL ANATOMY: Disc pain may be due to mechanical compression of nerve fibres in the periphery of the annulus fibrosis.

Muscles of the Trunk

The muscles producing movements of the neck (cervical spine) and of the head on the neck are considered on page 320; this section only considers muscles producing movements of the trunk (thoracic and lumbar regions) as a whole.

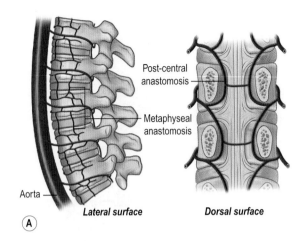

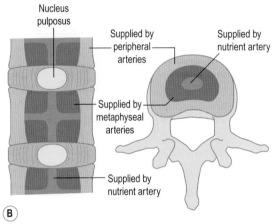

Fig. 3.18 (A) Anastomoses between the lumbar arteries and their branches. (B) Zoning of the blood supply to the intervertebral disc. (Adapted from Ratcliffe, J.F., 1980. The arterial anatomy of the adult human lumbar vertebral body: a microarteriographic study. J. Anat. 131, 57-79.)

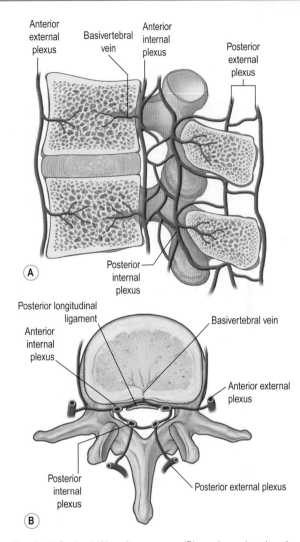

Fig. 3.19 Sagittal (A) and transverse (B) sections showing the venous drainage of the vertebral column.

The intrinsic muscles (erector spinae, semispinalis, multifidus, rotatores) of the vertebral column lie deep to superficial muscles (trapezius, latissimus dorsi, rhomboid major and minor); details of the superficial muscles can be found in Tables 5.1 and 5.2. Deep to the intrinsic muscles are two groups of segmental muscles: the levator costarum, which elevates the ribs, and the intertransversarii and interspinales, which stabilise adjacent vertebrae during movement; both groups are innervated by posterior primary rami of adjacent spinal nerves.

Working together both sets of intrinsic muscles extend the trunk; when one side only works, they can produce lateral flexion/bending and/or rotation. The largest and most superficial of the intrinsic muscles is erector spinae (Fig. 3.20A), deep to which are the semispinalis, multifidus and rotatores. Erector spinae have a distal attachment between the spinous and transverse processes extending as far as the angles of the ribs (Fig. 3.20A and B). Details of the attachments, action and nerve supply of all postvertebral muscles are given in Table 3.2.

Although attached to the front of the transverse process between the 12th rib and iliac crest, quadratus lumborum (Figs 3.20C and 3.21) extends the lumbar region

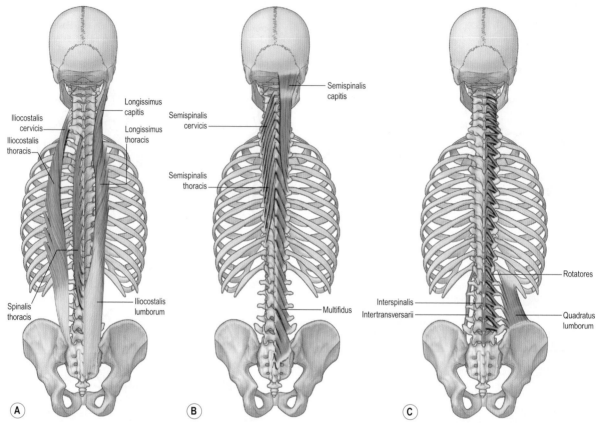

Fig. 3.20 (A) The position and attachments of the constituent parts of erector spinae. (B) The position and attachment of the right multifidus and semispinalis capitis. (C) The position and attachments of the right quadratus lumborum, rotatores and left interspinales and intertransversarii.

when both sides work together and produce lateral flexion/bending and/or rotation when acting individually.

Flexion of the trunk is produced by muscles of the anterior abdominal wall (rectus abdominis, external and internal oblique) and within the posterior abdominal cavity (psoas major). As with the postvertebral muscles working together, they produce flexion; however, contraction of right external oblique and left internal oblique produces rotation of the trunk to the left, and of left external oblique and right internal oblique rotation to the right. Details of the abdominal wall muscles can be found in Table 6.1 and of psoas major in Table 5.2.

The skin covering the vertebral column and back as far as the mid-axillary line is innervated by the posterior primary rami of spinal nerves; each nerve supplies a well-defined dermatome.

SPINAL CORD

The spinal cord is part of the central nervous system lying within the vertebral canal. In adults, it extends from just below the foramen magnum (page 242) to the L1/L2 intervertebral disc, approximately 45 cm in length. It is almost cylindrical with cervical and lumbar enlargements, due to large numbers of cell bodies, where it gives rise to the roots of the brachial (C5–T1) and lumbosacral (L1–S3) plexuses, respectively. The maximum diameter of the cervical enlargement lies opposite C5/C6 and of the lumbar enlargement opposite T12. The caudal end of the spinal cord tapers to a blunt pointed tip (conus medullaris).

The external surface has few named features (Fig. 3.22). On the anterior (ventral) surface in the midline is a marked depression (anterior median sulcus) dividing

TABLE 3.2	**The Attachments, Action and Innervation of Muscles Extending the Trunk**		
Muscle	**Attachments**	**Action**	**Nerve Supply (Root Value)**
Erector spinae: Iliocostalis (lumbar, thoracis, cervicis parts) the lateral column	From a thick, strong flat tendon along a U-shaped line around the origin of multifidus: the medial limb from the T11 to L5 spinous processes and lateral limb from the lateral and posterior sacral crest, sacrotuberous, sacrospinous and posterior sacroiliac ligaments. *Lumborum* attaches to the lower six ribs; *thoracis* to the upper six ribs and transverse process of C7; *cervicis* to the posterior tubercles of the transverse processes of C7–C4.	All three columns of both sides extend the vertebral column, as well as the head on the neck; they are also important in controlling flexion of the trunk. One side produces combined lateral flexion/bending and rotation. When standing on one leg the lower part on the non-weight-bearing side prevents the pelvis from dropping.	Posterior primary rami of adjacent spinal nerves
Longissimus (thoracis, cervicis, capitis parts) the intermediate column	*Thoracis* runs from the transverse processes of lumbar vertebrae and adjacent thoracolumbar fascia to the transverse processes of all 12 thoracic vertebrae and adjacent regions of the lower 10 ribs; *cervicis* from the transverse processes of T6–T1 to the posterior tubercles of the transverse processes of C6–C2; *capitis* from the transverse processes of T5–T1 and articular processes of C7–C4 to the posterior aspect of the mastoid process.		
Spinalis (thoracis, cervicis, capitis parts) the most medial column	*Thoracis* from the spinous processes of L2–T11 to those of T6–T1; *cervicis* and *capitis* are poorly developed often blending with adjacent muscles.		
Interspinales (best developed in cervical and lumbar regions)	Between adjacent spinous processes	Extends lumbar and cervical spine: stabilises vertebral column during movement	Posterior primary rami of adjacent spinal nerves

Continued

TABLE 3.2   The Attachments, Action and Innervation of Muscles Extending the Trunk—cont'd

Muscle	Attachments	Action	Nerve Supply (Root Value)
Semispinalis (thoracis, cervicis, capitis parts)	*Thoracis* from the transverse processes of T10–T6 to the spinous processes of T4–C6; *cervicis* from the transverse processes of T6–T1 to the spinous processes of C5–C2; *capitis* from the transverse processes of T6–T1 and articular processes of C7–C4 to an impression between the superior and inferior nuchal lines	Both sides produce extension of the thoracic and cervical parts of the vertebral column. Individually each produces rotation of the trunk and neck to the opposite side	Posterior primary rami of adjacent spinal nerves
Multifidus	From the back of the sacrum and fascia covering erector spinae, mammillary processes of lumbar vertebrae, transverse processes of all thoracic vertebrae and articular processes of C7–C4/3 to the spinous processes of L5–C2	Extension, rotation and lateral flexion/bending of the vertebral column at all levels; stabilises the vertebral column	Posterior primary rami of adjacent spinal nerves
Rotatores	From the transverse process of 1 vertebra to the lamina and spinous process of the vertebra above, being best developed in the thoracic region	Rotation between adjacent vertebrae; stabilises the vertebral column	Posterior primary rami of adjacent spinal nerves
Quadratus lumborum	From the iliac crest to the medial half of the lower border of the 12th rib, attaching to the lateral half of the anterior surface of the lumbar transverse processes	Together they extend the trunk; individually each laterally flexes/bends the vertebral column to the same side	Subcostal and lumbar nerves (T12 and L1–L4)

the spinal cord into right and left halves. Posteriorly, the dorsal surface is marked by several less pronounced longitudinal depressions: in the midline is the posterior median sulcus dividing the spinal cord into right and left halves; on the posterolateral aspects is the posterior lateral sulcus running the entire length of the spinal cord; between the posterior median and posterior lateral sulci is the posterior intermediate sulcus, being less prominent in the caudal half of the spinal cord. Rostrally between the posterior sulci are two slightly rounded prominences extending longitudinally: the medial (fasciculus gracilis) lies between the posterior median and posterior intermediate sulci, and lateral (fasciculus cuneatus) prominence between the posterior intermediate and posterior lateral sulci.

Meninges

The spinal cord is surrounded by three membranes (meninges) (Fig. 3.23) and bathed in cerebrospinal fluid. The outer meningeal covering (dura mater) is a tough fibrous layer enclosing the spinal cord; it extends from, and attaches to, the margins of the foramen

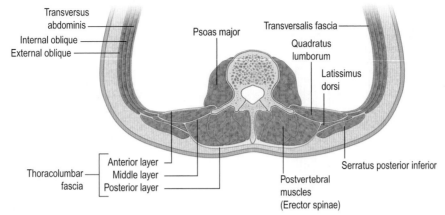

Fig. 3.21 Transverse section through the upper lumbar spine showing the attachment of the trunk extensors and formation of the thoracolumbar fascia.

magnum and terminates at the level of S2. Within the vertebral canal, the dural sac is relatively mobile, being loosely attached to the margins of the intervertebral foramina.

The middle meningeal covering (arachnoid mater) lines the deep surface of the dura mater (Fig. 3.23). Deep to the arachnoid mater is the subarachnoid space permeated by a network of threads connecting it to the pia mater; the space contains cerebrospinal fluid and is continuous with that surrounding the brain. Details of the cerebrospinal fluid can be found on page 261.

The subdural space is a potential space because the dura and arachnoid are closely apposed: it does not communicate with the subarachnoid space but continues for a short distance along the spinal nerves.

> **APPLIED ANATOMY:** Accidental subdural catheterisation can occur during epidural injections; the injected fluid may damage the spinal cord either through direct toxic effects or by the compression of blood vessels.

The inner thin transparent layer (pia mater) intimately invests the surface of the spinal cord; it extends caudally as a thin thread of tissue (filum terminale) devoid of neural tissue, which pierces the tip of the dural sac to attach to the coccyx (Fig. 3.23).

Crossing the subarachnoid space are a series of tooth-like extensions of the pia mater (denticulate ligaments) arising from the lateral aspect of the spinal cord; these anchor the spinal cord to the dural sac protecting

it from injury due to violent contact with the wall of the vertebral canal during movements of the trunk.

Epidural Space

This lies between the spinal dura and tissues lining the vertebral canal; it is closed superiorly by fusion of the dura with the margins of the foramen magnum and below by the posterior sacrococcygeal ligament closing the sacral hiatus. It contains loosely packed fat, blood vessels, lymphatics, and fibrous bands (meningovertebral ligaments) connecting the dural sac with tissues lining the vertebral canal; similar bands connect the nerve root sheaths within the intervertebral foramen.

> **CLINICAL ANATOMY:** Contrast media and other fluids injected into the epidural space can spread the whole length of the vertebral column. Local anaesthetics injected close to spinal nerves outside the intervertebral foramen can spread up or down to affect adjacent nerves or pass to the opposite side. The paravertebral spaces of each side communicate via the epidural space, especially in the lumbar region.

Blood Supply

Arterial supply. The arterial supply to the spinal cord is by three longitudinal arteries, one anterior and two posterior spinal and radicular arteries; all these anastomose in the pia mater before becoming end arteries to the spinal cord. The anterior spinal artery is formed by

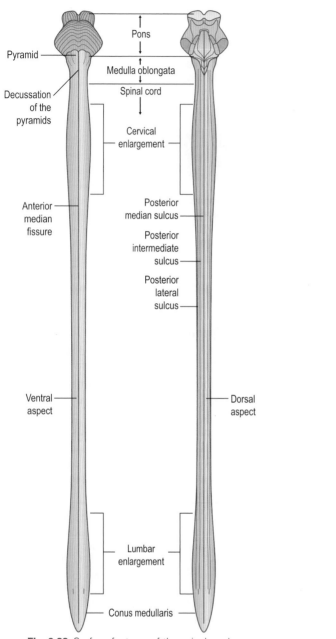

Fig. 3.22 Surface features of the spinal cord.

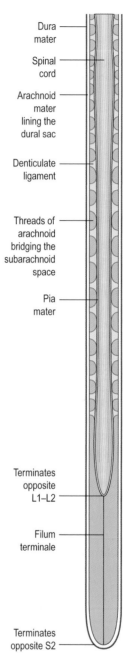

Fig. 3.23 Meningeal coverings of the spinal cord showing the denticulate ligaments (pia mater) holding the spinal cord in place.

a branch from the vertebral artery (page 266) on each side and supplies the anterior 2/3rd of the spinal cord; it descends anterior to the anterior median sulcus (Fig. 3.24). Each smaller posterior spinal artery arises from the vertebral artery and descends along the posterolateral aspect of the spinal cord behind the dorsal nerve roots (Fig. 3.24). At various levels along the spinal cord,

the anterior and posterior spinal arteries are reinforced by radicular arteries arising from vertebral, posterior intercostal and lumbar arteries which run along the ventral and dorsal nerve roots (Fig. 3.24).

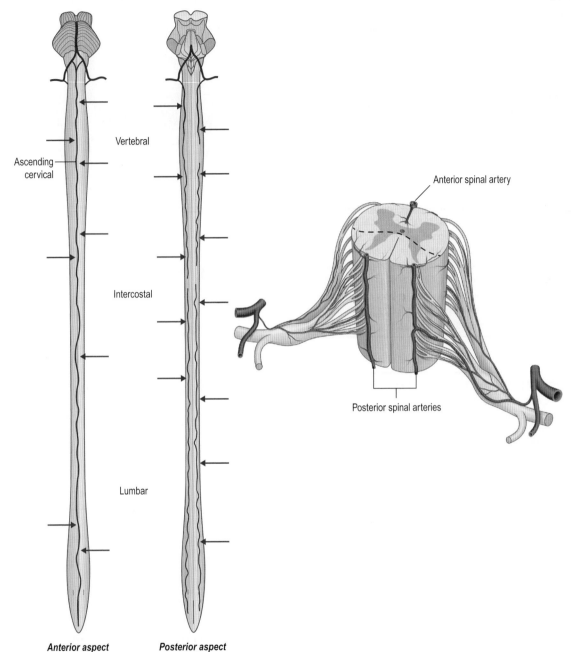

Ascending cervical

Vertebral

Intercostal

Lumbar

Anterior aspect

Posterior aspect

Anterior spinal artery

Posterior spinal arteries

Fig. 3.24 Arterial supply of the spinal cord: *arrows* indicate segmental reinforcement of the spinal arteries.

Venous drainage. The venous drainage of the spinal cord is by veins within the pia mater forming a plexus (venous vasa corona) consisting of six longitudinal venous trunks. One trunk accompanies the anterior spinal artery anterior to the anterior median sulcus, another lies behind the posterior median sulcus, one on each side behind the ventral roots and another on each side behind the dorsal roots. The longitudinal trunks communicate with the internal vertebral venous plexus between the dura mater and periosteum;

this communicates with the external vertebral venous plexus. The venous trunks are drained by veins that leave the vertebral canal through the intervertebral foramina to drain into vertebral, posterior intercostal, lumbar and lateral sacral veins. Superiorly, they are continuous with the basilar plexus of sinuses, inferior petrosal sinuses and inferior cerebellar veins within the skull.

> **APPLIED ANATOMY:** The anterior and posterior spinal arteries are only efficient in the upper cervical segments, whereas the radicular arteries are more significant in supplying other parts of the spinal cord. The lumbosacral segments of the spinal cord have the richest arterial supply, followed by the cervical and then thoracic segments. Each radicular artery supplies a single spinal segment; however, those at T1 and T11 may be enlarged forming arteria radicularis magna which supply several segments. The T11 artery is frequently referred to as the 'Artery of Adamkiewicz'; blockage may lead to softening of several segments of the spinal cord, especially those inferior to T11.

> **CLINICAL ANATOMY:** Occlusion of the anterior spinal artery is relatively common in the mid-thoracic region, resulting in acute thoracic cord syndrome with paraplegia and incontinence.

Internal Structure and Organisation

The spinal cord consists of grey matter internally, comprising nerve cells (neurons) and non-myelinated nerve fibres, surrounded by white matter, comprising myelinated nerve fibres, neuroglia (page 247) and blood vessels; the grey matter is arranged in an H-shape with ventral and dorsal horns (Fig. 3.25). Between the T1 and L2 spinal cord segments, an additional small horn of grey matter (lateral horn) projects laterally in the angle between the ventral and dorsal horns; it contains the cell bodies of neurons whose axons are part of the autonomic nervous system (page 223).

In transverse section, the spinal cord is almost completely divided into right and left symmetrical halves by the anterior and posterior median sulci and the central canal. The two halves are connected by three commissures: ventral (anterior) white commissure at the base of the anterior median sulcus; ventral grey commissure in front of the central canal connecting the ventral horns;

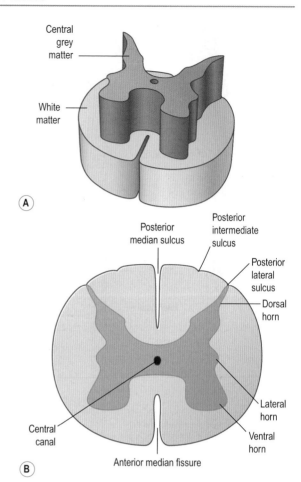

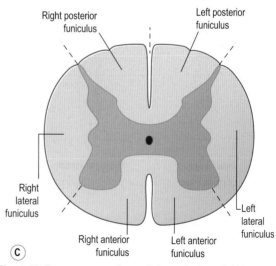

Fig. 3.25 Transverse sections of the spinal cord: (A) arrangement of the grey and white matter; (B) surface features; (C) position of major tracts.

TABLE 3.3 Regional Differences in Transverse Sections of the Spinal Cord

	Cervical	Thoracic	Lumbar	Sacral
Size of section	Large	Small	Largest	Small
Shape of section	Oval compressed anteroposteriorly	Oval to circular	Almost circular	Circular
White matter	Large amount	Relatively less	Very little	Very little
Anterior horns	Thick	Thin	Thick	Thick
Posterior horns	Thin and divergent	Thin and slightly divergent	Thick and parallel	Thick and parallel
Lateral horns	Absent	Prominent	Absent, except for upper two segments	Absent
Position of central canal	Nearer to ventral surface	Less close to ventral surface	Almost central	Central

and dorsal grey commissure behind the central canal connecting the dorsal horns. The amount of grey matter is increased in the cervical and lumbar enlargements, with the cell bodies being arranged in nuclei (collections of nerve cell bodies with a common function and pathway). Differences between regions of the spinal cord are given in Table 3.3.

Grey Matter

Lamination of the grey matter. Based on the cellular features of neurons in the grey matter, 10 laminae (layers of cells) are present from the dorsal to ventral surfaces of the grey matter, including the central canal; they extend throughout the length of the spinal cord. Laminae I to IV are the main receiving areas for cutaneous (exteroceptive) afferents; they are in the dorsal horn and give rise to long ascending tracts.

Lamina I: Waldeyer's layer corresponding to the posterior marginal nucleus.

Laminae II and **III**: correspond to the substantia gelatinosa of Rolandi.

Lamina IV: corresponds to the nucleus proprius.

Lamina V: receives afferent fibres from the superficial laminae and primary afferent and efferent fibres which form the contralateral spinothalamic tract.

Lamina VI: receives proprioceptive impulses; it is only present in spinal cord segments associated with the limbs.

Lamina VII: includes neurons of the nucleus dorsalis and the intermediomedial and intermediolateral (autonomic) nuclei.

Lamina VIII: receives afferent fibres from the reticulospinal and vestibulospinal (extrapyramidal) tracts, the medial longitudinal fasciculus (bundle) and contralateral lamina VIII; it has an excitatory effect on motor neurons in lamina IX.

Lamina IX: contains somatomotor nuclei (ventrolateral, ventromedial, dorsolateral, dorsomedial) which innervate skeletal muscle, as well as efferent neurons (>25 microns) to extrafusal muscle fibres causing contraction, and to efferent neurons (<25 microns) to intrafusal fibres controlling muscle tone.

Lamina X: part of the grey commissure located around the central canal.

Dorsal horn. The dorsal horn is sensory (somatic and visceral afferent); in its tip is a small posterior marginal nucleus which contains:

Substantia gelatinosa of Rolandi, a collection of small Golgi type II nerve cells at the apex of the dorsal horn which receive pain and temperature sensations; in the upper two cervical segments, it is continuous with the spinal nucleus of the trigeminal nerve. It corresponds to lamina II and part of lamina III of the grey matter and gives rise to the spinothalamic tract.

Nucleus proprius, a collection of large cells in the middle of the dorsal horn which receive proprioceptive sensations; it corresponds to lamina IV and gives rise to the dorsal spinocerebellar tract. Fibres from the nucleus proprius of the opposite side conveying proprioceptive impulses ascend to reach the inferior olivary nucleus via the spino-olivary tract, which then transmits them to the cerebellum.

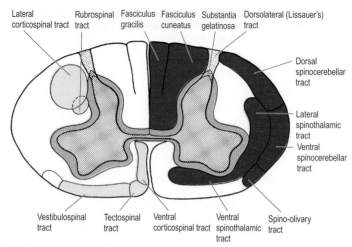

Fig. 3.26 Simplified diagram showing the positions of the ascending (*red*) and descending (*yellow*) tracts of the spinal cord: orange indicates the location of intersegmental tracts.

Nucleus dorsalis/thoracicus (Clarke's column), a collection of cells on the medial side of the root of the dorsal horn which are secondary sensory neurons carrying proprioceptive impulses to the cerebellum; it is present in the C8–L3 segments and corresponds to lamina VII.

Visceral afferent nucleus, lies lateral to the nucleus dorsalis in spinal segments C8–L3; its function is not clear but may receive visceral afferents (sensory) from nerve cells in the dorsal root ganglia.

Ventral horn. The ventral horn is somatosensory and contains five nuclei (ventromedial, dorsomedial, ventrolateral, dorsomedial, central) named according to their position.

Medial nuclei are present in all regions and supply muscles of the trunk.

Lateral nuclei supply muscles of the limbs and are present in cervical, lumbar and sacral regions.

The **central nucleus** is only present in cervical and lumbosacral segments. In the C3–C5 segments, it is known as the phrenic nucleus and gives rise to the phrenic nerves which innervate the diaphragm and also the spinal root of the accessory nerve: in lumbosacral segments, it is known as the lumbosacral nucleus.

Lateral horn. The lateral horn is autonomic and contains two groups of nuclei (intermediomedial, intermediolateral) corresponding to lamina VII. In spinal segments T1–L2, the cells give rise to the preganglionic sympathetic axons that pass through the ventral horns to the sympathetic trunk/chain via the white rami

communicantes. In spinal segments S2–S4, the cells give rise to the preganglionic parasympathetic axons (sacral parasympathetic outflow).

White Matter

A thick mantle surrounding the grey matter; it comprises ascending (short) and descending (long) tracts (parallel longitudinal bundles of myelinated nerve fibres). In transverse section, it is incompletely divided:

Posterior (dorsal) white column lies between the dorsal horn and posterior median septum; in cervical and upper thoracic segments, it is divided into medial and lateral parts by the posterior intermediate septum.

Lateral white column lies lateral to the dorsal and ventral horns: it is the widest.

Anterior (ventral) white column lies anteromedial to the ventral horn.

Afferent and Efferent Tracts

The nerves in the white matter are grouped into tracts, each of which has a specific origin, destination and function. Short (intersegmental axons) tracts begin and end in the spinal cord close to the grey matter, while long (projecting) tracts either end in (ascending tracts) or originate from (descending tracts) higher centres (Fig. 3.26).

Short tracts. These are associative in function and include the fasciculus proprius posterior, septomarginal tract, fasciculus interfascicularis (of Schaultz) and

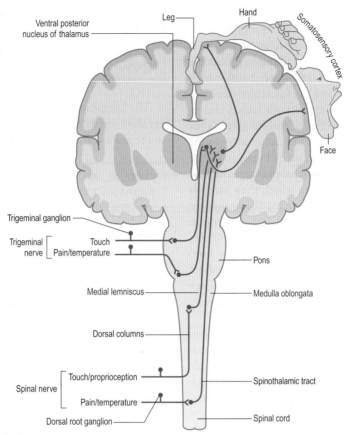

Fig. 3.27 Organisation of the general sensory pathways showing primary (1st), secondary (2nd) and tertiary (3rd) order neurons.

Lissauer's tract in the posterior white column; and the fasciculi proprius lateralis and anterior in the lateral white column.

The **fasciculi proprii posterior**, **lateralis** and **anterior** coordinate the function of the spinal cord in different regions.

The **septomarginal** and **fasciculus interfascicularis tracts** are descending fibres from the fasciculus gracilis and fasciculus cuneatus ending in the anterior horn cells; they are involved in the stretch reflex (page 217).

Lissauer's tract is present in all segments of the spinal cord. The cells are located in the posterior root ganglia from where the axons enter the spinal cord in the lateral part of the dorsal roots, where they either ascend or descend a few segments before relaying in cells of the substantia gelatinosa of Rolandi; axons of the latter cells cross to the opposite side anterior to the central canal to ascend as the lateral spinothalamic tract.

Long tracts. The long tracts are the ascending (sensory) tracts from the spinal cord to higher centres in the brain, and descending (motor) tracts from higher centres to the spinal cord.

In the following sections on ascending and descending tracts within the spinal cord, the reader is advised to refer to the relevant sections of the brain in Chapter 4 (Head and Neck).

Ascending (sensory) tracts. Ascending sensory projections related to the general senses consist of a series of three order neurons that extend from the peripheral receptor to the contralateral cerebral cortex; these are referred to as primary, secondary and tertiary (1st, 2nd, 3rd order) neurons (Fig. 3.27). The axons of primary neurons terminate by synapsing on cell bodies of ipsilateral secondary neurons. The ascending tracts (Fig. 3.26) arise from cells either in the dorsal root ganglion or in the posterior horn.

In the **posterior white (dorsal) column**, the fasciculi gracilis and cuneatus carry proprioceptive impulses concerning position, movement, pressure, vibration and fine touch. The fasciculus gracilis carries impulses from the lower limb and lower trunk which end in the gracile nucleus, and the fasciculus cuneatus from the upper trunk and upper limb which end in the cuneate nucleus. In the medulla oblongata, axons from the gracile and cuneate nuclei curve around the central grey matter (internal arcuate fibres), cross the midline and decussate with fibres of the opposite side to form the sensory decussation, which then ascends upwards (medial lemniscus) traversing the brainstem (medulla oblongata, pons, midbrain) to terminate in the thalamus (posterolateral ventral nucleus). From the thalamus, axons pass through the posterior limb of the internal capsule and then the corona radiata to reach the postcentral gyrus of the cerebral cortex where the body is represented upside down (sensory homunculus, page 258).

In the **lateral white column**, the *posterior (dorsal)* and *anterior (ventral) spinocerebellar tracts* carry proprioceptive impulses (muscle tone, coordination of muscle activity) and the *lateral spinothalamic tract* exteroceptive sensations (pain, temperature); the spinotectal and spino-olivary tracts also convey pain and temperature sensations.

> **APPLIED ANATOMY:** Some fibres of the anterior and lateral spinothalamic tracts leave the main tracts in the midbrain and pass to reach the superior colliculus (part of the tectum of the midbrain), forming the spinotectal tract which is concerned with spinovisual reflexes; stimuli ascending through these tracts lead to movement of the head and neck towards the source of stimulation.

The *posterior spinocerebellar tract* carries impulses from the same side of the body which ascend to the medulla oblongata, eventually reaching the cerebellum via the inferior cerebellar peduncle. The *anterior spinocerebellar tract* conveys non-discriminative (crude) touch and pressure sensations and consists of crossed and uncrossed fibres which ascend to the medulla oblongata, pons and midbrain, reaching the cerebellum via the superior cerebellar peduncle.

> **CLINICAL ANATOMY:** Destruction of the anterior and posterior spinocerebellar tracts leads to incoordination of muscle activity and disturbances of muscle tone (Friedreich's ataxia).

The *lateral spinothalamic tract* carries pain and temperature sensations from the opposite side of the body to the thalamus and sensory area of the cortex.

> **CLINICAL ANATOMY:** As the lateral spinothalamic tract ascends in the spinal cord, it becomes more superficial and lateral, where it is possible to incise the tract (cordotomy) to relieve pain on the opposite side of the body below the level of the incision; it can be undertaken without interfering with proprioceptive sensations.

> **CLINICAL ANATOMY:** Destruction of the lateral spinothalamic tracts leads to loss of exteroceptive sensation over the whole of the opposite side of the body below the level of the lesion.

In the **anterior white column**, the *anterior spinothalamic tract* conveys the exteroceptive sensation of crude touch.

Descending (motor) tracts. The descending tracts (Fig. 3.26) arise from the precentral gyrus of the cerebral cortex, where the body is represented upside down (motor homunculus), and brainstem and terminate in the ventral and lateral horn cells of the spinal cord; they control movement, muscle tone, spinal reflexes and spinal autonomic functions. The tracts influence activity in the lower motor neurons by separate pathways (pyramidal, extrapyramidal). The pyramidal pathways contain fibres which originate in the cerebral cortex, while the extrapyramidal system contains fibres originating from the basal ganglia in the midbrain, pons and medulla oblongata (page 247) and cerebellum (page 252), although the basal ganglia and cerebellum do have connections with the cerebral cortex.

Descending tracts consist of upper and lower motor neurons: upper motor neurons refer collectively to all descending pathways which impinge on the activity of lower motor neurons but are usually restricted to those related to the pyramidal tracts; lower motor neurons

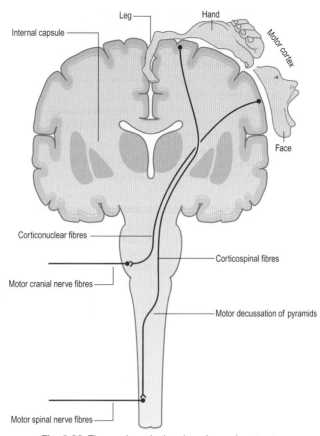

Fig. 3.28 The corticospinal and corticonuclear tracts.

are located in either the brainstem or spinal cord and directly innervate specific skeletal muscles.

> **CLINICAL ANATOMY:** Lower motor neuron lesions cause paralysis or paresis of specific muscles due to loss of direct innervation; there is loss or reduction of tendon reflex activity and reduced muscle tone: spontaneous muscular contractions occur with affected muscles atrophying over time. Upper motor neuron lesions cause paralysis or paresis of movements due to the loss of higher control, there is increased tendon reflex activity and muscle tone, a positive plantar (Babinski) reflex, but without muscle atrophy: spasticity is the combination of paralysis, increased tendon reflex activity and hypertonia.

The **pyramidal system** comprises the corticospinal and corticonuclear (corticobulbar) tracts (Fig. 3.28): the corticospinal tract is concerned with the initiation and control of discrete skilled voluntary movements, especially of the distal parts of the limbs, while the corticonuclear tract fibres terminate on cranial nerve nuclei in the brainstem and are therefore concerned with innervating muscles associated with the cranial nerves (e.g., muscles controlling eye movements) (page 300).

Corticospinal tract fibres originate from pyramidal (Betz) cells in the motor area in the precentral gyrus and the premotor area of the cerebral cortex. The axons pass downwards in the cerebral cortex as the corona radiata running in the anterior 2/3rd of the posterior limb of the internal capsule, then descend in the intermediate 2/5th of the crus cerebri (midbrain), basis pontis (pons) and pyramid of the medulla oblongata. In the lower medulla, most fibres (70%–90%) cross to the opposite side, with the remainder remaining uncrossed. The crossed fibres form the lateral corticospinal tract which runs in the lateral white column, and the uncrossed fibres in the ventral corticospinal tract which runs in the anterior white column; the uncrossed fibres cross to the opposite side at their segmental level. All axons, therefore, synapse with cells in the anterior horn of the opposite side of the spinal cord. Approximately 55% of corticospinal neurons terminate at cervical levels, 20% at thoracic levels and 25% at lumbosacral levels.

> **APPLIED ANATOMY:** Each cerebral hemisphere controls movements of the opposite side of the body.

Corticonuclear tract fibres cross the midline and terminate on the motor nuclei of cranial nerves: those to the nuclei of the 5th, 7th, 9th, 10th, 11th and 12th cranial nerves form the lateral corticonuclear tract, and those to the 3rd, 4th and 6th cranial nerves the medial corticonuclear tract.

> **APPLIED ANATOMY:** All corticonuclear fibres terminate around the motor nuclei of both sides except the lower half of the 7th, 11th and 12th nuclei, which receive fibres from the opposite side only.

The **extrapyramidal system** comprises the rubrospinal (Monakow's), vestibulospinal, lateral and medial reticulospinal, tectospinal and olivospinal tracts; they originate inferior to the level of the cerebral cortex.

The *rubrospinal tract* originates from cells in the red nucleus in the midbrain. The axons cross the tegmentum of the midbrain, descend through the reticular formation of the pons, medulla oblongata and then to the lateral white column terminating on anterior horn cells in the cervical and thoracic regions: they exert control over muscle tone of the limb flexors.

> **APPLIED ANATOMY:** The red nucleus receives afferents from the motor cortex and cerebellum representing a non-pyramidal route by which both can influence spinal motor activity.

The *tectospinal tract* originates from cells in the superior colliculus of the midbrain. The axons decussate in the tegmentum of the midbrain descending through the brainstem and anterior white column, terminating on anterior horn cells in the cervical region of the spinal cord.

> **APPLIED ANATOMY:** Through the tectospinal tract the visual reflex centre in the superior colliculus is functionally connected with lower motor neurons so that vision is correlated with body movements.

The *vestibulospinal tract* originates from cells in the lateral vestibular nucleus in the pons; the axons run in the anterior white column to synapse with anterior horn cells, with the majority of fibres remaining uncrossed.

> **APPLIED ANATOMY:** In the pons, the vestibulospinal tract receives input from the labyrinth (page 316) via the vestibular nerve (part of the 8th cranial nerve) and from the cerebellum. Impulses regarding body balance from the labyrinth are conveyed to lower motor neurons, serving as a reflex correlation of equilibrium with body movements.

The *lateral* and *medial reticulospinal tracts* originate in cells of the reticular nuclei in the pons and medulla; axons from the pons descend ipsilaterally forming the medial reticulospinal tract, while those from the medulla descend bilaterally forming the lateral reticulospinal tract. Both tracts lie in the anterior white column terminating around cells in the anterior and lateral horns of the spinal cord.

> **APPLIED ANATOMY:** The reticulospinal tracts influence voluntary movement, reflex activity and muscle tone by controlling activity in the lower motor neurons. They also have a pressor and depressor effect on the circulatory system, as well as being involved in the control of breathing.

The *olivospinal tract* originates in cells of the inferior olivary nucleus in the medulla oblongata; the axons synapse on anterior horn cells in the cervical region of the spinal cord. It carries fibres from the cerebellum and corpus striatum (basal ganglia) to the spinal cord.

Although its fibres do not enter the spinal cord, the *corticopontocerebellar pathway* enables the cortex to exert functional control over the cerebellum in the coordination of movement. The upper neurons are in the association areas of the cerebral cortex (frontal, temporal, occipital, parietal), descend in the internal capsule to the medial (frontopontine part) and lateral (temporopontine part) 1/5th of the crus cerebri in the midbrain. On reaching the pons, the fibres synapse with the nuclei pontis forming the parietopontine and occipitopontine fibres, which cross the midline to constitute the middle cerebellar peduncle to reach the cerebellum.

Spinal Reflexes

Connections between the spinal cord and brainstem underlie a number of reflexes in which the response to stimulation of peripheral structures is influenced and modulated, essentially automatically, by descending connections. A so-called reflex arc comprises an afferent neuron and an efferent neuron, usually connected by an interneuron; simple reflex arcs may not have an intervening interneuron. Reflexes can be confined to a single spinal cord segment (intrasegmental) or involve several segments (intersegmental); they are relatively fixed.

Spinal reflexes are influenced and modulated by descending connections from both the brainstem and cerebral cortex. Pathology of the descending supraspinal pathways results in abnormalities of spinal reflex activity, which can be tested for in neurological examinations: absent (areflexia), diminished (hyporeflexia) or exaggerated (hyperreflexia) reflexes.

Muscle stretch reflex. The muscle stretch (tendon, deep tendon) reflex is the mechanism by which stretch applied to a muscle elicits its reflex contraction: it is the simplest form of reflex (monosynaptic, myotatic) involving single afferent and efferent neurons. Stretch receptors (annulospiral endings) within the intrafusal muscle fibres (page 41) give rise to primary afferent fibres which enter the spinal cord and make direct contact with α motor neurons innervating the same muscle, causing it to contract. At the same time, the α motor neurons of antagonistic muscles are inhibited by collateral connections (reciprocal innervation) to inhibitory interneurons (Fig. 3.29).

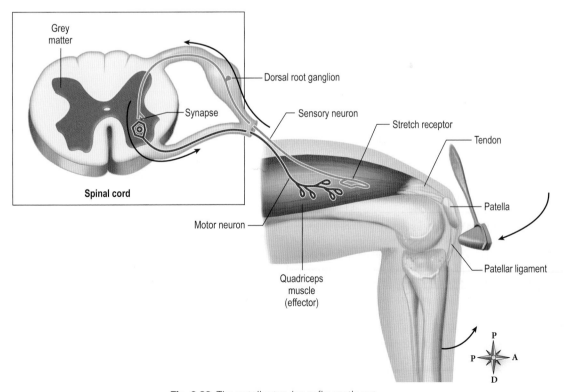

Fig. 3.29 The patellar tendon reflex pathway.

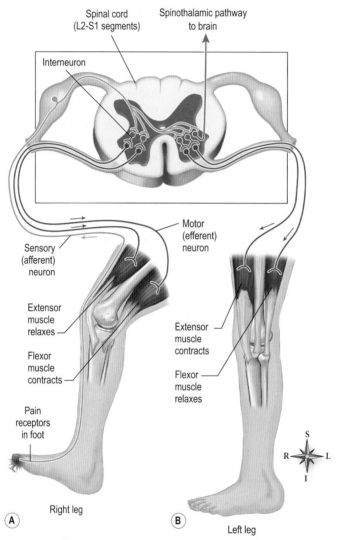

Spinal cord
(L2-S1 segments)

Spinothalamic pathway
to brain

Interneuron

Motor
(efferent)
neuron

Sensory
(afferent)
neuron

Extensor
muscle
relaxes

Extensor
muscle
contracts

Flexor
muscle
contracts

Flexor
muscle
relaxes

Pain
receptors
in foot

Right leg

Left leg

(A)

(B)

Fig. 3.30 The flexor (A) and crossed extensor (B) reflex pathways.

APPLIED ANATOMY: Extrafusal muscle fibres receive both α and δ motor neurons; the latter innervating intrafusal fibres. Activation of δ motor neurons (δ reflex) increases the sensitivity of the intrafusal fibres to stretch, which has a profound effect on the stretch reflex and on muscle tone. Changes in muscle tone and in the activity of the stretch reflex are commonly found in disorders of both the central and peripheral nervous systems due to the influence of descending pathways on the δ motor neurons.

Flexor reflex and crossed extensor reflex. Painful stimulation of a limb leads to flexion withdrawal via a polysynaptic reflex, in which nociceptive primary afferents cause activation of the limb flexor motor neurons (Fig. 3.30A); at the same time, collateralisation of fibres to adjacent spinal segments mediates limb flexion at several joints depending on the intensity of the stimulus. Decussating connections to the contralateral side of the spinal cord activate δ motor neurons innervating the corresponding extensor muscles, producing a crossed extensor reflex (Fig. 3.30B).

Spinal Cord Lesions

Compression due to trauma (vertebral burst fracture) or pathology (tumour in the epidural space) and secondary ischaemic trauma can cause irreversible damage and spinal cord disease (myelopathy), with the site (upper or lower cervical, thoracic, lumbosacral) and extent of the lesion (isolated, partial or complete transection) determining the presenting clinical syndrome. The time course of spinal cord disease is important, as it can suggest possible causes as the rate of progression depends on the aetiology. Disorders with a rapid or sudden onset are usually caused by trauma or stroke; development over days may be due to an inflammatory disorder (multiple sclerosis); neoplastic lesions (meningioma) as well as degeneration (amyotrophic lateral sclerosis, motor neuron disease) often progress over months or years (hereditary spastic paraparesis).

Complete transection. **High cervical cord transection** (above C4) causes spastic quadriplegia (tetraplegia) with hyperreflexia, extensor plantar responses (upper motor neuron lesion), incontinence, sensory loss below the level of the lesion and sensory ataxia (loss of proprioception (joint position sense)) resulting in poorly judged movements, with the incoordination increasing when the eyes are closed.

Lower cervical cord transection causes weakness, wasting and fasciculation (small local muscle contractions) and areflexia of the upper limbs (lower motor neuron lesion), paraplegia, hyperreflexia and extensor plantar responses (upper motor neuron lesion) in the lower limbs, incontinence, sensory loss below the level of the lesion and sensory ataxia.

Thoracic cord transection causes paraplegia, hyperreflexia and extensor plantar responses (upper motor neuron lesion), incontinence, sensory loss below the level of the lesion and sensory ataxia.

Lumbar cord transection causes weakness, wasting and fasciculation of muscles, paraplegia, areflexia of the lower limbs (lower motor neuron lesion), incontinence, sensory loss below the level of the lesion and sensory ataxia.

Hemisection. Gives rise to Brown-Séquard syndrome, characterised by ipsilateral upper motor neuron signs (hemiplegia/monoplegia) due to damage to the ventral horn cells, as well as loss of proprioception due to damage to dorsal horn cells. Below the level of hemisection, there is an ipsilateral motor neuron lesion (spastic paralysis) due to damage to the lateral corticospinal tract, as well as loss of proprioception and fine touch due to damage to the dorsal column tracts; contralaterally, there is loss of pain and temperature due to damage to the lateral spinothalamic tract. There is no loss of crude touch or pressure as these are conveyed by two routes.

Selective lesions. **Syringomyelia** (abnormal widening of the central canal) in the lower cervical and upper thoracic regions leads to the destruction of fibres in the white commissure crossing anterior to the canal. There is loss of pain and temperature sensation from skin supplied by the affected segments, although touch is not markedly affected (dissociate sensibility). This is due to the pain and temperature fibres crossing to the opposite side close to where they enter the dorsal roots, while touch fibres cross to the opposite side through the dorsal roots; fine touch is conveyed in posterior column tracts.

Poliomyelitis is caused by a virus that damages the anterior horn cells (spinal type) or motor nuclei (bulbar type) giving isolated lower motor neuron lesion paralysis, with no loss of sensation.

Tabes dorsalis is caused by degeneration of the posterior nerve roots of the fasciculi gracilis and cuneatus (dorsal column); it presents as loss of deep sensations below the level of the lesion on the same side. Lesion to both sides leads to tabes dorsalis, which manifests as loss of position and movement sense, tactile localisation and discrimination, vibration sense, and the ability to understand the form and nature of objects (astereognosis); crude touch, pain and temperature sensations are preserved as they are carried by the spinothalamic tract. There is hypotonia and loss of tendon reflexes due to interruption of the stretch reflex arc, as well as sensory ataxia with a positive Romberg sign (inability to stand upright with the eyes closed due to interruption of proprioception reaching the cerebellum).

Anterior spinal artery occlusion manifests as bilateral flaccid paralysis, loss of pain and temperature below the level of the lesion (upper motor neuron lesion), with the preservation of proprioception and touch.

Subacute combined degeneration is usually associated with pernicious anaemia, due to a lack of intrinsic factor which is essential for the absorption of vitamin B12. In this condition, bilateral degeneration of white fibres of the dorsal and lateral columns of the spinal cord occurs, especially involving the lumbosacral segments. Its manifestations include loss of position and

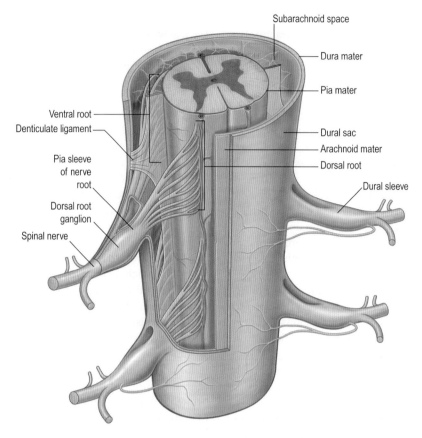

Subarachnoid space
Dura mater
Pia mater
Ventral root
Denticulate ligament
Dural sac
Arachnoid mater
Dorsal root
Pia sleeve of nerve root
Dural sleeve
Dorsal root ganglion
Spinal nerve

Fig. 3.31 The formation of a spinal nerve from ventral and dorsal roots and its subsequent division into ventral and dorsal rami. Also shown are the dorsal root ganglion and the relationship of the meningeal sheaths of the spinal nerves.

vibration sense of the lower extremities, as well as signs of upper motor neuron lesions, such as bilateral spasticity, exaggerated tendon reflexes and positive Babinski sign.

Spinal Nerves

The spinal nerves are the junction between the central (spinal cord) and peripheral (somatic, page 221) nervous systems; the spinal cord gives rise to 31 pairs of spinal nerves named according to the vertebra they are related to at birth, with the region giving attachment to a pair of spinal nerves being a segment. There are 8 cervical segments, 12 thoracic, 5 lumbar, 5 sacral and 1 coccygeal segment; the cervical spinal nerves each lie above the correspondingly numbered cervical vertebra, except C8 which lies below C7; the thoracic, lumbar, sacral and coccygeal nerves all lie below their correspondingly numbered vertebra.

> **APPLIED ANATOMY:** The 1st to 4th sacral nerves leave through the anterior and posterior sacral foramina, while the 5th sacral and coccygeal nerves leave via the hiatus sacralis to enter the pelvis again.

Each spinal nerve arises by ventral and dorsal roots; the ventral root carries motor fibres from the ventral horn and preganglionic fibres from the lateral horn, while the dorsal root consists of sensory fibres which are processes of the cells in the dorsal root ganglion (Fig. 3.31). The dorsal root ganglion contains pseudounipolar cells, where the peripheral processes pass into the spinal nerve and the central processes pass towards the spinal cord.

The spinal nerve is very short and lies in the intervertebral foramen with the dorsal root ganglion; there is mixing of the motor and sensory fibres in the spinal nerve before it divides into ventral and dorsal rami. The ventral rami carry motor and sensory fibres to the anterior aspect of the body; they form the cervical (page 320) and brachial (page 398) plexuses, the intercostal nerves (page 79), lumbar (page 578), and lumbosacral (page 580) plexuses. Between T1–L2 and S2–S4 the ventral rami are connected to the sympathetic trunk by white rami communicans from the spinal cord. All ventral rami are connected to the sympathetic trunk by a grey ramus communicans through which the autonomic fibres are distributed along the ventral and dorsal rami to reach organs, sweat glands, blood vessels and arrectores pilorum. The dorsal rami carry motor fibres to the muscles and sensory fibres from the skin of the back.

CLINICAL ANATOMY: The subarachnoid space between L2 and S3 contains the cauda equina and filum terminale suspended in cerebrospinal fluid. Cerebrospinal fluid can therefore be taken from the subarachnoid space by inserting a hollow needle into the space between L3 and L4 or L4 and L5 (lumbar puncture). This can be done for diagnosis of certain diseases or injuries; injection of substances into the subarachnoid space (anaesthetic drugs, air); and relief of increased fluid pressure in the central nervous system (haemorrhage).

In the early development of the central nervous system, the spinal cord is the same length as the vertebral column, each spinal nerve running transversely from the spinal cord to the corresponding intervertebral foramen (Fig. 3.32). As the foetus develops, differential growth of the vertebral column and spinal cord results in the vertebral column becoming much longer than the spinal cord. The dural sac grows to accommodate this difference; in adults, it terminates at the level of S2, whereas the spinal cord ends opposite the L1/L2 intervertebral disc. However, the spinal nerves retain their original relationship with their respective intervertebral foramen, with their roots remaining attached to their respective spinal cord segments. This is achieved by elongation of the more caudal nerve roots having an increasingly oblique course within the dural sac (Fig. 3.32); the leash of nerves hanging free within the dural sac is the cauda equina, with each nerve root surrounded by its own sleeve of pia mater and bathed in cerebrospinal fluid.

APPLIED ANATOMY: At 3 months the spinal cord extends the whole length of the vertebral canal: at birth, it ends at the level of L3; in adults, it ends at the L1/L2 intervertebral disc. In adults, the relationship between spinal segments and vertebral levels is the C8 segment lies opposite the C6 vertebra; the T6 segment lies opposite the T4 vertebra; the T12 segment lies opposite the T9 vertebra; and lumbar and sacral segments lie between the T9 and L2 vertebrae.

Nerve Root Sheaths

To reach the somatic nervous system the spinal nerves must penetrate the meninges. When they leave the spinal cord, the proximal ends of the spinal nerve roots are invested by the pia mater, which spreads over the surface of each nerve from its point of attachment to the spinal cord as far as where it leaves the vertebral canal. On leaving the dural sac, the nerve roots take a funnel-shaped extension of the dura and arachnoid mater with them (dural sleeves), which extends as far as the spinal nerve (Fig. 3.31); throughout their entire length, the spinal nerve roots are surrounded by cerebrospinal fluid.

Somatic Nervous System

The somatic (peripheral) nervous system comprises peripheral branches of the spinal nerves conveying motor axons to the muscles of the body and sensory fibres to the central nervous system: the cranial nerves (page 270) are also part of the peripheral nervous system.

On emerging from the intervertebral foramen, the spinal nerve divides into anterior (ventral) and posterior (dorsal) rami (Fig. 3.33), which then branch further; except for the C1 and C2 spinal nerves, the anterior rami are substantially larger than the posterior.

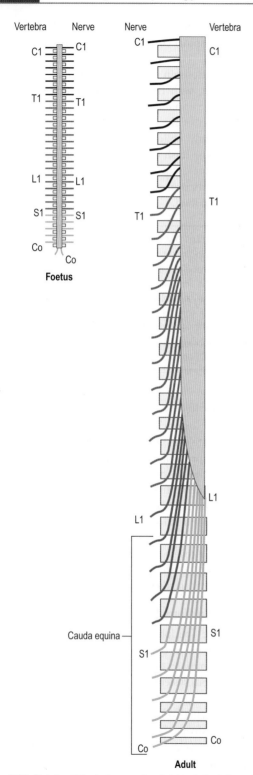

Fig. 3.32 Relationship between the intervertebral foramina, spinal nerves and spinal cord in the foetus and adults.

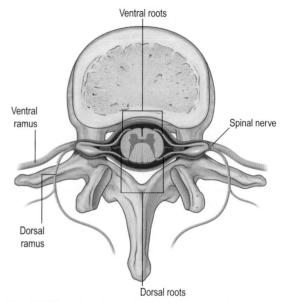

Fig. 3.33 Dorsal and ventral rami of a typical spinal nerve.

All posterior rami pass posteriorly into tissues of the back innervating the back muscles, as well as the ligaments and joints associated with the vertebrae; most also give cutaneous branches to skin over the posterior aspect of the head, neck, trunk and pelvic girdle, and the dermatomes of the spinal nerves are shown in Figs 4.6, 5.25 and 7.81). The posterior rami of C1, L4 and L5 lack cutaneous branches, while those of C4–C6 are inconstant; however, they convey sensory information from the muscles, ligaments and joints they supply.

The ventral rami innervate the sides and anterior aspects of the body wall, the limbs and the perineum. In the thoracic region, the ventral rami have a simple arrangement, with all except T1, forming a typical intercostal nerve which passes laterally from the intervertebral foramen under the rib of the same segment (Fig. 2.14). The main part of T1 passes over the 1st rib to join in the formation of the brachial plexus (page 398). Each intercostal nerve innervates muscles of its intercostal space and the overlying skin; the lower six intercostal nerves extend into the anterior abdominal wall segmentally supplying muscles of the anterior abdominal wall and overlying skin.

At cervical, lumbar and sacral levels the simple segmental arrangement is modified as the ventral rami form plexuses. A plexus is a network of interconnections between adjacent ventral rami allowing them to exchange nerve fibres before forming discrete peripheral nerves; there are five named plexuses on each side of the vertebral column (Fig. 3.34).

Cervical plexus (C1–C4): peripheral nerves distributed to the prevertebral muscles, levator scapulae, sternomastoid, trapezius, diaphragm, and skin of the anterior and lateral aspects of the neck from the shoulder to the lower jaw and external ear (Fig. 4.83B). Further details can be found on page 320.

Brachial plexus (C5–T1): innervation of the muscles and joints of the pectoral girdle and upper limb, and skin of the upper limb. Further details can be found on page 398.

Lumbar plexus (T12/L1–L4): smaller branches innervate muscles of the lower anterolateral abdominal wall, skin of the groin, lateral thigh and external parts of the external genitalia; larger branches (femoral and obturator nerves) innervate muscles and skin of the thigh. Further details can be found on page 578.

Lumbosacral plexus (L5–S3): innervation of muscles and skin of the lower limb. Further details can be found on page 580.

Sacral plexus (S3–S5): innervation of the pelvic floor and perineum. Further details can be found on page 556.

Knowledge of the distribution of the major nerves is important in the diagnosis and assessment of peripheral nerve injuries and neurological disorders in clinical practice.

Autonomic Nervous System

The autonomic nervous system comprises neurons located within both the central and peripheral nervous systems that are concerned with control of the internal environment through the innervation of secretory glands and cardiac and smooth muscle; its functions are closely integrated with those of the somatic nervous system. On topographical, anatomical, pharmacological and physiological grounds, it is considered in two parts (sympathetic, parasympathetic), although in practice it constitutes an integrated system underlying visceral and homeostatic neural regulation.

Topographically, the two systems differ in their connections with the central nervous system; parasympathetic nerves emerge from the central nervous system in cranial nerves III, VII, IX and X and the S2–S4 spinal

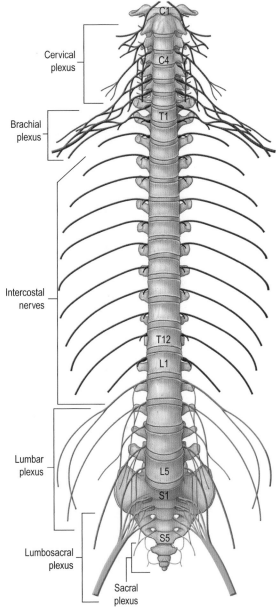

Fig. 3.34 The position of the major somatic nerve plexuses arising from the spinal cord.

nerves (craniosacral outflow), while sympathetic nerves emerge from spinal cord segments T1–L2 (thoracolumbar outflow).

Anatomically, in both systems, the target organ/structure is connected to the central nervous system by two neurons in series. The axon of the first nerve emerges from the central nervous system and synapses

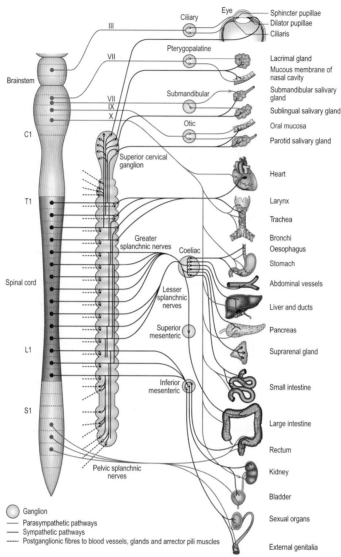

Fig. 3.35 Efferent pathways of the autonomic nervous system.

with the cell body of a second neuron at a ganglion (collection of cell bodies); parasympathetic ganglia lie close to the target organ and sympathetic ganglia further away (Fig. 3.35). Axons joining the central nervous system to ganglia are *preganglionic axons* and those from ganglia to the target organ/structure are *postganglionic axons*; postganglionic parasympathetic axons are short, while postganglionic sympathetic axons are longer.

Pharmacologically, the two systems differ in that the neurotransmitter in sympathetic and parasympathetic preganglionic neurons is acetylcholine, while the neurotransmitter

in parasympathetic postganglionic neurons is also acetylcholine, in sympathetic postganglionic neurons it is noradrenaline. While acetylcholine and noradrenaline are the primary neurotransmitters, many other substances in autonomic nerves fulfil the criteria for a neurotransmitter or neuromodulator. The principal co-transmitters in sympathetic nerves are adenosine 5′-triphosphate (ATP) and neuropeptide Y, and in parasympathetic nerves vasoactive intestinal polypeptide (VIP).

Physiologically, the autonomic nervous system exerts a variety of effects on different types of tissues; in general, these effects are exerted due to the contraction or relaxation of smooth muscle or myoepithelial cells in exocrine glands. Acetylcholine secreted by parasympathetic neurons generally excites smooth muscle causing it to contract. Noradrenaline can either excite or inhibit smooth muscle depending on the molecular receptors present on the smooth muscle membrane: α-receptors cause contraction and β-receptors relaxation. Different tissues have either α- or β-receptors; some have both types of receptors in different regions or even in the same region. It is these variations which give rise to the diversity of autonomic nervous system effects.

Parasympathetic Nervous System

The cell bodies of preganglionic parasympathetic neurons are located in the brainstem, associated with the nuclei of the oculomotor (III), facial (VII), glossopharyngeal (IX) and vagus (X) cranial nerves and in the intermediate grey matter of the S2–S4 sacral segments. Associated with each cranial nerve is a discrete peripheral ganglion: ciliary ganglion with III; pterygopalatine and submandibular ganglia with VII; and otic ganglion with IX. The distribution of the cranial preganglionic parasympathetic fibres is shown schematically in Fig. 3.36.

The ciliary ganglionic is located at the back of the orbit close to the optic nerve; the postganglionic neurons innervate the sphincter pupillae and ciliary muscles, causing them to contract narrowing the pupil and increasing the refractive (focusing) power of the lens, respectively.

The pterygopalatine ganglion is located in the pterygopalatine fossa receiving preganglionic fibres from the facial nerve. When stimulated, the postganglionic neurons innervate mucous glands of the nose and the lacrimal gland causing nasal and palatine secretions and lacrimation, respectively.

The submandibular ganglion is located in the submandibular region (page 321) receiving preganglionic fibres from the facial nerve via the chorda tympani (page 277); the postganglionic neurons innervate the submandibular and sublingual glands.

The otic ganglion lies just below the foramen ovale in the infratemporal fossa (page 287) receiving the majority of its preganglionic fibres from the glossopharyngeal nerve, with some from the facial nerve; postganglionic neurons innervate the parotid gland (page 312).

The parasympathetic fibres in the vagus are distributed to the heart, larynx, trachea, small intestine, liver,

biliary tract, pancreas and large intestine as far as the splenic flexure (page 475). Postganglionic fibres innervating the sinoatrial node arise from ganglia lying on the surface of the heart, while those of the respiratory, digestive and urinary tracts are embedded within the tract walls.

The descending and sigmoid colon, rectum and pelvic viscera are innervated by postganglionic neurons arising from the S2 to S4 segments of the spinal cord. Their ventral rami emerge from the anterior sacral foramina with the parasympathetic axons passing directly to the target viscera as the pelvic splanchnic nerves (Fig. 3.37). Preganglionic fibres destined for pelvic viscera pass directly into them, synapsing on postganglionic neurons located in their walls; those for the descending and sigmoid colon pass upwards out of the pelvis across the left posterior abdominal wall to reach the descending colon or enter the sigmoid mesocolon to reach the sigmoid colon.

Actions. The parasympathetic system slows activity in the sinoatrial node decreasing heart rate, at the same time causing contraction of bronchial musculature. There is contraction of smooth muscle in the digestive and urinary tracts and relaxation of their sphincters causing them to empty, as well as secretion of mucous and acid. There is also secretion of fluid from the salivary and lacrimal glands, vasodilation of blood vessels in the urogenital system enabling erection of the penis and clitoris, and vasodilation of blood vessels of the internal and external carotid circulation.

Sympathetic Nervous System

Details of the formation of the sympathetic chains (trunks) can be found on page 90 Although the majority of postganglionic axons joining the ventral ramus continue distally within it, some take a short recurrent course to enter the dorsal ramus. Postganglionic axons use the ventral and dorsal rami to reach blood vessels in the tissues they supply; some follow the course of cutaneous branches of somatic nerves to reach sweat glands and the arrectores pilorum muscles in the skin.

Because the skin and deep tissues in the head are supplied by cranial rather than spinal nerves, the postganglionic axons form plexuses around, and travel with, the common, internal and external carotid arteries and their branches to reach their destination. A modification to this is the sympathetic innervation of the eye; postganglionic axons leave the internal carotid

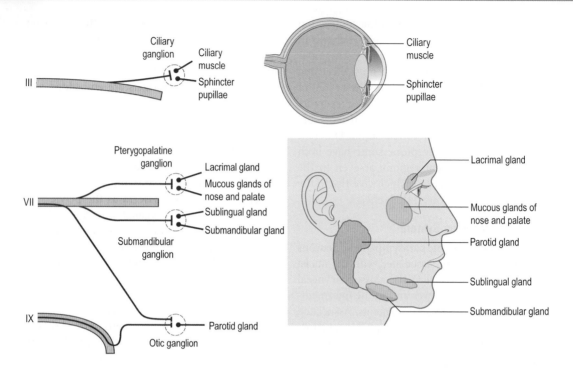

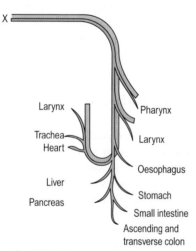

Fig. 3.36 Distribution of parasympathetic fibres in the oculomotor (III), facial (VII), glossopharyngeal (IX) and vagus (X) nerves.

plexus to join the ophthalmic branch of the trigeminal nerve (page 275) entering its nasociliary branch. The axons reach the eye either through the short ciliary branches of the ciliary ganglion or along the long ciliary branches of the nasociliary nerve; within the eye,

they are distributed to the dilator pupillae and blood vessels.

Sympathetic nerves to thoracic, abdominal and pelvic viscera pass directly from the sympathetic chain as splanchnic nerves; those to the heart and lungs are

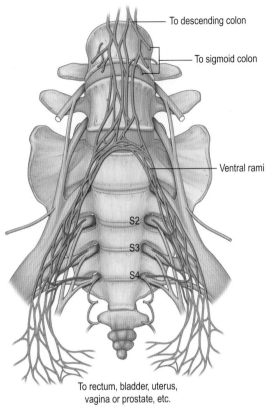

To descending colon

To sigmoid colon

Ventral rami

S2

S3

S4

To rectum, bladder, uterus,
vagina or prostate, etc.

Fig. 3.37 The pelvic splanchnic nerves.

formed by postganglionic axons arising from the upper four thoracic sympathetic ganglia (Fig. 2.23) and reach their destination by forming plexuses around the coronary arteries and bronchi.

The abdominal viscera are innervated by the greater, lesser and least splanchnic nerves (Fig. 2.23) with variable origins from the lower seven or eight thoracic segments of the spinal cord; they comprise preganglionic axons which pass through the sympathetic chain without synapsing. They enter the abdominal cavity by piercing the ipsilateral crus of the diaphragm (page 73) forming dense plexuses around the abdominal aorta, coeliac and renal arteries (Fig. 2.25), where they synapse in coeliac and aorticorenal ganglia. The postganglionic axons reach the abdominal viscera by forming plexuses around the arteries supplying the organ. An exception to this is the sympathetic innervation of the adrenal gland; embryologically the adrenal

medulla has the same origin as the sympathetic nervous system; consequently, its cells are equivalent to postganglionic neurons. The adrenal gland is therefore innervated directly by preganglionic and not postganglionic axons from the coeliac plexus.

Pelvic viscera receive their sympathetic innervation from postganglionic axons from the abdominal aortic plexus, which is supplemented by postganglionic axons from lumbar splanchnic nerves arising from lumbar sympathetic ganglia. The abdominal aorta terminates at the level of L4, after which the sympathetic plexus continues onto the anterior surface of L5 and promontory of the sacrum as the superior hypogastric plexus (Fig. 2.25). Leashes of nerves from this plexus descend either side of the sacrum with the internal iliac arteries, joining the pelvic splanchnic nerves to form the inferior hypogastric plexuses; postganglionic axons enter the bladder, rectum and other pelvic viscera.

Actions. The sympathetic system stimulates the sinoatrial node increasing heart rate, as well as directly stimulating cardiac muscle increasing the force of cardiac contraction. In the peripheral vasculature, the effects are variable: acting on α-receptors it causes vasoconstriction and on β-receptors vasodilation. In the digestive tract, it relaxes smooth muscle but stimulates its sphincters to contract; in the respiratory tract it relaxes bronchial smooth muscle; it causes the bladder sphincter to contract and mediates ejaculation in males by causing smooth muscle contraction in the vas deferens, seminal vesicle and prostate gland (page 535); in the eye it causes dilation of the pupil; it causes the hair of the skin to stand on end and sweating.

The effects of the sympathetic system are those that would be evident in the functions of fright, flight, fight and fill. The reaction to fright is seen as an increased heart rate, sweating, pupillary dilation and hair 'standing on end'; flight (running away) and fight involve increased heart rate, increased circulation (vasodilation) to muscles with blood being diverted away from (vasoconstriction) the digestive tract; fill refers to relaxation of bronchial smooth muscle increasing the entry of air into lungs: all these actions are mediated by the sympathetic system. Smooth muscle relaxation and contraction of the sphincters of the digestive tract result in filling of its lumen.

SELF-TEST QUESTIONS

1. How many free vertebrae are there?
   a. 12
   b. 19
   c. 24
   d. 27
   e. 33

2. Which of the following is NOT a function of the vertebral column?
   a. Haemopoiesis
   b. Absorbs impacts
   c. Supports the thoracic cage
   d. Protects the spinal cord
   e. Dissipates forces from other parts of the body

3. Concerning scoliosis, which of the following is the most common?
   a. Idiopathic
   b. Neuromuscular
   c. Congenital
   d. Metabolic
   e. Genetic

4. How many cervical spinal nerves are there?
   a. 6
   b. 7
   c. 12
   d. 14
   e. 16

5. Which of the following features is NOT associated with thoracic vertebrae?
   a. Short transverse processes
   b. Long spinous process
   c. Costal facets
   d. Heart-shaped body
   e. Laminae

6. Which of the following movements is NOT possible in the lumbar spine?
   a. Flexion
   b. Rotation
   c. Right lateral flexion
   d. Extension
   e. Left lateral flexion

7. How much of vertebral column length is accounted for by the intervertebral discs?
   a. 10%
   b. 15%
   c. 20%
   d. 25%
   e. 30%

8. Concerning the intervertebral disc, which of the following statements is NOT correct?
   a. The annulus fibrosis consists of concentric bands of collagen fibres.
   b. There is no clear distinction between the nucleus pulposus and annulus fibrosis.
   c. Proteoglycans are responsible for the hydrophilic properties of the nucleus pulposus.
   d. From middle age, the nucleus pulposus contains approximately 70% water.
   e. The cartilage end plates act as impermeable membranes.

9. Which of the following ligaments only attaches to the intervertebral discs and adjacent margins of the vertebral bodies?
   a. Posterior longitudinal
   b. Anterior longitudinal
   c. Intertransverse
   d. Ligamentum flavum
   e. Ligamentum nuchae

10. Concerning the blood supply of the spinal cord, which of the following statements is NOT correct?
    a. The single posterior spinal artery is formed by branches from the vertebral artery.
    b. The vertebral venous plexuses communicate with veins in other regions.
    c. Occlusion of the anterior spinal artery at mid-thoracic levels can lead to acute thoracic cord syndrome.
    d. Radicular arteries enter the vertebral canal via the intervertebral foramen.
    e. The anterior spinal artery is a direct branch of the vertebral artery.

11. Between which spinal cord levels is sympathetic outflow?
    a. C1–S4
    b. C1–L2
    c. T1–L1
    d. T1–L2
    e. T2–L1

12. Which of the following muscles is NOT an intrinsic muscle of the back?
    a. Semispinalis
    b. Quadratus lumborum
    c. Multifidus
    d. Rotatores
    e. Erector spinae

13. Which of the following cranial nerves contains parasympathetic fibres?
    a. IV
    b. V
    c. VI
    d. VII
    e. VIII
14. At which intervertebral level is a lumbar puncture usually performed?
    a. T12–L1
    b. L1–L2
    c. L2–L3
    d. L3–L4
    e. L5–S1
15. Which of the following features divides the spinal cord into right and left halves?
    a. Posterior lateral sulcus
    b. Medial prominence
    c. Anterior median sulcus
    d. Posterior intermediate sulcus
    e. Lateral prominence
16. The filum terminale is an extension of the:
    a. Dura mater
    b. Grey matter of the spinal cord
    c. White matter of the spinal cord
    d. Arachnoid mater
    e. Pia mater
17. Concerning the epidural space, which of the following statements is NOT correct?
    a. It lies between the dura mater and the tissues lining the vertebral canal.
    b. It is closed inferiorly by the posterior sacrococcygeal ligament.
    c. Fluids injected into it can spread throughout the length of the vertebral column.
    d. Local anaesthetics injected close to spinal nerves outside the intervertebral foramen do not spread to adjacent nerves.
    e. The paravertebral spaces on each side of the vertebral column communicate via the epidural space.
18. Which of the following is located in the dorsal horn of the spinal cord?
    a. Substantia gelatinosa
    b. Central nucleus
    c. Nucleus proprius
    d. Nucleus dorsalis
    e. Visceral afferent nucleus

19. Which of the following is NOT an ascending (sensory) tract of the spinal cord?
    a. Rubrospinal tract
    b. Lateral spinothalamic tract
    c. Posterior spinocerebellar tract
    d. Fasciculus gracilis
    e. Spino-olivary tract
20. Which of the following tracts is associated with the pyramidal system?
    a. Tectospinal
    b. Rubrospinal
    c. Corticospinal
    d. Olivospinal
    e. Vestibulospinal
21. Concerning spinal reflexes, which of the following statements is NOT correct?
    a. They are modulated by descending connections from the brainstem.
    b. Exaggerated reflexes can be indicative of pathology of supraspinal pathways.
    c. Intrafusal muscle fibres are innervated by α and β motor neurons.
    d. The flexion withdrawal reflex is polysynaptic.
    e. The simplest form of tendon reflex is monosynaptic.
22. Which of the following is NOT a selective lesion of the spinal cord?
    a. Poliomyelitis
    b. Tabes dorsalis
    c. Syringomyelia
    d. Hemisection
    e. Subacute combined degeneration
23. Concerning spinal nerves, which of the following statements is correct?
    a. Each spinal nerve arises by ventral and dorsal rami.
    b. The ventral root carries sensory fibres.
    c. There are six sacral spinal nerves.
    d. All spinal nerves contain parasympathetic fibres.
    e. They leave the vertebral canal via the intervertebral foramen.
24. Concerning the somatic nervous system, which of the following is NOT correct?
    a. It is part of the peripheral nervous system.
    b. The T1 nerve passes deep to the 1st rib.
    c. The lower six intercostal nerves pass into the anterior abdominal wall.
    d. The lumbosacral plexus is formed by the L5–S3 nerves.

e. Posterior rami supply structures of the back.

25. Which of the following is NOT a neurotransmitter associated with sympathetic nerve fibres?
   a. Noradrenaline
   b. Adenosine 5′-triphosphate (ATP)
   c. Neuropeptide Y
   d. Vasoactive intestinal peptide (VIP)
   e. Acetylcholine

26. Concerning the autonomic nervous system, which of the following statements is NOT correct?
   a. Parasympathetic innervation slows heart rate.
   b. Parasympathetic fibres are carried in the facial nerve.
   c. Preganglionic sympathetic fibres synapse in ganglia close to the target organ/structure.
   d. Parasympathetic fibres innervate glands in the nasal cavity.
   e. The splanchnic nerves arise from the sympathetic chain.

27. Concerning the ascending (sensory) tracts, which of the following statements is NOT correct?
   a. The posterior spinocerebellar tract carries impulses from the opposite side of the body.
   b. The lateral spinothalamic tract carries pain and temperature sensations.
   c. The anterior spinocerebellar tract conveys non-discriminative touch and pressure sensations.
   d. Destruction of the spinocerebellar tracts leads to disturbances of muscle tone.
   e. The spinotectal tract is concerned with spinovisual reflexes.

28. Concerning descending (motor) tracts, which of the following statements is NOT correct?

a. Lower motor neuron lesions cause paralysis of specific muscles.
b. Upper motor neuron lesions are associated with increased tendon reflex activity.
c. The extrapyramidal pathways contain fibres originating in the basal ganglia, pons and midbrain.
d. Each hemisphere controls movements of the opposite side of the body.
e. All corticonuclear fibres terminate around the nuclei of both sides of the body.

29. Concerning spinal cord lesions, which of the following statements is NOT correct?
   a. High cervical cord transection causes spastic quadriplegia.
   b. Lumbar cord transection is not associated with incontinence.
   c. Thoracic cord transection causes paraplegia.
   d. Below the level of hemisection there is ipsilateral spastic paralysis.
   e. Syringomyelia is an abnormal widening of the central spinal canal.

30. Concerning the spinal cord, which of the following statements is NOT correct?
   a. The lateral horn contains two groups of nuclei.
   b. The anterior white column lies anteromedial to the ventral horn.
   c. The lateral white column is the narrowest.
   d. The posterior white column lies between the dorsal horn and the posterior median septum.
   e. The fasciculi proprii coordinate the function of the spinal cord in different regions.

Head and Neck

CONTENTS

Key Concepts, 232
Learning Outcomes, 233
Overview, 234
Skull, 234
  Growth of the Skull, 235
  External Features, 236
    Skull Vault, 236
    Posterior Aspect, 239
    Lateral Aspect, 239
    Anterior Aspect, 240
    Base, 242
  Cranial Cavity, 242
    Anterior Cranial Fossa, 242
    Middle Cranial Fossa, 242
    Posterior Cranial Fossa, 243
Brain, 243
  Glial Cells, 247
  Adult Morphology, 247
    Brainstem, 247
    Cerebellum, 252
    Diencephalon, 253
    Cerebrum, 256
    Base of the Brain, 262
  Motor System, 263
  Sensory System, 263
  Limbic System, 263
  Meninges, 264
  Arterial Supply, 264
    Vertebral Artery, 266
    Basilar Artery, 266
    Internal Carotid Artery, 266
    Cerebral Arteries, 267
    Summary of the Arterial Supply to the Brain, 269
  Venous Drainage, 269
    Cerebral Veins, 269
    Intracranial Venous Sinuses, 270

Cranial Nerves, 270
  Olfactory Nerve (I), 272
    Olfactory Pathway, 272
  Optic Nerve (II), 272
    Visual Pathway, 272
  Oculomotor Nerve (III), 273
  Trochlear Nerve (IV), 273
  Trigeminal Nerve (V), 274
    Ophthalmic Division (V_1), 275
    Maxillary Division (V_2), 275
    Mandibular Division (V_3), 275
  Abducens Nerve (VI), 276
  Facial Nerve (VII), 276
  Vestibulocochlear Nerve (VIII), 277
    Vestibular Part, 277
    Cochlear Part, 277
  Glossopharyngeal Nerve (IX), 277
  Vagus Nerve (X), 279
  Accessory Nerve (XI), 280
  Hypoglossal Nerve (XII), 280
Mandible, 282
  Growth of the Mandible, 282
  Temporomandibular Joint, 283
    Movements, 286
  Infratemporal Fossa, 287
Face, 287
  Blood Supply and Innervation, 287
    Arterial Supply, 287
    Venous Drainage, 290
    Lymphatic Drainage. 290
    Innervation, 292
  Muscles of the Face, 292
    Muscles of the Forehead, 292
    Muscles Around the Eye, 292
    Muscles Around the Nose, 294
    Muscles Around the Mouth, 294

Orbit, 294
  Orbital Fascia and Ligaments, 295
  Vessels and Nerves Within the Orbit, 295
  Eyeball, 297
  Movement of the Eyeball, 300
External Nose, 304
Nasal Cavity, 304
  Paranasal Sinuses, 304
  Blood and Nerve Supply, 308
Oral Cavity, 308
  Lips, 309
  Teeth and Gums, 309
  Tongue, 311
  Salivary Glands, 312
  Palate, 313
  Oropharyngeal Isthmus, 314
Ear, 314
  External Ear, 314
  Middle Ear, 314
  Inner Ear, 316
Neck, 317
Cervical Vertebrae, 317
Regions, 317
  Posterior Triangle, 319
  Anterior Triangle, 320
  Compartments, 325
  Hyoid, 325
  Pharynx, 326
  Larynx, 328
  Thyroid Gland, 331
  Root of the Neck, 331
Endocrine System, 333
Hormones, 334

Endocrine Glands, 334
Pituitary Gland, 335
  Growth Hormone, 337
  Disorders of the Pituitary Gland, 339
Thyroid Gland, 340
  Regulation of Secretion, 341
  Function of Thyroid Hormones, 341
  Calcitonin, 342
Parathyroid Glands, 342
Adrenal (Suprarenal) Glands, 343
  Adrenal Cortex, 343
  Mineralocorticoids, 344
  Glucocorticoids, 345
Adrenal Medulla, 347
Islets of Langerhans, 347
  Insulin, 347
  Glucagon, 348
  Blood Glucose Regulation, 349
Gonads, 351
  Testes, 351
  Ovaries, 356
  Pregnancy, Parturition and Lactation, 361
Pineal Gland, 368
Kidneys, 368
Heart, 368
Thymus, 369
Hypothalamus, 369
Local Hormones, 369
  Local Hormones Produced in Tissues, 369
  Local Hormones Produced in Blood, 370

KEY CONCEPTS

- The skull consists of the cranium and facial skeleton.
- The cranium encloses and protects the brain.
- The face increases in size with the development of the paranasal sinuses.
- The brain is part of the central nervous system and is surrounded by meninges.
- The dura mater encloses venous sinuses and forms folds separating parts of the brain.

- Nerve fibres and cell bodies form grey matter and myelinated axons white matter.
- The cerebral and cerebellar cortex are grey matter and the medulla is white matter.
- Glial cells support and bind neurons together.
- The brain comprises cerebral hemispheres, diencephalon, cerebellum and brainstem.
- Thalamic nuclei are relay nuclei for all sensory inputs except smell.

- The cerebral hemispheres communicate across the midline via the corpus callosum.
- The surface of each cerebral hemisphere has ridges (gyri) and grooves (sulci).
- The central sulcus separates the primary motor and primary somatosensory cortices.
- Each cerebral hemisphere controls/receives input from the opposite side of the body.
- The limbic system influences behaviour, memory, motivation, emotion and learning.
- The ventricles contain cerebrospinal fluid.
- Cerebrospinal fluid bathes the brain regulating intracranial pressure.

- Branches of the vertebral and internal carotid arteries supply the brain.
- There are 12 pairs of cranial nerves.
- The trigeminal nerve is sensory to facial skin: the facial nerve innervates facial muscles.
- Fascia divides the neck into discrete compartments.
- The root of the neck is the transition between the thorax, neck and upper limb.
- The endocrine system regulates all physiological activities.
- The pituitary gland is the 'master' gland of the endocrine system.
- Puberty represents the onset of adult sexual maturity.

LEARNING OUTCOMES

At the end of this chapter, you should be able to:

- Identify and palpate individual bones of the skull and facial skeleton through the skin.
- Appreciate the influence of pathology and/or trauma on the skull and face.
- Identify, palpate and examine the mandible and hyoid.
- Describe, assess and examine movements, and their restraints, of the mandible.
- Appreciate the influence of pathology and/or trauma on the temporomandibular joint.
- Describe the organisation of brain tissue into grey and white matter and what each comprises.
- Describe the arrangement of the brain into the cerebrum (cerebral hemispheres), cerebellum, and brainstem (midbrain, pons, medulla oblongata).
- Describe the location of the lobes of the cerebral hemispheres and outline the major function of each.
- Describe the location and function of the cerebellum.
- Describe the location and function of each component of the brainstem.
- Describe the major ascending motor and descending sensory pathways/tracts.
- Describe the location and function of the thalamus.
- Describe the organisation and function of the meninges and their roles.
- Describe the arterial supply and venous drainage of the brain.

- Appreciate the influence of pathology and/or trauma to individual parts of the brain.
- Describe the origin, course, distribution and function of each cranial nerve.
- Appreciate the influence of pathology and/or trauma on each cranial nerve.
- Describe the organisation, location and function of structures within the orbit, nasal and oral cavities.
- Describe the structural organisation and function of the external, middle and inner ear.
- Appreciate the influence of pathology and/or trauma to the ear.
- Describe the structural organisation of the eye and the function of each layer of the eyeball.
- Describe the role of the extraocular muscles in altering the direction of gaze.
- Appreciate the influence of pathology and/or trauma on the eye.
- Describe the organisation of the neck into fascial compartments, and the structures, and their function, within each.
- Describe the processes of fertilisation, pregnancy, parturition and lactation.
- Describe the role of the limbic and endocrine systems.
- Describe the location and function of each endocrine gland.
- Appreciate the influence of pathology and/or trauma on each endocrine gland.

OVERVIEW

This chapter considers the anatomy and physiology of the head and neck, including the brain and cranial nerves, and neck, which houses the upper parts of the respiratory and digestive tracts. It is organised into five major sections: skull; brain and cranial nerves; face, including the mandible; neck, which includes the upper parts of the digestive and respiratory systems and root of the neck, an important transition area between the neck, thorax and upper limb enabling structures to pass between these regions; and endocrine glands.

SKULL

The skull forms the skeleton of the head and comprises a large cranial cavity, enclosing and protecting the brain, projecting anteriorly over the facial skeleton. The adult skull consists of 21 immobile bones (the paired parietal, temporal, zygomatic, maxillae, lacrimal, nasal, palatine and inferior conchae, and the individual occipital, frontal, ethmoid, sphenoid and vomer), together with the mandible. The bones of the skull ossify in membrane (intramembranous ossification, page 31), being joined edge to edge by fibrous interlocking joints (sutures, page 35); they comprise plates of bone with an outer and inner layer of compact bone (page 32) enclosing a central region (diploe) of cancellous bone (page 32).

> **CLINICAL ANATOMY:** Valveless diploic veins within the diploe of the flat bones of the skull communicate with the meningeal veins and intracranial venous sinuses (page 270): frontal veins join the supraorbital veins and/or superior sagittal sinus; anterior temporal veins join the sphenoparietal sinus; posterior temporal veins join the transverse sinus; and the large occipital veins join the transverse sinus or confluence of sinuses, although they can pass extracranially to join the occipital veins.

The vault and most of the sides of the skull are formed by the two large parietal bones, which articulate along their medial borders at the sagittal suture (Fig. 4.1); the parietal eminence is the most convex part of the parietal bone. The remainder of each side of the cranial cavity is formed by the squamous part of the temporal bone and part of the greater wing of the sphenoid: the junction of the frontal, parietal, temporal and sphenoid bones is the pterion. Passing medially and slightly anteriorly from the squamous part of the temporal bone is the petrous part of the temporal bone, which forms the floor of the middle cranial fossa (see Fig. 4.9B): it contains and protects the organs of hearing and balance.

> **CLINICAL ANATOMY:** The anterior branch of the middle meningeal artery passes deep to the region of the pterion; it may rupture following a severe blow to the side of the head and lead to an epidural haematoma. Pressure caused by the haematoma on the underlying brain can be released by making an opening 4 cm above the middle of the zygomatic arch 4 cm from the frontozygomatic suture.

Anteriorly the skull is formed by the frontal bone (Fig. 4.1), which joins the parietal bones at the coronal suture; the bregma is the area where the coronal and sagittal sutures meet. The frontal bone forms the forehead and separates the orbits from the anterior cranial fossa; it forms the roof of each orbit and the floor of the anterior cranial fossa.

> **CLINICAL ANATOMY:** The frontal bone develops in two parts, being separated by the metopic suture which usually completely disappears by age 6 but may persist in 9% of adults; in 6% of the population, a single frontal bone may still show evidence of a metopic suture.

The most posterior part of the cranial cavity is formed by the occipital bone (Fig. 4.1), which joins the posterior border of each parietal bone at the lambdoid suture; the lambda is where the sagittal and lambdoid sutures meet. The occipital bone curves forwards to surround the foramen magnum (see Fig. 4.9B), projecting anteriorly as the basilar part to join the body of the sphenoid at the spheno-occipital synchondrosis, which closes during adolescence, with closure in females being 2 years earlier than in males.

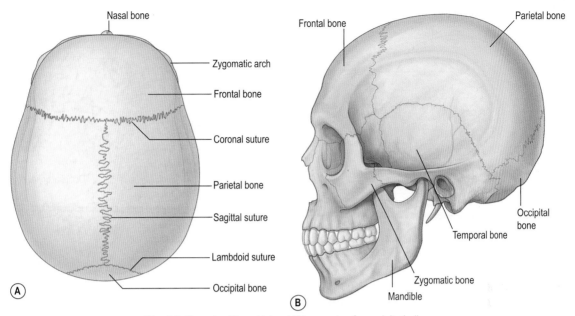

Fig. 4.1 Superior (A) and lateral (B) aspects of an adult skull.

Growth of the Skull

At birth, the cranial cavity is large and the face small (Fig. 4.2): the face comprises one-eighth of the whole skull, whereas in adults it is one-third. The individual bones of the skull vault are separated by sutures, which facilitates adaptation of the skull vault during childbirth, as well as the growth and development of the individual bones. Viewed from above anterior and posterior fontanelles are apparent (Fig. 4.2), while from the side can be seen the sphenoidal (anterolateral) fontanelle, at the pterion, and the mastoid (posterolateral) fontanelle, at the asterion.

The paranasal sinuses are rudimentary with the upper jaw and nasal cavities being small; the teeth are not also fully formed. Individual bones of the face are joined by cartilage, with ossification progressing with increasing age. The mastoid process is rudimentary so that the styloid process and stylomastoid foramen lie closer to the side of the head. The maxillae are shallow because they have no sinuses and consist mainly of alveolar bone and the developing teeth. The forehead appears prominent as there is no bridge to the nose (due to flat nasal bones) and the absence of superciliary arches. The orbits are relatively large with the nasal cavity lying almost completely between them.

After birth, the skull grows rapidly until age 7, with the greatest increase in the size of the cranial cavity being during the 1st year. As the mastoid process starts to develop the styloid process and stylomastoid

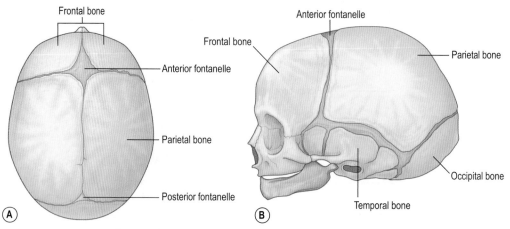

Fig. 4.2 Superior (A) and lateral (B) aspects of a foetal skull.

foramen begin to lie deeper. By age 7 the orbits are almost adult-sized; the petrous part of the temporal bone, body of the sphenoid and foramen magnum have all reached adult size. The maxillae and mandible have enlarged in preparation for eruption of the permanent teeth. There is slower skull growth after age 7, except during puberty when there is a rapid growth in all directions, especially in the facial and frontal regions accompanying expansion of the paranasal sinuses. From the early 20s to middle age there is gradual fusion of the sutures, beginning with the sagittal suture.

> **CLINICAL ANATOMY:** The shape and size of the skull, especially the skull vault, are partly determined by pressure exerted by the underlying brain during its growth and development.

> **CLINICAL ANATOMY:** A skull fracture may be of little consequence; however, it needs to be assessed to minimise the extent of primary brain injury and to treat potential secondary complications: significant fractures are depressed, compound and pterion fractures. *Depressed fractures* occur when a bony fragment is depressed below the normal skull convexity; it can lead to primary brain injury, as well as secondary arterial and venous bleeding with haematoma formation. *Compound fractures* occur when there is a fracture which breaches the overlying skin (often associated with scalp lacerations) and can lead to infection, with meningitis being a potential complication; intracranial infections following trauma may involve the paranasal sinuses and be a potential cause of morbidity. *Pterion fractures* (page 234).

> **APPLIED ANATOMY:** With increasing age, the bone of the skull vault tends to become thinner and therefore more liable to trauma.

External Features
Skull Vault

Apart from being wider posteriorly, the skull vault has few distinguishing features; its roundness means that the effects of a blow to the head, unless extremely violent, are dissipated and minimised.

Scalp. The multi-layered scalp (Fig. 4.3) extends from the supraorbital margins anteriorly to the external occipital protuberance and superior nuchal lines posteriorly, and as far laterally as the superior temporal line on the temporal bone. The outer three layers are firmly bound together and move as a single unit; it may be torn away in 'scalping' injuries.

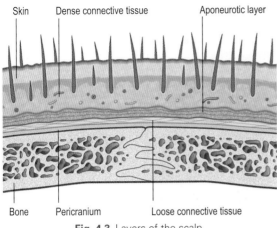

Skin   Dense connective tissue   Aponeurotic layer

Bone   Pericranium   Loose connective tissue

Fig. 4.3 Layers of the scalp.

Its layers are defined by the acronym:

Skin: similar to that elsewhere in the body, except that it has an abundance of hair.

Connective tissue: dense and fibrous containing blood vessels and nerves.

Aponeurosis: connecting the bellies of occipitofrontalis.

Loose areolar tissue: separating the aponeurotic layer from the skull vault.

Pericranium (periosteum): the outer surface of the skull vault.

Blood supply. The arterial supply to the scalp is from five branches on each side (Fig. 4.4): supratrochlear and supraorbital (from the ophthalmic branch of the internal carotid artery), superficial temporal, posterior auricular and occipital (from the external carotid artery).

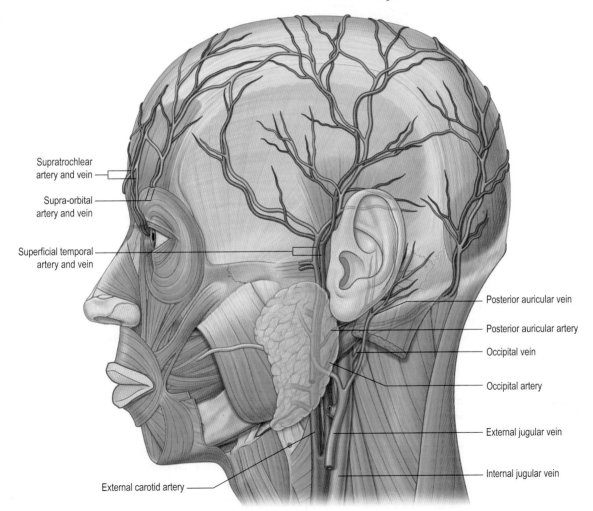

Supratrochlear artery and vein

Supra-orbital artery and vein

Superficial temporal artery and vein

External carotid artery

Posterior auricular vein

Posterior auricular artery

Occipital vein

Occipital artery

External jugular vein

Internal jugular vein

Fig. 4.4 Blood supply to the scalp.

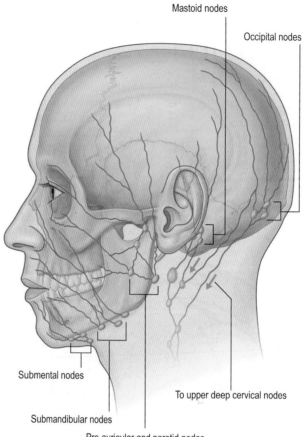

Mastoid nodes

Occipital nodes

Submental nodes

Submandibular nodes

Pre-auricular and parotid nodes

To upper deep cervical nodes

Fig. 4.5 Lymphatic drainage of the scalp.

The venous drainage generally corresponds to the arterial supply; the supratrochlear and supraorbital veins form the anterior facial vein at the medial angle of the eye, but also communicate with the superior ophthalmic vein; the superficial temporal vein joins the maxillary vein to form the retromandibular vein; the posterior auricular vein joins the posterior division of the retromandibular vein to form the external jugular vein; the occipital vein usually drains into the occipital venous plexus, but may communicate with the superior sagittal and/or sigmoid venous sinuses via emissary veins.

CLINICAL ANATOMY: Lacerations to the scalp bleed profusely as the dense connective tissue surrounding the vessels holds them open; in contrast, infections tend to localise in the loose connective tissue.

Lymphatic drainage. The lymphatic drainage tends to follow the pattern of the arterial supply. Anterior to the vertex, drainage is to preauricular and parotid nodes (Fig. 4.5); from the forehead, some lymph may drain to submandibular nodes via efferent vessels accompanying the facial vein. Posterior to the vertex, drainage is to retroauricular and posterior auricular (mastoid) nodes, with efferent vessels draining to upper deep cervical nodes (Fig. 4.5). In the occipital region, drainage is to occipital nodes and then to upper deep cervical nodes (Fig. 4.5).

Sensory innervation. Each side of the scalp is innervated by four nerves anterior to the external acoustic meatus, all branches of the divisions of the trigeminal nerve (V), and four nerves posterior, all of which are branches of C2 and/or C3 (Fig. 4.6). The anterior branches are supratrochlear and supraorbital

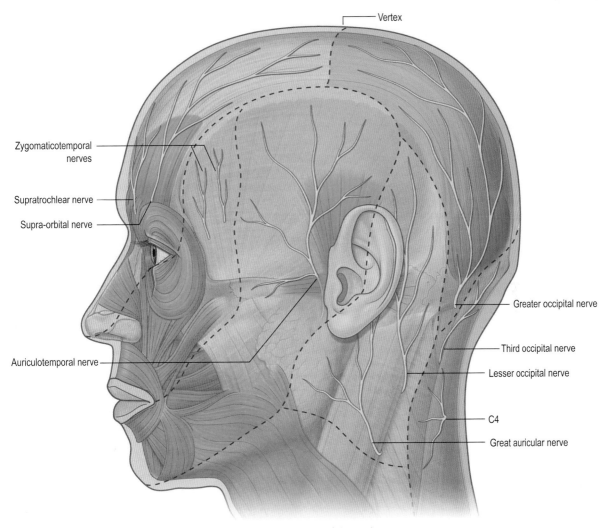

Fig. 4.6 Innervation of the scalp.

branches of the frontal nerve (ophthalmic division); zygomaticotemporal (maxillary division); and auriculotemporal (mandibular nerve). The posterior branches are the greater auricular nerve (C2/C3); lesser occipital nerve (C2); greater occipital nerve (C2); and 3rd cervical nerve (C3).

Posterior Aspect

Posteriorly midway between the lambda and foramen magnum is the external occipital protuberance; the most prominent part of which is the inion, running from the lower part of protuberance to the foramen magnum in the midline is the external occipital crest. The superior nuchal line passes laterally from the external occipital protuberance towards the mastoid process: below and above the superior nuchal line are the inferior nuchal and highest nuchal lines, respectively.

Lateral Aspect

Centrally is the temporal bone articulating superiorly with the greater wing of the sphenoid anteriorly, posteriorly the parietal bone, posteroinferiorly the occipital bone and inferiorly the head of the mandible (Fig. 4.1B). The external acoustic meatus lies in its postero-inferior part, above which the zygomatic arch projects forwards. The mastoid and styloid processes project

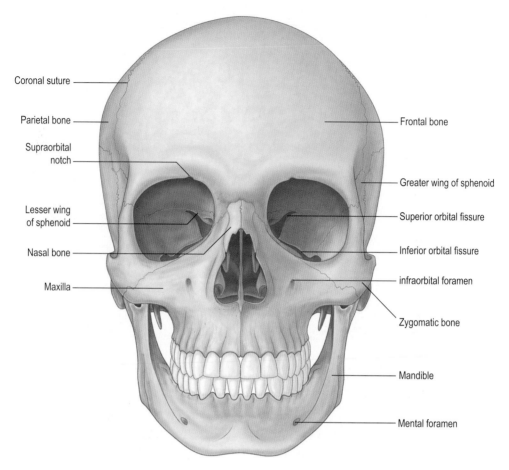

Coronal suture

Parietal bone

Supraorbital notch

Lesser wing of sphenoid

Nasal bone

Maxilla

Frontal bone

Greater wing of sphenoid

Superior orbital fissure

Inferior orbital fissure

infraorbital foramen

Zygomatic bone

Mandible

Mental foramen

Fig. 4.7 Anterior aspect of an adult skull.

inferiorly from the temporal bone into the infratemporal fossa (page 287), a space containing muscles, nerves and blood vessels.

> **APPLIED ANATOMY:** The asterion is the site of union of the parietal, occipital and mastoid parts of the temporal bones.

Anterior Aspect

Anteriorly, the forehead comprises the upper one-third of the skull, formed by the frontal bone and parts of the parietal, sphenoid and temporal bones, deep to which is the anterior cranial fossa. Below the forehead are the large orbital cavities/orbits (page 294), with the nasal cavity (page 304) lying below and medial to each orbit. Just above the superior rim of each orbit is the raised superciliary arch (more prominent in males), between which is a small depression (glabella); on the medial part of the superior rim of each orbit is the supraorbital foramen/notch. On the anterior surface of the maxillae below the inferior rim of the orbit is the infraorbital foramen. In the lower one-third of the face are the maxillae and mandible (page 282) and their respective teeth (Fig. 4.7). Either side of the symphysis menti of the mandible is the mental foramen.

The structures passing through the named opening on the front of the face, including the mandible, are shown in Table 4.1.

TABLE 4.1 Structures Passing Through Openings in the Anterior Aspect of the Skull and Mandible

Opening	Communicates With	Structures Passing Onto Face
Supraorbital foramen	Orbit	Supraorbital nerve and vessels[a]
Infraorbital foramen	Pterygopalatine fossa	Infraorbital nerve[b]
Mental foramen	Infratemporal fossa (via body and ramus of the mandible)	Mental branch of the inferior alveolar nerve[c]

[a]Branch of the frontal nerve, itself a branch of the ophthalmic division (V_1) of the trigeminal nerve (V).
[b]Branch of the maxillary division (V_2) of the trigeminal nerve (V).
[c]Branch of the mandibular division (V_3) of the trigeminal nerve (V).

CLINICAL ANATOMY: Midface fractures involving the maxillae and surrounding structures are known as Le Fort fractures, of which there are three types: as the classification increases (type I to type III) the anatomic level of the fractures ascends from inferior to superior with respect to the maxillae (Fig. 4.8). All Le Fort fractures involve disruption of the pterygoid plates. A *Le Fort I* (horizontal, floating palate) fracture results from a force applied to the alveolar margin or teeth in a downward direction; it involves the pterygoid plates, lateral margin of the nasal cavity, medial and lateral walls of the maxillary sinus and inferior nasal septum (Fig. 4.8A). There is swelling of the upper lip, ecchymosis beneath the zygomatic arch, malocclusion and mobility of the teeth; an impacted fracture may show little mobility. A *Le Fort II* (pyramidal) fracture results from a force applied to the lower or mid part of the maxilla; it involves the inferior orbital rim and extends from the bridge of the nose at or below the nasofrontal suture through the superior medial wall of the maxilla, inferolaterally through the lacrimal bones and inferior orbital margin near the infraorbital foramen on each side (Fig. 4.8B). There is gross oedema of the soft tissues of the midface, bilateral circumorbital ecchymosis and subconjunctival haemorrhage, diplopia, and enophthalmos. A *Le Fort III* (transverse, craniofacial dissociation) fracture results from a force applied to the upper maxilla or bridge of the nose; it usually involves the zygomatic arch. The fracture begins at the nasofrontal or frontomaxillary suture, extending posteriorly along the medial wall of the orbit, through the nasolacrimal groove and ethmoidal air cells, along the orbital floor and infraorbital fissure, lateral orbital wall to the zygomaticofrontal junction and zygomatic arch (Fig. 4.8C); within the nose the fracture continues through the base of the perpendicular plate of the ethmoid and vomer. As with a Le Fort II fracture, there is gross oedema of the soft tissues of the midface, bilateral circumorbital ecchymosis and subconjunctival haemorrhage, diplopia, and enophthalmos; cerebrospinal fluid may also be leaking from the nose.

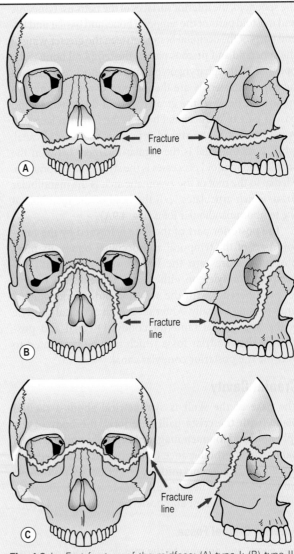

Fig. 4.8 Le Fort fracture of the midface: (A) type I; (B) type II; (C) type III.

Base

The facial skeleton lies below the anterior one-third of the cranial cavity, being limited posteriorly by the posterior border of the hard palate, whose anterior and lateral margins have sockets for the teeth; between the margins are the maxillae anteriorly and palatine bones posteriorly (Fig. 4.9A). Immediately behind the anterior margin is the incisive foramen, while medial to the 3rd molar tooth on each side are the greater and lesser palatine foramina.

The middle part of the base is formed by the body, lateral and medial pterygoid plates and the greater wings of the sphenoid, the inferior surfaces of the petrous, tympanic and mastoid parts of the temporal bone, and basilar and lateral parts of the occipital bone. Between the greater wing of the sphenoid and petrous part of the temporal bone is the opening of the pharyngotympanic (auditory, eustachian) tube: posterolaterally are the foramen ovale and foramen spinosum. Between the greater wing of the sphenoid and basilar part of the occipital bone is the foramen lacerum. Anteromedial to the styloid process is the carotid canal, while posteromedial is the jugular foramen; between the styloid and mastoid processes is the stylomastoid foramen. Medial to the root of the zygomatic arch is the mandibular fossa, which articulates with the head of the mandible at the temporomandibular joint (Fig. 4.9A).

The posterior part of the base is formed by the mastoid part of the temporal and occipital bones: its most obvious features are the foramen magnum with the occipital condyles on either side, the external occipital protuberance with the superior and inferior nuchal lines passing laterally. Anterior to each occipital condyle is the hypoglossal (anterior condylar) canal and posteriorly the condylar fossa which may be perforated to become the posterior condylar canal.

Cranial Cavity

The base of the skull is symmetrical about a sagittal plane, with the crista galli anteriorly, the body of the sphenoid and foramen magnum centrally, and the internal occipital protuberance posteriorly. It is divided into three fossae (anterior, middle, posterior) by prominent ridges; each fossa lies at a different level, with the anterior being the highest and posterior lowest (Fig. 4.9B).

Anterior Cranial Fossa

Lies above and anterior to the middle cranial fossa separated from it by the posterior concave edge of the lesser wings of the sphenoid and anterior clinoid processes (Fig.

4.9B); the frontal lobe of the brain occupies this region. The walls and most of the floor are formed by the frontal bone, with the posterior part formed by the lesser wings and body of the sphenoid. Between the two sides is an elongated hollow in the sagittal plane, in the centre of which is the crista galli with the perforated cribriform plates on either side: the foramen caecum lies just anterior to the crista galli. The floor of the anterior cranial fossa separates the frontal lobes of the brain from the orbital cavities and sphenoidal air cells. Attached to the crista galli and the internal occipital protuberance posteriorly is a sagittal fold of dura mater, falx cerebri (page 264), which passes between the right and left cerebral hemispheres (page 257).

The structures passing through each of the named openings in the anterior cranial fossa are shown in Table 4.2, together with the region each opening communicates with.

Middle Cranial Fossa

Lies behind and below the anterior cranial fossa, with the raised median part being formed by the body of the sphenoid and each lateral part by the greater wing of the sphenoid and petrous part of the temporal bone; the greater wing of the sphenoid forms the anterior wall of the lateral aspects, over which project the lesser wings of the sphenoid, and with the squamous part of the temporal bone it turns upwards to form the lateral wall of the skull (Fig. 4.9B). The lateral parts of the fossa contain the temporal lobes of the brain. The body of the sphenoid has a smooth hollow depression superiorly, the pituitary (hypophyseal) fossa housing the pituitary gland (page 335); from the back of the hollow project the posterior clinoid processes. Attached to the clinoid process is a horizontal fold of dura mater, tentorium cerebelli (page 264), separating the cerebral and cerebellar hemispheres (pages 252 and 257).

Between the greater wing of the sphenoid and (i) lesser wing of the sphenoid is the superior orbital fissure, with the optic canal being medial to the anterior clinoid process; (ii) maxilla is the inferior orbital fissure; (iii) petrous part of the temporal bone is the foramen lacerum. Below the superior orbital fissure close to the body of the sphenoid is the foramen rotundum, while lateral to the foramen lacerum in the greater wing of the sphenoid are the larger foramen ovale (medial) and smaller foramen spinosum (lateral).

The structures passing through each of the named openings in the middle cranial fossa are shown in Table 4.3, together with the region each opening communicates with.

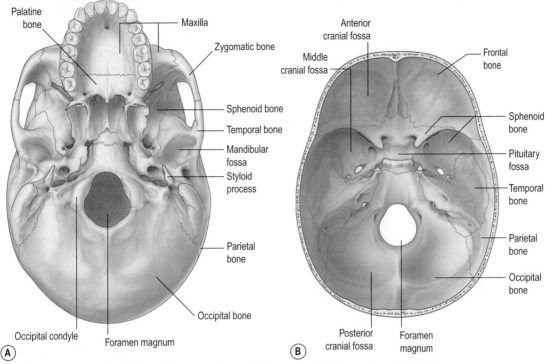

Fig. 4.9 External (A) and internal (B) aspects of the base of an adult skull.

		TABLE 4.2 Structures Passing Through Openings in the Anterior Cranial Fossa	
Opening	Communicates With	Structures Passing Into Anterior Cranial Fossa	Structures Passing Out of Anterior Cranial Fossa
Foramen caecum	Nasal cavity	Emissary vein	
Perforations in cribriform plate	Nasal cavity		Olfactory nerve (I) fibres from the olfactory bulb, which sits on the cribriform plate

Posterior Cranial Fossa

The largest and deepest cranial fossa, with the floor and most of the posterior wall formed by the concave surface of the occipital bone; a small part of the posterior wall is formed by the parietal bone. The anterolateral wall is formed by the posterior surface of the petrous part of the temporal bone, with the body of the sphenoid and basilar part of the occipital bone forming the anterior wall (Fig. 4.9B). It houses the cerebellum (page 252).

Grooves housing parts of the dural venous sinus system are also present along the superior border of the petrous part of the temporal bone, horizontally around the lateral and posterior walls, and descending towards the jugular foramen; details of the dural venous sinuses can be found on page 270.

The structures passing through each of the named openings in the posterior cranial fossa are shown in Table 4.4, together with the region each opening communicates with.

BRAIN

The brain, together with the spinal cord, comprises the central nervous system (CNS); it is formed by aggregations of bundles of axons and clusters of nerve cell bodies supported by glial cells, which constitute almost half the total volume. The brain is housed within the cranial cavity and protected by the skull vault. Details of the organisation of the spinal cord can be found on page 210.

TABLE 4.3   Structures Passing Through Openings in the Middle Cranial Fossa

Opening	Communicates With	Structures Passing Into Middle Cranial Fossa	Structures Passing Out of Middle Cranial Fossa
Superior orbital fissure	Orbit	Superior and inferior ophthalmic veins	From lateral to medial: lacrimal,[a] frontal,[a] trochlear (IV), superior and inferior divisions of the oculomotor (III), nasociliary[a] and abducens (VI) nerves
Optic canal	Orbit		Optic nerve (II) and ophthalmic artery
Foramen lacerum	Infratemporal fossa	Internal carotid artery and surrounding sympathetic plexus, meningeal branch of ascending pharyngeal artery, emissary vein	
Foramen rotundum	Pterygopalatine fossa		Maxillary nerve (V₂)[b]
Foramen ovale	Infratemporal fossa	Accessory meningeal artery, emissary vein	Mandibular nerve (V₃),[b] middle meningeal vein, lesser petrosal nerve
Foramen spinosum	Infratemporal fossa	Middle meningeal artery, nervus spinosus	

[a]Branches of the ophthalmic nerve (V₁).
[b]Division of the trigeminal nerve (V).

TABLE 4.4   Structures Passing Through Openings in the Posterior Cranial Fossa

Opening	Communicates With	Structures Passing Into Posterior Cranial Fossa	Structures Passing Out of Posterior Cranial Fossa
Internal acoustic meatus	Internal ear		Facial (VII) and vestibulocochlear (VIII) nerves, labyrinthine vessels
Carotid canal	Infratemporal fossa	Internal carotid artery and surrounding sympathetic plexus	
Jugular foramen	Infratemporal fossa	Meningeal branches of the occipital and ascending pharyngeal arteries	Sigmoid and inferior petrosal sinuses becoming the internal jugular vein, glossopharyngeal (IX), vagus (X) and accessory (XI) nerves
Hypoglossal (anterior condylar) canal	Neck		Hypoglossal (XII) nerve
Posterior condylar canal (when present)	Neck	Emissary vein	
Foramen magnum	Vertebral canal	Vertebral arteries and veins, spinal part of the accessory (XI) nerve	Medulla oblongata, anterior and posterior spinal arteries, internal vertebral venous plexus

The outer part of the brain is formed by nerve fibres and cell bodies and appears grey in transverse sections; the inner part mainly consists of myelinated axons and appears white in transverse sections (Fig. 4.10). Areas of the CNS formed mainly of axons are referred to as white matter, while areas formed by cell bodies are referred to as grey matter.

A collection of cell bodies forming a prominent (usually rounded) swelling is a ganglion, while clusters of axons forming a recognised bundle within the CNS is a fasciculus (Fig. 4.11); bundles of axons forming a raised bump or convex contour, typically in the spinal cord, are referred to as a funiculus. These terms refer to the topographic appearance of collections of cell bodies and axons without regard to their function; a cluster of axons with a similar function is a tract, while a collection of cell bodies with a similar function is a nucleus or ganglion (Fig. 4.11).

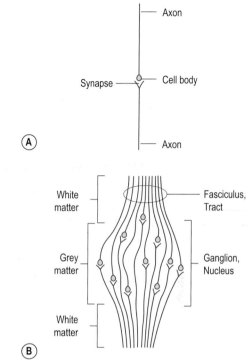

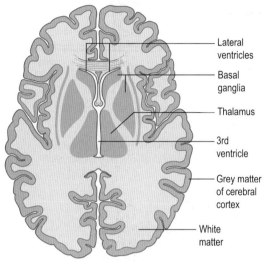

Fig. 4.10 Transverse section of the brain showing the arrangement of white and grey matter.

Fig. 4.11 (A) In the central nervous system, neurons are connected in series with the axon of one neuron synapsing with the cell body of the next neuron. (B) Formation of a nucleus/ganglion in the grey matter.

DEVELOPMENT: The CNS develops from a single tubular structure (neural tube) which forms along the dorsal surface of the embryo from the site of the future head to the tail. It has head (rostral, cephalic) and tail (caudal) ends, and ventral (facing the belly of the embryo) and dorsal (facing the back of the embryo) surfaces; these descriptions apply to the adult CNS (Fig. 4.12). Along its length the neural tube maintains a narrow cavity; however, the thickness of its walls increases as the cells multiply and grow in some regions. Most of the caudal part simply grows in length and diameter, its walls getting thicker but the cavity remaining narrow: this becomes the spinal cord. The rostral end undergoes several changes, including dilations (Fig. 4.12), with the walls of these regions becoming thicker due to cell proliferation. The most rostral end of the neural tube is the prosencephalon, which divides into the telencephalon (containing the lateral ventricle) and diencephalon (surrounding the 3rd ventricle), the mesencephalon (surrounding the cerebral aqueduct) more caudally and then the rhombencephalon, which divides into the metencephalon (surrounding the 4th ventricle) and myelencephalon; the prosencephalon is the forebrain, the mesencephalon the midbrain and the rhombencephalon the hindbrain. The telencephalon enlarges and grows rostrally, but mainly laterally and caudally covering and burying the diencephalon (Fig. 4.13); the telencephalon becomes the cerebrum and the diencephalon the thalamus. The dorsal part of the metencephalon becomes the cerebellum and the ventral part the pons: the myelencephalon (medulla oblongata) remains relatively undifferentiated connecting the pons to the spinal cord (medulla). Collectively the midbrain, pons and medulla oblongata form a single structural unit (brainstem) connecting the spinal cord to the diencephalon, with the cerebellum attached dorsally.

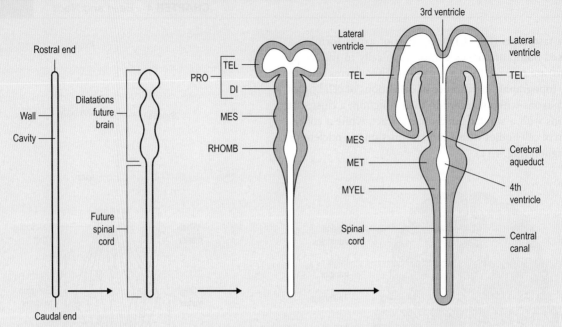

Fig. 4.12 Coronal sections (viewed dorsally) showing stages of development of the central nervous system. *DI,* Diencephalon; *MES,* mesencephalon; *MET,* metencephalon; *MYEL,* myelencephalon; *PRO,* prosencephalon; *RHOMB,* rhombencephalon; *TEL,* telencephalon.

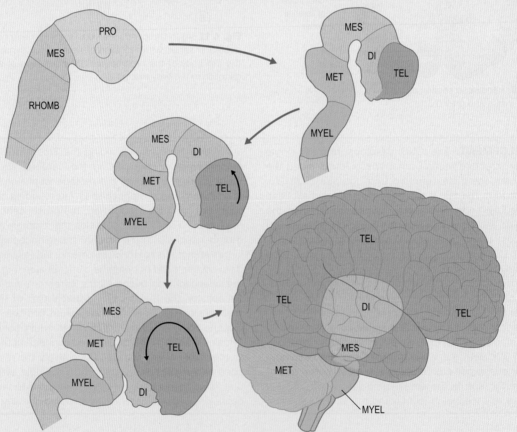

Fig. 4.13 Right lateral aspect of the developing brain. *DI,* Diencephalon; *MES,* mesencephalon; *MET,* metencephalon; *MYEL,* myelencephalon; *PRO,* prosencephalon; *RHOMB,* rhombencephalon; *TEL,* telencephalon.

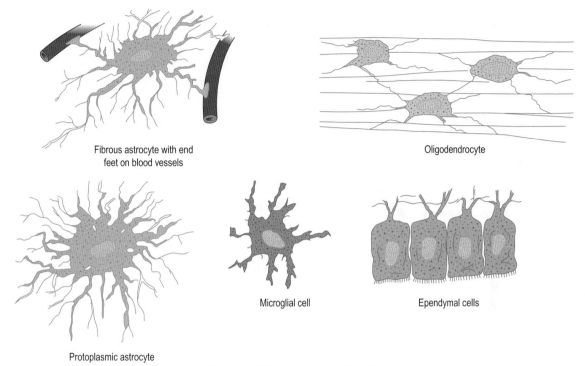

Fibrous astrocyte with end
feet on blood vessels

Oligodendrocyte

Protoplasmic astrocyte

Microglial cell

Ependymal cells

Fig. 4.14 Different types of glial cells.

Glial Cells

There are four types of glial cells in the CNS: oligodendrocytes, microglia, ependymal cells and astrocytes (protoplasmic, fibrous) (Fig. 4.14). Oligodendrocytes are responsible for myelination, as well as holding axons together as they myelinate several parallel axons. Microglia are the macrophages of the CNS, responsible for removing foreign matter and cellular debris. Ependymal cells are exclusively found lining the internal surface of the ventricles of the brain; they are epithelial cells arranged side-by-side forming a barrier between the nervous system and fluid in the ventricles. Protoplasmic astrocytes have thick processes that branch repeatedly and weave between cell bodies holding them together, some processes also attach to small blood vessels: they occur mainly in grey matter. Fibrous astrocytes have fewer but longer processes; they are mainly found in the white matter. The principal role of astrocytes is to provide a framework for the CNS by holding the cell bodies and axons in place relative to one another; they also have an important role in the nutrition and metabolic activities of neurons by regulating the exchange of chemicals between them and blood vessels.

Adult Morphology

The cerebellum fills the posterior cranial fossa with the brainstem lying on the clivus; the cerebrum occupies the anterior and middle cranial fossae (Fig. 4.15), with the thalamus lying deep within the cerebrum in the middle cranial fossa.

Brainstem

The brainstem comprises the medulla oblongata, pons and midbrain (Fig. 4.16); it is continuous inferiorly with the spinal cord and superiorly with the diencephalon. On the ventral surface of the brainstem is a thick bundle of transversely running nerve fibres (pons), rostral to which is the midbrain and caudal the medulla oblongata.

Medulla oblongata. The lower part of the brainstem is continuous inferiorly with the spinal cord and superiorly with the pons; the lower part contains a central canal (closed medulla), while the upper part is related to the 4th ventricle (open medulla).

The ventral surface has three elevations on each side of the anterior median sulcus, which is continuous inferiorly with the anterior median sulcus of the spinal cord; medially, the pyramid formed by fibres of the corticospinal

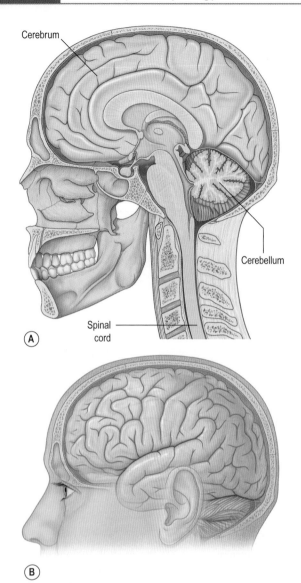

(B)

Fig. 4.15 (A) Sagittal section of the head showing the brain within the skull. (B) Left lateral aspect of the brain with the skull removed.

cerebello-olivary, spino-olivary and strio-olivary afferent fibres and sends efferent olivocerebellar (to the inferior cerebellar peduncle) and olivospinal fibres.

Laterally, the inferior cerebellar peduncle is a compact mass of white matter connecting the medulla oblongata and cerebellum (Fig. 4.16A). It receives afferent dorsal spinocerebellar, olivocerebellar, vestibulocerebellar, and dorsal and ventral external arcuate fibres and sends efferent cerebello-olivary, cerebellovestibular and cerebelloreticular fibres.

The glossopharyngeal (IX), vagus (X), accessory (XI) and hypoglossal (XII) cranial nerves emerge from the ventral surface of the medulla oblongata; XII in the anterolateral sulcus between the pyramid and olive, XI, X and IX (from below upwards) in the posterolateral sulcus between the olive and inferior cerebellar peduncle (Fig. 4.17).

On the dorsal surface of the closed medulla, the gracile tract and tubercle lie adjacent to the posterior median sulcus; the tract terminates superiorly in the gracile nucleus, which produces the tubercle (Fig. 4.16C). Lateral and parallel to the gracile tract are the cuneate tract and tubercle; the tract terminates in the cuneate nucleus which produces the tubercle (Fig. 4.16C). The gracile and cuneate nuclei are responsible for processing sensory information concerning pressure, touch and position senses that pass from the spinal cord to the brainstem and thalamus; see also page 254. The dorsal surface of the open medulla forms the lower part of the floor of the 4th ventricle, separated from the upper pontine part by the medullary stria; these comprise fibres passing to the cerebellum.

CLINICAL ANATOMY: Injury to the respiratory and vasomotor centres, which lie in the lower part of the floor of the 4th ventricle, leads to death. Lesion of the *pyramidal tract* leads to crossed hemiplegia (upper motor neuron lesion in the opposite side of the body); *spinothalamic tract* leads to loss of exteroceptive sensations (pain, temperature) on the opposite side of the body; *medial lemniscus* leads to loss of proprioception on the opposite side of the body; *inferior cerebellar peduncle* and *spinocerebellar tract* leads to incoordination of the same side arm and leg; *descending connection between the hypothalamus* and *cervical sympathetic fibres* (formed in the reticular formation) leads to Horrner's syndrome (ptosis, myosis, anhidrosis, enophthalmos) on the same side of the body; *hypoglossal nerve nucleus* with paralysis of the muscles of the tongue of the same side; and *glossopharyngeal, vagus* and *accessory nerve nuclei* leads to paralysis of the muscles supplied by these nerves, as seen in difficulty in swallowing.

(pyramidal) tract. The pyramidal decussation lies near the lower end of the medulla oblongata, being the site of crossing of the corticospinal fibres. Dorsal to the pyramid the medial lemniscus, formed by fibres from the gracile and cuneate tracts after their decussation, carries proprioceptive fibres and tactile impulses to the posterolateral ventral nucleus of the thalamus.

The olive lies lateral to the pyramid and marks the position of the inferior olivary nucleus, which has four parts (inferior, medial and lateral in the medulla oblongata, superior in the pons); their axons cross the midline to form the olivocerebellar tract. The nucleus receives

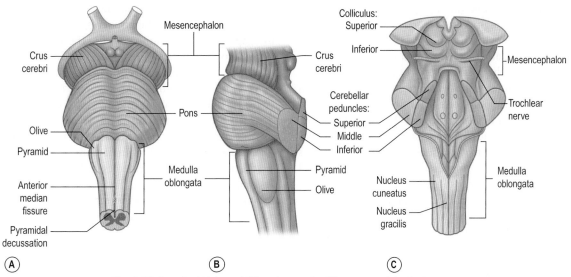

Fig. 4.16 Anterior (A); lateral (B) and posterior (C) aspects of the brainstem.

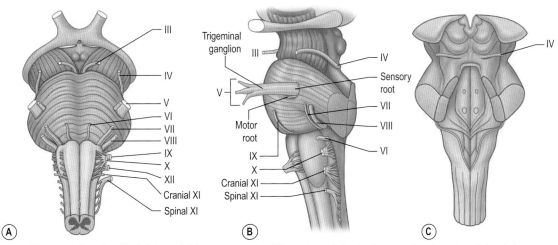

Fig. 4.17 Anterior (A); left lateral (B) and posterior (C) aspects of the brainstem showing the origin of the cranial nerves.

Pons. The pons lies anterior to the cerebellum bulging anteriorly more than the medulla oblongata and midbrain; in the midline anteriorly is a wide groove (basilar groove) for the basilar artery. On the ventral surface are transverse streaks formed by transverse pontocerebellar fibres. The middle cerebellar peduncle, containing pontocerebellar fibres, extends laterally connecting the pons with the cerebellum. From the lateral surface of the middle peduncle, the sensory and motor roots of the trigeminal nerve emerge, between the lower border of the pons and upper border of the pyramid the abducens nerve emerges, and between the lower border of the pons and inferior cerebellar peduncle (cerebellopontine angle), the facial (medial) and vestibulocochlear (lateral) nerves emerge (Fig. 4.17). The dorsal surface of the pons forms the upper part of the floor of the 4th ventricle.

The pons is divided into a large ventral (basilar) and smaller dorsal (tegmentum) part. The ventral part is composed of longitudinal nerve bundles, the corticospinal (pyramidal) tracts separated by transverse pontine fibres, which pass inferiorly to form the pyramid, and corticopontine fibres which terminate in the nuclei pontis; transverse pontocerebellar fibres, most of which cross the midline to join uncrossed fibres of the opposite side to form the middle cerebellar peduncle; and irregular masses of grey matter (nuclei pontis) whose axons form the transverse pontocerebellar fibres, and the 2nd neuron of the corticopontocerebellar pathway connecting the cerebral cortex and cerebellum.

The dorsal part is composed of cranial nerve nuclei (trigeminal, abducens, facial, vestibulocochlear); ascending lemnisci (medial, trigeminal, spinal, lateral); descending tracts (pyramidal, extrapyramidal); decussations of the trapezoid body; and the medial longitudinal bundle.

CLINICAL ANATOMY: Lesions of the: *medial segment of the lower pons* leads to spastic hemiplegia of the opposite side of the body, loss of deep sensations, and lower motor neuron lesions of the abducens and facial nerves of the same side; the *lateral segment of the lower pons* leads to loss of exteroceptive sensations, hearing, and Horner's syndrome; *middle pons* leads to loss of all sensations of the same side of the face and paralysis of the motor part of the trigeminal nerve; *lateral segment of the upper pons* leads to loss of all sensations of the opposite half of the body and face, and Horner's syndrome; the *medial segment of the upper pons* leads to hemiplegia of the opposite side of the body, and upper motor neuron lesion of the facial nerve with paralysis of the face below the eye on the opposite side.

CLINICAL ANATOMY: The most common lesions of the pons are Millard-Gubler syndrome (Gubler hemiplegia/paralysis, Millard-Grubler paralysis), a unilateral lesion involving the abducens and facial nerves and fibres of the corticospinal tract causing paralysis of the face of the same side (accompanied by paralysis of lateral movement of the eye) and paralysis of the limbs of the opposite side (crossed hemiplegia); and pontine haemorrhage, which is invariably fatal, being manifest by contralateral hemiplegia, deep coma, hyperpyrexia and pinpoint pupil.

Midbrain. The midbrain connects the pons and diencephalon and cerebral hemispheres; it passes through the gap in the tentorium cerebelli. The ventral surface shows two thick pillars (cerebral peduncles, crus cerebri) extending anterolaterally from the upper border of the pons (Fig. 4.16A and B); they contain the large ascending (sensory) and descending (motor) nerve tracts that run between the cerebrum and pons. The interpeduncular fossa lies between the peduncles, anterior to which are the mammillary bodies and infundibulum of the hypophysis; the oculomotor nerve emerges in the interpeduncular fossa medial to the peduncle (Fig. 4.17A and B).

Within the midbrain is a narrow canal (cerebral aqueduct (of Sylvius)) connecting the 3rd and 4th ventricles; an imaginary line across the aqueduct divides the midbrain into ventral and dorsal parts. The ventral part comprises the cerebral peduncle, substantia nigra and tegmentum, and the dorsal part, the tectum, comprising the superior and inferior colliculi.

The anterior part of the cerebral peduncle consists of bundles of fibres descending from the internal capsule: medial and lateral corticobulbar fibres to cranial nerve nuclei; frontopontine fibres from the frontal cortex to the nuclei pontis; corticospinal fibres; corticobulbar fibres; temporopontine fibres from the temporal cortex to the nuclei pontis, which are accompanied by a few fibres from the parietal and occipital cortex.

The substantia nigra is a thin layer of pigmented grey matter situated between the peduncle and tegmentum. It consists of afferent and efferent connections with the corpus striatum and forms part of the extrapyramidal system.

The tegmentum is continuous inferiorly with the tegmentum of the pons; it is the posterior part of the peduncle. It contains the ventral and dorsal tegmental decussations, the decussation of the superior cerebellar peduncle, lemnisci (medial, lateral, spinal, trigeminal), fibres/tracts (tectospinal, rubrospinal), red nucleus, cranial nerve III and IV nuclei and the medial longitudinal bundle.

The ventral tegmental decussation is in the superior part of the midbrain level with the superior colliculi; it consists of rubrospinal fibres. The dorsal tegmental decussation is also at the level of the superior colliculi, but posterior to the ventral decussation; it consists of tectospinal fibres. The superior cerebellar peduncles (dentatorubral fibres) decussate in the lower part of the midbrain at the level of the inferior colliculi; they continue superiorly to terminate in the thalamus via dentatothalamic fibres.

The red nucleus is a relay station and extrapyramidal centre in the medial part of the tegmentum at the level of the superior colliculus. It receives afferent fibres from the dentate nucleus of the cerebellum by dentatorubral fibres; frontal cortex by frontorubral fibres; corpus striatum (globus pallidus) by striorubral fibres; subthalamic nucleus; hypothalamus and tectum. It sends efferent fibres to the anterior grey column of the spinal cord, after decussating in the ventral tegmental decussation, by rubrospinal fibres; reticular formation of the brainstem to the anterior horn of the spinal cord by rubroreticular fibres; cranial nerve III, IV and VI nuclei by rubrobulbar fibres; lateral nucleus of the thalamus; and substantia nigra, which mediates impulses from the cerebellum to higher centres in the brain and lower centres in the spinal cord and as such influences motor functions of the medulla oblongata and spinal cord.

The cranial nerve nuclei include that for the: oculomotor (III) nerve, which lies close to the median plane at the level of the superior colliculus where it divides into several parts, being connected to the red nucleus, pyramidal tract and medial longitudinal bundle; and trochlear (IV) nerve, which lies close to the median plane at the level of the inferior colliculus, the trochlear nerves decussate in the tectum and emerges from the dorsal surface below the inferior colliculus: it is connected to the pyramidal tract and medial longitudinal bundle. The general visceral efferent (GVE) Edinger-Westphal nucleus is a group of cells immediately dorsal to the upper end of the motor part of the oculomotor nucleus; fibres from the nucleus run in the oculomotor nerve and synapse in the ciliary ganglion, with the parasympathetic postganglionic fibres passing to the ciliary muscles and constrictor pupillae; and trigeminal (V) nerve, which is known as the mesencephalic nucleus. It is situated along the anterolateral aspect of the periaqueductal grey matter and lies ventral to the inferior colliculi; it extends to the pons in the midbrain and receives fibres carrying proprioceptive information from the face.

The dorsal surface of the midbrain (tectum) is marked by four rounded projections (colliculi) arranged in pairs (superior and inferior) on each side (Fig. 4.16C). The superior colliculus is formed of alternating layers of grey and white matter; it is the reflex centre for vision, being involved in turning the head and eyes in response to visual stimuli. It receives afferent fibres from the spinal cord by the spinotectal tract, the retina and visual area of the cortex by the superior brachium quadrigeminum, the contralateral superior and ipsilateral inferior colliculi, and sends efferent fibres to the spinal cord by the tectospinal tract, the brainstem by the tectobulbar tract, the medial longitudinal bundle, the contralateral superior and ipsilateral inferior colliculi. The superior brachium quadrigeminum connects the superior colliculus to the lateral geniculate body and comprises fibres from the optic tract and occipital cortex passing to the superior colliculus. Deep to the upper lateral part of the superior colliculus is the pretectal nucleus, which receives afferent fibres via the superior brachium quadrigeminum from the optic tract (subserving the pupillary light reflex, page 273) and occipital cortex, and sends efferent fibres to the Edinger-Westphal nuclei of both sides.

The inferior colliculus is the reflex centre for hearing; it comprises the nucleus of the inferior colliculus, which is encapsulated by fibres of the lateral lemniscus. It receives afferent fibres from the lateral lemniscus, the auditory area of the temporal cortex by the inferior brachium quadrigeminum, the ipsilateral superior colliculus and contralateral inferior colliculus, and sends efferent fibres to the spinal cord by the tectospinal tract, the brainstem by the tectobulbar tract, the contralateral inferior and ipsilateral superior colliculi, and both medial geniculate bodies. The inferior brachium quadrigeminum connects the inferior colliculus to the medial geniculate body and comprises fibres from the lateral lemniscus and temporal cortex passing to the inferior colliculus.

CLINICAL ANATOMY: Lesion of the crus cerebri of the ventral part of the midbrain leads to Weber's syndrome (Weber's paralysis), which manifests as paralysis of the ipsilateral extraocular muscles producing ptosis, strabismus together with loss of the light and accommodation reflexes (page 273), accompanied by contralateral spastic hemiplegia with increased reflexes and loss of superficial reflexes: there is no sensory loss.

CLINICAL ANATOMY: Lesion of the dorsal part of the midbrain (tectum) leads to tegmental syndrome (Benedikt syndrome), which manifests as ipsilateral oculomotor paralysis and ataxia, accompanied by contralateral hyperkinesia, tremor and paresis; there is a loss of all general sensations contralaterally.

Medial longitudinal bundle. A band of fibres extending the whole length of the brainstem lying close to the median plane and the nuclei of the oculomotor, trochlear, abducens and hypoglossal nerves. Its short ascending and descending afferent fibres are from the vestibular nuclei (equilibrium), lateral lemniscus (hearing) and superior colliculus (vision), as well as from the interstitial nucleus of Cajal and commissural nucleus (extrapyramidal nucleus). It sends efferent fibres to the oculomotor, trochlear, abducens, spinal accessory and hypoglossal nuclei, and anterior horn cells of the spinal cord.

The fibres of the medial longitudinal bundle connect the oculomotor, trochlear and abducens nuclei with each other and with the motor nuclei of the facial, glossopharyngeal and hypoglossal nerves, ensuring coordinated action of the lips and tongue in speech. The bundle acts as an association tract for the coordination of eye and neck movements in relation to vestibular, auditory and visual stimuli.

Cerebellum

The cerebellum (Fig. 4.15A) is the largest component of the hindbrain located on the dorsal aspect of the brainstem overlying the 4th ventricle. It comprises two cerebellar hemispheres connected by a median vermis; it has a posterior notch occupied by the falx cerebelli (fold of dura mater) and an anterior notch lodging the brainstem. Two transverse fissures divide the cerebellum into three lobes; the primary fissure on the superior surface separates the smaller anterior and larger middle lobes, and the posterolateral fissure on the inferior surface separates the posterior (flocculonodular) lobe anteriorly and middle lobe posteriorly. The anterior lobe forms the anterior part of the superior surface, the middle lobe the posterior part of the superior and greater part of the inferior surfaces and the flocculonodular lobe the remainder of the inferior surface.

The cerebellum has an outer cortex of grey matter and an inner medulla of white matter (Figs 4.15A and 4.19), which extend into the folia forming white cores covered by a uniform layer of grey matter (arbor vitae cerebelli); the white matter contains nuclei (fastigial, globus, emboliform, dentate) of grey matter, which receive afferent fibres from outside the cerebellum (inferior olivary, vestibular, reticular and pontine nuclei) and within the cerebellum (cerebellar cortex).

Each cerebellar hemisphere controls the same side of the body and is entirely motor; its principal function is the control of posture, repetitive movements and geometrical accuracy of voluntary movements, as well as the coordination of muscle activity during movement. The archicerebellum (flocculonodular lobe and fastigial nucleus) is involved in the maintenance of equilibrium, the control of the axial musculature, bilateral movements and locomotion. The paleocerebellum (vermis, anterior lobe, globus and emboliform nuclei) controls muscle tone, posture and crude movements of the limbs. The neocerebellum (middle lobe and dentate nucleus) regulates fine movements of the body.

Inferior, middle and superior peduncles connect the cerebellum to the brainstem (Fig. 4.16B and C). Between the two superior cerebellar peduncles is the superior velum, which has a median ridge (frenulum veli) at its upper part; the trochlear nerve pierces the velum lateral to the frenulum veli. An inferior velum stretches between the inferior cerebellar peduncles: it is deficient inferiorly due to the presence of the median aperture of the 4th ventricle (foramen of Magendie).

The inferior cerebellar peduncles pass caudally into the dorsolateral aspect of the medulla oblongata and connect the cerebellum to the medulla oblongata and spinal cord. It receives afferent fibres from the posterior spinocerebellar tract, an uncrossed tract that conveys proprioceptive impulses from the ipsilateral limbs; olivocerebellar tract which crosses to the opposite side to reach the contralateral cerebellar hemisphere; vestibulocerebellar tract conveying vestibular stimuli, either directly from the vestibular nerve or indirectly via vestibular nuclei, to the ipsilateral cerebellar hemisphere; dorsal external arcuate fibres conveying proprioceptive impulses from the ipsilateral accessory cuneate nucleus; ventral external arcuate fibres conveying proprioceptive impulses from both sides; and reticulocerebellar fibres from reticular nuclei in the medulla oblongata to the ipsilateral cerebellar hemisphere. It sends efferent fibres to the flocculonodular lobe and fastigial nucleus to vestibular nuclei by cerebellovestibular fibres; the dentate nucleus to the contralateral inferior olivary nucleus by cerebello-olivary fibres; and the fastigial nucleus to the reticular formation in the pons and medulla oblongata by cerebelloreticular fibres.

The middle cerebellar peduncle passes around the lateral aspect of the brainstem and is directly continuous with the pons; it contains mainly afferent fibres which form part of the corticopontocerebellar pathways. It receives afferent fibres from pontine nuclei which cross the midline to terminate in the contralateral cerebellar hemisphere; it is by these pontocerebellar fibres that the cerebellum has a functional relationship with the cerebellum of the opposite side.

The superior cerebellar peduncle passes rostrally into the dorsal aspect of the midbrain and connects the cerebellum to the rostral portion of the brainstem and thalamus; it contains mainly efferent fibres with some afferent fibres. It receives afferent fibres from the: nucleus dorsalis to the cortex of the vermis of the anterior lobe by the anterior spinocerebellar tract; and tectum of the midbrain by the tectocerebellar tract. It sends efferent fibres to the: dentate nucleus which cross the midline to reach and relay in the red nucleus of the midbrain, after decussating the impulses are relayed inferiorly to the opposite side of the spinal cord either directly by the rubrospinal tract or indirectly by the reticulospinal tract (decussation brings each cerebellar hemisphere into a functional relationship with the same side of the body); and dentate nucleus, either directly or indirectly after relaying in the red nucleus, to the lateral nucleus of the thalamus by the dentatothalamic tract, from where the impulses are relayed to the motor and premotor cortex of the cerebrum constituting a pathway through which the cerebellum coordinates its activities with that of the cerebral cortex.

> **CLINICAL ANATOMY:** A midline (archicerebellum) lesion leads to the loss of postural control. A unilateral cerebellar hemisphere (neocerebellum) lesion results in an unsteady gait and ipsilateral incoordination of the arm (intention tremor) and leg. Bilateral dysfunction of the cerebellum leads to slowness and slurring speech (dysarthria), incoordination of both arms and a staggering wide-base unsteady gait; it is caused by hypothyroidism, inherited cerebellar degeneration (ataxia), as well as alcoholic intoxication.

Diencephalon

Thalamus. The largest part of the diencephalon consisting of a collection of nuclei, which also includes the metathalamus, epithalamus, hypothalamus and subthalamus; each thalamus lies within the middle of the cerebrum and is continuous caudally with the midbrain and separated from the opposite thalamus by the 3rd ventricle (Fig. 4.18). An oval mass of grey matter, covered by white matter, the external medullary lamina laterally and internal medullary lamina partly divide the grey matter into several nuclei (anterior, medial, lateral, posterior).

Anterior nuclei receive afferent fibres from the mammillothalamic tract and send efferent fibres to the gyrus cingula; they form part of the limbic system (page 263) and have an important role in autonomic visceral activities.

Medial nuclei, of which there are several, with the most important being the nucleus medialis dorsalis and centromedian nucleus; the nucleus medialis dorsalis has connections with the hypothalamus and frontal lobe cortex, and centromedian nucleus with other thalamic nuclei, the putamen and caudate nucleus.

Lateral nuclei are divided into ventral (anterior ventral, intermediate ventral, posterior ventral) and dorsal (dorsolateral, dorsomedial) nuclei. The *anterior ventral nucleus* receives afferent fibres from the globus pallidus (extrapyramidal), reticular formation and non-specific thalamic nuclei and sends efferent fibres to the premotor area of the cerebral cortex; it also forms connections with the corpus striatum. The *intermediate ventral nucleus* receives afferent fibres from the dentate nucleus of the cerebellum and sends efferent fibres to the motor and premotor areas of the frontal cortex. The *posterior ventral nucleus* is further subdivided into the *posterolateral ventral nucleus* which receives the main sensory pathways (medial, spinal, lateral lemnisci) and sends efferent fibres to the sensory area of the cerebral cortex, and *posteromedial ventral nucleus* which receives the trigeminal lemniscus and taste fibres and sends efferent fibres to the sensory area of the cerebral cortex and *dorsal nuclei,* where they form connections with the cortex of the parietal and temporal lobes.

Posterior nuclei receive afferent fibres from other thalamic nuclei and send efferent fibres to the cortex anterior to the visual area (parastriate cortex), auditory and parietal cortex, and nuclei (centromedian nucleus, reticular nucleus of the thalamus, midline nuclei) associated with the reticular formation: they receive reticulothalamic fibres from the reticular nuclei of the brainstem and send efferent fibres to the cerebral cortex of both sides. They are also connected to thalamic and hypothalamic nuclei and to

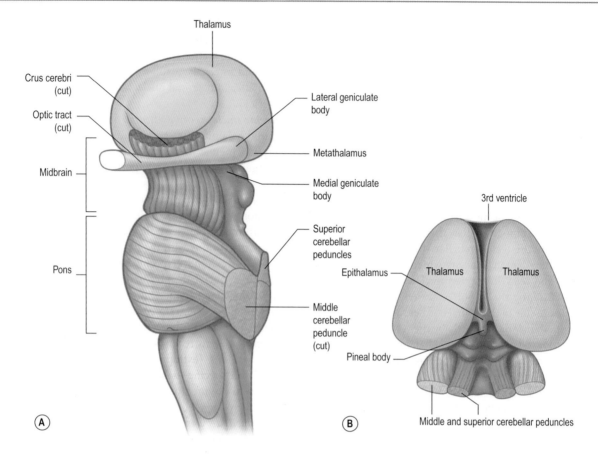

Fig. 4.18 (A) Left lateral aspect of the brainstem and thalamus, with the crus cerebri, optic tract and cerebellar peduncles cut (see also Fig. 4.16). (B) Superior aspect of the thalami on either side of the brainstem.

the corpus striatum and participate in arousal reactions of the brain.

CLINICAL ANATOMY: The blood supply to the thalamus is from branches of the posterior cerebral artery, some of which enter its posterolateral aspect supplying the dorsal part and others entering the base supplying the ventral part; due to its double blood supply, some thalamic lesions can lead to impaired sensation over the trunk and lower limb while the face remains unaffected.

Function: All sensory inputs (except olfaction) relay directly in the thalamus, where they are integrated and sent to cortical centres. It is considered to be a higher centre for pain and extremes of temperature stimuli, and an associative centre with connections between the cerebral cortex, cerebellum, hypothalamus, substantia nigra and basal ganglia. The connections with the frontal cortex are important in mood and emotions.

Metathalamus. Two prominences (medial and lateral geniculate bodies) projecting from the posterior, lateral and inferior surface of each thalamus (Fig. 4.18A). The medial geniculate body is an oval elevation lateral to the superior colliculus and is a centre for auditory sensation; it is connected to the inferior colliculus by the inferior brachium. It receives auditory sensations and fibres from both inferior colliculi via the lateral lemniscus and sends efferent fibres to the auditory area of the cortex in the temporal lobe via the acoustic (auditory) radiation. The lateral geniculate body is a small oval elevation anterolateral to the medial geniculate body inferior to the thalamus and is the centre concerned with visual sensation. It receives afferent fibres concerned with vision via the optic tract

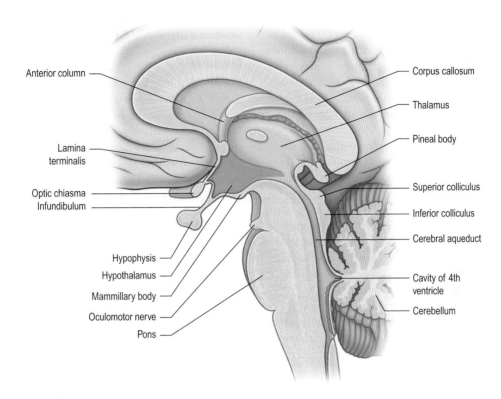

Fig. 4.19 Sagittal section of the brain and brainstem showing the location of the hypothalamus.

and sends efferent fibres to the visual area of the cerebral cortex via the optic radiation.

Epithalamus. A strip of tissue connecting the posterior medial ends of the two thalami (Fig. 4.15B); it forms part of the limbic system (page 263). The pineal body (epiphysis cerebri) projects from its posterior edge between the superior colliculi; it may be calcified in the elderly. It produces hormones that have an important regulatory influence on other endocrine organs (anterior and posterior pituitary gland, thyroid and parathyroid glands, adrenal cortex and medulla, and gonads (ovaries, testes)).

Hypothalamus. A thin layer of tissue hanging from the ventromedial surface of the thalamus (Fig. 4.19); it blends with the opposite hypothalamus in the midline forming a sling of neural tissue across the floor and lateral wall of the 3rd ventricle. It is divided into anterior (optic), tuberal (pars tuberalis), posterior (mammillary) and lateral parts; the optic part includes the preoptic, supraoptic, anterior and paraventricular nuclei; the tuber-

al part the ventromedial, dorsomedial and infundibular nuclei; the mammillary and posterior nuclei; and the lateral part the lateral nucleus, small parts of the supraoptic, lateral tuberal and tuberomammillary nuclei.

It has numerous afferent connections from: the olfactory cortex to the hypothalamic area by the medial forebrain bundle; the hippocampus to the mammillary nuclei by the fornix; the globus pallidus to the ventromedial nucleus by pallidohypothalamic fibres; the brainstem to the lateral mammillary nucleus by the mammillary peduncle; the thalamus by thalamohypothalamic fibres; and the amygdaloid nucleus by the stria terminalis.

Efferent connections are by fibres from the supraoptic nucleus to the neurohypophysis by the supraopticohypophyseal tract; the paraventricular nucleus to the neurohypophysis by the paraventriculohypophyseal tract; the mammillary nuclei to anterior thalamic nuclei by the mammillothalamic tract; and the mammillary nuclei to the tegmentum of the midbrain by the mammillotegmental tract. In addition, the dorsal longitudinal fasciculus carries fibres to the brainstem which terminates on the autonomic nuclei of the cranial nerves and motor cranial nerves, except the ocular motor nuclei.

There are also neural and vascular connections between the hypothalamus and pituitary gland; nerve fibres descend from the hypothalamus to the neurohypophysis (posterior lobe), while portal blood vessels connect the hypothalamus with the adenohypophysis (anterior lobe).

Functions: *Endocrine control*: regulates the secretion of thyrotropin (TSH), corticotropin (ACTH), somatotropin (STH), prolactin, luteinising hormone (LH), follicle-stimulating hormone (FSH) and melanocyte-stimulating hormone via its connection with the pituitary. *Neurosecretion*: oxytocin and vasopressin (antidiuretic hormone (ADH)) are transported to the neurohypophysis. *General autonomic effects*: the anterior hypothalamus mainly mediates parasympathetic activity and the posterior sympathetic activity.

The hypothalamus is also involved in the control of emotion, fear and pleasure, as well as the regulation of temperature, food and water intake, sexual behaviour and reproduction, and the biological clocks governing sleep and wakefulness.

Further details of the endocrine function of the pituitary gland can be found on page 335.

CLINICAL ANATOMY: Sham rage reaction is a severe rage reaction in response to minor stimuli; it can be produced by (i) lesion in the ventromedial thalamic nucleus, and (ii) stimulation of the amygdaloid nucleus. The reaction has sympathetic (tachycardia, a rise in blood pressure, piloerection, pupillary dilation) and somatic (biting, clawing, hissing, spitting, growling) effects.

Subthalamus. Lying between the midbrain and thalamus medial to the internal capsule and globus pallidus, the subthalamus consists of grey and white matter. The grey matter comprises the cranial ends of the red nucleus and substantia nigra, and the white matter the cranial ends of the lemnisci, superior cerebellar peduncle (dentatothalamic tract) together with rubrothalamic fibres, ansa lenticularis with fibres from the globus pallidus entering its anterior surface, and the fasciculus lenticularis dorsally with fibres from the globus pallidus also entering anteriorly. The subthalamic nucleus is considered an extrapyramidal centre being connected by efferent and afferent fibres to the globus pallidus, red nucleus and substantia nigra.

Cerebrum

It is divided into left and right halves (cerebral hemispheres) by the longitudinal fissure (Fig. 4.20); deep within the fissure the hemispheres are connected by a large body of transversely running fibres (corpus callosum). Separating the hemispheres their medial surfaces can be seen, as well as the cut surface of the corpus callosum (Fig. 4.20B). Each cerebral hemisphere is divided into four lobes (frontal, parietal, occipital, temporal) according to the bones of the skull to which each is most closely related (Fig. 4.20C). The anterior and posterior ends of each hemisphere are the frontal pole and occipital pole: the anterior end of the temporal lobe is the temporal pole.

The surface (cortex) of each hemisphere is a thin layer (2–5 mm) of grey matter containing the cell bodies of neurons responsible for various cerebral functions. Deep to the cortex is a large mass of white matter consisting of the axons of the neurons in the cortex, as well as those that enter the cerebrum from the brainstem and diencephalon. The surface is thrown into a series of ridges (gyri: singular gyrus) separated by depressions (sulci: singular sulcus); some gyri and sulci are important because they divide the cerebral hemispheres into topographical and functional regions.

The lateral sulcus separates the temporal lobe from the frontal and parietal lobes, while the central sulcus separates the frontal and parietal lobes (Fig. 4.20C). The parieto-occipital sulcus separates the parietal and occipital lobes; on the medial aspect of the hemisphere, the lower end of the parieto-occipital sulcus merges with the calcarine sulcus, either side of which the occipital lobe is responsible for vision. The parietal lobe is separated from the temporal lobe by the posterior end of the lateral sulcus; no feature delineates the junction between the temporal, parietal and occipital lobes.

The sulcus anterior to the central sulcus is the precentral sulcus, anterior to which is the precentral gyrus, which when stimulated elicits contraction of voluntary muscles. This is the motor cortex which contains a detailed topographically organised map (motor homunculus) of the opposite side of the body, with the head represented most laterally and the leg and foot most medially (Fig. 4.21A); the disproportionate representation of body

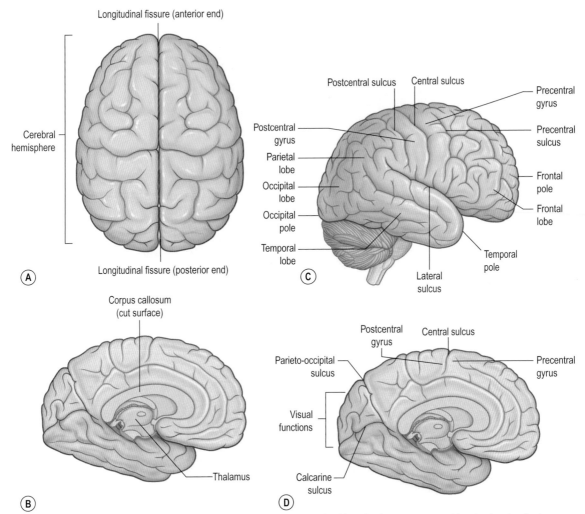

Fig. 4.20 (A) Superior aspect of the brain showing the cerebral hemispheres separated by the longitudinal fissure. (B) Medial aspect of the left cerebral hemisphere showing the sectioned surface of the corpus callosum. (C) Lateral aspect of the right cerebral hemisphere showing its subdivision into lobes and principal sulci. (D) Medial aspect of the left hemisphere showing the principal sulci and gyri.

parts (muscles of the face and hand) in relation to their physical size indicates areas capable of finely controlled movements. Posterior to the central sulcus is the postcentral sulcus, behind which is the postcentral gyrus, which receives sensory information from the brainstem and thalamus. This is the primary somatosensory cortex which contains within it a topographical map of the opposite side of the body; the face, tongue and lips are represented inferiorly, the trunk and upper limb on the superolateral aspect and the lower limb on the medial side of the hemisphere (Fig. 4.21B).

While the occipital lobe is associated with vision, the parietal lobe is, in general, associated with sensory functions (touch, pressure, position sense), as well as more sophisticated functions (three-dimensional perception, visual image analysis, language, geometry, calculations). The frontal lobe is associated with motor functions, as well as the expression of intellect and personality. The upper part of the temporal lobe opposite the postcentral gyrus is associated with the perception of sound, while the remainder is concerned with memory and emotion (Fig. 4.22).

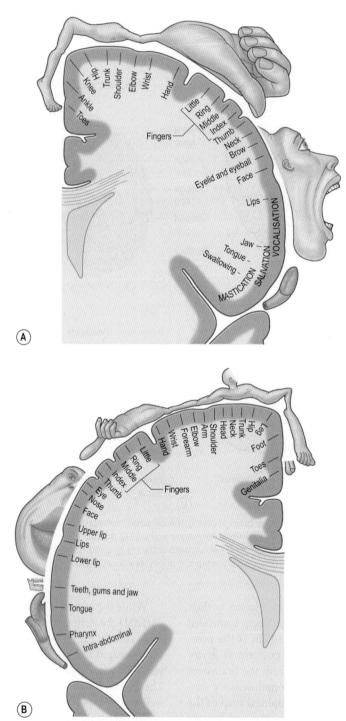

Fig. 4.21 (A) The motor homunculus showing the proportional somatotopical representation in the main motor area. (B) The sensory homunculus showing somatotopical representation in the somaesthetic cortex.

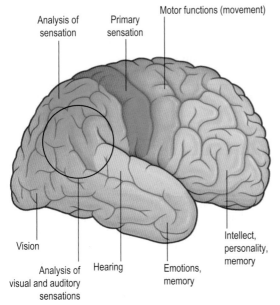

Fig. 4.22 Lateral aspect of the right hemisphere showing the principal functions of different regions of the cerebrum.

Cerebral medulla. Each hemisphere consists of an outer layer (cortex) of grey matter surrounding a mass of white matter (medulla), basal ganglia, and a lateral ventricle.

The white matter comprises association, commissural and projection fibres. **Short association fibres** connect close areas of grey matter within the hemisphere, while **long association fibres** are bands of white matter connecting distant areas of grey matter within a hemisphere. The *superior longitudinal bundle* passes from the frontal lobe to the occipital and temporal lobes; the *inferior longitudinal bundle* passes between the occipital and temporal poles; the *fasciculus uncinatus* connects the frontal and temporal lobes; and the *cingulum* passes from the frontal lobe to the uncus of the temporal lobe.

The **commissural fibres** connect corresponding areas of the two hemispheres via the corpus callosum: the anterior commissure connects the olfactory bulbs, piriform area and anterior part of the temporal lobes; the posterior commissure connects the superior colliculi,

CLINICAL ANATOMY: An injury to the head caused by a fall, blunt force trauma, sports injury or associated with a car/motorcycle accident can give rise to a non-penetrating traumatic brain injury, referred to as coup, contrecoup and coup-contrecoup injuries (Fig. 4.23); coup and contrecoup injuries are related to concussion injuries. Coup injuries present directly below the site of impact and can be mild to severe including bruising, brain swelling and haemorrhage; contrecoup injuries occur on the opposite side of the brain from the impact site and can be overlooked, long-term risks may result if not identified; coup-contrecoup injuries occur at the site of impact as well as on the opposite side where the brain comes into contact with the skull, the risk of permanent brain damage is high if both sites are not identified. The most common sites of contrecoup injury is to the lower part of the frontal lobes and front of the temporal lobes: coup-contrecoup injuries can tear or twist axon bundles and rupture blood vessels. Injury involving the *frontal lobe* can result in: impulsiveness; poor judgement; memory loss; problems with concentration; language difficulties (aphasia); behavioural and personality changes; and difficulties with problem solving and decision making. Injury involving the *parietal lobe* include numbness; poor hand-eye coordination; difficulty differentiating right from left with loss of direction; abnormal perception of pain; and difficulty with reading and writing. Injury involving the *occipital lobe* include partial and/or temporary loss of vison with decreased peripheral vision and visual hallucinations; word blindness; and poor visual recognition and attention. Injury involving the *temporal lobe* include hearing and memory loss; difficulty recognising faces and objects; difficulty in understanding spoken language and finding the correct words to say; and changes in emotional behaviour. Additional signs and symptoms include intense headache; dizziness; seizures; loss of consciousness; sensitivity to light and loud noises; nausea; slurred speech; muscle weakness; and difficulty with swallowing. In severe injuries, fragments of bone can penetrate brain tissue and increase intracranial pressure.

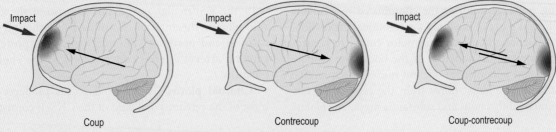

Fig. 4.23 Coup, contrecoup and coup-contrecoup injuries to the brain following a blow to the head: *arrows* represent the point of impact and *red* regions the area of injury.

transmitting corticotectal fibres and fibres from the pretectal nucleus to the Edinger-Westphal nucleus of the opposite side; the hippocampal commissure (commissure of the fornix) connects the crura of the fornix and hippocampal formations; the habenular commissure connects the habenular nuclei; and the hypothalamic commissures, which include the anterior hypothalamic commissure (of Ganser), the ventral supraoptic commissure (of Gudden) and the dorsal supraoptic commissure (of Meynert).

The **corpus callosum** (callosal commissure) is a wide thick nerve tract spanning the longitudinal fissure connecting the right and left cerebral hemispheres. It consists of a number of separate nerve tracts (subregions of the corpus callosum) which connect different parts of the hemispheres: the main ones being known as the genu, rostrum, trunk (body) and splenium. Each hemisphere controls movement and sensation in the opposite side of the body, as well as processing information, including language. Physical coordination and assessing complex information require both sides of the brain to work together; the corpus callosum acts as the connector.

The **projection fibres** connect the cerebral cortex to other parts of the CNS (brainstem, spinal cord) and comprise ascending afferent fibres (thalamic, optic and auditory radiations) and descending efferent fibres (pyramidal (corticospinal, corticobulbar)), corticopontine, corticothalamic, corticorubral tracts.

The **basal ganglia** are intracerebral masses of grey matter which form part of the extrapyramidal system; they include the corpus striatum, which is divided into the caudate and lentiform nuclei, with the lentiform nucleus further divided into a larger, darker lateral part (putamen) and smaller, lighter medial part (globus pallidus); the amygdaloid body, which is part of the limbic system; and claustrum, a thin plate of grey matter between the lentiform nucleus and insula.

The *corpus striatum* regulates muscle tone, controls automatic associative movements (swinging of the arms during walking), controls the coordinated movements of different parts of the body for emotional expression, and influences the precentral motor cortex to control the extrapyramidal activities of the body. The caudate nucleus and putamen are afferent nuclei which receive most of their afferent fibres from the cerebral cortex, thalamus, subthalamus and substantia nigra. The globus

pallidus is an efferent nucleus sending fibres to the thalamus, subthalamus, hypothalamus, substantia nigra and red nucleus; it gives rise to most of the efferent fibres of the corpus striatum.

CLINICAL ANATOMY: Lesion of the corpus striatum leads to hypertonicity, loss of automatic associative movements and facial expression, and involuntary movements such as tremors.

Ventricular system. The spaces (ventricles) within the brain are continuous with the central canal of the spinal cord: it comprises the lateral, 3rd and 4th ventricles and their connections. Each lateral ventricle is the space within each cerebral hemisphere; it is located mainly in the parietal lobe and has an anterior horn extending into the frontal lobe, a posterior horn extending into the occipital lobe, and an inferior horn extending into the temporal lobe. The lateral ventricles are continuous across the midline deep to the corpus callosum; each lateral ventricle communicates with the 3rd ventricle by the interventricular foramen (of Munro). The 3rd ventricle communicates with the 4th ventricle by the cerebral aqueduct and with the medulla by the central canal. The 3rd ventricle is the cavity within the diencephalon and the 4th the cavity within the hindbrain (medulla oblongata, pons and cerebellum) (Fig. 4.24).

The tela choroidea is a double-layered fold of pia mater found within each ventricle. That in the 3rd ventricle, together with the ventricular ependyma, forms the roof of the 3rd ventricle: it sends a lateral extension through the choroid fissure into the lateral ventricle. The tela choroidea in the 4th ventricle lies between the cerebellum and the lower part of the roof. In the lateral ventricle vascular folds invaginate the ventricular ependyma to form the choroid plexus; in the 3rd ventricle two vascular fringes from the lower fold invaginate the roof to form the choroid plexus; and in the 4th ventricle the anterior layer of the fold, together with the ventricular ependyma, constitute the choroid plexus. The anterior choroidal (from the internal carotid) and posterior choroidal (from the posterior cerebral artery) arteries convey blood to the choroid plexuses.

Choroid plexus. The choroid plexus produces the most of the cerebrospinal fluid of the CNS: it consists of

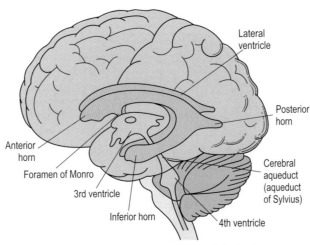

Fig. 4.24 The ventricular system of the brain.

modified ependymal cells surrounded by a core of capillaries and loose connective tissue, with the epithelium of the choroid plexus being continuous with the ependymal cell (ventricular) layer lining the ventricles. The choroid plexus epithelial layer has tight junctions (page 22) between the cells facing the ventricle, preventing the majority of substances from crossing the cell layer to the cerebrospinal fluid; the choroid plexus acts as a blood-cerebrospinal fluid barrier. Cerebrospinal fluid is formed as plasma is filtered from blood through the epithelial cells; choroid epithelial cells also actively transport sodium ions into the ventricles, with water following the resultant osmotic gradient.

> **CLINICAL ANATOMY:** Variations in the structure or function of the choroid plexus may be associated with cysts and other congenital malformations. Excess production of cerebrospinal fluid, or a reduction/blockage of its drainage into the venous system, leads to an increase in the size of the ventricles (especially the lateral) and enlargement of the cerebral hemispheres, pushing them against the bones of the skull vault and the development of hydrocephalus.

Cerebrospinal fluid. A modified tissue fluid, cerebrospinal fluid circulates within the ventricular system of the brain and subarachnoid space surrounding the brain and spinal cord. The majority is produced by the choroid plexuses of the lateral ventricles with smaller amounts being produced by the choroid plexuses of the 3rd and 4th ventricles; some may be produced by capillaries on the surface of the brain and spinal cord.

Cerebrospinal fluid is produced by the ependyma covering the choroid plexuses at the rate of 20 mL/h (4800 mL/day). From the lateral ventricles cerebrospinal fluid passes through the interventricular foramen to the 3rd ventricle, then to the 4th ventricle by the cerebral aqueduct. A small amount passes into the central canal of the spinal cord, with the majority passing into the subarachnoid space by a median (foramen of Magendie) and lateral (foramen of Luschka) apertures; the cerebellomedullary cistern. Most cerebrospinal fluid entering the subarachnoid space ascends slowly on the surface of the cerebellum and cerebral hemispheres via the tentorial notch, with only a small amount surrounding the spinal cord. From the subarachnoid space cerebrospinal fluid returns to the venous system by way of arachnoid granulations and villi (extensions of arachnoid mater), which pierce the inner layer of the dura mater (Fig. 4.26) to drain into the superior sagittal sinus (page 265).

Cerebrospinal fluid functions to regulate intracranial pressure and provides a fluid cushion protecting the CNS from shocks and trauma; it is the equivalent of lymph within the CNS. It can undergo rapid adjustments to accommodate an increased blood flow into the cranial cavity by increasing the flow of cerebrospinal fluid into the venous system.

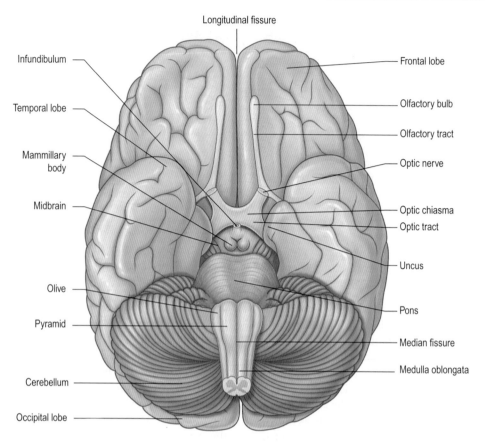

Longitudinal fissure

Infundibulum

Temporal lobe

Mammillary body

Midbrain

Olive

Pyramid

Cerebellum

Occipital lobe

Frontal lobe

Olfactory bulb

Olfactory tract

Optic nerve

Optic chiasma

Optic tract

Uncus

Pons

Median fissure

Medulla oblongata

Fig. 4.25 Base of the brain.

The production and composition of cerebrospinal fluid are regulated by the choroid plexus. It helps nourish the CNS and removes waste products, as well as regulating the composition of electrolytes and immune cells. The blood-cerebrospinal fluid barrier (created by the choroid plexus and meninges) helps protect the brain from infectious organisms, as well as controlling the flow of substances into and out of the brain; its permeability determines the ability of medications and drugs to enter the brain.

CLINICAL ANATOMY: Biochemical analysis of cerebrospinal fluid can be used as a diagnostic tool in many diseases. Cerebrospinal fluid can be obtained by lumbar, cisternal or ventricular puncture, with lumbar puncture being the easiest and most common; it is achieved by passing a needle into the subarachnoid space through the L3/L4 interspace with the vertebral column flexed.

Base of the Brain

Formed largely by the ventral surfaces of the frontal, temporal and occipital lobes (Fig. 4.25); the medial edge of the temporal lobe is the uncus, which is associated with the perception of smell.

Anteriorly, the hemispheres are separated by the longitudinal fissure, caudal to which is the floor of the 3rd ventricle. Most posteriorly, the brainstem projects caudally from the inferior surface of the diencephalon lying deep to the cerebral hemispheres. Projecting in the midline from the floor of the 3rd ventricle is the infundibulum connecting the hypothalamus to the pituitary gland; the infundibulum consists of axons from cells in the hypothalamus which regulate oxytocin and ADH secretion by the pituitary. Caudal to the infundibulum are two small prominences (mammillary bodies): their function is not fully understood.

The x-shaped structure with rostral and caudal limbs on the ventral surface of the diencephalon is the optic chiasma, the region where the medial fibres from each optic nerve cross the midline. The rostral limbs are the terminal ends of the optic nerves transmitting visual information from the retina of the eye (page 299); the caudal limbs are the optic tracts conveying visual information from one half of the visual field to the ipsilateral lateral geniculate body (Fig. 4.18).

Motor System

The motor system is a combination of central and peripheral structures that support and produce movement; central structures include the cerebral cortex, brainstem, spinal cord and pyramidal system (upper and lower motor neurons, extrapyramidal system, cerebellum) and peripheral structures include skeletal muscles and their neural connections.

The pyramidal system (pyramidal/corticospinal tract) starts in the precentral gyrus of the cerebral cortex, with the impulses originating in the giant pyramidal cells (of Betz); these are the upper motor neurons. Their axons pass to the corona radiata and internal capsule to descend through the midbrain and medulla oblongata. In the lower part of the medulla oblongata, the majority (90%–95%) of axons decussate and descend in the white matter of the lateral funiculus of the spinal cord on the opposite side, with the remainder passing to the same side; all fibres destined for the limbs pass to the opposite side. Fibres in the corticospinal tract terminate at different levels in the anterior (ventral) horn of the grey matter of the spinal cord, synapsing on lower motor neurons. Peripheral nerves then carry the motor impulses to the skeletal (voluntary) muscles.

The extrapyramidal system is involved in the modulation and regulation of lower motor neurons without directly innervating them. Extrapyramidal tracts (rubrospinal, reticulospinal, lateral vestibulospinal, tectospinal, olivospinal) are mainly found in the reticular formation of the pons and medulla and target lower motor neurons involved in reflexes, locomotion, complex movements and postural control; these tracts are modulated by the CNS, including the nigrostriatal pathway, basal ganglia, cerebellum, vestibular nuclei and different sensory areas of the cerebral cortex.

Sensory System

The different sensory systems are best covered with the organs mediating the sensation.

Limbic System

The limbic system comprises a set of cortical structures located at the boundary between the cerebral hemispheres and brainstem on either side of the thalamus, immediately beneath the medial part of the temporal lobe; it supports a variety of functions that regulate visceral autonomic processes, including the emotional processing of sensory inputs, behaviour, long-term memory and olfaction. It includes cortical areas (limbic lobe; orbitofrontal cortex involved in decision making; piriform cortex, part of the olfactory system; entorhinal cortex, related to memory and associative components; hippocampus and associated areas, which play a central role in the consolidation of memories; fornix, connecting the hippocampus to the mammillary bodies and septal nuclei), subcortical areas (septal nuclei, considered to be the 'pleasure zone'; amygdala, which is associated with a number of emotional processes; nucleus accumbens, involved in reward, pleasure and addiction) and structures within the diencephalon (hypothalamus, which is connected to the frontal lobes) septal nuclei and brainstem reticular formation via the medial forebrain bundle and to the thalamus by the mammillothalamic fasciculus, which is considered a limbic centre regulating many autonomic processes; mammillary bodies (part of the hypothalamus) receiving afferent fibres from the hippocampus via the fornix and projecting them to the anterior nuclei of the thalamus, where they are involved in the processing of memories.

The limbic system can be considered as the interface between subcortical structures and the cerebral cortex, operating by influencing the endocrine and autonomic nervous systems: as such it is involved in motivation, emotion, learning and memory. It is connected with the nucleus accumbens, which plays a role in sexual arousal, as well as the 'high' associated with recreational drugs; these responses are modulated by dopaminergic projections from the limbic system. The limbic system also interacts with the basal ganglia, which receives afferent fibres from the cerebral cortex and sends efferent fibres to the brainstem; the striatum of the basal ganglia control posture and movement.

> **CLINICAL ANATOMY:** An inadequate supply of dopamine in the striatum can lead to the symptoms of Parkinson's disease.

Meninges

Although glial cells hold the CNS neurons together and provide protection against metabolic insults, the brain is nevertheless a soft cellular mass vulnerable to external mechanical insults, which could arise if it were freely mobile within the skull (or vertebral canal in the case of the spinal cord). To help protect against such insults, the CNS is surrounded by three membranes (Fig. 4.26), the dura, arachnoid and pia mater (the meninges) and bathed in cerebrospinal fluid (page 261), which acts as a fluid cushion: details of the meninges associated with the spinal cord are given on page 206.

The **dura mater** is a thick membrane protecting the brain; it consists of two layers, which for the most parts are connected to each other, but in places are separate enclosing the intracranial venous sinuses (page 270). The outer (endosteal, cranial) layer lines the cranial cavity forming the endosteum of its inner surface; it is firmly adherent to the skull base and sutures and loosely attached to the vault. At the foramen magnum, it is continuous with the endosteum lining the vertebral canal, while at all other foramina, it is continuous with the periosteum on the outer surface of the skull; except in cases of trauma, there is no extradural space.

The inner (meningeal, cerebral) layer of the dura is duplicated in places forming reflections (falx cerebri, falx cerebelli, tentorium cerebelli, diaphragma sellae) projecting into the cranial cavity dividing it into compartments (see Fig. 4.30); it also has sleeve-like extensions around the cranial nerves as they leave the skull.

The *falx cerebri* projects from the roof of the skull vault, from the crista galli anteriorly to the internal occipital protuberance posteriorly, in the median plane into the longitudinal fissure; it is sickle-shaped in profile.

The *falx cerebelli*, also in the median plane, projects forwards between the cerebellar hemispheres.

The *tentorium cerebelli* projects from the anterior, lateral and posterior walls of the posterior cranial fossa in a transverse plane, forming a partial roof (see Fig. 4.30); the central notch transmits the midbrain from the posterior cranial fossa to the diencephalon. It separates the occipital and temporal lobes from the cerebellum. Posteriorly in the midline, the posterior end of the falx cerebri fuses with the upper surface of the tentorium cerebelli.

The *diaphragma sellae* is a fold of dura overlying the pituitary fossa; it has a central opening through which the infundibulum (pituitary stalk) passes from the neurohypophysis (posterior lobe of the pituitary gland) to the hypothalamus.

The dura lining the anterior cranial fossa and skull vault, the falx cerebri and tentorium cerebelli are all innervated by the ophthalmic division of the trigeminal nerve, that of the middle cranial fossa by the maxillary and mandibular divisions of the trigeminal nerve, and that of the posterior cranial fossa by the glossopharyngeal and vagus nerves.

The **arachnoid mater** is a delicate membrane loosely surrounding the brain lining the dura mater: it is separated from the dura by the subdural space and pia by the subarachnoid space, which contains cerebrospinal fluid. Small finger-like projections of arachnoid tissue (arachnoid villi) project into the cranial venous sinuses (mainly superior sagittal sinus) enabling cerebrospinal fluid to drain into the venous system (Fig. 4.26B); with increasing age, the villi form pedunculated tufts (arachnoid granulations), which can produce depressions in the skull vault adjacent to the sagittal suture.

APPLIED ANATOMY: A potential (subdural) space exists between the dura and arachnoid mater containing a small amount of fluid: it continues for a short distance along the cranial nerves. The optic nerve sheath of dura extends along the whole length of the nerve as far as the back of the eyeball.

The **pia mater** is a thin vascular membrane closely investing the brain following every convolution of its surface giving it a smooth appearance. It is more prominent around the brainstem, where it provides sheaths for the cranial nerves, merging with the epineurium surrounding them. The sheaths also provide perivascular sheaths for the minute vessels entering and leaving the brain substance; some folds enclose the choroid plexus arising from the tela choroidea.

Arterial Supply

The arterial supply to the brain is from the paired internal carotid and vertebral arteries (Fig. 4.27).

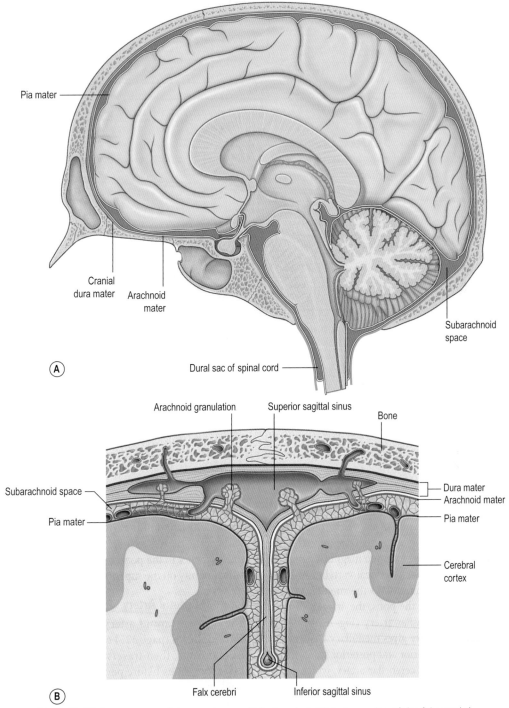

Pia mater

Cranial
dura mater

Arachnoid
mater

Subarachnoid
space

Dural sac of spinal cord

(A)

Arachnoid granulation Superior sagittal sinus Bone

Subarachnoid space

Pia mater

Dura mater
Arachnoid mater

Pia mater

Cerebral
cortex

(B) Falx cerebri Inferior sagittal sinus

Fig. 4.26 (A) Arrangement of the meninges within the skull. (B) In the region of the falx cerebri.

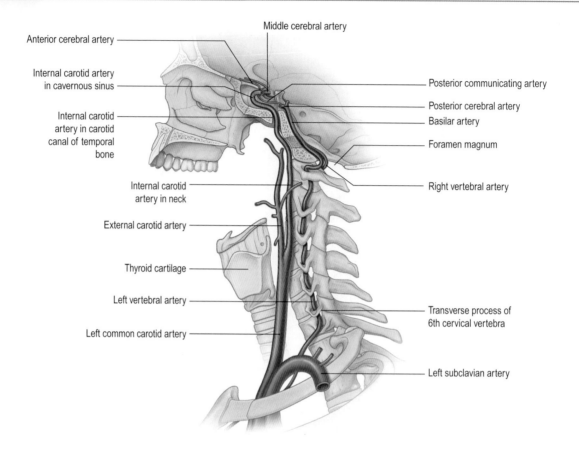

Fig. 4.27 The left internal carotid and vertebral arteries entering the skull to supply the brain.

Vertebral Artery

The vertebral artery (branch of the 1st part of the subclavian artery (page 319)) ascends in the neck through the foramina transversaria of the upper six cervical vertebrae. It enters the skull through the foramen magnum penetrating the dura just above the 1st cervical vertebra to enter the subarachnoid space. Anterior to the medulla oblongata at the lower border of the pons, the arteries of both sides unite, forming the basilar artery (Fig. 4.28). Before uniting, each vertebral artery gives medullary branches to the medulla oblongata; anterior and posterior spinal arteries; and a posterior inferior cerebellar artery, which ramifies over the posteroinferior surface of the cerebellum.

Basilar Artery

The basilar artery ascends in the basilar groove of the pons, terminating at its superior border by dividing into posterior cerebral arteries (Fig. 4.28), which supply the occipital lobe. Before dividing, it gives anterior inferior cerebellar arteries, which ramify on the anteroinferior surface of the cerebellum; labyrinthine arteries, which pass into the internal acoustic meatus to supply the vestibular labyrinth; pontine branches to the pons; and superior cerebellar arteries, which ramify on the superior surface of the cerebellum.

Internal Carotid Artery

The internal carotid artery ascends in the neck in the carotid sheath (page 325) entering the skull through the carotid canal, then traverses the foramen lacerum and cavernous sinus before penetrating the dura and arachnoid mater medial to the anterior clinoid process, to enter the subarachnoid space: it terminates by dividing into anterior and middle cerebral arteries lateral to the optic chiasma (Fig. 4.28). Before dividing, it gives the: ophthalmic artery supplying the orbit; posterior communicating artery, which joins the posterior cerebral

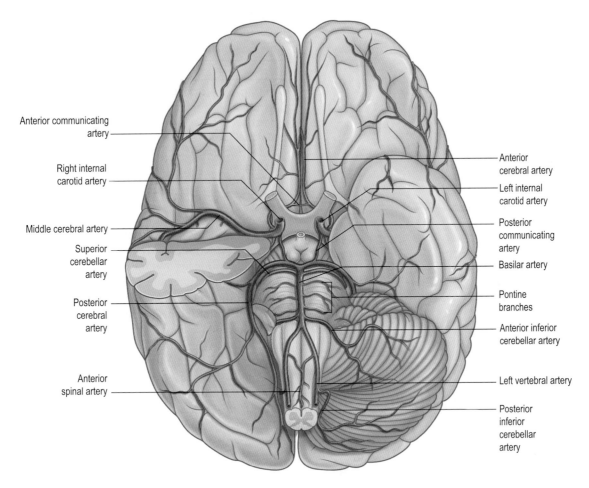

Fig. 4.28 Inferior aspect of the brain and brainstem showing the position of the vertebral and internal carotid arteries.

artery; and anterior choroidal artery, which passes to the choroid plexus of the lateral ventricle.

> **CLINICAL ANATOMY:** An arterial anastomosis (circle of Willis) between branches from the vertebral and the terminal branches of the internal carotid arteries exists around the hypothalamic region of the base of the brain. It acts to equalise pressure in the contributing vessels, as well as providing an alternative route of blood supply should a vessel become occluded; blood can flow in either direction depending on local pressures. The vessels involved in the anastomosis, from anterior to posterior, are: anterior communicating artery, which connects the two anterior cerebral arteries; right and left anterior cerebral arteries; right and left internal carotid arteries; right and left posterior communicating arteries; and right and left posterior cerebral arteries (Fig. 4.28).

Cerebral Arteries

Each cerebral hemisphere is supplied by anterior, middle and posterior cerebral arteries (Fig. 4.29); the anterior cerebral artery runs superior to the optic nerve into the longitudinal fissure on the medial side of the hemisphere passing above the corpus callosum; the middle cerebral artery passes into the lateral sulcus between the temporal and frontal lobes on the lateral surface of the hemisphere; and the posterior cerebral artery curves around the lateral surface of the midbrain to its dorsal surface to reach the inferior surface of the hemisphere to run in the calcarine sulcus.

Anterior cerebral artery. A terminal branch of the internal carotid artery (Fig. 4.29), the anterior cerebral artery runs anteromedially above the optic chiasm towards the longitudinal fissure, then curves anteriorly, where it is joined to the opposite anterior cerebral artery by the anterior communicating artery (Fig. 4.28). It then ascends in

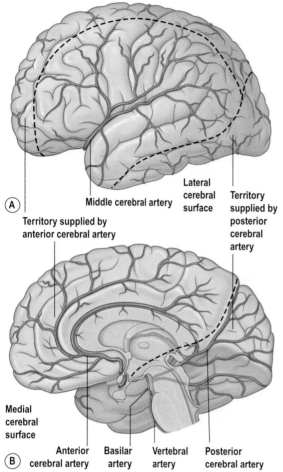

(A) Middle cerebral artery — Lateral cerebral surface — Territory supplied by posterior cerebral artery

Territory supplied by anterior cerebral artery

Medial cerebral surface

(B) Anterior cerebral artery   Basilar artery   Vertebral artery   Posterior cerebral artery

Fig. 4.29 Distribution of the anterior, middle and posterior cerebral arteries. (A) lateral aspect of the left cerbral hemisphere; (B) medial aspect of the right cerebral hemisphere.

> **APPLIED ANATOMY:** The anterior cerebral artery supplies the motor and sensory areas of the lower limb in the paracentral lobule.

> **CLINICAL ANATOMY:** Obliteration of the blood supply to the corpus callosum leads to the inability to perform purposeful movements in spite of an intact musculature (apraxia). Loss of the blood supply to the septal region of the septum lucidum may lead to prolonged unconsciousness.

Middle cerebral artery. A terminal branch of the internal carotid artery (Fig. 4.29), the middle cerebral artery passes laterally in the stem of the lateral sulcus, then turns posterosuperiorly in the posterior ramus of the lateral sulcus crossing over the insula, where it terminates by dividing into numerous branches. During its course it gives cortical branches which supply the whole of the lateral surface of the hemisphere, except a narrow strip along the superior border and frontal pole (supplied by the anterior cerebral artery) and the lateral surface of the occipital lobe and a narrow strip on the lateral surface of the temporal lobe close to the inferior border (supplied by the posterior cerebral artery); and central branches, many of which are striate arteries, arising near its origin supply the corpus striatum (lentiform and caudate nuclei) and posterior half of the anterior limb and anterior part of the posterior limb of the internal capsule.

> **APPLIED ANATOMY:** One of the central branches is larger than the others (artery of cerebral haemorrhage, Charcot's artery); it is the most susceptible artery to rupture of all those supplying the brain.

> **APPLIED ANATOMY:** The middle cerebral artery supplies the motor and sensory areas for the whole body, the auditory area in the superior temporal gyrus, and the motor speech area in the inferior frontal gyrus.

> **CLINICAL ANATOMY:** Obstruction of the blood supply to the internal capsule leads to hemiplegia.

the longitudinal fissure to reach the medial surface of the cerebral hemisphere, where it passes above the corpus callosum terminating anterior to the parieto-occipital fissure. During its course it gives cortical branches which supply the medial surface of the hemisphere from the frontal pole to the parieto-occipital sulcus, the superior 2.5 cm of the superolateral surface and superior end of the parieto-occipital sulcus, and medial half of the medial surface of the frontal lobe; central branches which supply the anterior part of the corpus callosum, anterior limb of the internal capsule and septal region of the septum lucidum; and callosal branches which supply all parts of the corpus callosum except the splenium, which is supplied by the posterior cerebral artery.

Posterior cerebral artery. A terminal branch of the basilar artery at the superior border of the pons (Figs. 4.28 and 4.29), the posterior cerebral artery curves posterolaterally around the cerebral peduncle of the midbrain parallel to the superior cerebellar artery. It then passes inferior to the corpus callosum on the medial surface of the hemisphere to enter the anterior part of the calcarine sulcus, where it terminates by dividing into two branches which run in the parieto-occipital and posterior part of the calcarine sulcus. During its course it gives: cortical branches which supply the tentorial surface of the temporal lobe, the medial and lateral surfaces of the occipital lobe and a narrow strip on the lateral surface of the temporal lobe along its inferior border; and central branches, of which the short medial group supply the cerebral peduncles, mammillary bodies, subthalamic region and anterior part of the thalamus, and the long lateral group the geniculate bodies, posterior part of the thalamus and pineal body; and the posterior choroidal artery which supplies the tela choroidea of the lateral and 3rd ventricles.

> **APPLIED ANATOMY:** The posterior cerebral artery supplies the centre for smell in the uncus, as well as the whole of the visual cortex.

Summary of the Arterial Supply to the Brain

Cerebral cortex
Medial surface: anterior cerebral artery from the frontal pole to the parieto-occipital sulcus; posterior cerebral artery from the parieto-occipital sulcus to the occipital pole; middle cerebral artery, the cortex of the temporal pole.

Lateral surface: anterior cerebral artery, an area 2.5 cm wide adjoining the superomedial border extending posteriorly to the parieto-occipital sulcus; posterior cerebral artery, the occipital lobe and a narrow strip adjoining the lower border; middle cerebral artery the remainder.

Inferior surface: anterior cerebral artery, the medial part of the orbital surface; middle cerebral artery, the temporal pole and lateral part of the orbital surface; posterior cerebral artery the remainder.

Cerebral projections
Motor and sensory areas: middle cerebral artery, except the upper superior parts (legs) supplied by the anterior cerebral artery.

Auditory and motor speech areas: middle cerebral artery.
Visual area: posterior cerebral artery.
Internal capsule: central branches from the middle cerebral artery; anterior cerebral artery; anterior communicating artery.
Corpus striatum: mainly by central branches from the middle cerebral artery; anterior cerebral artery; anterior communicating artery.
Thalamus: mainly by central branches from the posterior cerebral artery; posterior communicating artery.

Cerebellum
Superior surface: superior cerebellar branches of the basilar artery.
Anterior part of the inferior surface: anterior inferior cerebellar branches from the basilar artery.
Posterior part of the inferior surface: posterior inferior cerebellar artery (branch of the vertebral artery).

Brainstem
Midbrain: branches from the posterior cerebral arteries.
Pons: pontine branches from the basilar artery.
Medulla oblongata: medullary branches from the vertebral artery; branches of the posterior inferior cerebellar artery.

Choroid plexuses
Lateral and 3rd ventricles: anterior (from the internal carotid artery) and posterior (from the posterior cerebral artery) choroidal arteries.
4th ventricle: a branch of the posterior inferior cerebellar artery.

Venous Drainage
Cerebral Veins
The valveless cerebral veins are devoid of muscular walls; few veins arise from within the brain. External cerebral veins: 6–12 superior cerebral veins drain the superolateral surface of each hemisphere and terminate in the superior sagittal sinus; superficial middle cerebral veins drain the area around the posterior ramus of the lateral sulcus and terminate in the cavernous sinus; deep middle cerebral veins drain the surface of the insula and terminate in the basal vein; inferior cerebral veins, of which the orbital veins terminate in the superior cerebral veins or superior sagittal sinus, and the temporal veins drain into the cavernous (or adjacent venous sinuses).

Terminal veins are the great cerebral vein which drains into the straight sinus: the great cerebral vein has tributaries from the cerebral peduncle, interpeduncular structures, tectum of the midbrain and parahippocampal gyrus, while the straight sinus receives the basal veins, veins from the pineal body, the colliculi, cerebellum and adjoining part of the occipital lobes. The basal vein on each side is formed by the union of the deep middle cerebral, anterior cerebral and striate veins, which join the great cerebral vein.

> **CLINICAL ANATOMY:** A blow to the head may rupture the superior cerebral veins as they pass through the arachnoid and dura mater to enter the superior sagittal sinus, separating the two membranes. The increasing accumulation of blood gradually compresses the underlying brain; this is a subdural haematoma.

Intracranial Venous Sinuses

The intracranial (dural) venous sinuses are vascular channels found at constant sites along the internal surface of the skull; most are contained between the endosteal and meningeal layers of the dura mater, while others (inferior sagittal and straight sinuses) are located entirely within specific folds of dura mater. An intracranial venous sinus lacks the adventitial and muscular layers found in veins, being replaced by dura mater, with venous blood being separated from the surrounding tissues by a layer of endothelial cells.

The major intracranial venous sinuses are the paired cavernous, transverse, sigmoid, superior and inferior petrosal sinuses, and the single straight, occipital, superior and inferior sagittal sinuses (Fig. 4.30).

The superior sagittal sinus runs posteriorly in the attached edge of the falx cerebri (Figs 4.26 and 4.30); it drains blood from the external surfaces of the cerebral hemispheres via the superior cerebral veins and reabsorbs cerebrospinal fluid through the arachnoid granulations. The inferior sagittal sinus is enclosed within the free edge of the falx cerebri.

The straight sinus is located along the line of fusion of the falx cerebri and tentorium cerebelli: it receives the great cerebral vein and inferior sagittal sinus (Fig. 4.30). The superior sagittal, straight and occipital sinuses usually meet at the internal occipital protuberance (confluence of sinuses) where the transverse sinuses begin.

From the internal occipital protuberance each transverse sinus passes around the posterior and lateral walls of the posterior cranial fossa (Fig. 4.30); the right transverse sinus is usually continuous with the superior sagittal sinus, and the left with the straight sinus. The transverse sinuses receive veins from the cerebral and cerebellar surfaces, as well as the superior petrosal sinus (from the cavernous sinus) at their anterior ends. Each transverse sinus is directly continuous with the sigmoid sinus located in a groove on the mastoid part of the temporal bone; as it leaves the skull through the jugular foramen, the sigmoid sinus is joined by the inferior petrosal sinus (from the cavernous sinus) to form the internal jugular vein.

Smaller venous sinuses are located along the edges of bones projecting into the middle and posterior cranial fossae (superior and inferior petrosal sinuses) (Fig. 4.30); the sphenoparietal sinus runs along the lesser wing of the sphenoid and the occipital sinus along the internal occipital crest.

The cavernous sinus is formed by separation of the dura from the lateral side of the body of the sphenoid on either side of the pituitary fossa (Fig. 4.31); each is a narrow space filled with a dense plexus of venous channels. The oculomotor and trochlear nerves, together with the ophthalmic and maxillary divisions of the trigeminal nerve, are associated with the lateral wall between the dura mater and endothelial lining of the sinus, while the abducens nerve and internal carotid artery pass between the endothelium and bony floor of the sinus. The cavernous sinus mainly receives venous blood from the sphenoparietal sinus and superior ophthalmic vein, which drain the orbit, as well as the middle meningeal vein and veins from the cerebral hemisphere.

The majority of blood in the intracranial venous sinuses drains to the internal jugular veins, although some may drain through emissary veins that pass through bones of the skull at specific sites to communicate with veins outside the skull.

> **CLINICAL ANATOMY:** Emissary veins provide a potential route for the spread of infection from outside the skull into the cranial cavity.

CRANIAL NERVES

Certain nerves project from the cranial portion of the CNS within the skull connecting the brainstem and diencephalon with structures and tissues in the head and

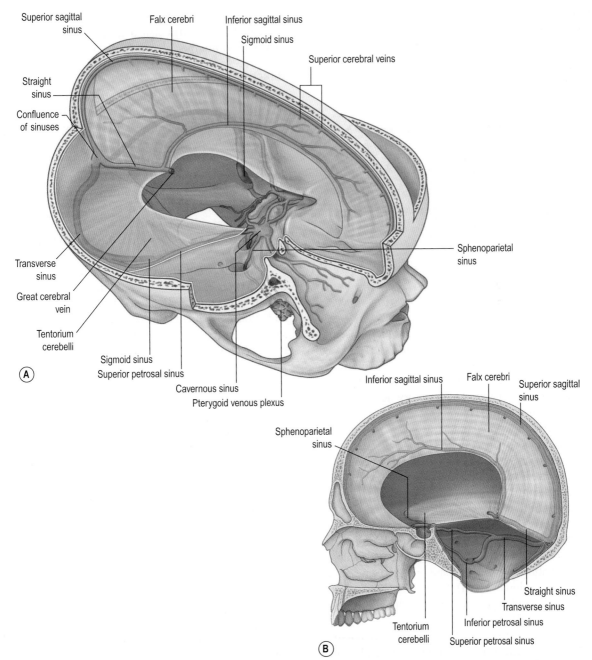

Fig. 4.30 Arrangement of the intracranial venous sinuses within the skull, as well as the dura mater and its reflections. (A) oblique view; (B) seen in sagittal section.

neck, and some thoracic and abdominal viscera: these are the cranial nerves (Figs 4.17 and 4.25). Once the cranial nerves have exited the skull, they become part of the peripheral nervous system. The 12 pairs of cranial nerves are referred to by number or name, with the name reflecting the form, function or distribution of the nerve.

Within the brainstem are seven functional columns of fibres which are associated with cranial nerve nuclei: *General somatic afferent (GSA)* associated with the perception of touch, pain and temperature: trigeminal (V), facial (VII), glossopharyngeal (IX) and vagus (X) nerve nuclei are associated with this column.

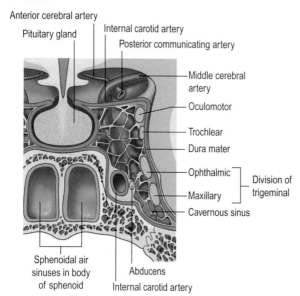

Anterior cerebral artery
Pituitary gland
Internal carotid artery
Posterior communicating artery
Middle cerebral artery
Oculomotor
Trochlear
Dura mater
Ophthalmic ⎤
            ⎬ Division of trigeminal
Maxillary ⎦
Cavernous sinus
Sphenoidal air sinuses in body of sphenoid
Abducens
Internal carotid artery

Fig. 4.31 Coronal section through the cavernous sinus.

General visceral afferent (GVA) associated with sensory input from viscera: glossopharyngeal (IX) and vagus (X) nerve nuclei are associated with this column.

Special visceral afferent (SVA) associated with the perception of smell and taste: olfactory nerve nuclei are associated with this column.

Special somatic afferent (SSA) associated with vision, hearing and balance: optic (II), facial (VII), vestibulocochlear (VIII), glossopharyngeal (IX) and vagus (X) nerve nuclei are associated with this column.

General somatic efferent (GSE) associated with the innervation of skeletal muscle: oculomotor (III), trochlear (IV), abducens (VI) and hypoglossal (XII) nerve nuclei are associated with this column.

General visceral efferent (GVE) associated with the innervation of smooth and cardiac muscle and glands: oculomotor (III), facial (VII), glossopharyngeal (IX) and vagus (X) nerve nuclei are associated with this column.

Special visceral efferent (SVE) associated with the innervation of skeletal muscle derived from pharyngeal (branchial) arches: trigeminal (V), facial (VII), glossopharyngeal (IX), vagus (X) and accessory (XI) nerve nuclei are associated with this column.

Olfactory Nerve (I)

Olfactory nerve fibres mediate the perception of smell; these are short nerves that pass from the olfactory

epithelium in the roof of the nasal cavity projecting through the cribriform plate of the ethmoid to the olfactory bulb within the anterior cranial fossa.

Olfactory Pathway

Each olfactory nerve synapses on cell bodies in the olfactory bulb, with their axons forming the olfactory tract (Fig. 4.25), which also carries commissural fibres connecting the two olfactory bulbs. The olfactory tracts terminate by dividing into medial and lateral olfactory stria; the medial stria passes across the anterior commissure carrying the commissural fibres, while the lateral stria carries fibres to the primary (periamygdaloid and prepiriform areas of the cerebral cortex) and secondary olfactory cortex (uncus), which receives axons from the primary cortex.

As well as being involved in olfaction the periamygdaloid cortex also has a role in olfaction, with recent studies suggesting that it may be involved in opiate addiction, assessment of negative emotions, and depression. Together with the amygdala, the periamygdaloid cortex conducts cognitive evaluation of the olfactory input it receives and projects it back to the olfactory bulbs.

> **APPLIED ANATOMY:** The olfactory pathway is the only sensory pathway reaching the cerebral cortex without passing through the thalamus.

> **CLINICAL ANATOMY:** Anosmia is associated with trauma to the olfactory epithelium or damage to the cribriform plate.

Optic Nerve (II)

The optic nerve transmits visual information from the retina to the optic chiasma (Fig. 4.25): it passes from the orbit through the optic canal to the middle cranial fossa.

Visual Pathway

This includes the structures concerned with the reception, transmission and perception of visual impulses: the impulses start in the receptors (rods and cones) in the retina, then pass in the optic nerve (axons of ganglion cells of the retina), optic chiasm, optic tract and optic radiation to the visual cortex. At the optic chiasma temporal (lateral) fibres in each optic nerve pass uncrossed to the ipsilateral optic tract and nasal (medial) fibres decussate and pass in the contralateral optic tract: macular fibres partially decussate and run in both tracts. Each optic tract consists of temporal fibres of the same side and nasal fibres of the opposite side, together with macular fibres of both sides. The tracts terminate by dividing into a smaller medial root comprising commissural fibres between the right and left medial geniculate bodies which terminate in the medial geniculate body, and a lateral root carrying the visual sensory fibres, which terminate in the lateral geniculate body, and visual reflex fibres, which pass to the superior branchial quadrigemina to terminate in the superior colliculus and pretectal nucleus of both sides. Axons of cells in the lateral geniculate body form the optic radiation, which passes anterolaterally in the internal capsule above the inferior horn of the lateral ventricle, and then on the lateral side of the posterior horn of the lateral ventricle to reach the visual cortex. The visual cortex lies inferior to the calcarine sulcus and around the postcalcarine sulcus where it extends posteriorly to the occipital pole (Figs 4.20D and 4.22).

CLINICAL ANATOMY: Lesions of the visual pathway and their effect on the visual field are shown in Fig. 4.32.

Light reflex pathway. Afferent light impulses are mediated through the retina to the optic nerve, optic chiasma and optic tract. The impulses leave the optic tract terminating in the superior colliculus and pretectal nucleus in the midbrain, where their axons convey the impulses to the Edinger-Westphal nucleus of the oculomotor nerve, then to the oculomotor nerve, ciliary ganglion, short ciliary nerves and sphincter pupillae producing constriction of the pupil. Focussing a light on one eye causes constriction of both pupils (consensual reflex) due to the bilateral connection of the pretectal nucleus with the Edinger-Westphal nucleus.

Accommodation reflex pathway. Constriction of the pupil occurs when focussing on near objects; this is mediated through the retina, optic nerve, optic chiasma, optic tract, lateral geniculate body, optic radiation, the visual area of the cortex, superior longitudinal association tract, frontal eye field, oculomotor nucleus, oculomotor nerve, ciliary ganglion, ciliary muscles and sphincter pupillae.

CLINICAL ANATOMY: Lesion involving the pretectal nucleus leads to loss of the light reflex, but with pupil constriction remaining intact (Argyll-Robertson pupil).

Oculomotor Nerve (III)

The oculomotor nerve contains general somatic and GVE fibres. The general somatic fibres originating in the oculomotor nucleus innervate levator palpebrae superioris, superior, medial and inferior rectus and inferior oblique, which are all involved in moving the eyeball; the general visceral fibres have their origin in the Edinger-Westphal nucleus and innervate the sphincter pupillae (pupillary constriction) and ciliary muscles (accommodation of the lens for near vision). The oculomotor nerve emerges from the ventral aspect of the midbrain at the level of the superior colliculus immediately medial to the crus cerebri on each side (Figs 4.20 and 4.17A, B). It reaches the orbit by passing through the lateral wall of the cavernous sinus (Fig. 4.31), where it divides into superior and inferior divisions, and the superior orbital fissure (Fig. 4.33) within the tendinous ring.

CLINICAL ANATOMY: Lesion of the oculomotor nerve leads to inferior and lateral movement of the eye, a dilated pupil, ptosis and loss of a normal pupillary reflex; it can occur as a result of pressure from an aneurysm of the posterior communicating, posterior cerebral or superior cerebellar artery, pressure from a herniating cerebral uncus, or a cavernous sinus mass or thrombosis.

Trochlear Nerve (IV)

The trochlear nerve contains GSE fibres which innervate superior oblique: the fibres originate in the trochlear nucleus. It emerges from the dorsal aspect of the midbrain immediately below the inferior colliculus (Figs 4.20 and 4.17A, C), then winds around the crus cerebri to appear on the ventral aspect of the brainstem. It reaches the orbit by passing under the free edge of the tentorium cerebelli and then through the lateral wall of the cavernous sinus (Fig. 4.31) and superior orbital fissure (Fig. 4.33) outside the tendinous ring.

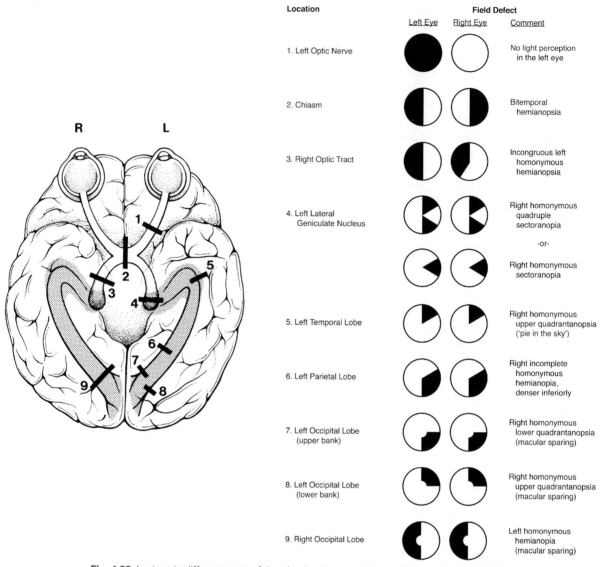

R   L

Location	Field Defect		
	Left Eye	Right Eye	Comment
1. Left Optic Nerve			No light perception in the left eye
2. Chiasm			Bitemporal hemianopsia
3. Right Optic Tract			Incongruous left homonymous hemianopsia
4. Left Lateral Geniculate Nucleus			Right homonymous quadruple sectoranopia -or- Right homonymous sectoranopia
5. Left Temporal Lobe			Right homonymous upper quadrantanopsia ('pie in the sky')
6. Left Parietal Lobe			Right incomplete homonymous hemianopia, denser inferiorly
7. Left Occipital Lobe (upper bank)			Right homonymous lower quadrantanopsia (macular sparing)
8. Left Occipital Lobe (lower bank)			Right homonymous upper quadrantanopsia (macular sparing)
9. Right Occipital Lobe			Left homonymous hemianopia (macular sparing)

Fig. 4.32 Lesions in different parts of the visual pathway and their effect on the visual field.

CLINICAL ANATOMY: Lesion of the trochlear nerve leads to an inability to look inferiorly when the eye is adducted; it can occur as a result of trauma to the nerve along its course around the brainstem or fracture of the orbit.

Trigeminal Nerve (V)

The trigeminal nerve arises from one motor and three sensory nuclei: the *motor nucleus* gives SVE fibres which innervate muscles derived from the 1st pharyngeal (branchial) arch; the *main sensory nucleus* receives GSA fibres conveying tactile impulses from the face and head, and sends efferent fibres, which cross the midline, to join the trigeminal lemniscus which ascends to the thalamus; the *spinal nucleus* receives GSA fibres conveying pain and temperature sensations from the face and head and sends efferent fibres, which cross the midline, to join the trigeminal lemniscus which ascends to the thalamus (the superior part of the spinal nucleus receives fibres from the mandibular division, the middle part from the maxillary division and inferior part from the

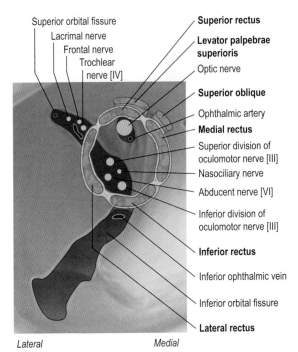

Superior orbital fissure
Lacrimal nerve
Frontal nerve
Trochlear
nerve [IV]

Superior rectus

Levator palpebrae superioris

Optic nerve

Superior oblique

Ophthalmic artery

Medial rectus

Superior division of oculomotor nerve [III]

Nasociliary nerve

Abducent nerve [VI]

Inferior division of oculomotor nerve [III]

Inferior rectus

Inferior ophthalmic vein

Inferior orbital fissure

Lateral rectus

Lateral   *Medial*

Fig. 4.33 The superior orbital fissure showing the structures passing through it, as well as the origin of the muscles moving the eyeball.

ophthalmic division); the *mesencephalic nucleus* receives GSA fibres conveying proprioceptive sensation from the face and head.

The trigeminal nerve exits the anterolateral surface of the pons (Figs 4.25 and 4.17A and B) as a large sensory and smaller motor root. The roots continue forward out of the posterior and into the middle cranial fossa by passing over the medial tip of the petrous part of the temporal bone, where the sensory root expands to form the trigeminal ganglion containing the cell bodies of the sensory neurons; the ganglion sits in a shallow depression (cavum trigeminale). The motor root lies below and is separated from the sensory root. The terminal divisions (ophthalmic, maxillary, mandibular) of the trigeminal nerve arise from the anterior border of the ganglion to exit the skull by the superior orbital fissure (ophthalmic division), foramen rotundum (maxillary division) and foramen ovale (mandibular division) (Fig. 4.34).

Ophthalmic Division (V₁)

The ophthalmic division contains sensory fibres only; it passes forward through the lateral wall of the cavernous sinus (Fig. 4.31), where it divides into the lacrimal,

frontal and nasociliary nerves, and superior orbital fissure (Fig. 4.33) to enter the orbit. It conveys sensory information from the eyes, conjunctiva, lacrimal gland and contents of the orbit, as well as from the nasal cavity, frontal sinus, ethmoidal cells, falx cerebri, dura mater of the anterior cranial fossa and superior parts of the tentorium cerebelli, upper eyelid, dorsum of the nose and anterior part of the scalp.

Maxillary Division (V₂)

The maxillary division contains sensory fibres only: it passes forward in the lower part of the lateral wall of the cavernous sinus (Fig. 4.31), leaving the skull through the foramen rotundum to enter the pterygopalatine fossa. It conveys sensory information from the dura mater of the middle cranial fossa, nasopharynx, palate, nasal cavity, upper teeth, maxillary sinus, and skin over the side of the nose, lower eyelid, cheek and upper lip.

Mandibular Division (V₃)

The mandibular division leaves the lower margin of the trigeminal ganglion exiting the skull through the foramen ovale to enter the infratemporal fossa: the sensory and motor roots remain separate as they pass through the foramen, uniting outside the skull.

It conveys sensory information from the skin of the lower face, cheek, lower lip, anterior part of the external ear, part of the external acoustic meatus and temporal region, lower teeth, mastoid air cells, mucous membranes of the cheek and mandible, and dura mater of the middle cranial fossa.

The motor fibres innervate temporalis, masseter, medial and lateral pterygoid (muscles of mastication), as well as tensor tympani in the middle ear, tensor veli palatini in the soft palate, the anterior belly of digastric and mylohyoid; all of these muscles are derived from the 1st pharyngeal (branchial) arch.

CLINICAL ANATOMY: The effects of lesion of the trigeminal nerve depend on the extent of the lesion, i.e., whether one or more divisions are affected, with loss of sensation and pain in the region of the face supplied by the division(s) affected; if the mandibular division is involved there will also be paralysis of the muscles of mastication on the side of the lesion. Lesions can occur in the region of the trigeminal ganglion or be the result of trauma/local masses around the foramina through which each division passes.

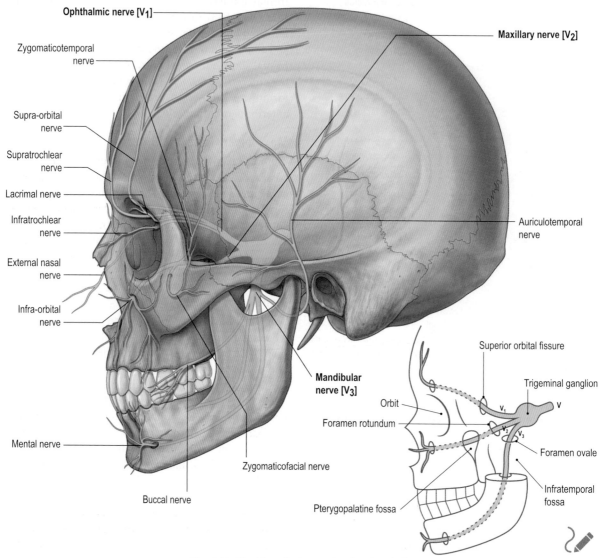

Ophthalmic nerve [V₁]

Zygomaticotemporal nerve

Supra-orbital nerve

Supratrochlear nerve

Lacrimal nerve

Infratrochlear nerve

External nasal nerve

Infra-orbital nerve

Mental nerve

Buccal nerve

Zygomaticofacial nerve

Mandibular nerve [V₃]

Maxillary nerve [V₂]

Auriculotemporal nerve

Superior orbital fissure

Trigeminal ganglion

Orbit

Foramen rotundum

V

Foramen ovale

Infratemporal fossa

Pterygopalatine fossa

Fig. 4.34 The trigeminal nerve leaving the skull.

Abducens Nerve (VI)

The abducens nerve consists of GSE fibres which innervate lateral rectus: the fibres originate in the abducens nucleus. It emerges from the brainstem at the junction of the pons and medulla; from here it crosses the superior edge of the petrous part of the temporal bone, contained within a dural sleeve, to enter and pass through the cavernous sinus (Fig. 4.31) and superior orbital fissure (Fig. 4.33) within the tendinous ring.

CLINICAL ANATOMY: Lesion of the abducens nerve leads to an inability to move the eye laterally; it can be the result of a brain lesion or thrombosis of the cavernous sinus compressing the nerve.

Facial Nerve (VII)

The facial nerve arises from three nuclei: the *motor nucleus* gives SVE fibres which innervate muscles derived from the 2nd pharyngeal (branchial) arch (facial muscles), stapedius, posterior belly of digastric and stylohyoid; the *superior salivary nucleus* receives SVA fibres conveying taste sensations from the anterior 2/3rd of the tongue; the *nucleus tractus solitarius* receives GSA fibres conveying sensory information from the external auditory meatus and deeper parts of the auricle of the ear, and gives GVE (preganglionic parasympathetic secretomotor) fibres to the lacrimal and salivary glands, and mucous membrane of the nasal cavity, and hard and soft palates.

The facial nerve leaves the lateral surface of the brainstem between the pons and medulla oblongata as a large motor and smaller sensory root (intermediate nerve); the motor root carries the SVE fibres and the sensory root all other fibres. The roots cross the posterior cranial fossa leaving the cranial cavity through the internal acoustic meatus with the vestibulocochlear nerve.

After entering the facial canal in the petrous temporal bone, the two roots unite forming the facial nerve: near this point the nerve enlarges (geniculate ganglion), which contains the cell bodies of the sensory neurons. The greater petrosal nerve arises at the geniculate ganglion and carries GVE (preganglionic parasympathetic secretomotor fibres) to the lacrimal gland, mucous glands of the nasal cavity, maxillary sinus and palate. The facial nerve then continues along the facial canal giving the nerve to stapedius and chorda tympani before leaving the skull through the stylomastoid foramen. The chorda tympani crosses the tympanic membrane before leaving the skull via the petrotympanic fissure (medial to the mandibular fossa) travelling a short distance in the infratemporal fossa before joining the mandibular division of the trigeminal nerve; it carries SVA fibres conveying taste sensation from the anterior two-third of the tongue.

On emerging from the stylomastoid foramen the facial nerve has a short extracranial course, giving branches to the posterior belly of digastric, posterior and superior auricular as well as stylohyoid, before entering the posterior aspect of the parotid gland, where it divides into its terminal branches; these branches emerge from the anterior border of the gland supplying muscles of the face (Fig. 4.35).

CLINICAL ANATOMY: Trauma to branches within the parotid gland (e.g., during parotid surgery) leads to paralysis of the facial muscles innervated by the affected branches; trauma to the temporal bone or inflammation of the nerve results in abnormal or loss of taste sensation from the anterior two-third of the tongue and dry conjunctiva; a brainstem lesion leads to paralysis of the contralateral facial muscles below the eye.

Vestibulocochlear Nerve (VIII)

The vestibulocochlear nerve emerges from the lateral surface of the brainstem between the pons and medulla; it crosses the posterior cranial fossa to enter the internal auditory meatus, where the two parts separate into their individual components (vestibular, cochlear) within the petrous part of the temporal bone.

Vestibular Part

The vestibular component arises from four vestibular (superior, inferior, medial and lateral) nuclei, which receive SSA fibres associated with balance and equilibrium: some afferent fibres pass directly to the cerebellum. Efferent fibres from the vestibular nuclei form the vestibulospinal and vestibulocerebellar tracts, as well as making connections with other cranial nerve nuclei through the medial longitudinal bundle.

Cochlear Part

The cochlear component arises from two cochlear (ventral and dorsal) nuclei, which receive SSA fibres associated with hearing.

Auditory pathway. Axons of the bipolar cells of the spiral ganglion form the cochlear nerve, reaching the pons lateral to the vestibular nerve, where it divides into ventral and dorsal roots which synapse on cells in the ventral and dorsal cochlear nuclei. Axons from these cells run transversely across the pons to synapse on cells in the ventral and dorsal trapezoid nuclei of both sides. From here fibres ascend in the brainstem as the lateral lemniscus, some fibres of which pass uninterrupted to the lateral lemniscus of the same side; all axons terminate in the inferior colliculus and medial geniculate body. The auditory radiation arises from the medial geniculate body through the internal capsule to terminate in the middle of the superior temporal gyrus, the auditory area of the cerebral cortex.

CLINICAL ANATOMY: A lesion at the cerebellopontine angle can result in progressive unilateral hearing loss and tinnitus.

Glossopharyngeal Nerve (IX)

The glossopharyngeal nerve arises from four nuclei (trigeminal sensory nucleus, nucleus tractus solitarius, nucleus ambiguus and inferior salivary nucleus): the *trigeminal sensory nucleus* receives GSA fibres conveying general sensations from the posterior one-third of

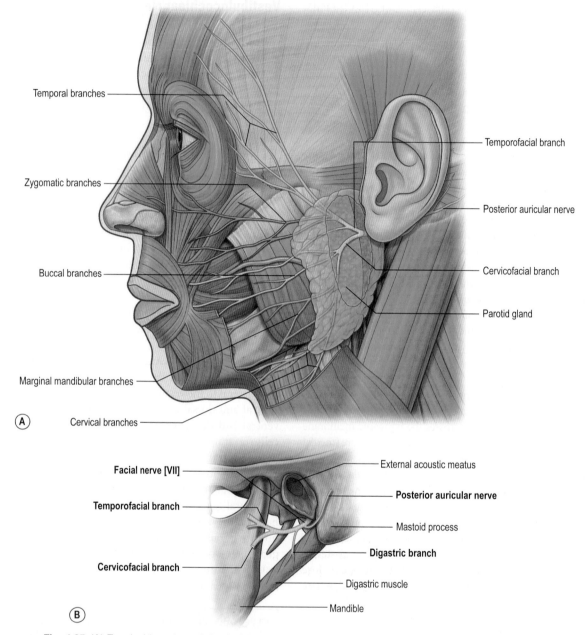

Fig. 4.35 (A) Terminal branches of the facial nerve on the face. (B) Branches prior to entering the parotid gland.

the tongue, palatine tonsils, oropharynx, and mucosa of the middle ear, pharyngotympanic (auditory, eustachian) tube and mastoid air cells; the *nucleus tractus solitarius* receives SVA fibres associated with the perception of taste from the posterior of the tongue, and GVA fibres from the carotid body (chemoreceptor), which detects changes in the composition of arterial blood (partial pressures of oxygen and carbon dioxide), blood pH and temperature, and sinus (baroreceptor), which detects changes in arterial blood pressure; the *inferior salivary nucleus* sends GVE (preganglionic parasympathetic secretomotor) fibres to the parotid gland; and the *nucleus ambiguus* sends SVE fibres which innervate stylopharyngeus (muscle of the 3rd pharyngeal arch).

The glossopharyngeal nerve emerges from the anterolateral surface of the medulla oblongata as a series of tiny rootlets above those for the vagus and accessory nerves (Fig. 4.17A and B); the rootlets cross the posterior cranial fossa before entering the jugular foramen with those of the vagus and accessory nerves. Associated ganglia (superior, inferior) near the jugular foramen contain the cell bodies of the sensory neurons. The tympanic branch arises after the glossopharyngeal nerve leaves the jugular foramen and re-enters the temporal bone to enter the middle ear where it participates in the formation of the tympanic plexus; the lesser petrosal nerve leaves the plexus and enters the middle cranial cavity to leave the skull again through the foramen ovale to synapse in the otic ganglion, from where fibres pass to the parotid gland. In the neck, the glossopharyngeal nerve passes forward between the internal and external carotid arteries (Fig. 4.36).

> **CLINICAL ANATOMY:** A brainstem lesion or penetrating neck wound can result in loss of taste from the posterior one-third of the tongue, as well as general sensation from the soft palate.

Taste (gustatory) pathway. Impulses from chemoreceptor cells located in the tongue and epiglottis are conveyed by SVA fibres to the cell bodies of neurons in the: geniculate ganglion of the facial nerve from the anterior two-third of the tongue; inferior ganglion of the glossopharyngeal nerve from the posterior one-third of the tongue; and inferior ganglion of the vagus from the root of the tongue and epiglottis. Cells in the rostral part of the solitary (gustatory) nucleus receive GVA fibres from the ganglion cells, which sends fibres in the ipsilateral central tegmental tract through the midbrain and subthalamus to the medial part of the ventral posterior nucleus of the thalamus. Fibres from the thalamus project to the cortical area for taste (adjacent to the general sensory area of the tongue extending into the insula).

Vagus Nerve (X)

The vagus nerve arises from four nuclei (trigeminal sensory nucleus, nucleus tractus solitarius, dorsal motor nucleus of the vagus and nucleus ambiguus): the *trigeminal sensory nucleus* receives GSA fibres conveying general sensation from the pharynx, larynx, trachea,

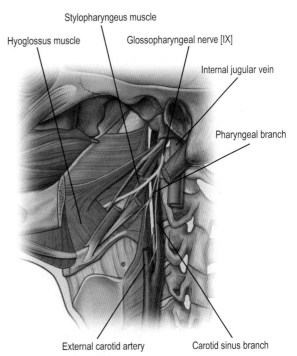

Fig. 4.36 The glossopharyngeal nerve in the neck.

oesophagus, part of the auricle and external auditory meatus; the *nucleus tractus solitarius* receives GVA fibres conveying sensory information from thoracic and abdominal viscera, GVA fibres from aortic bodies (chemoreceptors), which detects changes in the composition of arterial blood (partial pressures of oxygen and carbon dioxide) and blood pH, and aortic arch (baroreceptors), which detects changes in arterial blood pressure; the *dorsal motor nucleus of the vagus* sends, via the nucleus tractus solitarius, GVE fibres (preganglionic parasympathetic secretomotor) fibres to glands and smooth muscle in the pharynx, larynx, thoracic and abdominal viscera; the *nucleus ambiguus* sends SVE fibres to muscles of the soft palate (except tensor veli palatini), pharynx (except stylopharyngeus) and palatoglossus of the tongue.

The vagus emerges as a series of rootlets from the anterolateral surface of the medulla oblongata, below those of the glossopharyngeal nerve (Fig. 4.17A and B); the rootlets cross the posterior cranial fossa before entering the jugular foramen with those of the glossopharyngeal and accessory nerves. Within or immediately outside the foramen are two associated ganglia (superior/jugular, inferior/nodose) containing the cell bodies of the sensory neurons. Outside the skull the

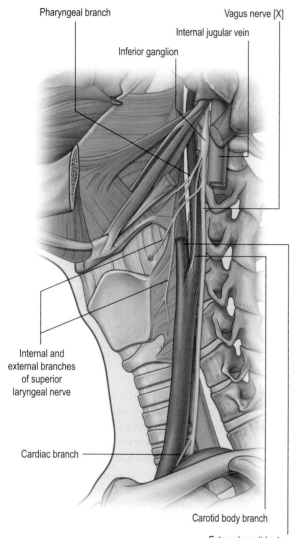

Pharyngeal branch

Vagus nerve [X]

Internal jugular vein

Inferior ganglion

Internal and external branches of superior laryngeal nerve

Cardiac branch

Carotid body branch

External carotid artery

Fig. 4.37 The vagus nerve in the neck.

vagus enters the carotid sheath, being medial to the internal jugular and posterior to the internal and common carotid arteries (Fig. 4.37). In the neck, the vagus gives a pharyngeal branch, a branch to the carotid body, the superior laryngeal nerve (which divides into internal (sensory) and external (motor) branches), as well as a cardiac branch.

> **CLINICAL ANATOMY:** A brainstem lesion or penetrating neck wound can result in deviation of the soft palate with deviation of the uvula to the normal side, and vocal cord paralysis.

Accessory Nerve (XI)

The accessory nerve has two parts (cranial and spinal roots): the cranial root arises from the *nucleus ambiguus* and carries SVE fibres to muscles of the soft palate and intrinsic muscles of the tongue, which are carried by the vagus; the spinal root arises from the C1 to C5 spinal cord segments and also carry SVE fibres to sternomastoid and trapezius.

The spinal fibres emerge from the lateral surface of the spinal cord, uniting as they ascend entering the cranial cavity through the foramen magnum; they pass through the posterior cranial fossa exiting through the jugular foramen. The spinal part crosses the floor of the posterior triangle of the neck, innervating sternomastoid and trapezius along the way (Fig. 4.38). The cranial root arises as a series of rootlets from the anterolateral surface of the medulla oblongata below those of the vagus; the rootlets cross the posterior cranial fossa before entering the jugular foramen with those of the glossopharyngeal and vagus nerves and the spinal root. Within the jugular foramen, the cranial root joins the vagus, with its fibres being distributed in its pharyngeal and laryngeal branches.

> **CLINICAL ANATOMY:** A penetrating wound to the posterior triangle of the neck can lead to paralysis of sternomastoid and trapezius.

Hypoglossal Nerve (XII)

The hypoglossal nerve arises from the *hypoglossal nucleus*: it carries GSE fibres which innervate all intrinsic and extrinsic muscles of the tongue, except palatoglossus. It leaves the cranial cavity through the hypoglossal canal to lie medial to the internal carotid artery and internal jugular vein; as it descends in the neck it passes between the two vessels (Fig. 4.39). As it continues forwards it passes over the occipital, internal and external carotid and lingual arteries, then deep to the posterior belly of digastric and stylohyoid and over the surface of the hyoglossus before passing deep to mylohyoid.

> **CLINICAL ANATOMY:** Penetrating wounds to the neck, as well as skull base pathology, can result in atrophy of the ipsilateral muscles of the tongue, accompanied by deviation to the affected side; because of the involvement of the tongue there may also be speech disturbances.

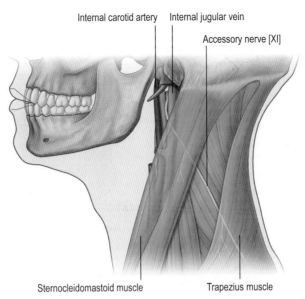

Internal carotid artery   Internal jugular vein

Accessory nerve [XI]

Sternocleidomastoid muscle   Trapezius muscle

Fig. 4.38 The accessory nerve crossing the floor of the posterior triangle of the neck.

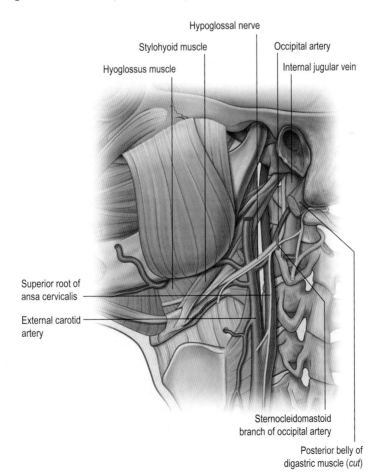

Hypoglossal nerve

Stylohyoid muscle   Occipital artery

Hyoglossus muscle   Internal jugular vein

Superior root of
ansa cervicalis

External carotid
artery

Sternocleidomastoid
branch of occipital artery

Posterior belly of
digastric muscle (*cut*)

Fig. 4.39 The hypoglossal nerve in the neck.

MANDIBLE

The mandible is a horseshoe-shaped bone of the lower jaw; the maxillae are the bones of the upper jaw. The mandible consists of a horizontal convex body, with two upward projecting rami posteriorly: the anterior border of each ramus ends as the thin coronoid process and the posterior border as the condylar process (head), below which is the neck (Fig. 4.40). The head articulates with the mandibular fossa of the temporal bone; it is broader transversely, being marked medially and laterally by prominent tubercles, than anteroposteriorly. Between the coronoid and condylar processes is the mandibular notch.

> **CLINICAL ANATOMY:** The maxillary artery and auriculotemporal nerve are intimately related to the medial side of the mandibular neck and are therefore liable to trauma in fractures of the neck and dislocation of the mandible at the temporomandibular joint.

The outer surface of the body is slightly concave from above down and markedly convex from side to side; a vertical midline depression may exist where the two halves fused, below which is a triangular elevation (symphysis menti) with raised areas on each side (mental tubercles). Towards the front of the body on each side is the mental foramen, which transmits the mental nerve and vessels; the upper border (alveolar margin) carries sockets for the teeth (maximum 16 (8 each side) in adults).

> **APPLIED ANATOMY:** In males, the mental tubercle is more prominent; the angle is rough and everted in males, but smooth and inverted in females.

The ramus is continuous with the body at the angle; its inner surface is marked by the mandibular foramen partly covered by the lingula to which is attached the sphenomandibular ligament. The inferior alveolar nerve and vessels enter the mandibular canal to run inside the body of the mandible; they supply the lower teeth. Passing from the mandibular foramen obliquely across the body is the mylohyoid line dividing it into upper and lower areas; anteriorly above the line is the sublingual fossa for the sublingual gland (page 313) and below in

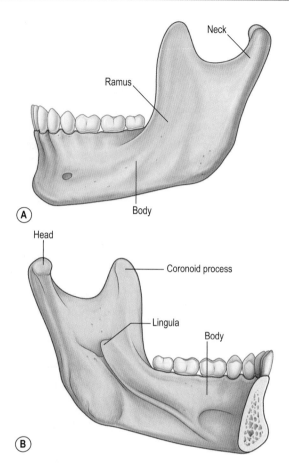

Fig. 4.40 Lateral (A) and medial (B) aspects of the mandible.

the middle one-third is the submandibular fossa for the submandibular gland (page 313).

Growth of the Mandible

At birth the mandible is in two parts: the body is a shell of alveolar bone surrounding the developing teeth. The ramus is short, making an angle with the body of 175 degrees so that the head is almost in line with the body (Fig. 4.41A); the mental foramen lies close to the lower border. During the 1st year, the two parts begin to fuse at the symphysis menti, which is completed by the end of the 2nd year. The ramus gradually enlarges, accompanied by a decrease in the angle between it and the body; by age 4 the angle is 140 degrees (Fig. 4.41B). Changes within the mandible continue, with the angle in adults being 110 degrees (Fig. 4.41C); the mental foramen lies midway between the alveolar margin and lower border.

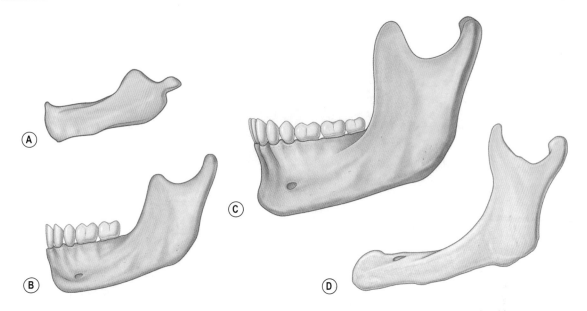

Fig. 4.41 Lateral aspect of the mandible at different ages: (A) birth; (B) age 4; (C) adult; (D) old age.

With loss of the teeth with increasing age, the alveolar sockets are absorbed, and the angle between the body and ramus increases to 140 degrees due to bone remodelling (Fig. 4.41D); the mental foramen lies close to the upper border. The head also becomes directed more posteriorly widening the mandibular notch.

There is also growth in width of the mandible between the angles, as well as in length, height and thickness; the head also grows superiorly, posteriorly and laterally contributing to its increase in length, height and width. Remodelling maintains the shape of the condyle and curves of the anterior margin of the ramus and coronoid process. In adults, the long axis of the head is directed posteromedially at an angle of 30 degrees with the frontal plane (Fig. 4.42); the angle is not always consistent from side to side. When prolonged the axes intersect in the median plane anterior at the anterior margin of the foramen magnum.

The length and height of the mandible can be readily palpated, with the angle being prominent, even though the lateral surface and posterior border of the ramus are covered by muscle and part of the parotid gland (page 312). The lateral tubercle of the head can be felt anterior to the tragus of the ear below the zygomatic arch; on opening and closing the mouth, the head can be felt moving forwards against the temporal bone.

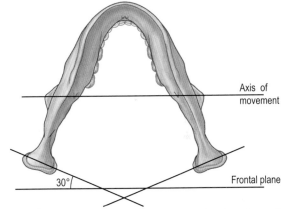

Fig. 4.42 Inferior aspect of the mandible showing the major axis of the head and the axis about which movement takes place.

Temporomandibular Joint

A synovial condyloid joint between the head of the mandible and mandibular fossa of the temporal bone; a complete intra-articular disc divides the joint space into upper and lower compartments facilitating the gliding and hinge actions possible at the joint. Movements at the joint take place about an axis passing between the lingulae (Fig. 4.42); this ensures that the

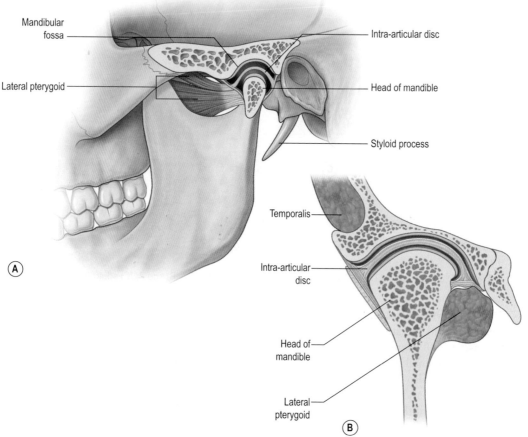

Fig. 4.43 Sagittal (A) and coronal (B) sections through the temporomandibular joint.

inferior alveolar nerve and vessels entering the mandibular foramen are not put under pressure during mandibular movements. The joint, together with the associated muscles, ligaments and occluding surfaces of the teeth, limits the forcible opposition of the jaws during biting; other aspects of normal function include mastication, suckling in infants, swallowing, yawning and speaking, although the latter involves little force at the joint.

The intra-articular disc is an avascular oval plate of fibrous tissue: flat at birth, becoming concavoconvex superiorly in adulthood to fit the mandibular fossa and articular eminence, and concave inferiorly over the mandibular head (Fig. 4.43). It is attached peripherally to the deep surface of the joint capsule and anteriorly

to the neck of the mandible, close to the attachment of lateral pterygoid.

A thin, loose but strong fibrous joint capsule encloses the joint; blending with and reinforcing the lateral aspect of the capsule is lateral ligament (Fig. 4.44). Accessory sphenomandibular and stylomandibular ligaments on the medial aspect of the joint help to control and limit joint movement.

The joint is relatively superficial, being covered only by skin and subcutaneous tissue. Anteriorly, the tendon of lateral pterygoid attaches to the neck and joint capsule; the tendon of temporalis passes deep to the zygomatic arch to attach to the coronoid process (Fig. 4.45). The superficial temporal artery crosses the zygomatic arch posteriorly in front of the external auditory

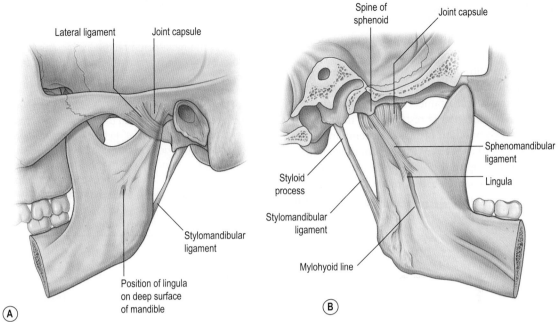

Fig. 4.44 Lateral (A) and medial (B) aspects of the temporomandibular joints showing their associated ligaments.

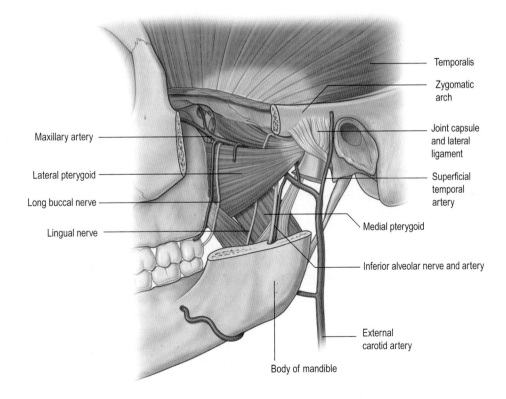

Fig. 4.45 Lateral aspect of the mandible and skull with part of the ramus removed showing the temporomandibular joint and its relations.

meatus; its pulse can be felt by applying pressure to the area. Posteromedial to the mandibular fossa is the root of the styloid process, with the carotid sheath (page 319) and its contents medial to it.

When the mouth is closed the teeth stabilise the mandible against the maxillae; backward dislocation is opposed by the lateral ligament and lateral pterygoid, while forward dislocation is restricted by the articular eminence and contraction of masseter, temporalis and medial pterygoid (Fig. 4.46). With the mouth open there is little to prevent upward dislocation through the thin roof of the mandibular fossa; this injury is rare as a blow to the drooping mandible usually causes the mouth to close or open more fully.

> **CLINICAL ANATOMY:** Forward dislocation, when one or both condyles move forward beyond the articular eminence, is the most common dislocation and can occur during yawning or opening the mouth too widely (Fig. 4.46A), reduction may be difficult/prevented by spasm of masseter. Dislocation of one side can be reduced by pulling downwards and backwards on the angle of the dislocated side releasing the condyle, which should then spring back into place; in bilateral dislocation both angles are pulled downwards and backwards with one hand while the other pushes the chin upwards releasing the condyles, which should then spring back into position. With the loss of the permanent dentition, the joint is less stable, with anterior dislocation occurring more readily; it is also more easily reduced.

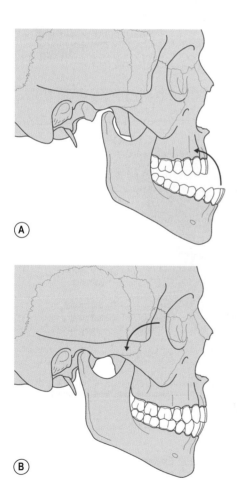

Fig. 4.46 Relationship between the head of the mandible and mandibular fossa in bilateral dislocation (A) and with the mouth closed (B).

Movements

There are four basic movements: protraction, pulling the mandible forwards so that the head articulates with the articular eminence; retraction, pulling the mandible backwards so that the head moves back into the mandibular fossa; elevation, closing the mouth; and depression, opening the mouth (Fig. 4.47). These movements are complex involving both compartments of the temporomandibular joint, as well as the coordinated action of the attached muscles.

Protraction and retraction occur in the upper compartment, with elevation and depression occurring in the lower compartment; combinations of these movements occur in chewing and grinding. Opening the mouth against resistance involves the infrahyoid muscles (page 323), which stabilises the hyoid and provides a firm base against which mandibular movements can be made.

With the mouth closed and the teeth are in contact (occluded) the upper incisors lie in front of the lower ones (Fig. 4.47A). When opening the mouth, the edges of the lower incisors pass downwards and forwards until the edges of both sets of incisors are directed towards each other. The downward and forward movement of the mandible is a combination of forward gliding and rotation, with rotation occurring about a transverse axis through the lingulae.

Details of the muscles involved in producing movements of the mandible are given in Table 4.5, with masseter, temporalis, and lateral and medial pterygoid shown in Fig. 4.48.

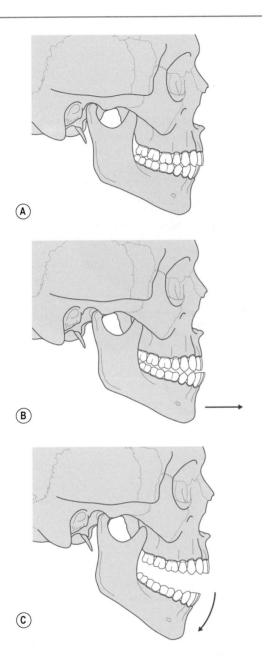

Fig. 4.47 The mandible retracted and elevated (A), i.e., the closed mouth; (B) protracted and (C) depressed.

Infratemporal Fossa

The infratemporal fossa is the space deep to the ramus of the mandible (Fig. 4.45). It is bounded superiorly by the infratemporal surface of the greater wing of the sphenoid; anteriorly by the posterior surface of the maxilla; medially by the lateral surface of the lateral pterygoid plate of the sphenoid; and laterally by the zygomatic arch, coronoid process and upper part of the ramus of the mandible: it has no posterior or inferior boundaries. The fossa contains muscles (medial and lateral pterygoid), nerves (maxillary, mandibular) and blood vessels (maxillary artery, pterygoid venous plexus).

APPLIED ANATOMY: The infratemporal fossa communicates with the temporal fossa via the space deep to the zygomatic arch; the pterygopalatine fossa via the pterygomaxillary fissure; the orbit via the inferior orbital fissure; and the middle cranial fossa via the foramen ovale and foramen spinosum.

FACE

The face is the anterior aspect of the head. It contains four openings (two orbits, nasal and oral cavities) housing the sense organs related to vision (eyes), smell (nose) and taste (mouth). Emotions are expressed through changes in facial shape; the face is essential for identity, with damage (scarring, developmental deformities) adversely affecting the individual's psyche. The face is clothed by muscles covered by elastic skin (vascular and rich in sebaceous and sweat glands), superficial fascia containing muscles, vessels, nerves and variable amounts of fat; there is no deep fascia except over the parotid gland, where it forms the parotid fascia, and over buccinator, where it forms the buccopharyngeal fascia.

Blood Supply and Innervation
Arterial Supply

The main artery of the face is the tortuous facial artery, a branch of the external carotid artery, reinforced by the transverse facial artery (branch of the superficial temporal artery) and arteries accompanying cutaneous branches of the trigeminal nerve (Fig. 4.49).

The facial artery enters the face by curving around the inferior border of the mandible anterior to masseter, where its pulse can be felt; it then runs anterosuperiorly towards the corner of the mouth, then

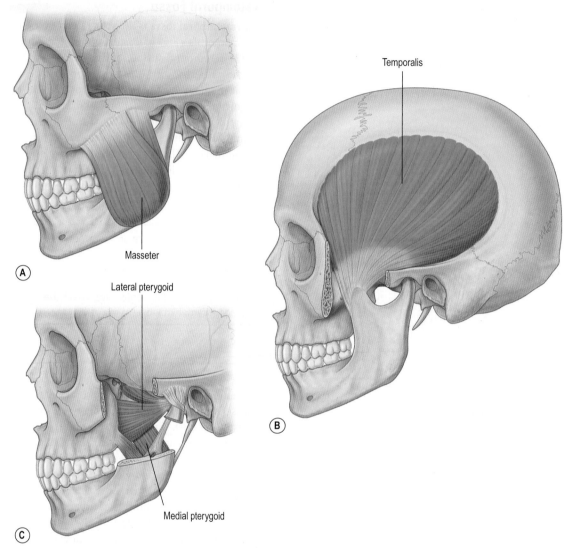

Fig. 4.48 (A) Lateral left aspect of the skull and mandible showing the muscles of mastication, with the part of the zygomatic arch removed in (B) and the zygomatic arch and ramus of the mandible removed in (C).

superomedially along the side of the nose terminating at the medial angle of the eye as the angular artery, which anastomoses with branches of the ophthalmic artery (Fig. 4.49A). Along its course, it gives inferior and superior labial and lateral nasal branches. The transverse facial artery runs between the zygomatic arch above and parotid duct below. Other arteries supplying the face are infraorbital, buccal and mental arteries, all branches from the maxillary artery (Fig. 4.49B); zygomaticofacial, zygomaticotemporal and

dorsal nasal arteries (Fig. 4.49A), all branches of the maxillary artery; and supratrochlear and supraorbital arteries (Fig. 4.49A) supplying the forehead and scalp, both branches from the ophthalmic artery.

> **CLINICAL ANATOMY:** The anastomosis between the superior and inferior labial arteries around the mouth provides an important connection between the facial and external carotid arteries on each side of the face.

TABLE 4.5 The Attachments, Actions and Innervation of the Muscles Involved in Movements of the Mandible

Muscle	Attachments	Action	Nerve Supply (Root Value)
Temporalis	From the temporal fossa of the temporal bone to the apex and deep surface of the coronoid process and anterior border of the ramus of the mandible: the posterior fibres run almost horizontally and anterior fibres almost vertically.	Retraction (posterior fibres) and elevation (anterior fibres) closing the mouth: the anterior fibres are constantly active to counter the effects of gravity.	Mandibular division (V_3) of the trigeminal nerve (V).
Masseter	From the zygomatic process of the maxilla and anterior two-third of the zygomatic arch (superficial part) and deep surface of the zygomatic arch (deep part) to the ramus and coronoid process of the mandible.	Elevation: the superficial fibres also aid protraction.	Mandibular division (V_3) of the trigeminal nerve (V).
Lateral ptery-goid	From the inferior surface of the greater wing of sphenoid (upper head) and lateral side of the lateral pterygoid plate (lower head) to the neck of the mandible, joint capsule and intra-articular disc of the temporomandibular joint.	Protraction: with medial pterygoid it produces slight rotation of the mandible towards the opposite side.	Mandibular division (V_3) of the trigeminal nerve (V).
Medial ptery-goid	From the medial side of the lateral pterygoid plate, pyramidal process of the palatine bone and maxillary tubercle to the rough triangular impression on the inner surface of the angle of the mandible.	Elevation and protraction: with lateral pterygoid it produces slight rotation of the mandible towards the opposite side.	Mandibular division (V_3) of the trigeminal nerve (V).
Digastric	Posterior belly from the medial surface of the mastoid process to an intermediate tendon which passes through the insertion of stylohyoid to the anterior belly which attaches to the digastric fossa on the lower border of the mandible.	With the hyoid fixed, it depresses the mandible to open the mouth against resistance. When the mandible is elevated, it aids retraction, and with the mandible fixed it raises the hyoid and with it the larynx (important in swallowing).	Posterior belly by the facial nerve (VII), anterior belly by the mandibular division (V_3) of the trigeminal nerve (V).
Mylohyoid	From the mylohyoid line on the inner surface of the body of the mandible with the fibres passing towards the midline and meeting in a midline raphe extending from the symphysis menti to the upper surface of the body of the hyoid.	Depression against resistance: elevation of the hyoid and raising the floor of the mouth. With the hyoid fixed it helps press the tongue against the roof of the mouth (important during swallowing).	Mandibular division (V_3) of the trigeminal nerve (V) by the nerve to mylohyoid.

TABLE 4.5	The Attachments, Actions and Innervation of the Muscles Involved in Movements of the Mandible (cont'd)		
Muscle	Attachments	Action	Nerve Supply (Root Value)
Geniohyoid	From the inferior genial (mental) spine on the posterior surface of the symphysis menti to the front of the body of the hyoid.	Depression of the mandible or elevation of the hyoid depending on which bone is fixed. Pulling the hyoid forwards shortens the floor of the mouth widening the pharynx in readiness to receive food.	Anterior primary ramus of C1 (the fibres travel with the hypoglossal nerve (XII)).
Platysma	From the skin and superficial fascia of the chest and shoulder to the lower border of the body of the mandible.	Depression of the mandible	Facial nerve (VII).

Venous Drainage

The face is mainly drained by the facial and retromandibular veins (Fig. 4.49), which receive all veins accompanying the arteries of the face. The anterior facial vein is formed by the union of the supratrochlear and supraorbital veins near the medial angle of the eye; it passes inferolaterally behind the facial artery as far as the inferior border of the mandible, where it passes superficial to the submandibular gland to pierce the deep fascia of the neck. It joins with the anterior division of the retromandibular vein, forming the common facial vein, which drains into the internal jugular vein. The retromandibular vein is formed within the substance of the parotid gland by the union of the superficial temporal and maxillary veins (or pterygoid venous plexus): within the gland, it lies deep to the facial nerve and superficial to the external carotid artery. At the inferior part of the parotid gland, the retromandibular vein divides into anterior and posterior divisions; the anterior joins the facial vein (see above) and posterior the posterior auricular vein to form the external jugular vein (Fig. 4.49A).

CLINICAL ANATOMY: The anterior and posterior divisions of the retromandibular vein provide a communication between the venous drainage of the face and the intracranial venous sinuses so that congestion involving the internal jugular vein can be accommodated by the external jugular vein, permitting continued venous drainage from the cranial cavity.

The facial vein has numerous connections with venous channels passing into deeper regions of the head (Fig. 4.50); at the medial corner of the eye with the superior and inferior ophthalmic veins; in the cheek with the infraorbital vein; by the deep facial vein with the pterygoid venous plexus.

CLINICAL ANATOMY: The deep communications of the facial vein have connections with the intracranial venous sinuses via emissary veins. As there are no valves in the facial vein or the venous sinuses within the head, blood can flow in any direction; infection from the face, especially in the triangular area above the mouth to the bridge of the nose ('danger area') has the potential to spread infection from the face to the intracranial region.

Lymphatic Drainage

The lymphatic drainage of the face is primarily to three groups of nodes: submental, draining the medial part of the lower lip and chin bilaterally; submandibular, draining an area from the medial corner of the orbit, most of the external nose, medial part of the cheek, upper lip and lateral part of the lower lip; and pre-auricular and parotid, draining the eyelids, the remainder of the external nose and lateral part of the cheek (Fig. 4.51). All groups of nodes drain into the deep cervical lymph nodes.

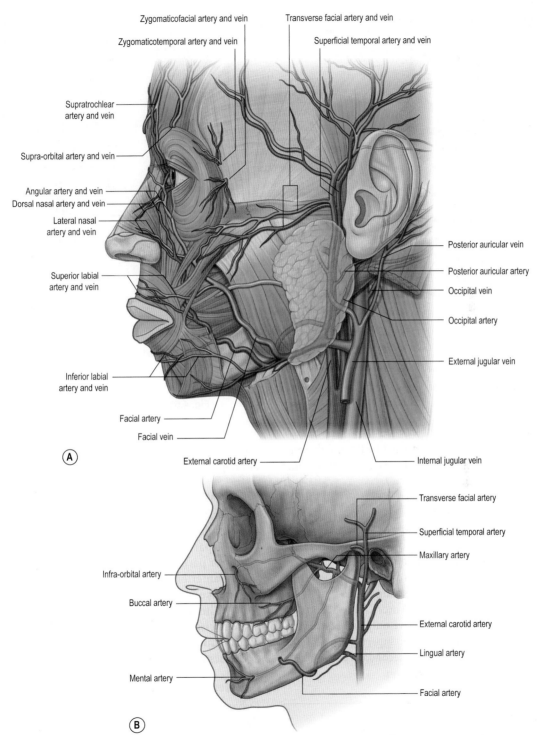

Zygomaticofacial artery and vein

Zygomaticotemporal artery and vein

Transverse facial artery and vein

Superficial temporal artery and vein

Supratrochlear artery and vein

Supra-orbital artery and vein

Angular artery and vein

Dorsal nasal artery and vein

Lateral nasal artery and vein

Superior labial artery and vein

Inferior labial artery and vein

Facial artery

Facial vein

External carotid artery

Posterior auricular vein

Posterior auricular artery

Occipital vein

Occipital artery

External jugular vein

Internal jugular vein

Infra-orbital artery

Buccal artery

Mental artery

Transverse facial artery

Superficial temporal artery

Maxillary artery

External carotid artery

Lingual artery

Facial artery

Fig. 4.49 Superficial (A) and deep (B) vasculature of the face.

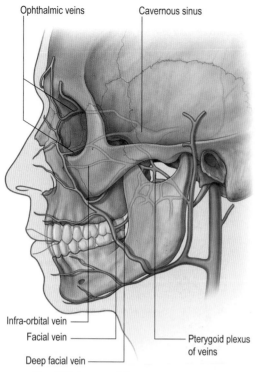

Fig. 4.50 Intracranial venous connections.

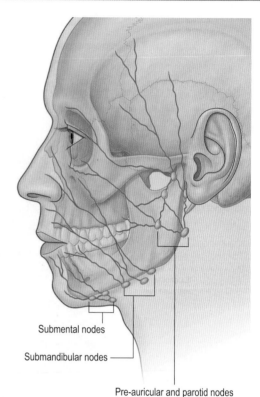

Fig. 4.51 Lymphatic drainage of the face.

Innervation

The skin over the face is innervated by the ophthalmic, maxillary and mandibular divisions of the trigeminal nerve (V) (Fig. 4.52).

Muscles of the Face

The primary action of the majority of facial muscles (Fig. 4.53) is to dilate (open) or constrict (close) the eyes, nose and mouth. In addition, buccinator plays an important role in mastication (chewing), while others are involved in forming and shaping sounds produced in the larynx into recognisable words. These actions are possible because the muscles have only one attachment to bone, the other being to the superficial fascia and skin; when they contract their secondary action has a profound effect on facial expression.

> **DEVELOPMENT:** All facial muscles are derived from the 2nd pharyngeal arch and are innervated by the facial nerve (VII). Damage to branches of the facial nerve results in loss of tone in the muscles supplied by that branch, accompanied by sagging of that part of the face.

The facial muscles are best considered in groups in relation to their action on the eyes, nose and mouth, although some muscles do not follow this plan.

Muscles of the Forehead

Occipitofrontalis is a two-part muscle united by the strong aponeurosis of the scalp (page 236): the larger anterior part pulls the scalp forwards and the smaller posterior part backwards. Acting from the aponeurosis, the anterior bellies raise the eyebrows together (as in surprise) or individually (as in a quizzical expression). The small corrugator supercilii blends with orbicularis oculi and pulls the eyebrows together (as in frowning). Procerus pulls the medial part of the eyebrows down.

Muscles Around the Eye

Orbicularis oculi is the most important muscle around the eye. It consists of three parts (orbital, palpebral and lacrimal) (Fig. 4.53). The orbital part surrounds the orbit and spreads onto the forehead, temple and cheek; it attaches to the medial margin of the orbit and medial palpebral ligament (page 300), with fibres from above

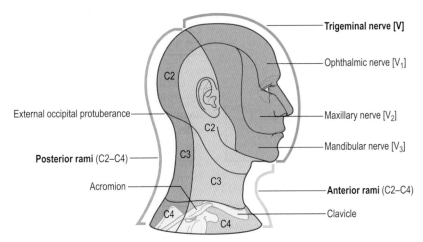

Fig. 4.52 Cutaneous distribution of the trigeminal nerve (V).

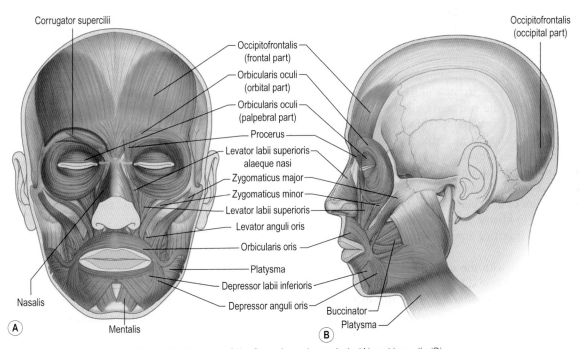

Fig. 4.53 Muscles of the face viewed anteriorly (A) and laterally (B).

the medial palpebral ligament passing elliptically around the orbit attaching again below it. The thinner palpebral part lies within the eyelids, while the lacrimal part arises from fascia behind the lacrimal sac (page 293) to attach to the tarsal plate of each eyelid.

The muscle as a whole has an important role in protecting the eye by bathing the eyeball with tears and firmly closing to protect the eye against insult and injury. The orbital part draws the skin of the forehead and cheek towards the medial angle of the orbit to screw the eye up tightly preventing light or dust from entering the eye. The palpebral part exerts fine control over the individual eyelids; by reflex or voluntary contraction it pulls the upper lid down and the lower lid up: small movements of the eyelids are important in non-verbal communication. Pulling the eyelids medially during blinking causes tears (produced by the lacrimal gland) to wash over the surface of the eyeball keeping it moist. The lacrimal part dilates the lacrimal sac.

> **CLINICAL ANATOMY:** Paralysis of orbicularis oculi results in the inability to close the eye, with the eyeball becoming red and inflamed.

Muscles Around the Nose

These muscles either dilate (nasalis, levator labii superioris alaeque nasi) or constrict (depressor septi) the nasal openings.

Muscles Around the Mouth

The most obvious muscle surrounding the mouth is orbicularis oris (Fig. 4.53); it has deep and superficial parts. The deep fibres attach to both the maxillae and mandible being continuous with buccinator, while the superficial fibres are derived from other muscles: some superficial fibres decussate similar to those of buccinator. Between the two parts, the intrinsic fibres of orbicularis oris run elliptically around the mouth; they have no bony attachment. Orbicularis oris has important roles in speech, by changing the shape of the mouth and lips, and mastication, by contracting against the teeth to keep food between the teeth during chewing. Contraction of orbicularis oris produces puckering of the lips, as in kissing and whistling, while contraction of muscles inserting into it change the shape of the mouth.

Continuous with the deep part of orbicularis oris, buccinator forms the substance of the cheek (Fig. 4.53); it has an extensive attachment to the maxillae and mandible opposite the molar teeth, the pterygoid hamulus and posterior part of the mylohyoid line and the intervening pterygomandibular raphe. Its medial fibres decussate posterolateral to the angle of the mouth, with the upper fibres passing into the lower lip and lower fibres to the upper lip; the interlacing of deep buccinators fibres with some superficial orbicularis oris fibres forms a palpable nodule (modiolus) at the angle of the mouth. Buccinator presses the cheek against the teeth preventing the accumulation of food in the vestibule of the mouth (page 308) during chewing.

> **CLINICAL ANATOMY:** Paralysis of buccinator results in accumulation of food in the vestibule of the mouth.

Levator labii superioris alaeque nasi, levator labii superioris, zygomaticus major and minor, and levator anguli oris (Fig. 4.53) act on the upper lip; when both sides contract the result is a smile, while contraction of one side only produces a sneer. Zygomaticus major and levator anguli oris raise and pull the angle of the mouth laterally as in laughing.

> **CLINICAL ANATOMY:** Paralysis of the upper lip muscles results in gradual drooping of the angle of the mouth on the affected side, leading to leakage of saliva and a constant dribble from the corner of the mouth.

Depressor anguli oris, depressor labii inferioris, risorius and mentalis (Fig. 4.53) act on the lower lip. The two depressors pull the mouth inferiorly as in sadness, while depressor labii inferioris curls the lower lip downwards; mentalis pulls the skin of the chin upwards resulting in protrusion of the lower lip as in pouting, with risorius pulling the angle of the mouth laterally.

> **CLINICAL ANATOMY:** Paralysis of the muscles on one side of the face (Bell's palsy) result in an inability to close the eye; a tendency for food to accumulate between the cheek, lips and teeth; drooping of the corner of the mouth; and, on smiling, the mouth is pulled towards the non-affected side.

Orbit

Pyramidal-shaped spaces situated below the forehead, each having an apex, base and four walls (medial, lateral, roof and floor). The base is the opening and has margins formed by the frontal bone superiorly, the frontal bone and maxilla medially, maxilla and zygomatic bone inferiorly, and zygomatic and frontal bones laterally (Fig. 4.54); the apex is at the optic canal, which communicates with the middle cranial fossa. The medial wall is formed by the frontal, lacrimal and part of the ethmoid bones; in its lower part is the lacrimal groove leading to the nasolacrimal canal, which communicates with the nasal cavity, while higher up are openings for the anterior and posterior ethmoidal neurovascular bundles, which leave the

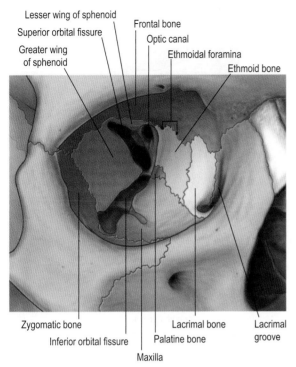

Lesser wing of sphenoid
Superior orbital fissure
Greater wing of sphenoid
Frontal bone
Optic canal
Ethmoidal foramina
Ethmoid bone
Zygomatic bone
Inferior orbital fissure
Palatine bone
Maxilla
Lacrimal bone
Lacrimal groove

Fig. 4.54 Bones of the orbit.

orbit to enter the nasal cavity. The lateral wall is formed by the zygomatic bone and the greater wing of the sphenoid. The thin roof is formed by the frontal bone and lesser wing of the sphenoid, separating the orbit from the anterior cranial fossa; the lacrimal fossa houses the lacrimal gland. The floor is formed by the maxilla and zygomatic bone; it contains the infraorbital groove and canal. The superior orbital fissure, which communicates with the middle cranial fossa, lies between the greater and lesser wings of the sphenoid, while the inferior orbital fissure lies between the greater wing of the sphenoid and the maxilla.

> **CLINICAL ANATOMY:** Orbital fractures are not uncommon and may involve the orbital margins as well as the walls, in which case they extend into the maxilla, frontal and zygomatic bones; they may be associated with complex facial fractures (Le Fort fractures, page 241). Fractures of the floor are one of the more common types of injury, tending to pull the inferior oblique muscle and associated tissues into the fracture line; individuals may not be able to direct their gaze upwards in the affected eye (upward gaze diplopia). Radiographs of medial wall fractures usually show air in the orbit, due to direct continuity between the orbit and ethmoidal paranasal sinuses; individuals may report a full sensation within the orbit when blowing the nose.

The orbit contains the eyeball, extraocular muscles (medial, lateral, superior and inferior rectus, superior and inferior oblique), sensory nerves (optic (II), ophthalmic (V_1)), motor nerves (oculomotor (III), trochlear (IV), abducens (VI)), the ciliary ganglion and blood vessels (ophthalmic artery and veins), all of which are surrounded and supported by periorbital fat.

Orbital Fascia and Ligaments

The orbital fascia (orbital periosteum) is a funnel-shaped sheath enclosing the orbital contents, except the infraorbital and zygomatic nerves; the apex is continuous with the dura mater at the optic canal and the base with the orbital septum (fibrous tissue stretching from the orbital periosteum to the tarsi of the eyelids). The bulbar fascia (Tenon's capsule) envelops the eyeball and extraocular muscles; the sheaths of the medial and lateral rectus give side expansions (check ligaments) to the medial and lateral walls of the orbit. The suspensory ligament of the eyeball extends between the medial and lateral walls below the eyeball.

Vessels and Nerves Within the Orbit

The arterial supply to structures within the orbit is from the ophthalmic artery (branch of the internal carotid artery) (Fig. 4.55), with venous drainage being to the cavernous sinus; some veins anastomose with veins on the face (Fig. 4.56).

Most nerves enter the orbit via either the superior orbital fissure or the optic canal (Fig. 4.33): the terminal branches of some nerves leave the orbit to supply the forehead (supraorbital, supratrochlear), face (infratrochlear) or nasal cavity (anterior and posterior ethmoidal). The position of the nerves and their branches within the orbit is shown in Fig. 4.57.

Ciliary ganglion: The small ciliary ganglion lies superior and lateral to the optic nerve; it is associated with the ophthalmic nerve (V_1). It receives fibres from three sources: parasympathetic fibres from the Edinger-Westphal nucleus in the midbrain via the inferior division of the oculomotor nerve, which synapse in the ganglion, with the postganglionic fibres passing in short ciliary nerves to supply sphincter pupillae and the ciliary muscles; sympathetic fibres from the plexus surrounding the internal carotid artery reaching the orbit via the nasociliary nerve; and sensory fibres from the nasociliary nerve, which pass through the ganglion without synapsing to supply the cornea and iris. The fibres leaving the ganglion form

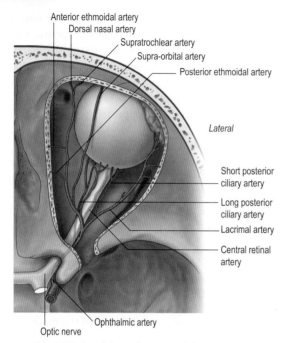

Fig. 4.55 Arterial supply to the orbit and eyeball.

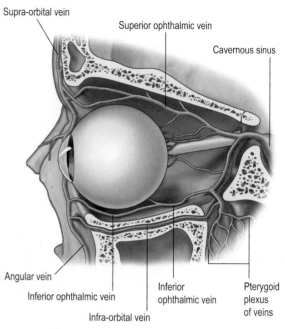

Fig. 4.56 Venous drainage of the orbit.

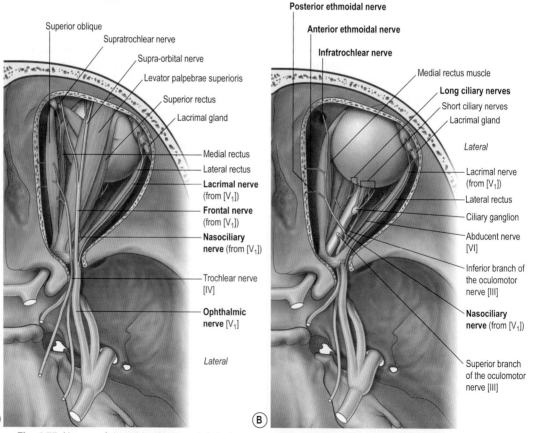

Fig. 4.57 Nerves of the orbit: (A) the ophthalmic nerve and its divisions; (B) other nerves within the orbit.

15 to 20 short ciliary nerves which pierce the sclera around the optic nerve.

Eyeball

The eyeball consists of three concentric layers: an outer fibrous supporting layer (sclera, cornea); a middle vascular pigmented layer (choroid); and an inner layer of nervous elements (retina). The interior is divided into two compartments (anterior and posterior) by the lens and its attachments, with the anterior compartment containing aqueous humour and the posterior the vitreous body (Fig. 4.58).

Surrounding the sclera is a thin fibrous sheet separating the eyeball from the other contents of the orbit: the eyeball is supported inferiorly by the suspensory ligament and surrounded and protected by extraocular fat. The two eyes look forwards: an imaginary line connecting the centre of the corneal curvature (anterior pole)

and centre of the scleral curvature (posterior pole) is the optic axis (Fig. 4.55B). The more important visual axis passes between the centre of the cornea and the fovea centralis (Fig. 4.55B) and represents the path taken by light from the centre point of vision: when looking at distant objects the visual axes are parallel, with the optic axes converging slightly posteriorly and the optic nerves markedly so.

In adults the eyeball is almost spherical, with a diameter of 25 mm; relative to body size the eyeball is much larger in infants and children as it completes the majority of its growth prior to birth, it is also slightly larger in females than males.

CLINICAL ANATOMY: The anteroposterior diameter might be greater or less than normal giving rise to myopia (short-sightedness) or hypermetropia (long-sightedness), respectively (Fig. 4.59).

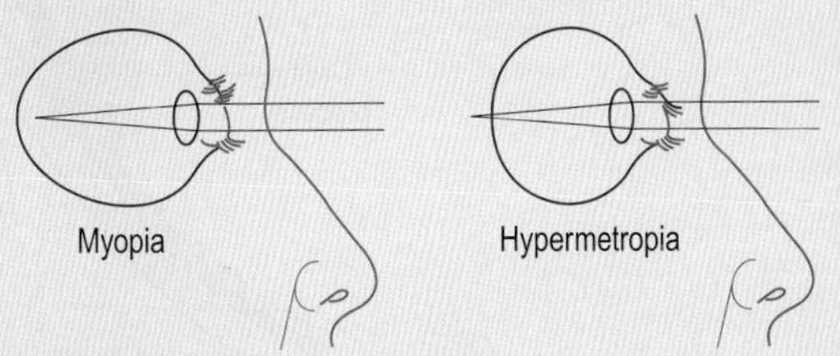

Myopia   Hypermetropia

Fig. 4.59 Schematic representation of myopia (short-sightedness) and hypermetropia (long-sightedness).

Outer fibrous layer. The sclera forms the posterior five-sixth of the circumference of the eyeball and is continuous with the cornea forming the anterior one-sixth; the anterior part of the sclera is covered by conjunctiva (the white of the eye). The sclera is thicker (1 mm) posteriorly than anteriorly (0.5 mm) and gives attachment to the extraocular muscles (page 300); posteriorly it is pierced by the optic nerve and accompanying vessels 3 mm medial to the fovea. The avascular cornea is continuous with the sclera at the dense uniformly thick (1 mm) corneoscleral junction and is covered by conjunctiva: it is richly innervated by the ophthalmic nerve, with abrasions of its surface being extremely painful.

The surfaces of the conjunctiva and cornea are kept moist and clean by a watery fluid secreted by the lacrimal gland (page 302). Constant blinking is an important part of the mechanism of fluid flow across the cornea; drying of the cornea causes serious damage to the surface cells.

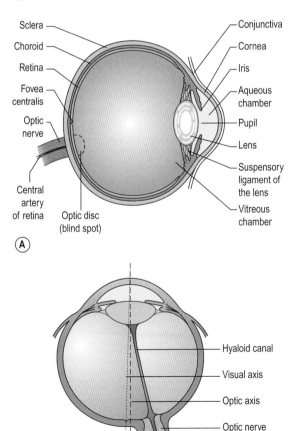

Sclera — Conjunctiva
Choroid — Cornea
Retina — Iris
Fovea centralis — Aqueous chamber
Optic nerve — Pupil
— Lens
— Suspensory ligament of the lens
Central artery of retina   Optic disc (blind spot) — Vitreous chamber

(A)

— Hyaloid canal
— Visual axis
— Optic axis
— Optic nerve

(B)

Fig. 4.58 (A) Horizontal section through the eyeball. (B) Visual and optic axes of the eyeball.

CLINICAL ANATOMY: The sensitivity of the cornea to touch is the basis of the corneal reflex resulting in reflex contraction of orbicularis oculi and closure of the eye.

APPLIED ANATOMY: The majority of the refraction of light takes place at the surface of the cornea: irregularities in its curvature interferes with the ability to form sharp images on the retina. When the cornea is more curved in one direction than the other the condition is astigmatism.

Middle vascular layer. The middle layer (uvea) comprises three parts (choroid, ciliary body and iris). The thin choroid lines the sclera as far as the corneoscleral junction, being loosely connected to the sclera except near where the optic nerve pierces, where it is firmly attached. It has two parts: an outer pigmented (brown) layer preventing light passing through the sclera and the scattering of light entering the pupil; and an inner vascular layer which is nutritive to the outer layer of the retina.

The ciliary body is a wedge-shaped ring connecting the choroid to the iris: it contains the ciliary muscle and ciliary processes and is lined by the ciliary part of the retina (Fig. 4.60A). The inward projecting part of the

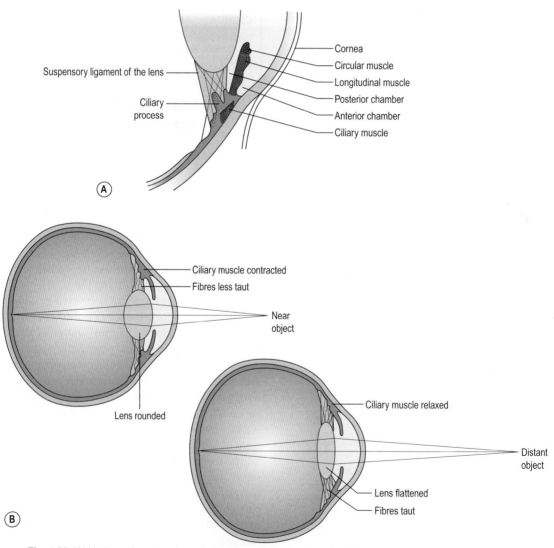

Fig. 4.60 (A) Horizontal section through the anterior eye showing the ciliary muscle and suspensory ligament of the lens. (B) The process of accommodation.

wedge is directed towards the lens, being connected to it by the suspensory ligament of the lens: the ciliary processes (60–80 radiating processes) give attachment to the suspensory ligament of the lens. The ciliary muscle consists of two sets of smooth muscle fibres (inner oblique, outer radial), both under parasympathetic control. Contraction of the ciliary muscle reduces tension in the suspensory ligament of the lens, allowing its inherent elasticity to increase its curvature enabling the eye to focus on near objects (Fig. 4.60B).

The biconvex lens (10 mm diameter, 4 mm thick) consists of concentric lamellae of lens fibres surrounded by a capsule firmly attached to the ciliary body by the suspensory ligament of the lens: both the lens and capsule are transparent and elastic. The shape of the lens is modified by the ciliary muscles as the eye focuses on objects at different distances (Fig. 4.60B).

> **CLINICAL ANATOMY:** The lens becomes thinner, less elastic and transparent after middle age: the loss of elasticity leads to presbyopia, an inability to focus on objects (accommodation), while the loss of transparency gives rise to cataracts.

Firmly attached to the periphery of the ciliary body is the iris, which lies in front of the lens and has a central opening (pupil); the colour of the iris is determined by pigmented cells in its posterior layer. In individuals with few pigment cells, the pupil appears pale blue, with increasing numbers of pigment cells the iris darkens and may become brown. The size of the pupil is controlled by inner sphincter pupillae (under parasympathetic control) and outer dilator pupillae (under sympathetic control) muscles.

Refracting media. The iris partly divides the region anterior to the lens into anterior and posterior chambers (Fig. 4.58A); both contain aqueous humour, a clear watery solution formed by the epithelium of the ciliary processes, with the fluid being resorbed at the iridocorneal angle into the sinus venosus to re-enter the circulation. Behind the lens and ciliary body is the posterior chamber containing vitreous humour, a transparent colourless semigelatinous material.

> **CLINICAL ANATOMY:** Interference with the resorption of aqueous humour results in an increase in intraocular pressure (glaucoma) and pressure on the retina; this affects the peripheral visual field.

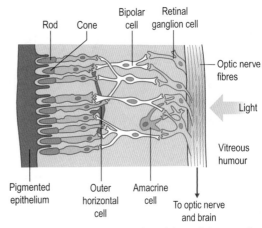

Fig. 4.61 Schematic representation of the cellular organisation of the retina.

Inner nervous layer. The light-sensitive layer (retina) extends onto the ciliary body and iris, but this region is nonfunctioning (contains no nerve elements); it comprises an outer pigmented epithelial layer and an inner transparent layer containing the light receptors (rods, cones) (Fig. 4.61). Within the inner layer, the rods and cones lie closest to the choroid so that light has to pass through most of the retina to reach them. The cones are used for colour discrimination, as well as in bright light: the macula only contains cones so that it functions in detailed vision so that when an object is specifically looked at it is always focused on the macula. Moving away from the macula the number of cones rapidly decreases; however, the number of rods increases, and rods are used in dim light. The pigment in rods is bleached out in bright light, but reforms in dim light so that objects not seen previously can be seen (dark adaptation); there are many more rods than cones in the retina.

Where the fibres of the optic nerve converge to pass through the choroid and sclera is the optic disc: it is insensitive to light (blind spot) as it contains no light receptors. The macula lies 3 mm lateral to the optic disc, with its central depression (fovea centralis) being where vision is most acute. Posteriorly the retina is 0.5 mm thick, thinning to 0.1 mm anteriorly; it is much thinner over the optic disc and fovea centralis.

Blood supply to the retina. This is from the central artery of the retina, a branch of the ophthalmic artery, which divides into four branches, each supplying a separate quadrant of the retina.

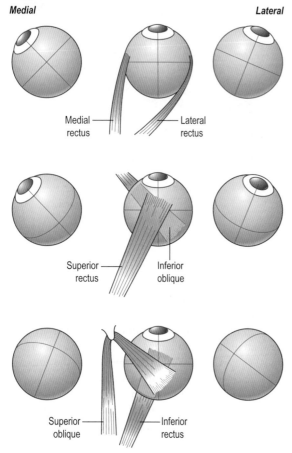

Medial   *Lateral*

Medial —   — Lateral
rectus   rectus

Superior —   — Inferior
rectus   oblique

Superior —   — Inferior
oblique   rectus

Fig. 4.62 Schematic representation of the extraocular muscles of the right eye and the effect each has on the direction of gaze.

CLINICAL ANATOMY: Each branch of the central artery of the retina is an end artery, consequently blockage results in blindness in the associated quadrant. The retina may also become detached from the choroid (either spontaneously or from a blow to the eye) impairing vision; tearing of the retina results in fluid passing outside the layer of rods and cones with vision being lost. In both cases, laser treatment can reattach the retina to prevent further tearing and separation.

Movement of the Eyeball

The direction of the gaze is controlled by the extraocular muscles. Medial and lateral rectus cause the eye to look horizontally medially and laterally (Fig. 4.62), respectively; however, because of the oblique course of superior and inferior rectus they tend to pull the eye medially in addition to turning it to look up and down

(Fig. 4.62), respectively. Superior and inferior oblique pull the eye laterally as well as moving it up and down (Fig. 4.62) because they attach behind the equator and pull on the back of the eyeball. In reality, most movements of the eyeball involve at least three muscles, with the coordination of movement between the eyes controlled by the brain.

Extraocular muscles. There are six extraocular muscles which move the eyeball and direct the gaze; details of their attachments, action and innervation are given in Table 4.6.

Protection of the eyeball. The eyes are protected by the eyebrows, eyelids and lacrimal apparatus; the eyebrows protect the eyes from injury and excessive light, with the hairs trapping sweat preventing it from running into the eyes.

Eyelids. The upper and lower eyelids, when closed, protect the anterior surface of the eyeball; the space between the eyelids when open is the palpebral fissure. The eyelids consist of a number of layers (from anterior to posterior): skin; subcutaneous tissue; muscle (palpebral part of orbicularis oculi, page 292); orbital septum; tarsus; and conjunctiva (Fig. 4.63).

CLINICAL ANATOMY: The thin layer of connective tissue, together with its loose arrangement allows the accumulation of blood (black eye) following injury or trauma.

The major support for each eyelid is the tarsus (plate of dense connective tissue) attached to the orbital walls by the medial and lateral palpebral ligaments; levator palpebrae superioris is attached to the tarsus in the upper eyelid, as well as the superior tarsal muscle (Fig. 4.63).

CLINICAL ANATOMY: Ptosis (drooping of the upper eyelid) results from the loss of function of either levator palpebrae superioris or the superior tarsal muscle.

Thin conjunctiva lines the eyelid and is reflected onto the outer surface (sclera) of the eyeball at the corneoscleral junction; a conjunctival sac is formed when the eyelids are closed.

Embedded in the tarsal plates are modified sebaceous (tarsal) glands, which secrete an oily substance increasing the viscosity of the tears decreasing their rate of evaporation from the surface of the eyeball.

TABLE 4.6 The Attachments, Action and Innervation of the Extraocular Muscles

Muscle	Attachments	Action	Nerve Supply
Superior rectus	From the common tendinous ring[a] above the optic canal and medial part of the superior orbital fissure to the sclera 6–8 mm from the corneoscleral junction anterior to the equator	Elevation and adduction of the eyeball	Superior division of the oculomotor nerve (III)
Inferior oblique	From the floor of the orbit lateral to the nasolacrimal canal, the tendon then runs inferolaterally to the eyeball then curves upwards and laterally to attach to the lateral sclera posterior to the equator of the eyeball	Elevation and abduction of the eyeball	Inferior division of the oculomotor nerve (III)
Inferior rectus	From the common tendinous ring[a] and medial part of the superior orbital fissure to the sclera 6–8 mm from the corneoscleral junction anterior to the equator	Depression and adduction of the eyeball	Inferior division of the oculomotor nerve (III)
Superior oblique	From the apex of the orbit medial to the optic canal the tendon passes forwards to hook around the trochlea and then curves posteriorly, inferiorly and laterally to the lateral surface of the sclera to attach behind the equator of the eyeball	Depression and abduction of the eyeball	Trochlear nerve (IV)
Medial rectus	From the common tendinous ring[a] and medial part of the superior orbital fissure to the sclera 6–8 mm from the corneoscleral junction anterior to the equator	Adduction of the eyeball	Inferior division of the oculomotor nerve (III)
Lateral rectus	From the common tendinous ring[a] and medial part of the superior orbital fissure to the sclera 6–8 mm from the corneoscleral junction anterior to the equator	Abduction of the eyeball	Abducens nerve (VI)
Levator palpebrae superioris[b]	From the roof of the orbit anterior to the optic canal to the skin of the upper eyelid, superior tarsus and superior fornix of the conjunctiva	Elevates the upper eyelid	Superior division of the oculomotor nerve (III)

[a]See Fig. 4.33.
[b]Although located within the orbit, it is not an extraocular muscle (Fig. 4.57A).

CLINICAL ANATOMY: The blink (corneal) reflex is an involuntary blinking of the eyelids elicited by stimulation of the cornea (touching, foreign body), although it can also be the result of a peripheral stimulus: stimulation of one cornea normally elicits a consensual response with both eyelids closing. The reflex protects the eyes from foreign bodies and bright light, as well as when sounds greater than 40–60 dB are made; use of contact lenses may diminish or abolish the reflex. The reflex occurs within 0.1 second; it is absent in infants under 9 months. The afferent limb of the reflex arc is via the nasociliary branch of the ophthalmic nerve (V_1); the central component is in the pons; and the efferent limb is via temporal and zygomatic branches of the facial nerve (VII). Examination of the reflex is part of some neurological examinations, especially when evaluating coma; damage to the ophthalmic nerve results in an absent reflex when the affected eye is stimulated.

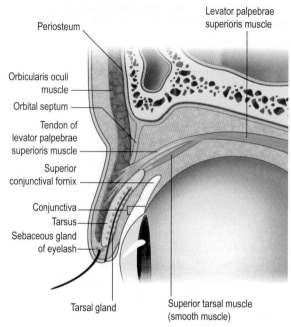

Periosteum

Levator palpebrae
superioris muscle

Orbicularis oculi
muscle

Orbital septum

Tendon of
levator palpebrae
superioris muscle

Superior
conjunctival fornix

Conjunctiva

Tarsus

Sebaceous gland
of eyelash

Tarsal gland

Superior tarsal muscle
(smooth muscle)

Fig. 4.63 Structure of the eyelids.

Lacrimal apparatus. The lacrimal apparatus (gland, ducts, canaliculi, sac, nasolacrimal duct) is involved in the production, movement and drainage of fluid across the surface of the eyeball (Fig. 4.64). The gland secretes a fluid which lubricates, protects and provides nutrients to the conjunctiva and cornea.

The lacrimal gland is located in the anterior superolateral aspect of the orbit in the lacrimal fossa; it comprises two connected lobes (orbital and palpebral) separated by the aponeurosis of levator palpebrae superioris. It secretes a clear fluid containing significant amounts of water to keep the surface of the eye moist, as well as dissolved elements necessary for normal cellular function; it also contains antimicrobial agents (phospholipase, lysozyme, peroxidase, lactoferrin, immunoglobulins) that provide defence against invading pathogens, proteins (retinol) and growth factors (epidermal, fibroblast, keratinocyte) involved in corneal regeneration and maintenance of corneal avascularity and transparency. Lacrimal fluid forms part of the three-layered covering (tear film) of the ocular surface of the eye: an inner mucin layer (from conjunctival goblet cells), a middle aqueous layer, and an outer lipid layer (from Meibomian glands). Given its constituents the tear film has a number of important functions: protecting the ocular surface from pathogens; removing debris and metabolic waste; creating an air-tissue interface for gaseous exchange to provide oxygen

to the avascular cornea; provide an even ocular surface for light transmission at the air-cornea interface; and provide the cornea with nutrients and metabolites.

Lacrimal fluid is continuously secreted from the gland into the lateral aspect of the superior conjunctival fornix via 6–8 lacrimal ducts. The fluid spreads over the entire ocular surface (from lateral to medial) with each blink. At the medial canthus, the fluid collects in a triangular space (lacrimal lake), from where it is drained by capillary action into the lacrimal canaliculi via the lacrimal puncta. From the canaliculi, the fluid drains medially into the lacrimal sac at the upper end of the nasolacrimal duct, which opens into the anterior part of the inferior meatus of the nasal cavity (page 304) and then into the nasopharynx (page 327) where it is swallowed.

The lacrimal nerve provides sensory innervation to the gland; it also receives sympathetic and parasympathetic innervation. Sympathetic stimulation (from the superior cervical ganglion) regulates blood flow through the gland and glandular secretions, while parasympathetic secretomotor stimulation is associated with the secretion of lacrimal fluid.

> **APPLIED ANATOMY:** Crying is associated with a number of emotional states which stimulate an increase in fluid production without the presence of an irritant.

CLINICAL ANATOMY: Irritation of the cornea and conjunctiva stimulates receptors that initiate the lacrimation reflex (increased secretion from the lacrimal gland), with the aim of washing out the cause of the irritation. The afferent limb of the reflex arc is via fibres in ciliary nerves to the nasociliary branch of the ophthalmic nerve (V_1); the cell bodies are in the trigeminal ganglion. The central component of the arc is the superior salivary nucleus of the facial nerve. The efferent limb of the arc involves preganglionic parasympathetic secretomotor fibres passing via the facial nerve to the pterygopalatine ganglion, from where postganglionic parasympathetic secretomotor fibres pass via the zygomaticotemporal branch of the maxillary nerve (V_2), which hitchhike along the lacrimal nerve to the lacrimal gland.

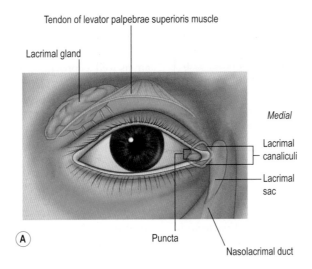

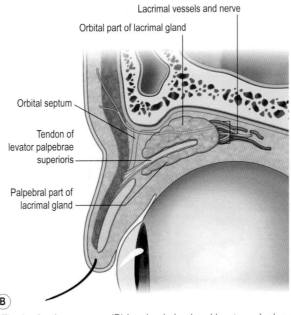

Fig. 4.64 (A) The lacrimal apparatus. (B) Lacrimal gland and levator palpebrae superioris.

External Nose

The external nose consists of the alae (flared parts lateral to the nares (nostrils)), the dorsum (ridge passing from the tip of the nose to the forehead) and the root of the nose (bridge) where it meets the forehead: the bridge has a part bony (nasal bones, frontal processes of the maxillae, nasal part of the frontal bone) and part cartilaginous (septal, lateral nasal and alar cartilages) skeleton (Fig. 4.65).

> **CLINICAL ANATOMY:** Because the nose is a prominent unprotected structure in the centre of the face it is vulnerable to trauma, with accidents and violence often resulting in a broken nose, which usually involves the nasal bones as well as the cartilages. Mild fractures are associated with swelling in and around the nose, with bruising around the eyes. In severe fractures the nose appears deformed or shifted out of its midline position and may be associated with severe bleeding, a blocked nostril or problems with airflow; occasionally there is a clear (cerebrospinal) fluid discharge.

Nasal Cavity

The nasal cavity communicates anteriorly with the external environment via the vestibule and nostrils (nares) of the mainly cartilaginous external nose, and posteriorly with the nasopharynx (page 327) via the choanae; it also communicates with the paranasal sinuses located within specific bones of the skull. It is divided into two cavities by the nasal septum, with each cavity having a floor, roof, and lateral and medial walls (Fig. 4.66); the medial wall separates the right and left nasal cavities. The floor

separates the nasal and oral cavities; it is formed by the hard palate (page 313). The narrower roof is formed (from anterior to posterior) by the nasal, frontal, ethmoid and sphenoid bones. The medial wall is the nasal septum (septal cartilage, perpendicular plate of the ethmoid, vomer), and the lateral wall consists of parts of the lacrimal, ethmoid, maxilla, palatine, sphenoid and inferior concha; conchae project medially from the lateral wall (Fig. 4.66B).

The conchae (superior, middle, inferior) are thin curved plates of bone projecting into the nasal cavity: the superior and middle are projections from the ethmoid, while the inferior is a separate bone (Fig. 4.67). Their function is to reduce turbulence of the incoming air, as well as providing a large surface area for respiratory epithelium to facilitate warming and humidifying the incoming air to prevent damage to the trachea and lungs.

Beneath and lateral to each concha is a space (meatus), each of which receives various openings: the space above the superior concha is the sphenoethmoidal recess (Fig. 4.68). The sphenoethmoidal recess receives the opening of the sphenoidal sinus; the superior meatus receives the posterior ethmoidal air cells; the middle meatus receives the frontal and maxillary sinuses, it also contains a small elevation (bulla ethmoidalis) onto which open the middle ethmoidal air cells, below which is a crescentic curve (hiatus semilunaris); and the inferior meatus receives the nasolacrimal duct.

Each nasal cavity has a vestibule, olfactory and respiratory regions. The vestibule is the dilation adjacent to the nostril lined with stratified squamous epithelium continuous with that of the skin of the face; it contains hairs (vibrissae) and sebaceous glands, which filter and trap large particles in the incoming air before they are carried into the rest of the nasal cavity. The stratified squamous epithelium of the vestibule thins posteriorly and undergoes a transition to pseudostratified ciliated (respiratory) epithelium.

Paranasal Sinuses

The paranasal sinuses (frontal, ethmoid, maxillary, sphenoid) communicate with the nasal cavity (Fig. 4.69); they are lined by mucoperiosteum covered with respiratory epithelium continuous with that of the nasal cavity. They act as resonating chambers during speech, reduce the weight of the skull anteriorly, and assist in warming and humidifying the inspired air.

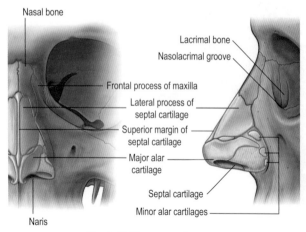

Nasal bone

Lacrimal bone

Nasolacrimal groove

Frontal process of maxilla

Lateral process of septal cartilage

Superior margin of septal cartilage

Major alar cartilage

Septal cartilage

Minor alar cartilages

Naris

Fig. 4.65 The external nose.

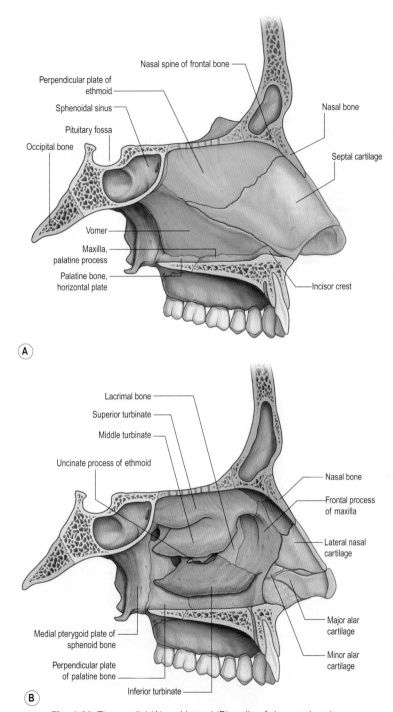

Fig. 4.66 The medial (A) and lateral (B) walls of the nasal cavity.

Frontal sinus. It is variable in size lying in the squamous and orbital parts of the frontal bone: anteriorly is the forehead; posterior and superior is the anterior cranial fossa; and inferiorly is the roof of the orbit.

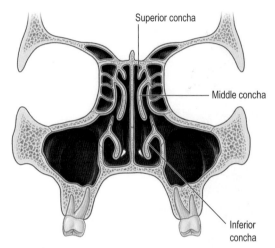

Fig. 4.67 Coronal section through the nasal cavity showing the position of the conchae.

Ethmoid sinus. Consists of numerous cells grouped together as anterior, middle and posterior ethmoidal air cells: medially is the nasal cavity; laterally is the orbit; and superiorly is the anterior cranial fossa.

Maxillary sinus. The largest of the sinuses lying within the body of the maxilla. The roof is the floor of the orbit and the medial wall is the lateral wall of the nasal cavity; the medial wall contains the opening of the sinus two-thirds the way up. Projecting into the floor and anterior wall are elevations produced by the roots of the teeth.

CLINICAL ANATOMY: Maxillary sinusitis is frequently accompanied by toothache because of the relationship of the roots of the upper teeth with the maxillary sinus. Tooth extraction may also cause infection of the maxillary sinus if the anterior and posterior walls are breached due to their thinness.

Sphenoid sinus. Lies within the body of the sphenoid; it is divided into right and left parts by a bony septum: anteriorly is the nasal cavity; posteriorly the pons in the posterior cranial fossa; superiorly the hypophyseal fossa,

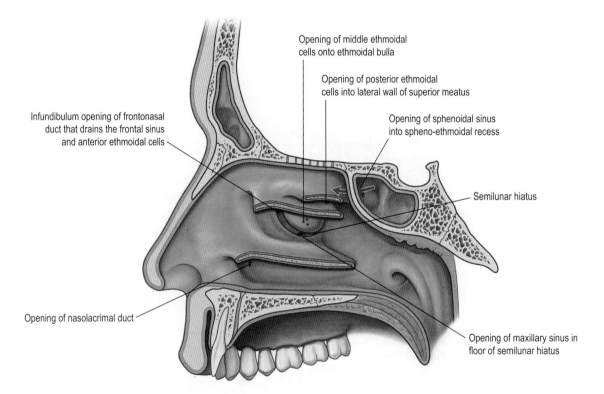

Fig. 4.68 Openings into the superior, middle and inferior meati and sphenoidal recess.

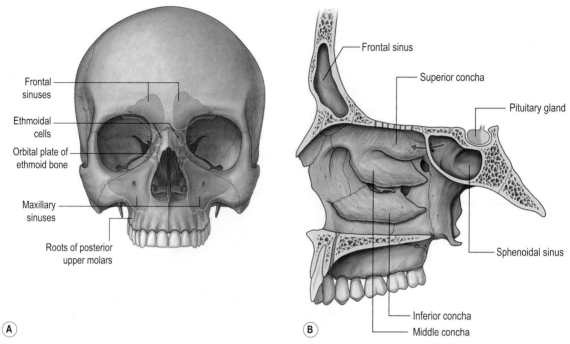

Fig. 4.69 Location of the paranasal sinuses: (A) frontal view; (B) parasagittal view of right nasal cavity.

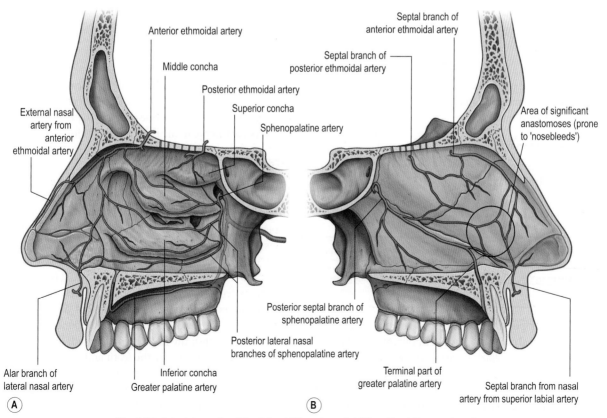

Fig. 4.70 Arterial supply of the lateral (A) and medial (B) walls of the nasal cavity.

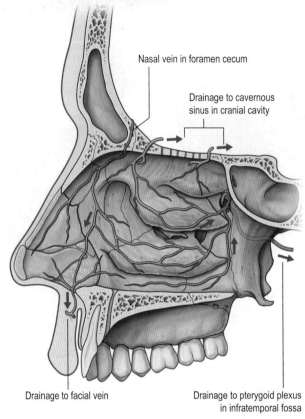

Nasal vein in foramen cecum

Drainage to cavernous
sinus in cranial cavity

Drainage to facial vein

Drainage to pterygoid plexus
in infratemporal fossa

Fig. 4.71 Venous drainage of the nasal cavity.

optic nerve and optic chiasma; inferiorly the nasal cavity and nasopharynx; and laterally the cavernous sinus and internal carotid artery.

Blood and Nerve Supply

The arterial supply to the nasal cavity is by branches of the ophthalmic, maxillary and facial arteries (Fig. 4.70), with the venous drainage being into the cavernous sinus, facial vein and pterygoid venous plexus (Fig. 4.71).

> **CLINICAL ANATOMY:** Nasal bleeding (epistaxis) occurs most frequently in the anterior part of the nasal septum anterior to the inferior concha (Little's/Kiesselbach's area).

The upper posterior parts of the lateral wall and septum of the nasal cavity are covered by olfactory epithelium, innervated by the olfactory nerve (I), while the remainder of the cavity is lined by respiratory epithelium, innervated by branches of the ophthalmic (V_1) and maxillary (V_2) nerves (Fig. 4.72). Parasympathetic secretomotor

innervation of mucous glands in the nasal cavity and paranasal sinuses is by fibres from the facial nerve (VII), which synapse in the pterygopalatine ganglion to join branches of the maxillary nerve in the pterygopalatine fossa.

Oral Cavity

The oral cavity consists of the vestibule between the lips and cheeks externally and gums and teeth internally, and the oral cavity proper (mouth). The vestibule is closed superiorly and inferiorly by mucous membrane reflections from its inner and outer boundaries; it communicates with the oral cavity proper behind the last molar tooth and has the opening of the parotid duct (conveying secretions from the parotid gland) on each side opposite the upper 2nd molar tooth. The roof of the mouth is formed by the hard (maxilla, palatine bones) and soft (muscular) palates; the floor by mylohyoid; laterally and anteriorly it is bounded by the teeth and gums: on either side of the frenulum are the openings of the submandibular ducts and those from the sublingual salivary glands (Fig. 4.73). The sublingual gland lies beneath the mucosa

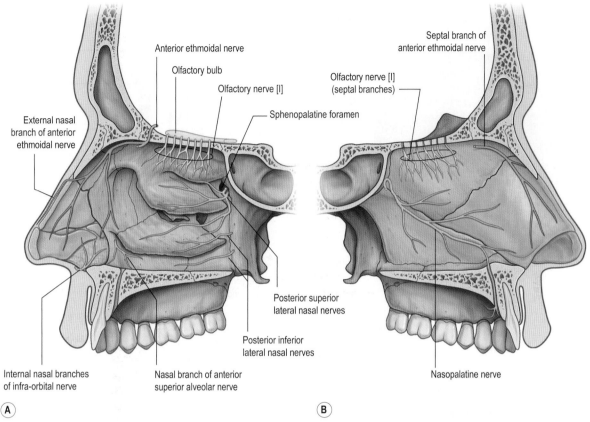

External nasal branch of anterior ethmoidal nerve

Anterior ethmoidal nerve

Olfactory bulb

Olfactory nerve [I]

Sphenopalatine foramen

Septal branch of anterior ethmoidal nerve

Olfactory nerve [I] (septal branches)

Posterior superior lateral nasal nerves

Posterior inferior lateral nasal nerves

Internal nasal branches of infra-orbital nerve

Nasal branch of anterior superior alveolar nerve

Nasopalatine nerve

(A)   (B)

Fig. 4.72 Innervation of the lateral (A) and medial (B) walls of the nasal cavity.

of the floor of the mouth on the upper surface of the mylohyoid; it is related laterally to the sublingual fossa on the medial surface of the body of the mandible. The mouth is continuous posteriorly with the oropharynx via the oropharyngeal isthmus (page 314).

The highly mobile upper and lower lips help retain saliva and food within the mouth, as well as changing their shape to produce different sounds during phonation. The cheek (buccinator) acts to prevent food from accumulating in the vestibule; its lining is continuous with that covering the gums (gingiva), which is continuous with the periosteum lining the alveolar sockets.

Lips

The gap between the lips is the oral fissure connecting the vestibule with the outside; it can be opened and closed, as well as change shape by the actions of the facial muscles associated with the lips and surrounding regions, and by movements of the mandible. The lips consist entirely of soft tissues lined by oral mucosa internally and covered by skin externally; a transition area exists externally between the thicker skin overlying the margins of the lips, which continues as oral mucosa onto their deep surface connecting the lips to the adjacent gum. Blood vessels close to the surface in areas of thinner skin result in the presence of a vermillion border at the margins of the lips. The upper lip has a shallow vertical groove (philtrum) between two vertical ridges.

Teeth and Gums

Each tooth has a crown above and a root below the gum margin (Fig. 4.74A), the greater part is formed by dentine covered by enamel over the crown and cementum over the root; within the dentine is the pulp cavity containing vessels and nerves. The upper (maxillary) teeth are innervated by superior alveolar nerves (branches of the maxillary nerve) and lower (mandibular) teeth by the inferior alveolar nerve (branch of the mandibular nerve); superior and inferior alveolar arteries (branches from the maxillary artery) accompany the nerves.

There are two sets of teeth (deciduous, permanent) whose components (incisor, canine, premolar, molar)

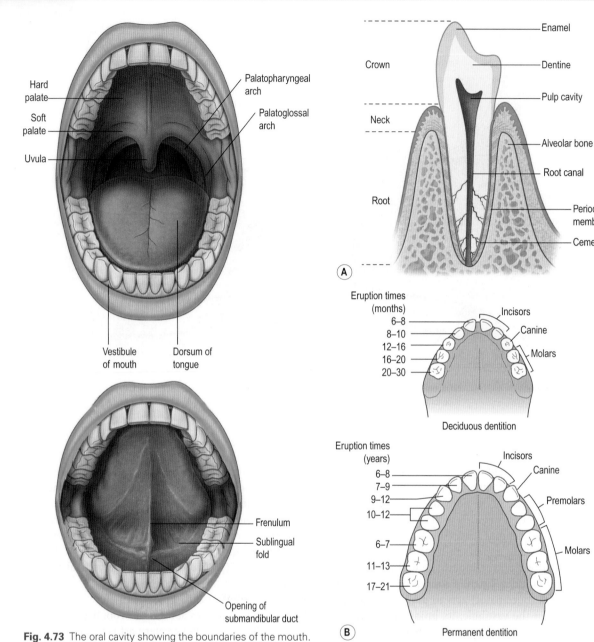

Fig. 4.73 The oral cavity showing the boundaries of the mouth.

Fig. 4.74 (A) Longitudinal section through a tooth. (B) The deciduous and permanent dentition, also showing the average eruption times for each tooth.

erupt at specific times (Fig. 4.74B); the 3rd molars may not erupt. As permanent teeth are lost with increasing age the surrounding alveolar bone is gradually resorbed, reducing the depth of the mandible (page 282).

The gingivae (gums) are specialised regions of oral mucosa surrounding the teeth and covering the adjacent regions of alveolar bone (gums). The gingiva associated with the upper teeth is innervated on the lingual surface by the nasopalatine and greater palatine nerves, and on

the buccal surface by the anterior, middle and posterior superior alveolar nerves. The gingiva on the lingual side of the lower teeth is innervated by the lingual nerve and on the buccal side by the inferior alveolar nerve. All nerves supplying the teeth and gingivae are branches of the trigeminal nerve (V). The arterial supply and venous drainage of the gingivae is by similarly named vessels: lymphatic drainage is mainly to submandibular, submental and deep cervical nodes.

> **CLINICAL ANATOMY:** Dental occlusion refers to the alignment of the teeth and the way the upper and lower teeth fit together: the upper teeth should fit slightly over the lower, with the points of the upper molars fitting in the grooves of the corresponding lower molars. Malocclusion occurs when the teeth do not fit together properly; it can be caused by differences in size of the upper and lower jaws; differences between the jaw and tooth size; the shape of the jaws or birth defects (cleft lip, cleft palate); childhood habits (thumb sucking, tongue thrusting); extra, lost, impacted or abnormally shaped teeth; ill-fitting dental fillings, crowns, dental appliances, retainers or braces; misalignment of jaw fractures following severe trauma; and tumours of the mouth and/or jaw. There are different classes of malocclusion: class I (most common), the bite is normal, but the upper teeth slightly overlap the lower teeth; class II (retrognathism or overbite) occurs when the upper jaw and teeth severely overlap the bottom jaw and teeth; class III (prognathism or underbite) occurs when the lower jaw protrudes or juts forward, causing the lower jaw and teeth to overlap the upper jaw and teeth. Inadequate overlap of the front teeth is an open bite; an overbite (deep bite) is excessive vertical overlap of the front teeth, it can be caused by disproportionate eruption of the front teeth or overdevelopment of the supporting bone; underbite is when the lower teeth bite in front of the upper teeth, it can be caused by undergrowth of the upper jaw, overgrowth of the lower jaw or a combination of both.

Tongue

The mobile muscular tongue lies partly in the mouth (anterior two-thirds) and partly in the oropharynx (posterior one-third), with the parts separated on the dorsum by the sulcus terminalis (Fig. 4.75); at the apex of the sulcus is the foramen caecum (site of origin of the thyroglossal duct) from which the thyroid gland descended into the neck. The tongue consists of extrinsic muscles (genioglossus, hyoglossus, styloglossus, palatoglossus), which attach to the skull and mandible, changing its position in the mouth, and intrinsic muscles, which change its shape: all muscles are innervated by the hypoglossal nerve (XII), except palatoglossus which is innervated by the vagus (X) via the pharyngeal plexus. The tongue plays an important role in chewing, swallowing, speech and taste.

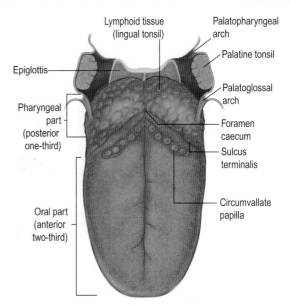

Fig. 4.75 Dorsum of the tongue showing its division into two parts by the sulcus terminalis.

The tip and margins of the tongue rest against the lower teeth and gums; the inferior surface lies entirely within the mouth and is covered by a thin transparent mucosa and is attached to the floor by the frenulum in the midline; the dorsal surface faces the palate. The rough anterior two-thirds is covered by numerous filiform (white conical) and fewer fungiform (red globular) papillae, the walls of which contain taste buds; a few rows of foliate papillae are located on the sides of the tongue anterior to the sulcus terminalis. A row of large rounded circumvallate papillae, whose walls also contain taste buds, lies anterior and parallel to the sulcus terminalis. The nodular appearance of the posterior one-third is due to the underlying aggregations of lymphoid tissue forming the lingual tonsil; it has no papillae but does have taste buds scattered over its surface. The posterior one-third is connected to the epiglottis by median and lateral glossoepiglottic folds.

Arterial supply, venous and lymphatic drainage and innervation

Arterial supply. The lingual artery supplies the tongue, arising from the external carotid artery close to the tip of the greater horn of the hyoid (page 325) it then passes deep to hyoglossus to enter the floor of the oral cavity (Fig. 4.76): it also supplies the sublingual gland, gingiva and oral mucosa of the floor of the oral cavity.

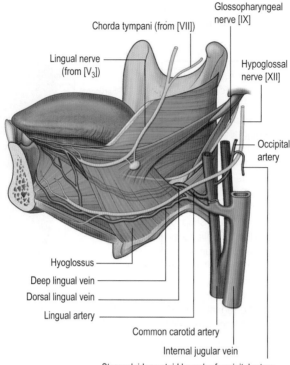

Fig. 4.76 The arteries, veins and nerves of the tongue.

Venous drainage. The dorsal lingual (visible through the mucosa on the undersurface of the tongue) and deep lingual veins drain the tongue; both drain into the internal jugular vein (Fig. 4.76).

Lymphatic drainage. The pharyngeal part of the tongue drains mainly into the jugulodigastric node of the deep cervical chain; the oral part drains directly into the deep cervical nodes and indirectly to these nodes via submental (below mylohyoid) and submandibular (below the floor of the oral cavity) nodes; the tip of the tongue drains into the submental nodes and then into the jugulo-omohyoid node of the deep cervical chain; the deep cervical chain lies along the internal jugular vein within the carotid sheath (Fig. 4.81).

Innervation. The general sensory innervation of the mucous membrane covering the dorsum reflects its development from the 1st and 3rd pharyngeal (branchial) arches: from the anterior two-thirds it is conveyed by the lingual branch of the mandibular nerve (V_3), while for the posterior one-third it is by the glossopharyngeal nerve (IX). Taste sensations from the anterior two-thirds are by the chorda tympani branch of the facial nerve (VII) and from the posterior one-third, including the circumvallate papillae, by the glossopharyngeal nerve.

Salivary Glands

These glands secrete their contents into the oral cavity; most are small glands in the submucosa/mucosa of the oral epithelium lining the tongue, palate, cheeks and lips opening directly via short ducts; in addition, there are three pairs of larger paired glands (parotid, submandibular, sublingual). The secretions (saliva) of the glands are a mixture of water, electrolytes, mucous, proteolytic enzymes (e.g., alpha-amylase, the initial step in the decomposition of starch), leukocytes, antibodies and lysozyme.

Parotid gland. The mainly serous parotid gland lies entirely outside the boundaries of the oral cavity (Fig. 4.35A), extending over masseter and the posterior belly of digastric; its duct (Stenson's duct) leaves the anterior border and passes over masseter, turns medially to pierce buccinator to open into the oral cavity opposite the upper 2nd molar tooth. It surrounds the external carotid artery, retromandibular vein and extracranial part of the

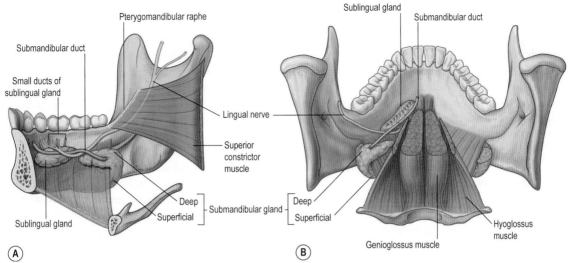

Fig. 4.77 The submandibular and sublingual glands viewed medially (A) and posteriorly (B).

facial nerve (VII). It receives its parasympathetic secretomotor innervation from the glossopharyngeal nerve (IX) via the otic ganglion and auriculotemporal branch of the mandibular nerve (V_3).

Submandibular gland. The mixed, but mainly serous, submandibular gland is partly outside (superficial part) and partly within (deep part) the mouth as it hooks around the posterior border of mylohyoid (Fig. 4.77): the superficial part lies in a shallow depression (submandibular fossa) on the medial side of the mandible below mylohyoid. The duct (Wharton's duct) leaves the deep part of the gland to open beside the base of the frenulum of the tongue; it has the lingual nerve looping around it during its course (Fig. 4.77). It receives its parasympathetic secretomotor innervation from the facial nerve (VII) via the chorda tympani and lingual branch of the mandibular nerve (V_3).

Sublingual gland. The small mixed, but mainly mucous, sublingual gland lies in the sublingual fossa on the medial surface of the anterior one-third of the mandible immediately lateral to the submandibular duct and lingual nerve in the floor of the mouth (Fig. 4.77); its numerous ducts open directly into the floor of the mouth. The parasympathetic secretomotor innervation is the same as for the submandibular gland.

Palate

The roof of the oral cavity is formed anteriorly by the hard palate and posteriorly by the soft palate (Fig. 4.73); the hard palate separates the mouth from the nasal cavity and is continuous with the soft palate posteriorly, which acts as a valve which can be depressed to help close the oropharyngeal isthmus or elevated to separate the nasopharynx from the oropharynx (page 326). The hard palate comprises the palatine process of the maxilla anteriorly and horizontal plate of the palatine bone posteriorly, while the soft palate is formed and moved by four pairs of muscles (tensor veli palatini, levator veli palatini, palatopharyngeus, palatoglossus) plus musculus uvulae in the midline. The soft palate is covered with mucous membrane continuous with that lining the pharynx, and oral and nasal cavities. Tensor and levator veli palatini tense and elevate the soft palate, respectively, while palatopharyngeus and palatoglossus depress it bringing the arches formed by each muscle towards the midline, as well as elevating the pharynx and back of the tongue, respectively.

Arterial supply, venous and lymphatic drainage and innervation

Arterial supply. By the greater palatine artery (branch of the maxillary artery), ascending palatine artery (branch of the facial artery) and palatine artery (branch of the ascending pharyngeal artery); the maxillary, facial and ascending pharyngeal arteries are all branches of the external carotid artery.

Venous and lymphatic drainage. Venous drainage is to the pterygoid venous plexus in the infratemporal fossa, while lymphatic drainage is to deep cervical nodes.

Innervation. The muscles of the soft palate are innervated by the vagus (X) via the pharyngeal plexus, except tensor veli palatini which is innervated by the mandibular branch (V_3) of the trigeminal nerve (V).

General sensation from the mucous membrane is by the greater and lesser palatine and nasopalatine nerves, which arise from the maxillary nerve (V_2) and pass through the pterygopalatine ganglion; the greater palatine nerve supplies the hard palate and gingiva as far as the 1st premolar, the nasopalatine nerve the mucosa and gingiva adjacent to the incisor and canines, and the lesser palatine nerve the soft palate.

Parasympathetic fibres to glands of the hard palate and taste from the soft palate are conveyed by a branch of the facial nerve (VII) via the pterygopalatine ganglion.

Oropharyngeal Isthmus

The opening between the mouth and oropharynx: it is formed by the palatoglossal arches laterally, the soft palate superiorly and the sulcus terminalis of the tongue inferiorly. It can be closed by elevation of the posterior part of the tongue, depression of the soft palate and medial movement of the palatoglossal arches towards the midline, together with medial movement of the palatopharyngeal arches; closing the isthmus is important for holding food and liquid in the mouth while breathing. Details of the pharynx can be found on page 326.

Ear

The ear has external, middle and inner parts, with the middle and inner parts being within the petrous part of the temporal bone; the auricle of the external ear is attached to the tympanic part of the temporal bone (Fig. 4.78).

External Ear

The external ear consists of the auricle and external auditory meatus (Fig. 4.78A). The auricle projects posterolaterally from the side of the head and collects the sound waves, conveying them towards the external auditory meatus and tympanic membrane; it is a single piece of cartilage, except for the fibrofatty lobule, covered with skin. Its shape is highly variable in adults, increasing three-fold in length from birth to adulthood; it also tends to increase in size and thickness in old age.

The external auditory meatus is cartilaginous in its outer one-third, being continuous with the auricle, and bony in its medial two-thirds, being formed by the tympanic part of the temporal bone: it is about 25 mm in length, with the inferior wall being 5 mm longer than the superior due to the obliquity of the tympanic membrane. The skin lining the meatus is firmly attached to the underlying tissue; the outer one-third contains numerous ceruminous (wax secreting) cells and hairs. The meatus lies behind the temporomandibular joint, with the mastoid air cells being immediately posterior.

Middle Ear

A narrow irregular air-filled space containing the three auditory ossicles (malleus, incus and stapes) is immediately medial to the tympanic membrane (Fig. 4.78A); for convenience, it can be considered a six-sided space. The space communicates with the nasopharynx (page 329) via the auditory (eustachian) tube opening into the anterior wall, and with the mastoid air cells via the aditus in the posterior wall (Fig. 4.78B).

The lateral wall is formed by the tympanic membrane, with the area above it being the epitympanic recess; the thin oval tympanic membrane forms the lateral wall of the middle ear and consists of three layers (modified skin externally; middle fibrous layer; inner mucous membrane). Its concave lateral surface is directed anteroinferiorly, with the umbo at the centre of the concavity; it has the malleus attached to its inner surface, conveying vibrations of the membrane to the auditory ossicles. The majority of the membrane is tense (pars tensa), except that part above the anterior and posterior malleolar folds (pars flaccida).

CLINICAL ANATOMY: The chorda tympani (branch of the facial nerve (VII)) conveys taste sensations from the anterior two-thirds of the tongue and preganglionic parasympathetic fibres to the submandibular ganglion; it lies between the external and middle layers of the tympanic membrane. Middle ear infections can create pressure on the tympanic membrane compressing the chorda tympani resulting in a temporary dulling or loss of taste.

In addition to the opening of the auditory tube, the anterior wall also has a blind-ending canal housing tensor tympani, which attaches to the malleus: tensor tympani is innervated by the mandibular nerve (V_3). The anterior wall is related inferiorly to the internal carotid artery.

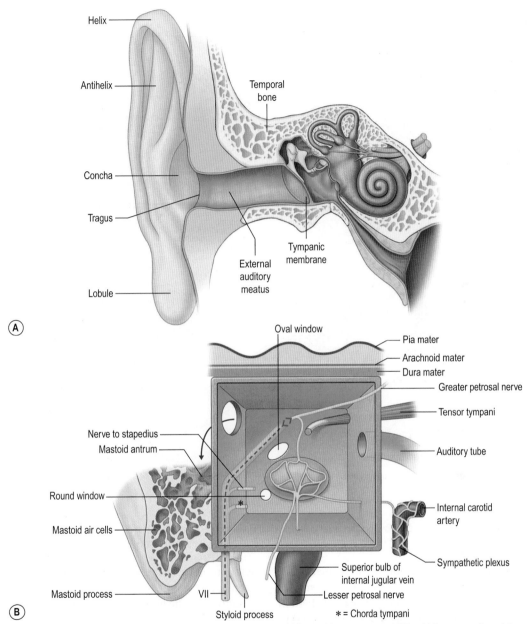

Fig. 4.78 Schematic representation of the (A) external, middle and inner ear; and (B) middle ear cavity with the tympanic membrane and auditory ossicles removed.

Separating the middle and inner ear is the medial wall, which has a rounded bulge (promontory), formed by the basal turn of the cochlea, and two openings (oval and round windows). On the surface of the promontory is the tympanic plexus derived from the tympanic branch of the glossopharyngeal nerve (IX), conveying preganglionic parasympathetic fibres, and sympathetic fibres from the internal carotid artery plexus. Above the promontory and oval window is the facial canal in which the facial nerve (VII) passes from the geniculate ganglion: the canal continues down the posterior wall to the stylomastoid foramen.

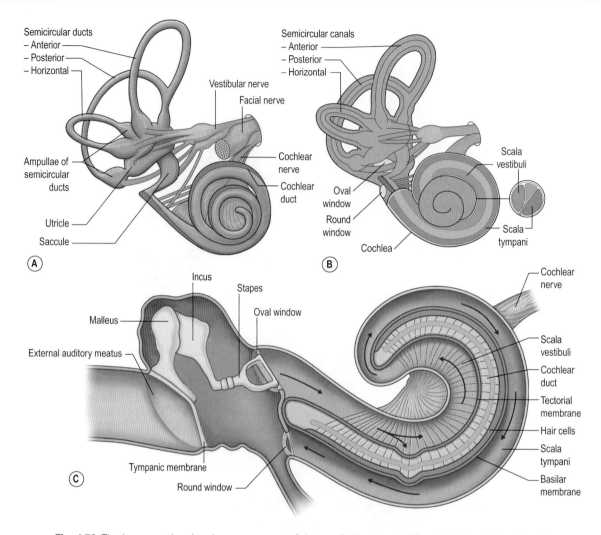

Fig. 4.79 The inner ear showing the arrangement of the vestibular system (A) and the labyrinth and spiral organ (B); (C) schematic representation of the conversion of sound waves into mechanical vibrations.

The posterior wall has the aditus and a small conical projection (pyramidal eminence), the inner surface of which gives attachment to stapedius, with its tendon emerging from the apex to attach to the stapes; stapedius is innervated by the facial nerve (VII).

> **APPLIED ANATOMY:** Tensor tympani and stapedius contract in response to loud noises reducing vibrations of the tympanic membrane and of stapes in the oval window.

The roof is formed by the thin tegmen tympani separating the middle ear from the middle cranial fossa and temporal lobe of the brain. The floor is formed by the jugular fossa of the temporal bone separating it from the beginning of the internal jugular vein (jugular bulb).

Inner Ear

The inner ear consists of a complex series of communicating bony chambers and spaces (vestibule, semicircular canals, cochlea), the bony labyrinth, lined by epithelium (membranous labyrinth) and filled with fluid (perilymph) (Fig. 4.79). Displacement of the fluid in the membranous labyrinth stimulates sensory endings in the lining epithelium. One part of the system of chambers and spaces is associated with maintaining balance and equilibrium (vestibule, semicircular canals) and the other with hearing (cochlea).

Balance and equilibrium. The vestibule, containing the utricle and saccule, and semicircular canals (anterior, posterior, horizontal) are associated with maintaining balance and equilibrium (Fig. 4.79A and B). The anterior and posterior semicircular canals are at right angles to each other and lie 45 degrees to the sagittal plane, with the anterior being anterior and lateral and the posterior being posterior and lateral; the horizontal canal lies horizontally. The membranous semicircular ducts are dilated at one end (ampulla) in which there is a thickening (ampullary crest) where the vestibular nerve endings terminate. The three ducts open into the utricle, which communicates with the cochlea. Thickenings of both the utricle and saccule (maculae) contain terminations of the vestibular nerve. The ampullary crests of the semicircular canals convey information about rotatory and angular movements of the head, whereas the maculae convey information about linear and tilting movements.

> **CLINICAL ANATOMY:** Diseases of the semicircular ducts, utricle and saccule give rise to varying degrees of giddiness.

Hearing. The bony cochlear consists of 2¾ turns of a spiral; it has a central supporting column of bone (modiolus) to which is attached a thin lamina of bone partly dividing the spiral into two parts, scala vestibuli above and scala tympani below (Fig. 4.79B and C). The membranous cochlear duct lines the bony cochlear, which is triangular in shape. The outer wall of the triangle is thickened forming the spiral ligament, the lower part of which is the basilar membrane and the upper part of the vestibular membrane. The specialised thickened spiral organ (organ of Corti) lies on the basilar membrane. Pulsations transmitted to the perilymph within the membranous cochlea by movement of the stapes in the oval window pass through the scala tympani and are transmitted to the fluid in the scala vestibuli, adjusted by compensatory movements of the membrane covering the round window; this causes movement of the basilar membrane stimulating hair cells of the spiral organ (Fig. 4.79C), resulting in auditory perception. Low-frequency sounds cause maximum activity in the basilar membrane, while high-frequency sounds are limited to the basal portion of the cochlea.

> **CLINICAL ANATOMY:** Hearing loss is a common problem often developing with increasing age or after prolonged exposure to loud noises; there are two main causes of hearing loss (conductive and sensorineural). Conductive hearing loss occurs when sounds are unable to pass from the tympanic membrane to the inner ear via the auditory ossicles, so that sounds are soft or muffled: it can be due to ear infections or allergies and is not always permanent. Sensorineural hearing loss is associated with damage to the inner ear or neural pathways, making sounds appear muffled or unclear; it can be due to birth defects, ageing, exposure to loud noises, trauma to the head, Meniere's disease (which also affects balance), acoustic neuroma, infections (measles, mumps, meningitis, scarlet fever) and is usually permanent.

NECK

Cervical Vertebrae

The seven cervical vertebrae provide the bony support for the neck; the upper two vertebrae are specialised supporting the head on the neck. Details of the cervical vertebrae can be found on page 193. The movements possible in the suboccipital and lower cervical regions of the neck, together with their associated ranges, can be found in Table 3.1.

In addition to the ligaments associated with the vertebral column, a number of small muscles help stabilise the head on the neck, as well as control the movements possible; to some extent, each of these small muscles acts as an extensible ligament.

Regions

The lateral and anterior aspects of the superficial neck are divided into posterior (Fig. 4.80A) and anterior triangles (Fig. 4.80B) by sternomastoid and further subdivided by other muscles, while deeper neck structures are contained within compartments, each surrounded by fascia (Fig. 4.81).

> **APPLIED ANATOMY:** Sternomastoid is the common boundary between the posterior and anterior triangles of the neck.

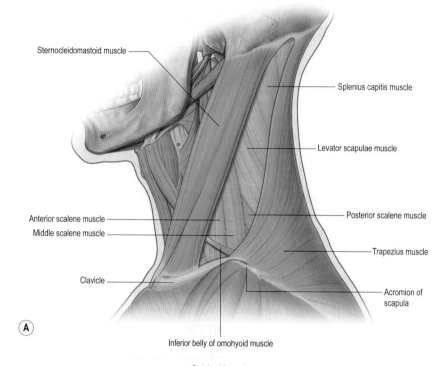

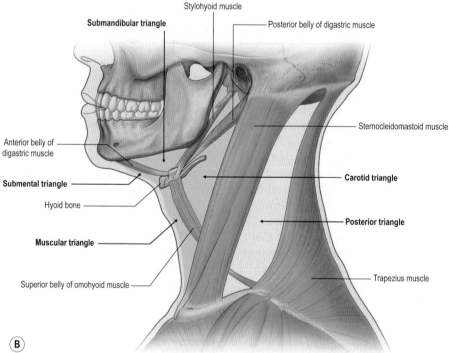

Fig. 4.80 The posterior (A) and anterior (B) triangles of the neck.

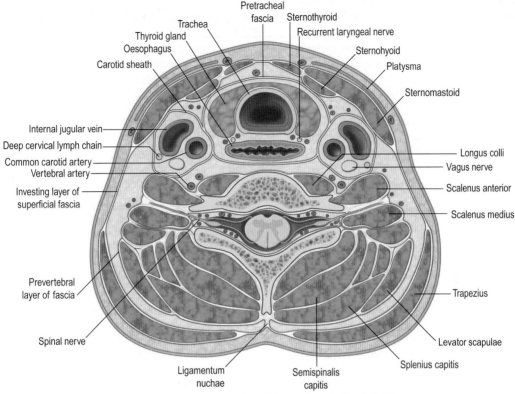

Fig. 4.81 Transverse section of the neck at the level of C6.

Posterior Triangle

The posterior triangle is bounded anteriorly by the posterior border of sternomastoid, posteriorly by the anterior border of trapezius, its base is the middle one-third of the clavicle and the apex is where sternomastoid and trapezius meet; it is subdivided by the inferior belly of omohyoid into occipital and supraclavicular (omoclavicular, subclavian) triangles. The muscular floor is covered by the deep fascia of the neck (prevertebral fascia) and the roof by the investing layer of deep fascia, which splits to enclose trapezius and sternomastoid; platysma, cutaneous branches of the cervical plexus and the external jugular vein all lies in the superficial fascia of the roof. From below upwards, the muscular floor comprises scalenus anterior, scalenus medius, scalenus posterior, levator scapulae, splenius capitis, and semispinalis capitis at the apex (Fig. 4.80A, Table 4.7).

Contents. The contents of the triangle lie between the prevertebral and investing layer of deep cervical fascia. The trunks of the brachial plexus and subclavian artery emerge

between scalenus anterior and medius in the lower part of the occipital triangle (Fig. 4.82); the upper and middle trunks lie above the artery and lower trunk posterior. Details of the brachial plexus can be found on page 398.

Arteries. The subclavian artery arises from the brachiocephalic trunk on the right and directly from the arch of the aorta on the left and passes over the 1st rib (Fig. 4.82) becoming the axillary artery at its lateral border. It is divided into three parts by scalenus anterior: the 1st part is medial and gives three branches (internal thoracic (mammary), vertebral artery, thyrocervical trunk); the 2nd part is behind and gives one branch (costocervical trunk, which divides into deep cervical and superior intercostal arteries); and the 3rd part is lateral and has no branches.

Other arteries in the lower part of the posterior triangle are the suprascapular and transverse cervical arteries both from the thyrocervical trunk; in the upper part of the triangle is the occipital artery (branch of the external carotid artery) which supplies the back of the skull.

TABLE 4.7   Muscles Associated With the Posterior Triangle of the Neck

Muscle	Attachments	Action	Innervation Root Value
Sternomastoid	From the upper part of the manubrium (sternal head) and upper surface of the medial one-third of the clavicle (clavicular head) to the lateral half of the superior nuchal line (sternal head) and lateral surface of the mastoid process (clavicular head)	Individually, it laterally flexes and rotates the head to the same side (bringing the ear to shoulder); together the sternal fibres flex the head and neck, while the clavicular fibres extend the head on the neck	The spinal part of the accessory nerve (XI), with proprioceptive fibres from C2, C3
Trapezius	See Table 5.1		
Semispinalis capitis	See Table 3.2		
Splenius capitis	From the lower part of the ligamentum nuchae and spinous processes of C7–T4 to the posterior aspect of the mastoid process and lateral one-third of the superior nuchal line	Individually extends the head and neck, laterally flexes the neck with rotation of the face to the same side; together they extend the head and neck	Posterior rami of C3–C5
Levator scapulae	See Table 5.1		
Scalenus posterior	From the posterior tubercles of C4–C6 to the outer surface of the 2nd rib	Individually each laterally flexes the neck to the same side; together they flex the neck	C6–C8
Scalenus medius	From the transverse processes of C1 and C2, posterior tubercles of C3–C7 to the upper surface of the 1st rib behind the subclavian groove	Individually each laterally flexes the neck to the same side; together they flex the neck	C3–C8
Scalenus anterior	From the anterior tubercles of C6–C3 to the scalene tubercle on the 1st rib	Individually each laterally flexes the neck to the same side; together they flex the neck	C4–C6
Omohyoid	See Table 4.8		

Veins. The subclavian vein lies anterior to scalenus anterior and the subclavian artery, situated mainly behind the clavicle, and joins with the internal jugular vein at the medial end of the clavicle to form the brachiocephalic vein; its only tributary is the external jugular vein. The external jugular vein is formed by the union of the posterior auricular vein and posterior division of the retromandibular vein (Fig. 4.83A) within the substance of the parotid gland, it receives the anterior jugular, transverse cervical and suprascapular veins; it pierces the deep fascia just above the clavicle.

Nerves. The cervical plexus has four cutaneous branches (greater auricular (C2, C3), lesser occipital (C2), transverse cervical (C2, C3), supraclavicular (C3, C4)), two sensory branches to muscles (sternomastoid (C2), trapezius (C3)), muscular branches to geniohyoid (C1), thyrohyoid (C1), rectus capitis lateralis (C1,C2), rectus capitis anterior (C1, C2), longus capitis (C1, C2, C3, C4), longus colli (C2, C3, C4), scalenus medius (C3, C4), levator scapulae (C3, C4), and via the ansa cervical (C1, C2, C3) to sternohyoid, sternothyroid and omohyoid; it also gives rise to the phrenic nerve (C3, C4, C5). The cutaneous nerves emerge around the posterior border of sternomastoid (Fig. 4.83B), while the accessory nerve (XI) passes obliquely across the floor of the posterior triangle on levator scapulae.

Anterior Triangle

The anterior triangle is bounded anteriorly by the midline of the neck, posteriorly by the anterior border of

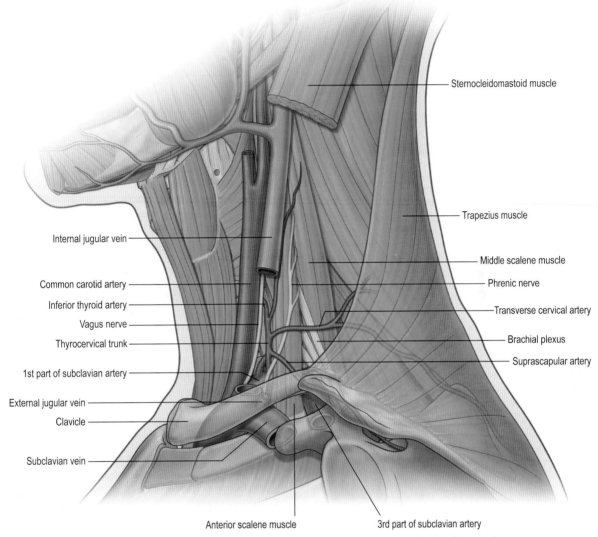

Internal jugular vein

Common carotid artery

Inferior thyroid artery

Vagus nerve

Thyrocervical trunk

1st part of subclavian artery

External jugular vein

Clavicle

Subclavian vein

Sternocleidomastoid muscle

Trapezius muscle

Middle scalene muscle

Phrenic nerve

Transverse cervical artery

Brachial plexus

Suprascapular artery

Anterior scalene muscle

3rd part of subclavian artery

Fig. 4.82 Major nerves and arteries associated with the posterior triangle of the neck.

sternomastoid, superiorly by the lower border of the mandible, with the apex at the medial end of the clavicle (Fig. 4.80B); it is subdivided into submental, submandibular (digastric), carotid and muscular triangles.

Submental triangle. Bounded inferiorly by the body of the hyoid, laterally by the anterior belly of digastric and medially by the midline of the neck, with the floor being mylohyoid (Fig. 4.84A, Table 4.8); it contains the submental lymph nodes, submental artery, nerve to mylohyoid and the beginning of the anterior jugular vein.

Submandibular triangle. Bounded superiorly by the lower border of the mandible, anteriorly and posteriorly by the anterior and posterior bellies of digastric, with the floor being mylohyoid anteriorly and hyoglossus posteriorly (Fig. 4.84A, Table 4.8); it contains the submandibular salivary gland and lymph nodes, facial artery and vein, hypoglossal nerve and nerve to mylohyoid.

Carotid triangle. Bounded anteroinferiorly by the superior belly of omohyoid, anterosuperiorly by the posterior belly of digastric and posteriorly by the anterior

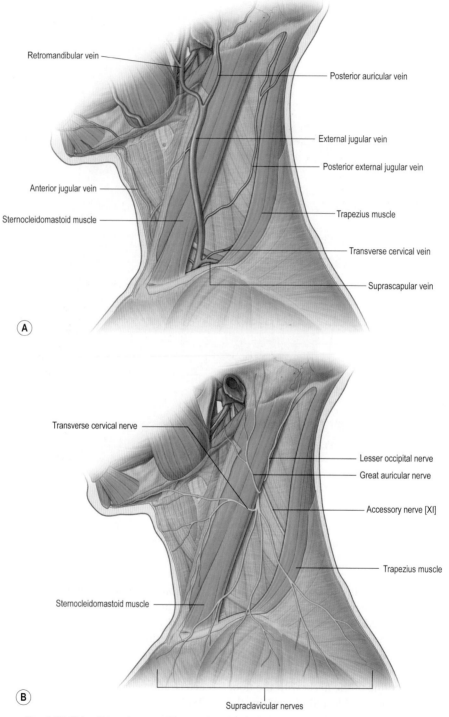

Retromandibular vein

Posterior auricular vein

External jugular vein

Posterior external jugular vein

Anterior jugular vein

Trapezius muscle

Sternocleidomastoid muscle

Transverse cervical vein

Suprascapular vein

(A)

Transverse cervical nerve

Lesser occipital nerve

Great auricular nerve

Accessory nerve [XI]

Trapezius muscle

Sternocleidomastoid muscle

Supraclavicular nerves

(B)

Fig. 4.83 Veins (A) and nerves (B) associated with the posterior triangle of the neck.

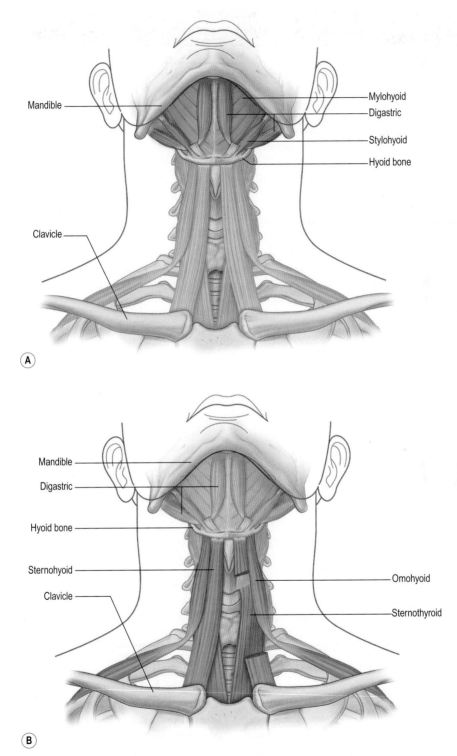

Fig. 4.84 Anterior aspect of the neck showing the suprahyoid (A) and infrahyoid (B) muscles.

TABLE 4.8   The Attachments, Action and Innervation of the Suprahyoid and Infrahyoid Muscles

Muscle	Attachments	Action	Innervation
Digastric	From the digastric fossa on the lower aspect of the medial side of the mandible (anterior belly) to the mastoid notch on the medial side of the mastoid process (posterior belly) via an intermediate tendon, which is bound by fascia to the body of the hyoid	Opens mouth by lowering mandible; raises hyoid bone	Anterior belly: nerve to mylohyoid (branch of the mandibular nerve (V_3) Posterior belly: facial nerve (VII)
Mylohyoid	From the mylohyoid line on the medial surface of the body of the mandible to the body of the hyoid: the fibres pass medially inserting into a midline raphe	Elevates the hyoid; supports and elevates the floor of the mouth	Nerve to mylohyoid (branch of the mandibular nerve (V_3))
Geniohyoid	From the inferior mental (genial) spine on the inner surface of the symphysis menti of the mandible to the anterior surface of the body of the hyoid	With the mandible fixed it elevates and pulls the hyoid forwards; with the hyoid fixed it pulls the mandible downwards and backwards	C1, which travels with the hypoglossal nerve (XII)
Stylohyoid	From the base of the styloid process to the lateral side of the body of the hyoid	Pulls hyoid upwards and backwards	Facial nerve (VII)
Omohyoid	From the transverse scapular ligament and adjacent border of the suprascapular notch (inferior belly) via an intermediate tendon (held down by a fascial sling to the clavicle and 1st rib) to the lower border of the body of the hyoid (superior belly)	Elevates hyoid or depresses mandible if hyoid is fixed	C1–C3 via the ansa cervicalis
Sternohyoid	From the back of the manubrium and medial end of the clavicle to the lower border of body of the hyoid	Depresses the hyoid during swallowing; fixes the hyoid during movements of the tongue	C1–C3 via the ansa cervicalis
Sternothyroid	From the back of the manubrium and 1st costal cartilage to the oblique ridge on lamina of the thyroid cartilage	Pulls the larynx down during the 2nd phase of swallowing	C1–C3 via the ansa cervicalis
Thyrohyoid	From the oblique ridge on the lamina of the thyroid cartilage to the lower border of the body of the hyoid	Depresses the hyoid; elevates the larynx when the hyoid is fixed	C1, which travels with the hypoglossal nerve (XII)

border of sternomastoid, with the floor being hyoglossus and thyrohyoid anteriorly and the middle and inferior constrictors of the pharynx posteriorly; it contains the common and internal carotid arteries, internal jugular vein, vagus (X) and deep cervical lymph chain enclosed within the carotid sheath (Fig. 4.82), and external carotid and its branches (superior thyroid, ascending pharyngeal, lingual, facial, occipital arteries), and the accessory (XI) and hypoglossal (XII) nerves outside the sheath.

Muscular triangle. Bounded anteriorly by the midline of the neck, posterosuperiorly by the superior belly of omohyoid, posteroinferiorly by the anterior border of sternomastoid; it contains the infrahyoid muscles (Fig. 4.84B, Table 4.8).

APPLIED ANATOMY: The ansa cervicalis is a loop of nerve fibres from C1 to C3 which lies outside, but around, the carotid sheath.

Compartments

Fascia. Superficial fascia completely surrounds the neck; it contains platysma (innervated by the facial nerve (VII)) which begins in the superficial fascia of the thorax, passes upwards to attach to the mandible and blends with the muscles of the face. The deep fascia is organised into a number of distinct layers (Fig. 4.81) by which the neck is organised into four longitudinal compartments. The investing layer of deep cervical fascia also completely surrounds the neck, splitting to enclose sternomastoid and trapezius; the prevertebral layer surrounds the vertebral column and its associated muscles; the pretracheal fascia encloses the viscera; and the carotid sheaths surround the neurovascular bundles either side of the neck (Fig. 4.81).

Investing layer. Attaches posteriorly to the ligamentum nuchae and C7 spine, anteriorly it merges with the fascia surrounding the infrahyoid muscles, superiorly to the external occipital protuberance and superior nuchal line, laterally to the mastoid process and zygomatic arch, and inferiorly to the spine of the scapula, acromion, clavicle and manubrium. It is pierced by the external and anterior jugular veins, and the lesser occipital, great auricular, transverse cervical and supraclavicular nerves.

Prevertebral layer. Attaches posteriorly to the ligamentum nuchae, superiorly to the external occipital protuberance and superior nuchal line, laterally to the mastoid process, and anteriorly to the basilar part of the occipital bone, the jugular foramen, carotid canal, anterior surfaces of the body and transverse process of C1–C7.

In the lower part of the posterior triangle the prevertebral layer extends from scalenus anterior and medius to surround the brachial plexus and subclavian artery as they pass into the axilla; this is the axillary sheath (page 398).

Pretracheal layer. A collection of fascias surrounding the larynx and trachea, pharynx and oesophagus and the thyroid gland. The pretracheal fascia encloses the infrahyoid muscles, thyroid gland (page 331) and covers the trachea: superiorly it begins at the hyoid and ends inferiorly in the upper thorax; posteriorly it is continuous with the fascia surrounding the oesophagus. Behind the pharynx it becomes the buccopharyngeal fascia separating the pharynx from the prevertebral layer; superiorly it begins at the base of the skull, merging with the fascia covering the oesophagus as it continues inferiorly into the thorax.

Carotid sheath. A fascial sheath surrounding the common and internal carotid arteries, internal jugular vein, vagus (X) and deep cervical lymph chain as they pass through the neck; it is in contact with the investing, prevertebral and pretracheal layers of fascia.

Fascial spaces. Between the fascial layers are spaces (pretracheal, retropharyngeal, within the prevertebral layer) which can provide a route for the spread of infection from the neck to the mediastinum (Fig. 4.85).

Pretracheal space. Lies between the investing layer on the posterior surface of the infrahyoid muscles and pretracheal fascia on the anterior surface of the trachea and thyroid gland; it passes between the neck and superior mediastinum.

Retropharyngeal space. Lies between the buccopharyngeal fascia on the back of the pharynx and oesophagus and the prevertebral fascia on the anterior surface of the bodies and transverse processes of the cervical vertebrae; it extends from the base of the skull to the upper part of the posterior mediastinum.

Space within the prevertebral layer. Lies in the prevertebral layer covering the anterior surface of the bodies and transverse processes of cervical vertebrae; it splits into two creating a space starting at the base of the skull extending through the posterior mediastinum to the diaphragm.

Hyoid

A U-shaped bone deficient posteriorly (Fig. 4.86) in the anterior neck between the tongue and larynx: it has a body and pairs of greater and lesser wings (horns, cornua). It is connected by muscles and ligaments to the tongue, mandible, styloid process, thyroid cartilage and sternum. The body is separated by cartilage from the greater wings until middle age and from the lesser wings until old age. By applying firm pressure, the greater horns can be felt through the skin below the mandible.

Being attached to the tongue it moves up and down during swallowing; because it is also firmly attached to the larynx by the thyrohyoid membrane when the hyoid moves upwards it carries the larynx with it.

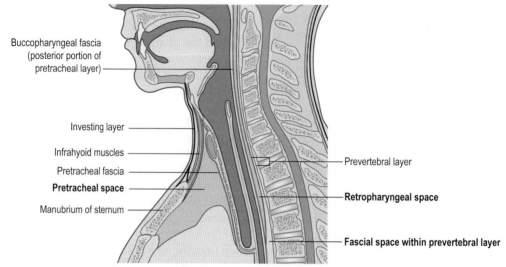

Fig. 4.85 Sagittal section showing the fascia and fascial spaces within the neck.

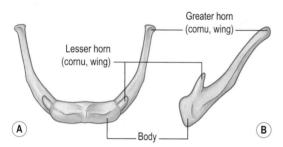

Fig. 4.86 Superior (A) and lateral (B) aspects of the hyoid.

Pharynx

A fibromuscular tube extending from the base of the skull to the cricoid cartilage (page 329) at the level of C6; the nasopharynx communicates anteriorly with the nasal cavity via the choanae, the oropharynx with the mouth via the oropharyngeal isthmus, and the laryngopharynx with larynx via the laryngeal inlet (Fig. 4.87). It is lined by respiratory epithelium (pseudostratified ciliated columnar) in the nasopharynx and stratified squamous epithelium in the oropharynx and laryngopharynx, outside which is the closely applied and supporting pharyngobasilar fascia, outside which is muscle enclosed within the buccopharyngeal fascia containing the pharyngeal plexus of nerves.

The mucous membrane lining the pharynx has different innervations in each region; in the nasopharynx it is by the maxillary nerve (V_2), in the oropharynx the glossopharyngeal nerve (IX), and in the laryngopharynx the vagus (X).

Pharyngeal muscles. There are three pairs of circularly arranged muscles (superior, middle and inferior constrictor) and three pairs of longitudinally arranged muscles (palatopharyngeus, stylopharyngeus and salpingopharyngeus). The constrictor muscles overlap from above downwards and when they contract push the bolus of food or liquid through the pharynx into the oesophagus; however, that part of inferior constrictor attached to the cricoid cartilage (cricopharyngeus) acts as a sphincter between the pharynx and oesophagus by maintaining tonic contraction. The longitudinal muscles act to raise the pharynx during swallowing. The pharyngeal muscles are innervated by the vagus (X) via the pharyngeal plexus, except stylopharyngeus which is innervated by the glossopharyngeal nerve (IX).

> **APPLIED ANATOMY:** Above superior constrictor the gap between it and the base of the skull is closed by the pharyngobasilar fascia through which the auditory tube passes. Stylopharyngeus and the glossopharyngeal nerve (IX) pass through the gap between superior and middle constrictor. The internal laryngeal nerve (branch of the vagus (X)) and superior laryngeal artery (branch of the superior thyroid artery) pass through the gap between middle and inferior constrictor.

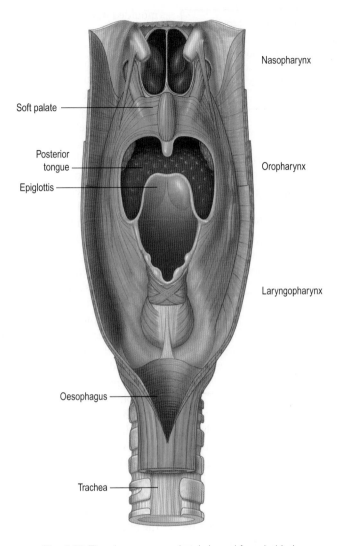

Fig. 4.87 The pharynx opened and viewed from behind.

Labels on figure:
Nasopharynx
Soft palate
Posterior tongue
Epiglottis
Oropharynx
Laryngopharynx
Oesophagus
Trachea

Nasopharynx. Extends from the base of the skull to the soft palate, functionally being part of the respiratory system and is always open: superiorly it is related to the body of the sphenoid and its sinus. It has the opening of the auditory (eustachian) tube opposite the inferior concha, which has a prominent elevation (tubal elevation) on its posterosuperior aspect; a vertical fold descends from the elevation, behind which is a narrow space (pharyngeal recess). Beneath the epithelium of the posterior wall is a collection of lymphoid tissue (pharyngeal tonsil, adenoids).

Auditory tube. A bony and cartilaginous tube connecting the nasopharynx and middle ear, which pierces the pharyngobasilar fascia at the base of the skull above superior constrictor; it enables the middle ear to maintain ambient air pressure. The cartilaginous anterior two-thirds lies in a groove at the skull base and opens into the nasopharynx; it is normally closed, being open only during swallowing and yawning by the actions of tensor and levator veli palatini attached to it. The bony posterior one-third lies in the petrous part of the temporal bone and opens into the middle ear cavity; it is always open.

CLINICAL ANATOMY: The auditory tube provides a path for the spread of respiratory infections and infections of the pharyngeal tonsils to the middle ear. Prior to age 10, the tube is almost horizontal, becoming more oblique in adulthood; middle ear infections tend to decrease after age 10.

Oropharynx. Extends from the soft palate to the upper border of the epiglottis anterior to the bodies of C2 and C3; it is shared by the respiratory and digestive systems conducting air during breathing and food and liquid during swallowing.

Palatine tonsil. An accumulation of lymphoid tissue in the tonsillar fossa between the palatoglossal and palatopharyngeal arches lying on superior constrictor: the internal carotid artery lies deep to the floor of the fossa.

CLINICAL ANATOMY: When enlarged, the palatine tonsil may impair breathing; it is prominent in children, regressing with age. Together with the pharyngeal and lingual tonsils, it forms a ring of lymphoid tissue (Waldeyer ring) at the entrance to the nasopharynx and oropharynx.

Laryngopharynx. Extends from the upper border of the epiglottis to the lower border of the cricoid cartilage where it becomes continuous with the oesophagus (page 87); it lies posterior to the larynx and anterior to C4, C5 and C6. The recess between the tongue and the epiglottis is the vallecular.

Piriform fossa. That part of the laryngopharynx lying lateral to the larynx; immediately lateral to the fossa is the carotid sheath. Food or foreign bodies may lodge in the fossa, with sharp objects (fish bones) potentially penetrating the wall and impinging on structures within the carotid sheath.

CLINICAL ANATOMY: The internal laryngeal nerve lies below the mucosa of the piriform fossa, where it can be anaesthetised.

Swallowing. Food is broken down into smaller fragments by the movements of the mandible and grinding of opposing teeth, as well as the action of salivary enzymes starting to digest the food so that it can be moulded into a soft manageable bolus that can be swallowed. Once a suitable consistency has been achieved the bolus is collected in the anterior part of the mouth by the tip of the tongue and pressed backwards between the tongue and hard palate towards the oropharynx, the floor of the mouth is raised by mylohyoid elevating the hyoid and pulling it forwards to widen the pharynx ready to receive the bolus. At the same time, the soft palate is tensed and elevated to prevent food and/or liquid from entering the nasopharynx and nasal cavity. When the bolus of food passes the palatoglossal arches, they are brought together closing the oropharyngeal isthmus preventing food from returning to the mouth. Once the bolus makes contact with the pharyngeal wall the swallowing reflex is initiated.

Elevation of the tongue and hyoid closes the laryngeal inlet preventing food from entering the airways: the bolus of food slides over the surface of the epiglottis into the piriform fossa of the laryngopharynx. Respiration is reflexly inhibited by closure of the nasopharynx above and laryngeal inlet below as the pharyngeal constrictors successively push the bolus of food towards the oesophagus, and the longitudinal pharyngeal muscles elevate the larynx and pharynx in readiness to receive the bolus: cricopharyngeus relaxes to allow the bolus to enter the oesophagus. When the bolus has passed the laryngeal inlet the hyoid and larynx are pulled down to their resting position: breathing is then resumed.

Swallowing liquids is essentially similar, except that in the initial stages the tongue forms a longitudinal furrow along which the fluid flows; it is forced backwards by the tongue to flow over the sides of the epiglottis into the piriform fossae.

APPLIED ANATOMY: Six cranial nerves are involved in the coordination of chewing and swallowing: mandibular nerve (V$_3$) innervates the muscles of mastication; hypoglossal nerve (XII) innervates muscles of the tongue; vagus (X) and accessory (XI) nerves innervate muscles of the soft palate and pharynx; facial (VII) and glossopharyngeal (IX) nerves convey taste from the anterior two-thirds and posterior one-third of the tongue.

Larynx

The larynx is formed by a framework of cartilages maintained by membranes and muscles (Fig. 4.88); it is firmly anchored to the hyoid. The intrinsic muscles act

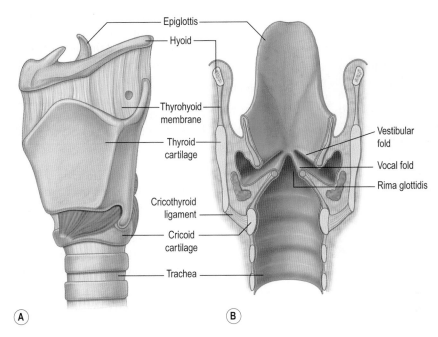

Fig. 4.88 (A) Components of the larynx. (B) Coronal section viewed posteriorly.

primarily as sphincters protecting the lower respiratory tract, as well moving the vocal chords (ligaments, folds) during respiration and speech (phonation); the vocal chords regulate the flow of air during speech and accommodate the normal variations associated with expiration and inspiration. The larynx is continuous inferiorly with the trachea (page 94).

The framework of the larynx comprises three large unpaired cartilages (epiglottis, thyroid and cricoid) and three pairs of smaller cartilages (arytenoid, corniculate and cuneiform).

Epiglottis. A leaf-shaped fibroelastic cartilage (Fig. 4.88B) attached to the posterior surface of the thyroid cartilage where the two laminae meet; it lies posterior to the root of the tongue and above the laryngeal inlet.

Thyroid cartilage. The largest cartilage with each lamina meeting anteriorly forming a V-shaped notch (90 degrees in males, 120 degrees in females); in males, the notch forms the midline laryngeal prominence which becomes more prominent after puberty (Adam's apple). Each lamina has a pair of horns (superior, inferior): the superior horn is connected to the greater horn of the hyoid by the thyrohyoid ligament and lateral thickening of the thyrohyoid membrane, the inferior horn articulates

with the cricoid cartilage by the synovial cricothyroid joint. It is attached superiorly to the hyoid by the thyrohyoid membrane and inferiorly to the cricoid by the cricothyroid ligament (Fig. 4.88). On the outer surface of each lamina is an oblique line for muscle attachments (inferior constrictor, sternothyroid, thyrohyoid).

Cricoid cartilage. Ring-shaped with a narrow anterior arch and wide posterior lamina (Fig. 4.89) lying at the level of C6; superiorly it is attached to the thyroid cartilage by the cricothyroid membrane and inferiorly to the 1st tracheal ring by the cricotracheal ligament. It articulates with the inferior horn of the thyroid cartilage by the synovial cricothyroid joint and by its lamina with the arytenoid cartilages by synovial cricoarytenoid joints (Fig. 4.89).

Arytenoid cartilages. Paired hyaline cartilages pyramidal in shape situated on the upper surface of the cricoid lamina: the apex is superior; the base inferior forming the synovial cricoarytenoid joint; the muscular process extends laterally from the base giving muscle attachments (posterior and lateral cricoarytenoid); the vocal process extends anteriorly from the base giving attachment to thyroarytenoid and the vocal ligament (Fig. 4.89).

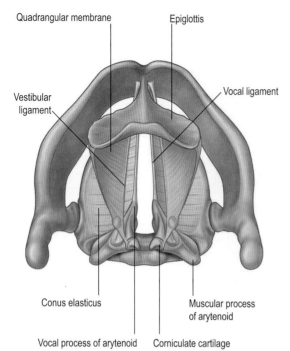

Fig. 4.89 Superior view of the laryngeal cartilages also showing the vestibular and vocal ligaments.

Corniculate and cuneiform cartilages. Small, paired cartilages within the aryepiglottic fold, with the cuneiform lying above the corniculate cartilage.

Membranes and ligaments

Thyrohyoid membrane. The tough fibrous thyrohyoid membrane, thickened in the midline (median thyrohyoid ligament), connects the upper border of the thyroid cartilage to the lower border of the hyoid; it is pierced by the internal laryngeal nerve (branch of the superior laryngeal nerve) and superior laryngeal artery (branch of the superior thyroid artery).

Cricothyroid membrane. Attached to the arch of the cricoid it extends superiorly deep to the thyroid cartilage between the mucous membrane and thyroarytenoid as the conus elasticus; it is thickened along its upper free border forming the **vocal ligament**, which attaches to the vocal process of the arytenoid cartilage and also contains the vocalis muscle.

Quadrangular membrane. Lies in the lateral margin of the epiglottis and anterolateral surface of the arytenoid cartilage of the same side (Fig. 4.88); it has free upper and lower margins, with the lower free border being thickened to form the vestibular ligament. Between

the vestibular and vocal ligaments is a gap (laryngeal vestibule) which extends anterosuperiorly between the vestibular fold and thyroid cartilage (laryngeal saccule); mucous secreted from cells within the saccules lubricate the vocal folds.

> **APPLIED ANATOMY:** When viewed from above the vestibular ligaments lie lateral to the vocal ligaments.

Muscles. The intrinsic muscles of the larynx function to close the laryngeal inlet and move the vocal cords to control the flow of air by opening and closing the rima glottidis: the regulation of airflow produces sounds. The rima glottidis is the interval between the paired vocal cords anteriorly and the arytenoid cartilages posteriorly; it is the narrowest part of the laryngeal cavity.

> **CLINICAL ANATOMY:** Obstruction of the laryngeal airway at the rima glottidis may result from aspirated food or oedema in the mucosa due to an allergic reaction. In emergencies, an opening can be made through the cricothyroid membrane to provide an airway below the level of the vocal cords.

The action of the intrinsic laryngeal muscles on the vocal cords is as follows:
- **Increased length/tension** by rotation of the thyroid cartilage anteroinferiorly with respect to the cricoid cartilage: **cricothyroid**
- **Decreased length/tension** by pulling the thyroid cartilage towards the arytenoid cartilages: **thyroarytenoid**
- Varying the **length/tension** and **thickness** of the vocal cords: **vocalis**
- **Abduction** and **external rotation** of the arytenoid cartilages on the upper surface of the cricoid lamina (increasing the size of the rima glottidis): **posterior cricoarytenoid**
- **Adduction** and **internal rotation** of the arytenoid cartilages on the upper surface of the cricoid lamina (decreasing the size of the rima glottidis: **lateral cricoarytenoid, transverse arytenoid, oblique arytenoid**

All intrinsic muscles are innervated by the recurrent laryngeal nerve (branch of the vagus (X)), except cricothyroid, which is innervated by the external laryngeal nerve (branch of the superior laryngeal nerve from the vagus (X)). Above the level of the vocal cords, the mucous membrane lining the larynx is supplied by the internal laryngeal nerve (branch of the superior laryngeal nerve) and below by the recurrent laryngeal nerve. The blood supply to the upper part of the larynx is from the superior laryngeal artery (branch of the superior thyroid artery from the external carotid artery), which anastomoses with the inferior laryngeal artery (branch of the inferior thyroid artery from the thyrocervical trunk of the subclavian artery).

Thyroid Gland

> **DEVELOPMENT:** The thyroid gland arises from the endodermal lining of the floor of the pharynx as a median outgrowth at the apex of the sulcus terminalis (foramen caecum); the thyroglossal duct marks the path of the thyroid gland to its final adult position. The duct usually disappears in early development; however, remnants may persist along its length (cyst presenting as a midline mass) or as a connection to the foramen caecum or anterior neck (fistula). Consequently, functional thyroid tissue may be associated with the posterior one-third of the tongue (lingual thyroid), anywhere along the path of migration of the gland, or project upwards from the gland along the path of the thyroglossal duct (pyramidal lobe).

The thyroid gland lies deep to the infrahyoid muscles in the anterior neck below and lateral to the thyroid cartilage enclosed within the pretracheal fascia (Fig. 4.81); because the pretracheal fascia is attached to the thyroid cartilage the thyroid gland moves upwards with the larynx during swallowing. It consists of two lateral lobes, covering the anterolateral surface of the trachea, cricoid cartilage and lower part of the thyroid cartilage, joined by an isthmus which lies anterior to the 2nd, 3rd and 4th tracheal rings (Fig. 4.90). On the posterior aspect of the gland are two pairs (superior, inferior) of parathyroid glands (Fig. 4.90B). Details of the endocrine function of the thyroid and parathyroid glands can be found on pages 341 and 343.

> **CLINICAL ANATOMY:** Enlargement of the thyroid (goitre) may indicate either hypothyroidism or hyperthyroidism. Hypothyroidism can be caused by insufficient dietary iodine or by an inherited autoimmune disease (Hashimoto thyroiditis); it is characterised by mental and physical sluggishness. Hyperthyroidism (Graves' disease) is caused by excessive amounts of thyroid hormones released into the circulation; it is characterised by weight loss, excessive sweating, tachycardia, nervousness, protrusion of the eyeballs and retraction of the eyelids, and an enlarged thyroid.

Arterial supply, venous and lymphatic drainage

Arterial supply. Two major arteries (superior and inferior thyroid) supply the thyroid gland; it is drained by three veins (superior, middle and inferior thyroid) (Fig. 4.90A). The superior thyroid artery (1st branch of the external carotid artery) descends towards the superior pole of the lateral lobe dividing into anterior and posterior branches: the anterior branches anastomose across the isthmus and posterior branches anastomose with branches of the inferior thyroid artery. The inferior thyroid artery (branch of the thyrocervical trunk from the subclavian artery) ascends behind the carotid sheath towards the inferior pole of the lateral lobe, where it divides into several branches (Fig. 4.90B). When a pyramidal lobe is present a small artery (thyroidea ima from the brachiocephalic trunk or aortic arch) ascends anterior to the trachea.

> **CLINICAL ANATOMY:** The external laryngeal nerve lies close to the superior thyroid artery, while the recurrent laryngeal nerve passes between the terminal branches of the inferior thyroid artery; these relationships are important when ligation of the arteries is necessary during thyroid surgery, as damage to the recurrent laryngeal nerve (even on one side) can have profound effects on the quality of the voice.

Venous drainage. The paired superior and middle thyroid veins drain into the internal jugular vein, and the single inferior thyroid vein drains the venous plexus associated with the isthmus into the left brachiocephalic vein.

Lymphatic drainage. To pretracheal nodes and deep cervical nodes below omohyoid along the internal jugular vein.

Root of the Neck

The root of the neck is the transition between the thorax, neck and upper limb, with structures passing from one region to another; it also contains an upward projection of the pleural cavity (apical part of the superior lobe of the lung) on each side.

Vessels. The subclavian arteries and veins on each side arch upwards out of the thorax into the neck giving off the vertebral artery, thyrocervical trunk, internal thoracic artery and costocervical trunk (Fig. 4.91); small veins accompany the arteries, while larger veins (internal and external jugular, brachiocephalic) form major drainage channels.

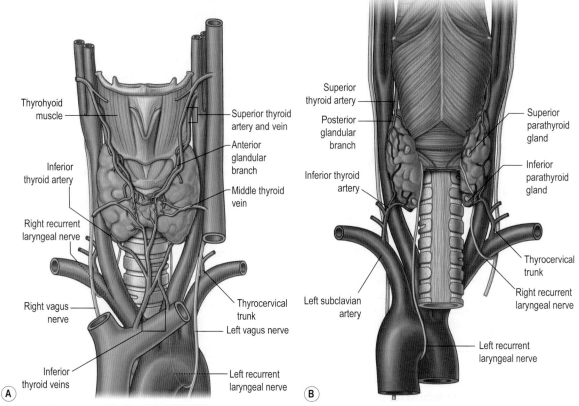

Thyrohyoid muscle

Superior thyroid artery and vein

Anterior glandular branch

Inferior thyroid artery

Middle thyroid vein

Right recurrent laryngeal nerve

Right vagus nerve

Thyrocervical trunk

Left vagus nerve

Inferior thyroid veins

Left recurrent laryngeal nerve

(A)

Superior thyroid artery

Posterior glandular branch

Inferior thyroid artery

Superior parathyroid gland

Inferior parathyroid gland

Left subclavian artery

Thyrocervical trunk

Right recurrent laryngeal nerve

Left recurrent laryngeal nerve

(B)

Fig. 4.90 Anterior (A) and posterior (B) views of the thyroid gland showing the associated blood vessels and nerves.

The thoracic duct on the left (Fig. 4.92) and right lymph trunk on the right drain into the junction of the internal jugular and subclavian vein; these are the major lymphatic vessels returning lymph from the whole of the body to the circulation.

Nerves. The phrenic nerves pass around the lateral border of scalenus anterior across its anterior surface passing between the subclavian artery (posterior) and subclavian vein (anterior) to enter the thorax (Fig. 4.93).

The vagus nerves (X) descend in the carotid sheath between the common carotid artery and internal jugular vein and enter the thorax by passing anterior to the subclavian artery and posterior to the subclavian vein (Fig. 4.93); during their course, they give off the recurrent laryngeal nerves supplying muscles of the larynx.

The sympathetic chain (Fig. 4.93) passes from the thorax into the neck lying posteromedial to the carotid sheath, while the trunks of the brachial plexus pass from

the neck into the upper limb in association with the subclavian artery (Fig. 4.92).

Other structures. Posteriorly are the oesophagus and trachea, as well as various muscles and ligaments associated with the vertebral column.

> **CLINICAL ANATOMY:** Penetrating wounds immediately above the clavicle can result in trauma to any of the structures above, some of which may be fatal.

> **CLINICAL ANATOMY:** The following structures can be felt in the midline of the neck from above downwards: mylohyoid raphe; body of the hyoid; thyrohyoid membrane; thyroid cartilage; cricothyroid ligament; cricoid cartilage; cricotracheal ligament; 1st tracheal ring (cartilage); isthmus of thyroid gland; suprasternal notch.

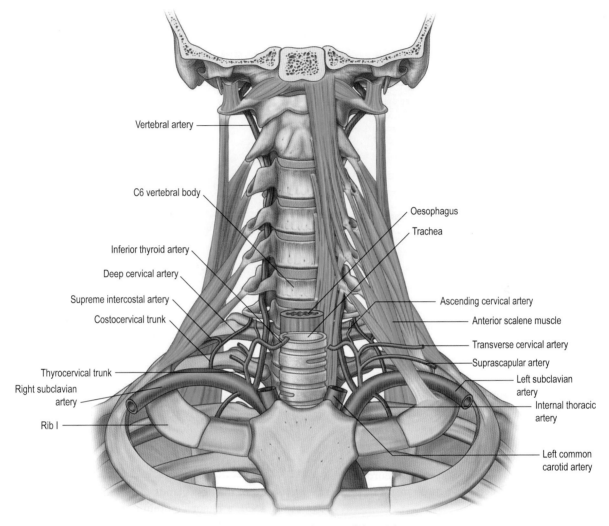

Vertebral artery

C6 vertebral body

Oesophagus

Trachea

Inferior thyroid artery

Deep cervical artery

Supreme intercostal artery

Costocervical trunk

Ascending cervical artery

Anterior scalene muscle

Transverse cervical artery

Suprascapular artery

Thyrocervical trunk

Right subclavian artery

Left subclavian artery

Internal thoracic artery

Rib I

Left common carotid artery

Fig. 4.91 Arteries in the root of the neck.

ENDOCRINE SYSTEM

All physiological activities of the body are regulated by either the nervous or endocrine systems, which interact, whereby cells communicate with each other; the endocrine system does this by secreting chemical substances (hormones). There are a number of ways in which communication between cells occurs. Intercellular communication (cell-to-cell signalling, cell signalling) occurs when information is transferred from one cell to another by chemical messengers, which are mainly secreted by endocrine glands, although some are secreted by nerve endings and cells of other tissues: the signalling (controlling) cells sends information to the target cells.

Chemical messengers are generally classified into two types (classical hormones secreted by endocrine glands; local hormones secreted by other tissues). They can also be considered as: endocrine messengers (e.g., growth hormone, insulin) are classical hormones; paracrine messengers (e.g., prostaglandins, histamine) are local hormones which diffuse from control to target cells through the interstitial fluid, with some substances entering the target cell through gap junctions; autocrine messengers (e.g., leukotrienes) are intracellular mediators which control the source cells which secrete them; and neurocrine messengers are neurotransmitters (e.g., acetylcholine, dopamine) carrying information between nerve cells or between nerve and muscle (or other

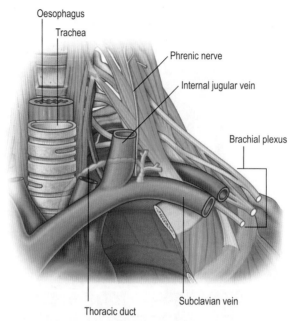

Oesophagus

Trachea

Phrenic nerve

Internal jugular vein

Brachial plexus

Subclavian vein

Thoracic duct

Fig. 4.92 Left side of the root of the neck showing the thoracic duct and brachial plexus associated with the subclavian artery.

tissue) cells, and neurohormones released by the nerve cell directly into the blood and transported to the target cells (e.g., oxytocin, ADH, hypothalamic-releasing hormone) (Fig. 4.94). Some substances act as more than one type of messenger: noradrenaline and dopamine function as classical hormones as well as neurotransmitters, while histamine acts as a neurotransmitter and as a paracrine messenger.

Hormones

Hormones are synthesised by endocrine glands and are of three types: steroid hormones are synthesised from cholesterol and its derivatives and secreted by the adrenal cortex, gonads and placenta; protein hormones are secreted by the pituitary, parathyroid glands, pancreas and placenta; and tyrosine (an amino acid) derivatives secreted by the thyroid and adrenal medulla. The classification of hormones depending on whether they are steroid or protein hormones or are derived from tyrosine is shown in Table 4.9.

Hormones bind with receptors (large proteins) present on the cell membrane, within the cytoplasm or within the nucleus of the target cells forming a hormone-receptor complex: depending on where the receptor is located the complex either alters the permeability of the cell membrane, activates intracellular enzymes or acts on genes; each receptor is specific for a single hormone.

ENDOCRINE GLANDS

A series of ductless glands form the endocrine system (Fig. 4.95), a major communicating system regulating and coordinating various body functions by synthesising and releasing hormones into the bloodstream; they play an important role in homeostasis and the control of various functions. The endocrine system comprises the pituitary (hypophysis), thyroid, parathyroid and adrenal (suprarenal) glands, the pancreas (islets of Langerhans) and gonads (testes in males, ovaries in females), with other regions (hypothalamus, kidneys, digestive tract, thymus, pineal gland) also having endocrine functions.

> **CLINICAL PHYSIOLOGY:** Hyperactivity or hypoactivity of an endocrine gland can lead to various disorders depending on the specific gland and its secretion(s): these changes often manifest themselves via signs and symptoms, which can then be addressed.

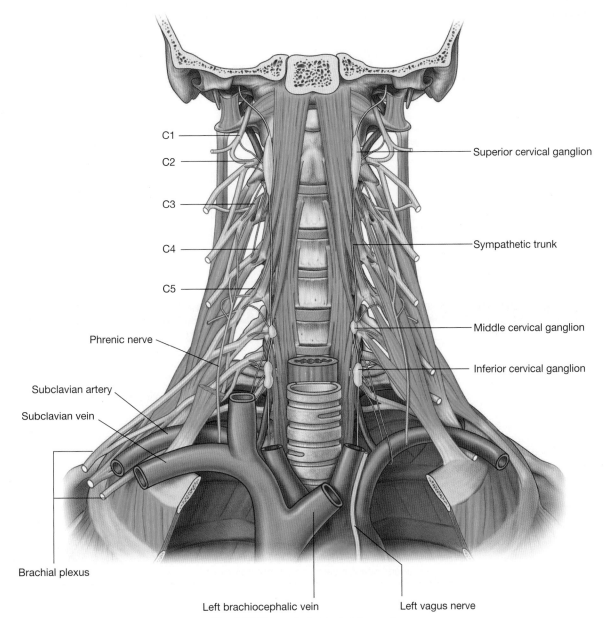

C1
C2
C3
C4
C5
Phrenic nerve
Subclavian artery
Subclavian vein
Brachial plexus

Superior cervical ganglion
Sympathetic trunk
Middle cervical ganglion
Inferior cervical ganglion

Left brachiocephalic vein   Left vagus nerve

Fig. 4.93 Nerves in the root of the neck.

Pituitary Gland

A small gland with two lobes (anterior (adenohypophysis) and posterior (neurohypophysis)) situated within the pituitary fossa on the superior surface of the body of the sphenoid; it is connected to the hypophysis by the infundibulum (Fig. 4.96A). Further details of the gross anatomy and neural connections of the pituitary gland can be found on page 255.

The hypothalamo-hypophyseal portal system of blood vessels (Fig. 4.96B) transports hormones from the hypothalamus to the anterior and posterior lobes, but hormones from the hypothalamus to the posterior lobe are transported by nerve fibres via the hypothalamo-hypophyseal tract (Fig. 4.96C). The two parts of the pituitary gland produce a number of different hormones which act on different target glands or cells;

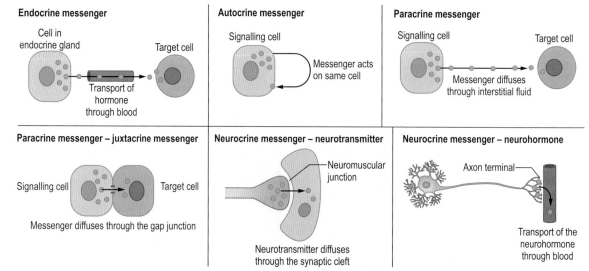

Fig. 4.94 Different types of chemical messengers.

TABLE 4.9 Hormone Classification According to Their Derivation		
Steroid Derivatives	**Protein Derivatives**	**Tyrosine Derivatives**
Aldosterone	Growth hormone (GH)	Thyroxine (T_4)
11-deoxycorticosterone	Thyroid-stimulating hormone (TSH)	Triiodothyronine (T_3)
Cortisol	Adrenocorticotropic hormone (ACTH)	Adrenaline/epinephrine
Corticosterone	Follicle-stimulating hormone (FSH)	Noradrenaline/norepinephrine
Testosterone	Luteinising hormone (LH)	Dopamine
Dihydrotestosterone	Prolactin	
Dehydroepiandrosterone	Antidiuretic hormone (ADH)	
Androstenedione	Oxytocin	
Oestrogen	Parathormone	
Progesterone	Calcitonin	
	Insulin	
	Glucagon	
	Somatostatin	
	Pancreatic polypeptide	
	Human chorionic gonadotropin (hCG)	
	Human chorionic somatomammotropin	

consequently, it is often considered the 'master' gland of the endocrine system.

The adenohypophysis contains two types of cells in equal proportions: chromophobe cells are precursors of chromophil cells, they do not secrete, while chromophil cells are secretory. There are five types of chromophil cells: somatotropes secrete growth hormone (GH); corticotropes secrete adrenocorticotropic hormone (ACTH); thyrotropes secrete thyroid-stimulating hormone (TSH); gonadotropes secrete follicle-stimulating hormone (FSH) and LH; and lactotropes secrete prolactin (PRL). GH stimulates the secretory activity of the liver and other tissues, while the remaining hormones all exert their effects on other endocrine glands.

The neurohypophysis consists of pituicytes (derived from glial cells, they do not secrete) and unmyelinated nerve fibres, as well as numerous blood vessels; antidiuretic hormone (ADH) and oxytocin released from the posterior pituitary are synthesised in the hypothalamus and transported to the neurohypophysis through the hypothalamo-hypophyseal tract.

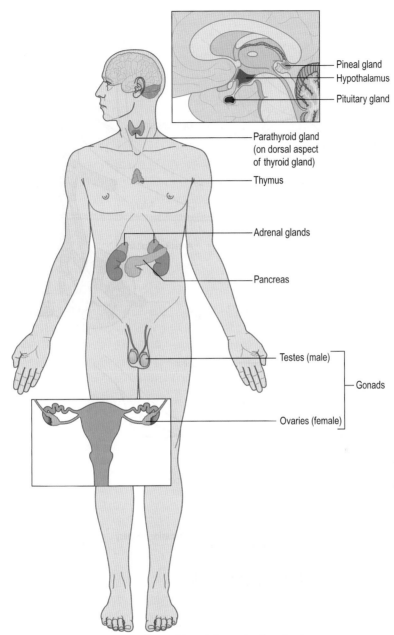

Fig. 4.95 The position of the endocrine glands.

The target organs/glands for each of the above hormones released by the pituitary gland, together with their action, are shown in Table 4.10.

Growth Hormone

As well as its effects on growth, achieved by increasing the size and number of cells by mitosis, GH also causes specific differentiation of certain cell types (bone, muscle), and influences the metabolism of the three major food types by increasing the synthesis of proteins, mobilising fats from adipose tissue, and conserves glucose in carbohydrates. In bone, GH: increases the synthesis and deposition of proteins by chondrocytes and osteogenic cells, as well as enhancing intestinal calcium absorption

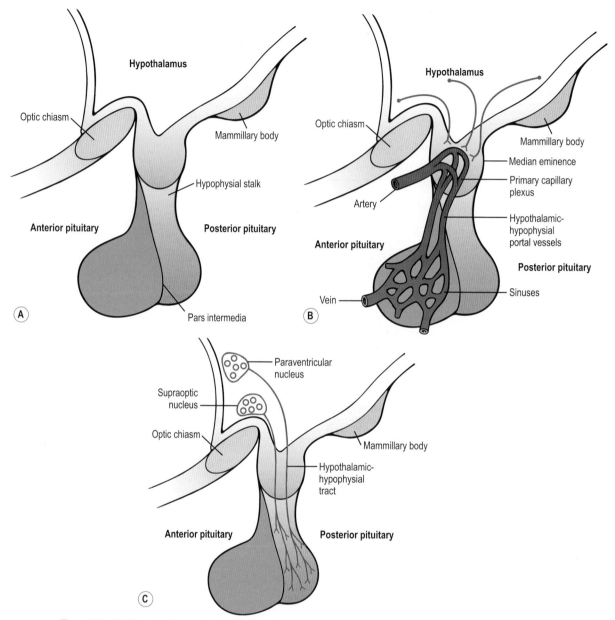

Fig. 4.96 (A) The pituitary gland. (B) Hypothalamo-hypophyseal portal system of blood vessels. (C) Hypothalamo-hypophyseal tracts.

to increase their numbers; promotes the conversion of chondrocytes into osteogenic cells; and makes calcium available for bone mineralisation.

Regulation of growth hormone secretion. Secretion is stimulated by hypoglycaemia, fasting, starvation, exercise, stress and trauma, and the initial stages of sleep, while it is inhibited by hyperglycaemia, increased free fatty acids in blood, and the later stages of sleep. It is regulated by various factors, with the hypothalamus and negative feedback mechanisms having important roles. The hypothalamus regulates secretion via: growth hormone–releasing hormone (GHRH) by stimulating the somatotropes in the adenohypophysis; growth hormone-releasing polypeptide (GHRP) by increasing

TABLE 4.10 The Target Organs/Glands for Each of the Hormones Secreted by the Pituitary Gland, Together With Its Action

Hormone	Target	Function
Adrenocorticotropic hormone (ACTH): also known as corticotrophin	Adrenal (suprarenal) glands	Stimulates the adrenal gland to produce cortisol.
Thyroid-stimulating hormone (TSH): also known as thyrotrophin	Thyroid	Stimulates the thyroid to secrete thyroxine.
Luteinising hormone (LH) and follicle-stimulating hormone (FSH): collectively known as gonadotropins. In males, LH is also known as interstitial cell stimulating hormone (ICSH).	Ovaries (females) and testes (males)	Controls reproductive functioning and secondary sexual characteristics; stimulates ovaries to produce oestrogen and progesterone and the testes to produce testosterone and sperm.
Prolactin (PRL)	Breasts	Stimulates the breasts to produce milk: it is secreted in large amounts during pregnancy and breastfeeding but is present at all times in both men and women.
Growth hormone (GH)	All cells	Stimulates growth and repair.
Anti-diuretic hormone (ADH): also known as vasopressin or arginine vasopressin (AVP)	Kidneys	Controls the amount of fluid in blood and the mineral levels in the body by affecting water retention by the kidneys.
Oxytocin	Uterus and breasts	Affects uterine contractions during pregnancy and parturition and the subsequent release of breast milk.

the release of GHRH and GH from the adenohypophysis; and GH-inhibitory hormone (GHIH) or somatostatin by decreasing GH secretion, somatostatin is also secreted by delta cells in the islets of Langerhans in the pancreas (page 347).

Disorders of the Pituitary Gland

These can arise from either hyperactivity or hypoactivity, mainly of the adenohypophysis as shown in Table 4.11.

Gigantism. Caused by an excess secretion of GH before puberty. General overgrowth leading to a huge stature with the limbs being disproportionately long, being associated with hypogonadism; individuals are hyperglycaemic and develop glycosuria and pituitary diabetes (10% of cases), with tumours of the gland often causing a constant headache and visual disturbances.

Acromegaly. Caused by an excess secretion of GH after puberty. Characterised by enlargement, thickening and broadening of bones, particularly in the limbs (hands, feet); kyphosis; thickening of the scalp; overgrowth of body hair, enlargement of the lungs, liver, heart and spleen; hyperactivity of the thyroid, parathyroid and

TABLE 4.11 Disorders of the Pituitary Gland

	Hyperactivity	Hypoactivity
Adenohypophysis	Gigantism Acromegaly Acromegalic gigantism Cushing disease	Dwarfism Acromicria Simmonds disease
Neurohypophysis	Syndrome of inappropriate hypersecretion of anti-diuretic hormone (SIADH)	Diabetes insipidus
Adenohypophysis and neurohypophysis		Dystrophia adiposogenitalis

adrenal glands; hyperglycaemia, glycosuria and diabetes; gynecomastia; hypertension; headache; and visual disturbances.

Acromegalic gigantism. A combination of the symptoms of acromegaly and gigantism; it can develop when increased GH secretion remains untreated.

Cushing's disease. Details can be found on page 346.

Dwarfism. Characterised by stunted growth, with the proportions of the body being almost normal. There is no decline in mental ability or reproductive function; however, in panhypopituitarism puberty is not reached due to the deficiency of gonadotropic hormones.

Acromicria. Rare disease of adults characterised by atrophy and thinning of the extremities (hands, feet), lethargy and loss of sexual functions. It is associated with hypothyroidism and hyposecretion of adrenocortical hormones.

Simmonds' disease/syndrome. Caused by destruction of the adenohypophysis from any cause leading to atrophy of the viscera, including the heart, liver, spleen, kidneys, thyroid, adrenal glands and gonads; it is more common between ages 20 and 45 and much more common in women than men. It is characterised by cachexia, premature senility, atrophy of the gonads and genitalia, amenorrhea and atrophy of the breasts (in women), loss of pubic and axillary hair, loss of libido, skin changes (mainly increased dryness), anorexia and constipation, hypotension and muscle weakness, hypoglycaemia, decreased sugar tolerance, lowered basal metabolism and depressed specific dynamic action of proteins, anaemia, lymphocytosis and occasional eosinophilia: death occurs if left untreated.

> **CLINICAL PHYSIOLOGY:** Sheehan's syndrome (postpartum hypopituitarism/postpartum pituitary insufficiency) can occur following severe uterine bleeding during childbirth; conditions increasing the risk of haemorrhage include multiple pregnancies (twins, triplets) and placental abnormalities.

Syndrome of inappropriate hypersecretion of antidiuretic hormone. Characterised by loss of sodium in the urine due to hypersecretion of ADH: it can be caused by cerebral and lung tumours secreting ADH. The signs and symptoms include loss of appetite, weight loss, nausea and vomiting, headache, muscle weakness/spasm/cramps, fatigue, restlessness and irritability; in severe conditions, the individual may die as a result of convulsions or coma.

Diabetes insipidus. Characterised by excess excretion of large quantities of dilute urine with increased frequency of voiding (polyuria), increased intake of water (polydipsia) and dehydration. Nephrogenic diabetes insipidus (a genetic disorder) is due to the inability of the renal tubules to respond to ADH.

Dystrophia adiposogenitalis (Frolich's syndrome). A rare childhood metabolic disorder characterised by obesity, growth retardation and retarded development of the genital organs; occurs more frequently in boys. It is associated with tumours of the hypothalamus resulting in increased appetite and decreased secretion of gonadotropin. There may be impaired vision due to the tumour impinging on the optic nerve.

> **CLINICAL PHYSIOLOGY:** Hypopituitarism, often caused by a benign tumour or by infections (meningitis), severe blood loss, head injury or rare diseases (sarcoidosis), results in underactivity of the gland; multiple pituitary hormone deficiency (MPHD) is when two or more hormones are not produced, with panhypopituitarism being when all hormones stop being produced. Typical symptoms include (depending on which hormone is affected): excessive tiredness, muscle weakness, reduced body hair, irregular periods (oligomenorrhea) or loss of normal menstrual function (amenorrhea), impotence in males, reduced fertility, decreased sex drive, weight gain, increased sensitivity to cold, constipation, dry skin, pale appearance, low blood pressure and dizziness on standing (postural hypotension), headaches, visual disturbances and diabetes insipidus.

Thyroid Gland

Details of the gross anatomy of the thyroid gland, including its blood supply, can be found on page 331.

The thyroid follicles are the functional and structural unit of the thyroid gland (Fig. 4.97), with each follicle being roughly spherical, filled with a secretory substance (colloid) and lined with cuboidal epithelial cells that secrete into their interior; the epithelium contains two types of cells (follicular (principle) and parafollicular (C)). Follicular cells are responsible for synthesising triiodothyronine (T_3) and thyroxine (T_4) and the parafollicular cells calcitonin (thyrocalcitonin). The major component of colloid is thyroglobulin containing the thyroid hormones. Once the secretions have entered the follicles, they are absorbed back through the follicular epithelium into the bloodstream before they can function in the body. Iodine is necessary for the production of thyroxine, it is absorbed by the gastrointestinal tract with most being rapidly secreted by the kidneys;

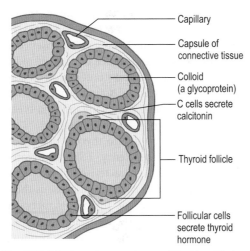

Capillary

Capsule of
connective tissue

Colloid
(a glycoprotein)

C cells secrete
calcitonin

Thyroid follicle

Follicular cells
secrete thyroid
hormone

Fig. 4.97 Microscopic appearance of the thyroid gland.

however, about 20% is selectively removed from the circulation by cells in the thyroid gland and used for synthesising thyroid hormones.

The thyroid gland secretes two major hormones (thyroxine (T_4), triiodothyronine (T_3)) which increase metabolic rate, with secretion being controlled mainly by TSH secreted by the adenohypophysis. Complete lack of thyroid secretion results in the metabolic rate falling to 40%–50% below normal, while extreme excesses of thyroid secretion can result in the metabolic rate increasing to 60%–100% above normal. Of the metabolically active hormones secreted 93% is T_4, with the remainder being T_3; however, almost all T_4 is converted to T_3 in the tissues. The function of the hormones is effectively the same differing only in the rapidity and intensity of their action: T_3 is more potent than T_4, but is present in blood in smaller quantities, it also persists for a shorter time than T_4.

CLINICAL PHYSIOLOGY: During pregnancy T_3 and T_4 both cross the placenta and are critical in the early stages of brain development. Thyroid hormone deficiency results in irreversible damage to the CNS with reduced numbers of neurons, defective myelination and intellectual disability: if maternal thyroid deficiency is present before development of the foetal thyroid the intellectual deficiency is severe.

Regulation of Secretion

The main factor controlling secretion is TSH (secreted by the adenohypophysis), which controls every stage in the formation and release of thyroid hormones.

The hypothalamus controls TSH through thyrotropic-releasing hormone transported via the hypothalamo-hypophyseal portal blood vessels. The thyroid hormones also regulate their own secretion through a negative feedback system.

Other factors increasing secretion include low basal metabolic rate, leptin, α-melanocyte-stimulating hormone and, in children, low body temperature; factors decreasing secretion include excess iodine intake, stress, somatostatin, glucocorticoids and dopamine.

Following synthesis, the thyroid hormones remain as vesicles within thyroglobulin which can be stored for up to 4 months. Release of the hormones involves the follicular cells sending out foot-like extensions (pseudopods) around the thyroglobulin-hormone complex converting it into small pinocytic vesicles; lysosomes then fuse with the vesicles which digest the thyroglobulin releasing the hormone, which diffuse through the base of the follicular cells to enter the capillaries, where it is transported by thyroxine-binding globulin, thyroxine-binding prealbumin or albumin.

Function of Thyroid Hormones

Thyroxine increases metabolic activity in most body tissues except the brain, retina, spleen, testes and lungs, by increasing tissue oxygen consumption. Thyroid hormones also increase protein metabolism in cells; stimulate most processes associated with carbohydrate metabolism (increased absorption of glucose from the gut, enhanced glucose uptake by cells, increased breakdown of glycogen into glucose, accelerated gluconeogenesis); decrease fat storage by mobilising fat deposits, thereby increasing free fatty acid levels in blood; decrease cholesterol, phospholipids and triglyceride levels in plasma and increases fat deposition in the liver (fatty liver), with increased secretion of cholesterol from the liver into bile; and increases the formation of enzymes, which can lead to vitamin deficiency.

CLINICAL PHYSIOLOGY: Hyposecretion of thyroxine increases plasma levels of cholesterol which can result in atherosclerosis.

Thyroid hormones increase heat production raising body temperature leading to sweating, and accelerates growth of the body, especially in children; lack of thyroxine arrests growth with early closure of the epiphyses (page 33).

Increased thyroxine secretion leads to a decrease in body weight (decreased secretion leads to an increase in body weight); accelerates erythropoietic activity and blood volume (polycythaemia is common in hyperthyroidism); increases the overall activity of the cardiovascular system (increased heart rate, force of contraction, blood pressure, vasodilation of blood vessels); increases the rate and force of respiration indirectly through the increased demand for oxygen and the formation of carbon dioxide; increases appetite and food intake, as well as increasing secretions and movements of the gastrointestinal tract; and increases the demand for secretion by other endocrine glands.

Thyroxine is essential for the development and maintenance of normal functioning of the CNS; the normal activity of skeletal muscles, with increases in thyroxine levels making muscles work with greater vigour; however, hypersecretion causes muscle weakness due to protein catabolism (thyrotoxic myopathy); normal sleep patterns; normal sexual function, in men hypothyroidism leads to complete loss of libido and hyperthyroidism to impotence, while in women hypothyroidism can lead to polymenorrhea or amenorrhea while hyperthyroidism leads to oligomenorrhea or amenorrhea.

Hyperthyroidism. Hyperthyroidism caused by increased secretion of thyroid hormones (Graves' disease, thyroid adenoma); details of Graves' disease can be found on page 331. The signs and symptoms are intolerance to heat due to increased basal metabolic rate; increased sweating; weight loss; diarrhoea due to increased gastrointestinal motility; muscle weakness; nervousness, extreme fatigue, inability to sleep; mild tremors in the hands; psychoneurotic symptoms (hyperexcitability, extreme anxiety or worry); toxic goitre; oligomenorrhea or amenorrhea; exophthalmos (protrusion of the eyeball), which can lead to blindness due to stretching of the optic nerve, and dryness of the cornea from an inability to close the eyes; polycythaemia; tachycardia and atrial fibrillation; systolic hypertension; and cardiac failure. Increased secretion of thyroid hormones caused by a thyroid tumour can lead to enlargement of the gland (toxic goitre).

Treatment is by antithyroid drugs (thiocyanate, thioureylenes, high concentrations of inorganic iodines) which suppress thyroid hormone secretion; or surgical removal.

Hypothyroidism. Caused by decreased secretion of thyroid hormones leading to cretinism in children and myxoedema in adults. Hypothyroidism is treated by administering thyroid extract or ingestion of thyroxine.

Cretinism. Occurs due to congenital absence of the thyroid gland, a genetic disorder or lack of iodine in the diet. It is characterised by stunted growth, sluggish movements and a 'croaking' sound when crying; the tongue tends to protrude producing guttural breathing that can cause choking.

Myxoedema. Occurs due to thyroid diseases, a genetic disorder, iodine deficiency, TSH or thyrotropin-releasing hormone: it is characterised by a generalised oedematous appearance. A common cause is the auto-immune disease Hashimoto's thyroiditis, prevalent in late middle-aged women. The signs and symptoms are facial swelling; bagginess under the eyes; non-pitting oedema; atherosclerosis leading to arteriosclerosis; anaemia; fatigue and muscular sluggishness; sleeping 14–16 h/day; menorrhagia and polymenorrhea; decreased cardiovascular function (reduced rate and force of contraction, cardiac output, blood volume); increased body weight; constipation; mental sluggishness; depressed hair growth; skin scaliness; husky voice; and cold intolerance.

Calcitonin

Calcitonin is secreted by parafollicular (C) cells; it is a physiological antagonist to parathyroid hormone (parathormone) and helps lower blood calcium levels by suppressing the resorptive action of osteoclasts and promoting calcium deposition in bones by increasing the rate of osteoid calcification: its secretion is regulated directly by blood calcium levels.

> **CLINICAL PHYSIOLOGY:** Calcitonin is secreted by a number of endocrine tumours; it is used as a tumour marker to monitor progress of recovery following surgical resection of the tumour. It can also be used to treat individuals with disorders associated with excess bone resorption (osteoporosis, Paget's disease).

Parathyroid Glands

Four small glands lying on or embedded in the posterior surface of the lobes of the thyroid gland close to the upper and lower poles: each gland consists of chief (produce parathyroid hormone/parathormone) and oxyphil cells. Oxyphil cells have no known function; however, they begin to appear at puberty and increase with age.

The major function of the parathyroid glands is to maintain the body's calcium and phosphate levels within narrow limits by secreting parathormone enabling the nervous and muscular systems to function properly; parathormone has antagonistic effects to those of calcitonin. Blood calcium levels in adults should be in the range of 8.5–10.5 mg/dL (2.125–2.625 mmol/L); parathormone directly stimulates osteoblasts and indirectly stimulates osteoclasts to breakdown bone and release calcium, it also increases gastrointestinal calcium absorption by activating vitamin D and promotes calcium resorption by the kidneys. Blood phosphate levels in adults should be 2.5–4.5 mg/dL (0.615–1.125 mmol/L); parathormone acts on the kidneys by inhibiting proximal tubular reabsorption of phosphorus, by activating vitamin D the absorption of intestinal phosphate is increased.

CLINICAL PHYSIOLOGY: Hyperparathyroidism can be considered as being: *primary* (excess circulating parathormone due to parathyroid gland tumour) causing bone pain and tenderness (generally managed by surgical removal of the abnormal gland), there may also be other symptoms (dehydration) associated with hypercalcemia; *secondary* (often associated with renal disease), when too much calcium is lost the parathyroid glands hypertrophy and respond by releasing parathormone; *tertiary* is a state of prolonged loss of calcium with the parathyroid glands becoming unresponsive to blood calcium levels and begin to autonomously release parathormone. Hypoparathyroidism is most commonly associated with damage to the parathyroid glands or their blood supply during thyroid surgery: removal of all parathyroid glands is followed by increased neuromuscular excitability and muscle spasms, eventually leading to death within a few days. Hypoparathyroidism may also be associated with rare genetic syndromes (DiGeorge syndrome).

CLINICAL PHYSIOLOGY: Occasionally an individual's tissues are resistant to the effects of parathormone (pseudohypoparathyroidism). The parathyroid glands are fully functional, but the hormone is not able to function resulting in decreased blood calcium levels; it can be treated with vitamin D analogues.

Adrenal (Suprarenal) Glands

The adrenal glands lie on the superior poles of their respective kidney; the right being triangular and left crescentic in shape. Each gland has two parts (cortex (80%) and medulla (20%)), which function as separate endocrine glands: the medulla secretes adrenaline (epinephrine) and noradrenaline (norepinephrine) in response to sympathetic stimulation, and the cortex secretes corticosteroids (mineralocorticoids, glucocorticoids) and small amounts of sex hormones (especially androgenic hormones).

Adrenal Cortex

The adrenal cortex is essential to life with interference in its function causing disruption of fluid and electrolyte balance, as well as carbohydrate metabolism and normal bodily reactions to stress; it consists of three relatively distinct layers (Fig. 4.98).

Zona glomerulosa. A thin layer of cells just below the capsule (15% of cortex) which secrete significant amounts of aldosterone; secretion is controlled by extracellular fluid concentrations of angiotensin II and potassium, both of which stimulate secretion.

Zona fasciculata. The widest layer (75% of cortex) secreting cortisol and corticosteroids, as well as small amounts of adrenal androgens and oestrogens; secretion is mainly controlled by the hypothalamic-pituitary axis via ACTH.

Zona reticularis. Deepest layer of the cortex secreting adrenal androgens (dehydroepiandrosterone (DHEA), androstenedione) as well as small amounts of oestrogens and some glucocorticoids; secretion is regulated by ACTH, as well as cortical androgen-stimulating hormone released from the pituitary.

CLINICAL PHYSIOLOGY: Aldosterone and cortisol secretion are regulated by independent mechanisms. Angiotensin II specifically increases the output of aldosterone with hypertrophy of the zona glomerulosa; it has no effect on the other two zones. ACTH increases secretion of cortisol and adrenal androgens with hypertrophy of the zona fasciculata and zona reticularis; it has little effect on the zona glomerulosa.

Of the adrenocorticoid hormones, 90%–95% of cortisol in plasma binds to plasma proteins slowing the elimination of cortisol from the plasma, in contrast only 60% of aldosterone combines with plasma proteins; both hormones are transported throughout the extracellular fluid compartments in both the combined and free forms. The binding to plasma proteins acts as a reservoir

Magnified section

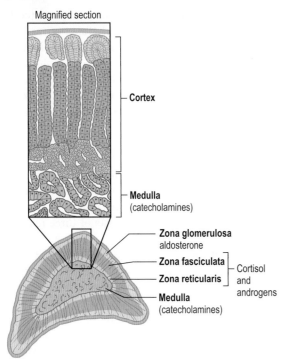

Cortex

Medulla
(catecholamines)

Zona glomerulosa
aldosterone

Zona fasciculata ⎤
                  ⎥ Cortisol
Zona reticularis ⎦ and
                    androgens
Medulla
(catecholamines)

Fig. 4.98 Section through the adrenal (suprarenal) gland showing the cortex and medulla, together with the secretions of each part. *CCK,* Cholecystokinin; *PYY,* peptide YY.

to lessen rapid fluctuations in free hormone concentration helping to ensure a relatively uniform distribution of the adrenal hormones to the tissues.

The hormones are mainly degraded in the liver and conjugated to glucuronic acid and sulphates, which are inactive. Approximately 25% of the conjugates are excreted in bile and then faeces, with the remainder entering the circulation where they are filtered by the kidneys and excreted in the urine.

> **CLINICAL PHYSIOLOGY:** Diseases of the liver depresses the rate of inactivation of adrenocortical hormones, and of the kidney reduces the excretion of the inactive conjugates.

The normal concentration of aldosterone in blood is 0.006 µg/100 mL, with an average secretion rate of 0.15 mg/day; however, blood concentration depends on several factors, including dietary intake of sodium and

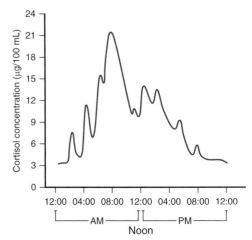

Fig. 4.99 The pattern of cortisol concentration in the blood during a 24-hour period.

potassium. The concentration of cortisol in blood averages 12 mg/mL, with an excretory rate of 15–20 mg/day; however, both concentration and secretion fluctuate during the day, rising in the early morning and declining in the evening (Fig. 4.99).

Mineralocorticoids

Aldosterone is the major mineralocorticoid, exerting 90% of mineralocorticoid activity of the adrenocortical secretions; however, cortisol also provides a significant amount of mineralocorticoid activity. Aldosterone increases the reabsorption of sodium simultaneously increasing the secretion of potassium by the renal tubular epithelial cells (principal cells of the collecting tubules) and osmotic absorption of water increasing extracellular fluid volume, and arterial pressure. The rise in arterial pressure increases kidney excretion of salt (pressure natriuresis) and water (pressure diuresis). A similar effect occurs in sweat and salivary glands as in the renal tubules.

Excess aldosterone stimulates transport of potassium from the extracellular fluid into most cells of the body, leading to hypokalaemia, with severe muscle weakness due to alteration of the electrical excitability of nerve and muscle fibre membranes preventing transmission of normal action potentials.

Regulation of aldosterone. The regulation of aldosterone secretion is almost entirely independent of the regulation of cortisol and androgens. A number of factors have essential roles: increased potassium ion and angiotensin II concentration in the extracellular fluid both increase aldosterone secretion; increased sodium ion concentration in the extracellular fluid slightly decreases aldosterone secretion. ACTH from the adenohypophysis is necessary for aldosterone secretion but has little effect in controlling the rate of secretion in most physiological conditions.

> **CLINICAL PHYSIOLOGY:** Total loss of adrenocortical secretion usually causes death within 3–14 days unless the individual receives extensive salt therapy or mineralocorticoid injections. Without mineralocorticoids, potassium ion concentration in the extracellular fluid rises markedly, sodium and chloride are rapidly lost from the body, accompanied by a reduction in total extracellular fluid and blood volume. There is reduced cardiac output progressing to a shock-like state, followed by death.

Glucocorticoids

The majority of the glucocorticoid activity (>95%) of the adrenocortical secretions results from the secretion of cortisol (hydrocortisone), with a small, but significant, amount provided by corticosterone. Cortisol and other glucocorticoids stimulate gluconeogenesis (formation of carbohydrates from proteins and other substances) by the liver through two main effects: increasing the enzymes required to convert amino acids into glucose in liver cells, and mobilising amino acids from extrahepatic tissues (mainly muscle). Increased gluconeogenesis results in an increase in glycogen storage in liver cells, allowing other glycolytic hormones (adrenaline, glucagon) to mobilise glucose in times of need (e.g., between meals). Increased gluconeogenesis also causes a rise in blood glucose concentrations, which in turn stimulates insulin secretion; however, high levels of glucocorticoid reduces the sensitivity of many tissues (skeletal muscle, adipose tissue) to the stimulatory effect of insulin on glucose uptake and utilisation. Excess secretion of glucocorticoids can cause disturbances in carbohydrate metabolism similar to the effects of excess levels of GH.

> **CLINICAL PHYSIOLOGY:** Blood glucose levels more than 50% above normal lead to adrenal diabetes, with insulin only moderately lowering blood glucose concentrations because the tissues are resistant to the effects of insulin.

A principal effect of cortisol on metabolism is a reduction in protein stores in all cells except liver cells, being caused by decreased protein synthesis and increased catabolism of protein in the cells. Both effects are partly due to decreased amino acid transport into extrahepatic tissues and partly due to depression of the formation of RNA and subsequent protein synthesis in many extrahepatic tissues (muscle, lymphoid tissue). With large excesses of cortisol, the muscles can become so weak that an individual may have difficulty in rising from a chair; the immunity function of lymphoid tissue also decreases.

Cortisol promotes amino acid mobilisation from muscle and of fatty acids from adipose tissue, increasing the concentration of free fatty acids in the plasma thereby increasing their utilisation for energy; it also enhances the oxidation of fatty acids in cells. Individuals with excess cortisol secretion develop excess fat deposition in the chest and head, giving a buffalo-like torso and round moon face; this type of obesity probably results from excess stimulation of food intake, with fat being generated in some tissues more rapidly than it is mobilised and oxidised.

Most types of stress (physical, neurogenic) cause an immediate increase in ACTH secretion by the adenohypophysis, followed within minutes by greatly increased adrenocortical secretion of cortisol.

Tissue damage (trauma, bacterial infection) results in tissue inflammation, which can be more damaging than the trauma or disease (e.g., rheumatoid arthritis); cortisol can block the inflammation or reverse many of the effects once it has begun.

> **APPLIED PHYSIOLOGY:** There are five main stages of inflammation: (1) release of chemical substances (histamine, bradykinin, proteolytic enzymes, prostaglandins, leukotrienes) from the damaged cells that activate the inflammation process; (2) increased blood flow to the inflamed area (erythema); (3) leakage of large amounts of plasma out of the capillaries into the damaged areas due to increased capillary permeability, followed by clotting of the tissue fluids (non-pitting oedema); (4) infiltration of the area by leukocytes and (5) ingrowth of fibrous tissue after days or weeks.

Cortisol prevents inflammation by stabilising lysosomal membranes, reducing the release of proteolytic enzymes; decreasing the permeability of the capillaries,

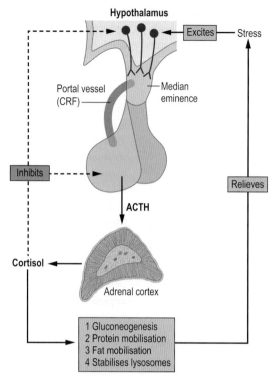

Fig. 4.100 The regulation of glucocorticoid secretion. *ACTH*, Adrenocorticotropic hormone; *CRF*, corticotrophin–releasing factor.

preventing loss of plasma into the tissues; decreasing migration of white blood cells into the inflamed area and phagocytosis of damaged cells; suppressing the immune system, decreasing lymphocyte reproduction; and attenuating fever by reducing the release of interleukin-1 from white blood cells.

Regulation of cortisol. Cortisol secretion is almost entirely controlled by ACTH secreted by the adenohypophysis; ACTH secretion is controlled by corticotrophin-releasing factor (CRF) secretion into the primary capillary plexus of the hypophyseal portal system and then carried to the adenohypophysis (Fig. 4.100). The key to control is excitation of the hypothalamus by different types of stress activating the system, causing rapid release of cortisol, which in turn initiates a series of metabolic effects directed towards relieving the stress.

Cortisol also feeds back directly to the hypothalamus and adenohypophysis decreasing cortisol concentrations in the plasma when the body is not experiencing stress; however, stress stimuli are more potent and can override the direct inhibitory feedback of cortisol, resulting in periodic rises of cortisol secretion during the day or prolonged cortisol secretion in times of chronic stress.

Abnormalities of adrenocorticoid secretion

Hypoadrenalism/adrenal insufficiency (Addison's disease). This is due to the inability of the adrenal glands to produce sufficient adrenocortical hormones, usually caused by primary atrophy or injury to the adrenal cortex; atrophy is caused by autoimmunity against the cortex (80% of cases). Hypoadrenalism can also be the result of tuberculous destruction of the adrenal glands or invasion of the cortex by cancer; however, it can be secondary to impaired function of the adenohypophysis to produce sufficient ACTH.

Left untreated, individuals with Addison's disease die within days to weeks due to weakness and circulatory shock; small quantities of mineralocorticoids and glucocorticoids administered daily can enable individuals to live for years.

Hyperadrenalism (Cushing's syndrome). Usually, the result of abnormal amounts of cortisol; however, excess secretion of androgens can also have important effects. Hypercortisolism can have multiple causes: adenoma of the adenohypophysis secreting large amounts of ACTH, resulting in adrenal hyperplasia and excess cortisol secretion; abnormal function of the hypothalamus causing high levels of corticotropin-releasing hormone, stimulating excess ACTH release; ectopic secretion of ACTH by a tumour (abdominal carcinoma); and adenoma of the adrenal cortex. Cushing's syndrome secondary to excess ACTH secretion by the adenohypophysis is Cushing's disease.

Treatment of Cushing's syndrome is removal of the adrenal tumour or decreasing the secretion of ACTH; if ACTH secretion cannot be decreased, partial/complete adrenalectomy is undertaken followed by administration of adrenal steroids to alleviate any insufficiencies.

Adrenal Medulla

The adrenal medulla secretes either adrenaline (epinephrine) or noradrenaline (norepinephrine). Adrenaline is released in response to stress, increasing heart rate, raising blood pressure and causing the release of sugar into the bloodstream from the liver; it is also a neurotransmitter in the brain associated with many functions including cardiovascular and respiratory responses. Noradrenaline has widespread effects including cardiac stimulation, blood vessel constriction, relaxation of the bronchioles and relaxation of the digestive tract. Within the brain, it is involved in regulating body temperature, food and water intake, and cardiovascular and respiratory control.

Islets of Langerhans

Details of the gross anatomy and relations of the pancreas can be found on page 482. The pancreas consists of two major types of tissue (Fig. 4.101): acini which secrete digestive juices into the duodenum, and islets of Langerhans which secrete insulin and glucagon directly into the blood; it also secretes amylin, somatostatin and pancreatic polypeptide.

Each islet is arranged around a small capillary into which its cells secrete their hormones; the islets contain three major cell types (alpha, beta, delta) and at least one other present in small numbers (PP cell). Beta cells (60% of all cells) are mainly in the middle of each islet and secrete insulin and amylin (a hormone often secreted in parallel with insulin); alpha cells (25% of all cells) secrete glucagon; and delta cells (10% of all cells) secrete somatostatin; PP cells (5% of all cells) secrete pancreatic polypeptide. The interrelations between the different cell types promote cell-to-cell communication and direct control of secretion of some hormones by others; insulin inhibits glucagon secretion; amylin inhibits insulin secretion; somatostatin inhibits both insulin and glucagon secretion.

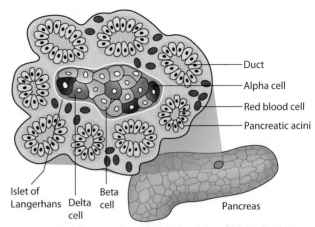

Fig. 4.101 Microscopic anatomy of an islet of Langerhans.

Insulin

An abundance of energy-giving foods in the diet (especially carbohydrates) increases insulin secretion, which has an important role in storing excess energy; excess carbohydrates are stored as glycogen in the liver and muscles, with any excess that cannot be stored converted into fats and stored in adipose tissue. Insulin also directly promotes amino acid uptake by cells and converts them into protein, at the same time inhibiting the breakdown of protein already in the cells.

To initiate its effects on cells insulin binds with and activates a membrane receptor protein, which then causes the subsequent effects. Within seconds the membranes of 80% of the body's cells increase their uptake of glucose, especially muscle and adipose tissue cells but not most neurons in the brain; the cell membrane becomes more permeable to amino acids, potassium and phosphate ions causing their increased transport into the cell. Slower effects occur during the next 10–15 minutes to change the activity levels of many intracellular enzymes, these slower effects continue to occur for several hours being the result of changed rates of translation of messenger RNA forming new proteins. It is this sequence of events that enables insulin to remould the cellular enzyme machinery to achieve its metabolic goals.

Effect on carbohydrate metabolism. Following a high carbohydrate meal, the increase in blood glucose results in rapid secretion of insulin causing rapid uptake, storage and use of glucose by almost all body tissues, especially muscles, adipose tissue and the liver. The most important effect is to cause most of the absorbed glucose to be stored in the liver as glycogen; when blood glucose levels decrease insulin secretion rapidly decreases and liver glycogen is split back into glucose, which is released back into the blood to prevent glucose levels falling too low.

During storage insulin inactivates liver phosphorylase preventing the breakdown of already stored glycogen; causes enhanced uptake of glucose from the blood by liver cells by increasing the activity of glucokinase, resulting in phosphorylation of glucose temporarily trapping it in the cells; and increases the activity of glycogen synthase promoting glycogen synthesis. When blood glucose levels fall insulin secretion decreases, reversing all the effects of storage by preventing the uptake of glucose by the liver. The lack of insulin and the increase of glucagon activate phosphorylase splitting glycogen into glucose phosphate, with glucose phosphatase causing phosphate to split from the glucose allowing free glucose to diffuse back into the blood.

> **CLINICAL PHYSIOLOGY:** Most brain cells, which normally only use glucose for energy, are permeable to glucose and can use it without the mediation of insulin; it is, therefore, important that blood glucose levels are maintained above a critical level. Blood glucose levels between 20 and 50 mg/100 mL result in symptoms of hypoglycaemic shock characterised by progressive nervous irritability, fainting, seizures and coma.

Effect on fat metabolism. Insulin promotes fatty acid synthesis, especially when more carbohydrates are ingested than can be used for immediate energy; almost all synthesis occurs in the liver cells, with the fatty acids being transported from the liver by blood lipoproteins to the adipose tissues for storage. Insulin has two effects essential for fat storage; it inhibits the action of lipase, which causes hydrolysis of the triglycerides stored in fat cells, thereby inhibiting fatty acid release from the adipose tissues into the blood, and increases the use of ketoacids by peripheral tissues; and it promotes glucose transport through the cell membrane into the fat cells in the same way that it promotes glucose transport into muscle cells. When insulin is not available, the storage of large amounts of fatty acids transported from the liver in lipoproteins is effectively blocked.

> **CLINICAL PHYSIOLOGY:** Long-term lack of insulin can result in atherosclerosis, often leading to a heart attack and cerebral stroke.

Effect on protein metabolism and growth. Insulin shares with GH the ability of increasing the uptake of amino acids into cells. It stimulates transport of many amino acids (valine, leucine, isoleucine, tyrosine, phenylalanine) into the cells; increases the translation of messenger RNA forming new proteins; increases the rate of transcription of selected DNA genetic sequences in the cell nuclei (this occurs over a longer time period); inhibits protein catabolism decreasing the rate of amino acid release from cells, especially muscle cells; and depresses the rate of gluconeogenesis in the liver, conserving the amino acids in the body's protein stores. Insulin has a direct effect on growth by stimulating the synthesis of macromolecules in tissues such as cartilage and bone and an indirect effect by stimulating the transcription of the related gene IGF-I and inhibiting the gene for one of the IGF-I binding proteins; this leads to an increase in IGF-I which enhances growth.

> **CLINICAL PHYSIOLOGY:** When insulin is not available, plasma amino acid concentration increases, with most excess amino acids being used directly for energy or as substrates for gluconeogenesis, leading to enhanced urea excretion in the urine. The resulting protein wasting is one of the most serious effects of severe diabetes mellitus; it can lead to extreme weakness and deranged functioning of many organs.

Control of secretion. A number of conditions/factors either increase or decrease insulin secretion. Those that cause an increase are blood glucose concentration greater than 90 mg/100 mL; increased concentrations of fatty acids and amino acids (arginine, lysine) in blood; gastrointestinal hormones (gastrin, secretin, cholecystokinin, gastric inhibitory peptide); glucagon, GH, oestrogen, progesterone, thyroxine, cortisol; blood minerals (potassium, calcium); parasympathetic stimulation and acetylcholine; B-adrenergic stimulation; insulin resistance and obesity; and sulfonylurea drugs (glyburide, tolbutamide). Those that cause a decrease are: insulin (negative feedback); decreased blood glucose levels; fasting; somatostatin; and α-adrenergic activity and leptin.

Glucagon

Glucagon enhances the availability of glucose to other organs by stimulating the breakdown of liver glycogen (glycogenolysis) and increasing gluconeogenesis in the liver. It can also activate adipose cell lipase making increased quantities of fatty acids available and inhibit the storage of triglycerides in the liver. In high concentrations it enhances the strength of the heart; increases blood flow in some tissues (kidneys); enhances bile secretion; and inhibits gastric secretion.

Control of secretion. The major factor controlling glucagon secretion is blood glucose concentration, being the opposite effect of glucose on insulin secretion. In hypoglycaemia glucagon is secreted in large amounts, greatly increasing the release of glucose from the liver thus correcting the hypoglycaemia. As with insulin, high concentrations of arginine and lysine stimulate the secretion of glucagon, promoting the rapid conversion of the amino acids to glucose making it more available to the tissues. Other factors, including strenuous exercise, β-adrenergic stimulation, stressful stimuli, and infection, can increase glucagon secretion.

Effect of somatostatin on insulin and glucagon secretion. Most factors related to food ingestion (increased blood glucose/amino acids/fatty acids, increased concentrations of gastrointestinal hormones released from the upper gastrointestinal tract) increase somatostatin secretion. Somatostatin has many inhibitory effects: it depresses both insulin and glucagon secretion by acting locally within the islets of Langerhans; decreases the motility of the stomach, duodenum and gallbladder; and decreases both secretion and absorption in the gastrointestinal tract.

> **CLINICAL PHYSIOLOGY:** Somatostatin is the same chemical substance as growth hormone inhibitory hormone (GHIH) secreted by the hypothalamus suppressing GH secretion by the adenohypophysis.

Blood Glucose Regulation

Normally blood glucose concentration is narrowly controlled (80–90 mg/100 mL); following a meal it can increase to 120–140 mg/100 mL, but feedback systems controlling blood glucose soon return the levels back to control levels; in starvation, gluconeogenesis in the liver provides the glucose needed to maintain fasting blood glucose levels.

This is achieved through a number of mechanisms: the liver acting as an important blood glucose buffer system; insulin and glucagon function as important feedback control systems for maintaining a normal blood glucose concentration; in severe hypoglycaemia the direct effect of low blood glucose on the hypothalamus stimulates the sympathetic nervous system to

secrete noradrenaline from the adrenal glands, further increasing the release of glucose from the liver; and over a longer time period (days, weeks) GH and cortisol are secreted in response to prolonged hypoglycaemia, both of which decrease the rate of glucose utilisation by most cells in the body, converting to a greater dependence on fat utilisation.

It is important to regulate blood glucose because glucose is the nutrient normally used by the brain, retina and germinal epithelium of the gonads in sufficient quantities. Most glucose formed by gluconeogenesis during fasting is used for metabolism in the brain; it is, therefore, important that the islets of Langerhans do not secrete any insulin during this time; otherwise, any available glucose would go to the muscles and other peripheral tissues starving the brain.

It is also important that blood glucose levels do not rise too high because glucose can exert large osmotic pressures in the extracellular fluid; if glucose concentration rises excessively, it can cause cellular dehydration. Excessively high blood glucose concentrations result in loss of glucose in the urine, causing osmotic diuresis by the kidneys depleting the body of its fluids and electrolytes. Long-term increases in blood glucose levels can damage blood vessels, with vascular damage being associated with uncontrolled diabetes mellitus and an increased risk of heart attack, stroke, end-stage renal disease and blindness.

Diabetes mellitus. Diabetes mellitus is a syndrome associated with impaired carbohydrate, fat and protein metabolism caused by either a lack of insulin secretion or decreased sensitivity of the tissues to insulin; type I diabetes (insulin-dependent diabetes mellitus, IDDM) results from a lack of insulin secretion, while type II diabetes (non-insulin-dependent diabetes mellitus, NIDDM) is initially caused by decreased sensitivity (insulin resistance) of target tissues to the metabolic effect of insulin. In both types, the effect is to prevent the efficient uptake and utilisation of glucose by most cells, except the brain. As blood glucose concentration increases, cell utilisation of glucose becomes lower, with the utilisation of fats and proteins increasing. The clinical characteristics of individuals with type I and type II diabetes are shown in Table 4.12.

Type I diabetes. Viral infections or autoimmune disorders can injure or impair insulin production by the beta cells, although hereditary it also has a role in determining the susceptibility of beta cells to destruction; it can occur abruptly, over a few days or weeks. Prolonged

TABLE 4.12 Differences Between and Characteristics of Individuals With Type I and Type II Diabetes Mellitus

	Type I	Type II
Age at onset	Usually before age 40	Usually after age 40
Major cause	Lack of insulin	Lack of insulin receptors
Insulin deficiency	Yes	Partial deficiency
Need for insulin	Always	Not initially, but possibly later
Insulin resistance	No	Yes
Immune destruction of β-cells	Yes	No
Involvement of other endocrine disorders	No	Yes
Hereditary cause	Yes	Possibly
Control by oral hypoglycaemic agents	No	Yes
Symptoms appear	Rapidly	Slowly
Body weight	Low (wasted) to normal	Obese
Stress-induced obesity	No	Yes
Plasma insulin	Low or absent	Normal to high initially
Plasma glucagon	High, but can be suppressed	High, resistant to suppression
Plasma glucose	Increased	Increased
Ketosis	Yes	Possibly
Insulin sensitivity	Normal	Reduced
Therapy	Insulin	Weight loss, metformin, insulin, thiazolidinediones, sulphonylureas

poor control of blood glucose concentrations leads to structural changes to blood vessels in many tissues, resulting in an inadequate blood supply to the tissues; this can lead to increased risk of heart attack, end-stage kidney disease, retinopathy and blindness, ischaemia and gangrene of the limbs. In addition, there may also be peripheral neuropathy and autonomic nervous system dysfunction (impaired cardiovascular reflexes, impaired bladder control, decreased sensation in the extremities) in chronic uncontrolled diabetes mellitus. Hypertension (secondary to renal injury) and atherosclerosis (secondary to abnormal lipid metabolism) may develop amplifying the tissue damage caused by the elevated glucose levels. Individuals with severe untreated diabetes mellitus suffer rapid weight loss and asthenia (lack of energy) despite eating large amounts of food (polyphagia); without treatment, this can cause severe wasting of the body tissues and death within a few weeks.

Type II diabetes. More common than type I, accounting for 90%–95% of all cases of diabetes mellitus; it develops gradually. It is associated with increased

plasma insulin concentrations (hyperinsulinaemia) as a compensatory response by beta cells for diminished sensitivity of target tissues to the metabolic effects of insulin (insulin resistance) impairing carbohydrate utilisation and storage, raising blood glucose levels. With prolonged and severe type II diabetes, increased levels of insulin are insufficient to maintain normal glucose regulation, resulting in the early stages in moderate hyperglycaemia following the ingestion of carbohydrates. In later stages, the beta cells become exhausted or damaged and are unable to produce enough insulin to prevent more severe hypoglycaemia, especially after a carbohydrate-rich meal. In the early stages, type II diabetes can be effectively treated with exercise, restricting calorie intake and weight reduction; later, drugs that increase insulin sensitivity (thiazolidinediones), suppress liver glucose production (metformin) and cause additional release of insulin by the pancreas (sulfonylureas) can be used.

Insulinoma (Hyperinsulinism). Rarer than diabetes, excessive insulin production can occur from an adenoma of an islet of Langerhans, 10%–15% of which are malignant with occasional spread of metastases throughout the body causing tremendous production of insulin by both the primary and secondary tumours.

Individuals with insulin-secreting tumours or who self-administer too much insulin may suffer from insulin shock. When blood glucose levels fall to 50–70 mg/100 mL the CNS becomes excitable because the hypoglycaemia sensitises neuronal activity, with extreme nervousness, whole-body trembling, sweating and sometimes hallucinations. As blood glucose levels fall to 20–50 mg/100 mL clonic seizures and loss of consciousness may occur. With further falls in glucose levels, the seizures stop and a state of coma remains.

> **CLINICAL PHYSIOLOGY:** It may be difficult by simple clinical examination to distinguish between diabetic coma resulting from insulin-lack acidosis and coma resulting from hypoglycaemia caused by excess insulin; the acetone breath and rapid deep breathing associated with diabetic coma are not present in hypoglycaemic shock.

Immediate intravenous administration of large quantities of glucose usually brings the individual out of shock within a few minutes. The administration of glucagon causes glycogenolysis in the liver rapidly increasing blood glucose levels. Without treatment, permanent damage to neuronal cells of the CNS occurs.

Gonads

Details of the gross anatomy of the reproductive organs in males and females can be found on pages 532 and 541, respectively. Steroid hormones are produced and secreted by the gonads (testes in males, ovaries in females) and are necessary for sexual development and the control of reproductive function. The most important hormones are androgens (testosterone, dihydrotestosterone) found predominantly in males, and progesterones (progesterone) and some oestrogens (oestradiol, oestrone, oestriol) found predominantly in females: they tend to act on the brain influencing sexual and other behaviour.

Androgens are necessary for the development of male genitalia in the foetus; during puberty, they promote development of secondary sexual characteristics (growth of the penis and testes, appearance of pubic, facial and body hair, increase in muscle strength, deepening of the voice); in adults, they are needed for producing sperm and maintaining libido.

Oestrogens are responsible for the development of female secondary sexual characteristics, as well as promoting sexual readiness and preparation of the uterus for implantation of the embryo. Progesterone is required for maintaining pregnancy and preparing the uterus for implantation; it also inhibits ovulation during pregnancy and prepares the breasts for lactation.

Testes

Spermatogenesis. In the embryo, primordial germ cells migrate into the testes and become immature germ cells (spermatogonia) lying in two or three layers on the inner surface of the seminiferous tubules (Fig. 4.102A). Spermatogenesis occurs within the coiled seminiferous tubules, beginning during puberty when they undergo mitotic division as a result of stimulation by the adenohypophyseal gonadotropic hormones; this continual proliferation and differentiation through definitive stages of development to form sperm continue throughout life: it markedly decrease in old age. In the initial stage, the spermatogonia migrate among Sertoli cells towards the central lumen of the tubule; the Sertoli cells have large amounts of cytoplasm which envelops the developing spermatogonia all the way to the central lumen (Fig. 4.102B).

Sertoli (sustentacular, nurse) cells: support and nourish the spermatogenic cells until the spermatozoa are released by them; secrete aromatase (an enzyme) which convert androgens into oestrogen; secrete androgen-binding protein essential for testosterone activity during spermatogenesis; secrete oestrogen-binding protein; secrete inhibin which inhibits FSH release from the adenohypophysis; secrete activin which increases FSH release from the adenohypophysis; and secretes Mullerian regression factor (Mullerian inhibiting substance) which is responsible for the regression of the Mullerian ducts during sexual differentiation.

Once spermatogonia cross the barrier into Sertoli cells they become progressively modified and enlarged, forming large primary spermatocytes (Fig. 4.103), each of which undergoes meiotic division to form two secondary spermatocytes; a few days later these also divide by meiosis forming spermatids that are eventually modified to become spermatozoa (sperm) (Fig. 4.103).

Several hormones have essential roles in spermatogenesis: LH (secreted by the adenohypophysis)

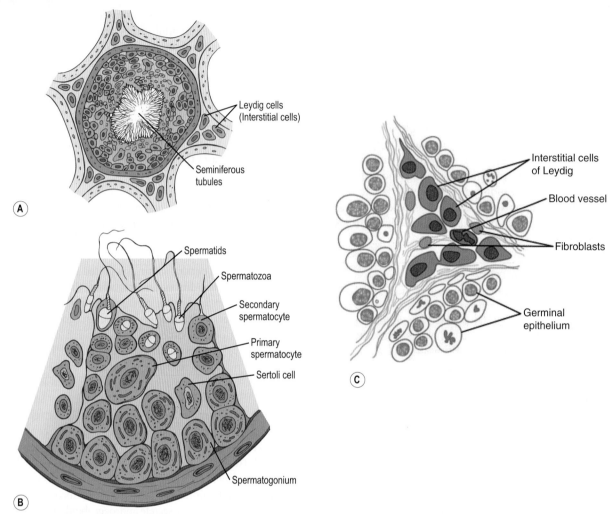

Fig. 4.102 (A) Cross-section of a seminiferous tubule. (B) Stages in the development of sperm from spermatogonia. (C) Leydig cells.

stimulates Leydig cells (Fig. 4.102A, C) to secrete testosterone in the 1st stage of sperm formation, it is essential for the growth and division of the testicular germinal cells; FSH (secreted by the adenohypophysis) stimulates Sertoli cells promoting the conversion of spermatids to sperm; oestrogens (formed from testosterone by Sertoli cells) are also essential for spermatogenesis; and GH controls the background metabolic function of the testes, specifically promoting early division of spermatogonia. Decreased thyroxin secretion inhibits spermatogenesis and promotes infertility.

APPLIED ANATOMY: Between the spermatocyte and spermatid stages, the 23 pairs of chromosomes are each divided, with 23 going to 1 spermatid and 23 to the other; this divides the chromosomal genes so that only half the genetic characteristics of the foetus come from the father, the other half coming from the mother (page 531). The gender of the foetus is determined by whether it is a sperm carrying the male Y chromosome or is carrying the female X chromosome: males have XY sex chromosomes and females XX sex chromosomes.

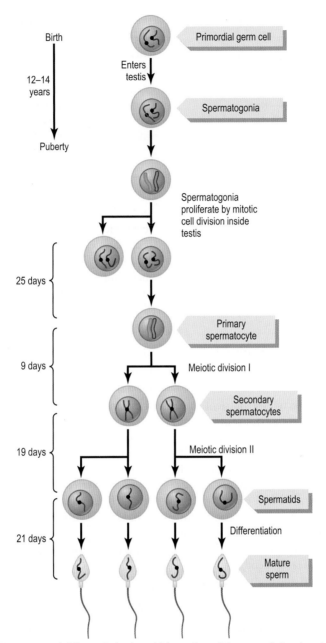

Fig. 4.103 The stages of differentiation by which a primordial germ cell develops into a sperm.

Initially, spermatids have the characteristics of epithelioid cells, but soon differentiate and elongate into spermatozoa (Fig. 4.104); each spermatozoon comprises a head and tail (flagellum). The acrosome contains hyaluronidase (to digest proteoglycan filaments) and proteolytic enzymes (to digest protein) enabling the sperm to enter the ovum and fertilise it. Flagellar movements

of the tail propel it forwards through the female genital tract to reach the ovum.

As sperm move along the male reproductive tract (rete testis, efferent ductules, epididymis, vas deferens), they develop the capability of motility and continue to mature; however, not until they are ejaculated does the process of full maturation occur. Sertoli cells and the

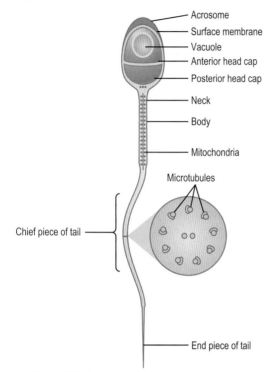

- Acrosome
- Surface membrane
- Vacuole
- Anterior head cap
- Posterior head cap
- Neck
- Body
- Mitochondria

Microtubules

Chief piece of tail

End piece of tail

Fig. 4.104 Structure of a human spermatozoa.

epithelium of the epididymis secretes a nutrient fluid containing hormones (testosterone, oestrogens) and enzymes necessary for maturation. It is only after ejaculation, when sperm comes into contact with fluids in the female genital tract, that changes occur to activate it ready for fertilisation (capacitation); inhibitory factors suppressing sperm activity are washed away by fluid in the uterine and Fallopian tubes; excess cholesterol vesicles are lost, weakening the membrane covering the head of the sperm (acrosome); calcium enters the sperm through the more permeable membrane, changing the activity of the flagellum, the leading edge of the acrosome releases enzymes (hyaluronidases, proteolytic enzymes) enabling the sperm to penetrate the granulosa cell mass surrounding the ovum as it attempts to penetrate the zona pellucida. Without these changes, fertilisation cannot occur.

When the sperm reaches the zona pellucida, its anterior membrane binds with receptor proteins in the zona pellucida following which the acrosome dissolves, releasing all acrosomal enzymes, thus opening a pathway for the sperm head through the zona pellucida to the inside of the ovum. Within a very short time, the sperm head and oocyte fuse forming a single cell, with

the genetic material of both sperm and ovum combining to form a new cell genome with an equal number of chromosomes and genes from each parent; this is fertilisation, following which the embryo begins to develop.

> **APPLIED PHYSIOLOGY:** Once the 1st sperm has penetrated the zona pellucida, calcium ions diffuse inward through the oocyte membrane resulting in the exocytotic release of numerous cortical granules from the oocyte preventing the binding of additional sperm.

Testosterone. One of a number of hormones collectively called androgens (testosterone, dihydrotestosterone, androstenedione) secreted by the testis, testosterone is formed by Leydig cells (interstitial cells of Leydig). Leydig cells are numerous in newborn males for a few months and after puberty, but almost non-existent during childhood. Testosterone (<5%) is also produced by the zona fasciculata and zona reticularis of the adrenal glands (page 343). Following secretion, 97% of testosterone becomes loosely bound with plasma albumin or tightly bound with beta globulin (sex hormone-binding globulin) and circulates in the blood for a limited time (minutes to hours), after which it is transferred to the tissues or degraded into inactive products that are excreted. Most testosterone fixed to tissues is converted within the cells to dihydrotestosterone, especially in the prostate in adult males and external genitalia in male foetuses. Testosterone not fixed to tissues is converted (mainly in the liver) into androsterone and DHEA and conjugated as glucuronides or sulphates and excreted via bile into the gut or urine by the kidneys.

> **APPLIED PHYSIOLOGY:** During pregnancy human chorionic gonadotropin (hCG) is secreted by the placenta; if the foetus is male it causes the secretion of testosterone.

Small amounts of oestrogens are found in males, being converted from testosterone by Sertoli cells in the seminiferous tubules into oestradiol, where it is necessary for spermatogenesis, and in the liver into androstanediol.

> **APPLIED PHYSIOLOGY:** X-ray treatment or excessive heat can destroy the germinal epithelium of the testes; Leydig cells are less easily destroyed and are often able to continue producing testosterone. Leydig cell tumours secrete large amounts of testosterone.

Functions. Testosterone is responsible for the development of male sexual characteristics, being formed in the testes at about the 7th week of embryonic life. The SRY (sex determining region Y) gene encodes the testis determining factor (SRY protein), which in turn initiates a cascade of gene activations causing the genital ridge cells to differentiate into cells that secrete testosterone and become the testes; in contrast, female chromosomes cause the ridge to develop female sexual organs. Testosterone secreted by the genital ridges and later by the foetal testes is responsible for the development of male body characteristics (formation of the penis, scrotum, prostate gland, seminal vesicles, male genital ducts) rather than the formation of female genital organs (clitoris, vagina, uterus, Fallopian tubes).

Testosterone causes descent of the testes into the scrotum in the later stages of gestation. At the onset of puberty, testosterone production rapidly increases under the stimulation of adenohypophyseal gonadotropic hormones, which lasts throughout most of the remainder of life (Fig. 4.105).

During puberty, the penis, scrotum and testes enlarge, with male secondary sexual characteristics also developing: growth of body hair (pubis, upward along the line alba (page 454), face, chest); deepening of the voice by enlargement of the larynx and hypertrophy of the laryngeal mucosa; increases in skin thickness, protein formation and development of the musculature, bone growth and calcium retention, basal metabolic rate, numbers of red blood cells, and blood and extracellular fluid volumes in relation to body weight.

APPLIED PHYSIOLOGY: The lack of non-functioning testes in foetal life leads to no male sexual characteristics developing; instead, female organs are formed because the basic genetic characteristic of the foetus is to form female sexual organs. It is the presence of testosterone which induces male organs.

For the most part, the control of sexual function in males (and females) begins with the secretion of gonadotropin-releasing hormone (GnRH) by the hypothalamus (Fig. 4.106), which in turn stimulates the adenohypophysis to secrete gonadotropic hormones (LH, FSH); LH is the main stimulus for testosterone secretion by the testes, while FSH primarily stimulates spermatogenesis.

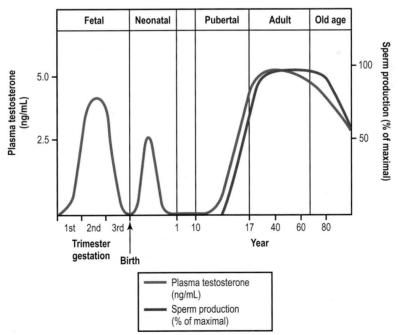

Fig. 4.105 Average plasma testosterone concentration (*red line*) and sperm production (*blue line*) throughout life. (Modified from Griffin JF, Wilson JD. The testis. In: Bondy PK, Rosenberg LE, eds. Metabolic control and disease. 8th ed. Philadelphia, PA: WB Saunders; 1980.)

APPLIED PHYSIOLOGY: If the testes are removed (extirpated) before puberty, the individual continues to have infantile sexual characteristics throughout life (eunuchism): the bones are weak and thin, muscles are weak, secondary sexual characteristics fail to develop, the voice fails to deepen, the sexual organs remain child-like, there is abnormal fat deposition on the buttocks, hip, pubis and breast resembling the female distribution. If removed immediately after puberty, some secondary sexual characteristics revert to those of a child, while others are retained. When the testes are removed in adulthood there is no loss of secondary sexual characteristics; however, the accessory sexual organs (seminal vesicles, prostate) start to degenerate and although erection is possible ejaculation is rare.

Hypergonadism. A condition characterised by the hypersecretion of sex hormones, being mainly due to tumour of the Leydig cells; it is common in prepubertal males who develop pseudopuberty. There is a rapid growth of bones and muscles, but height is less due to early fusion of the epiphyses with the shaft, excess development of the external genitalia and secondary sexual characteristics, as well as enlargement of the breasts (gynaecomastia) due to the secretion of oestrogen.

Hypogonadism. Hypogonadism can be due to a number of testicular abnormalities: congenital non-functioning testes; underdeveloped testes due to the absence of human chorionic gonadotropin in foetal life; cryptorchidism, associated with partial or total testicular degeneration; castration; absence of androgen receptors in the testes; disorder of the gonadotrope cells in the adenohypophysis; or a hypothalamic disorder.

CLINICAL PHYSIOLOGY: When caused by testicular disorders increasing gonadotropin secretion, it is known as hypergonadotropic hypogonadism; when due to a deficiency in gonadotropins (pituitary or hypothalamic disorder), it is known as hypogonadotropic hypogonadism.

Ovaries

Details of the female reproductive tract can be found on page 541.

During foetal life, the outer surface of the ovary is covered by germinal epithelium, derived from the germinal ridge epithelium, with primordial ova differentiating

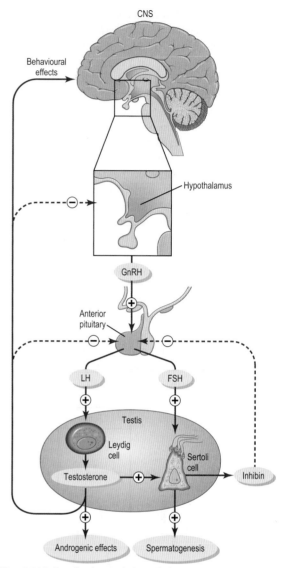

Fig. 4.106 Feedback regulation of the hypothalamic-pituitary-testicular axis in males. *CNS,* Central nervous system; *FSH,* follicle-stimulating hormone; *GnRH,* gonadotropin-releasing hormone; *LH,* luteinising hormone.

from this epithelium and migrating into the substance of the ovarian cortex. Each ovum collects around it a layer of spindles (granulosa cells) from the ovarian stroma; the ovum and single layer of granulosa cells is a primordial follicle (Fig. 4.107). Between 400 and 500 primordial follicles develop sufficiently to expel their ova (1/month) during the female's reproductive years, with the remainder degenerating; following menopause any remaining primordial follicles also degenerate.

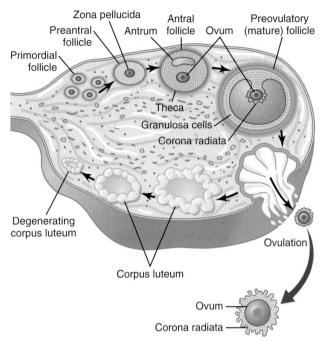

Fig. 4.107 Stages of follicular growth in the ovary; also shown is the formation of the corpus luteum.

Reproductive hormones. Throughout the reproductive period, there are rhythmical changes in the rates of secretion of female hormones (Fig. 4.108) and corresponding changes in the ovaries and other sexual organs: the female menstrual cycle averages 28 days. Within each cycle, a single ovum is normally released and the uterine endometrium is prepared in advance for implantation of the fertilised ovum.

The ovarian changes are entirely dependent on gonadotropic hormones (FSH, LH) secreted by the adenohypophysis; the ovaries remain inactive without these hormones. During puberty, the adenohypophysis starts to secrete progressively more of both hormones; there is a cyclical increase and decrease causing cyclical ovarian changes. With the secretion of FSH and LH some primordial follicles start to grow, seen initially as enlargement of the ovum followed by the growth of additional layers of granulosa cells in some follicles, resulting in primary follicles (Fig. 4.107). When the concentrations of both FSH and LH increase, there is accelerated growth of 6–12 primary follicles each month, accompanied by rapid proliferation of the granulosa cells, with spindle cells (derived from the ovary interstitium) outside

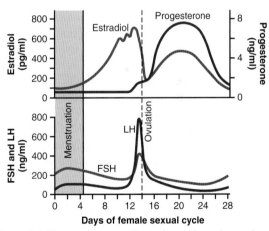

Fig. 4.108 Plasma concentrations of gonadotropins and ovarian hormones during the female sexual cycle. *FSH*, follicle-stimulating hormone; *LH*, luteinising hormone.

the granulosa cells forming the theca, which divides into two layers. Theca interna cells develop the ability to secrete additional steroid sex hormones (oestrogen, progesterone), while the theca externa cells develop into a highly vascular connective tissue capsule of the developing follicle.

Following the proliferative phase, the granulosa cells secrete a follicular fluid containing high concentrations of oestrogen, causing an antrum to appear within the mass of granulosa cells (Fig. 4.107). Once growth of the antral cells begins, the ovum also enlarges. After a week of growth, but before ovulation one follicle outgrows the rest, with the remainder involuting (atresia) becoming atretic; the single follicle is large (10–15 mm diameter) and is now a mature follicle. Prior to ovulation the protruding outer wall of the follicle rapidly swells leaving a small area in the centre of the capsule (stigma) protruding, fluid oozes through the stigma which then ruptures allowing more viscous fluid to evaginate; the viscous fluid carries with it the ovum surrounded by numerous granulosa cells (corona radiata). A surge in LH is required for the final follicular growth and ovulation, without it the follicle will not progress to the stage of ovulation, even when large quantities of FSH are present; the presence of LH converts the granulosa and theca cells to become progesterone-secreting cells.

Ovulation. Following the rapid secretion of follicular steroid hormones containing progesterone, two events occur: the theca externa cells release proteolytic enzymes from lysosomes causing dissolution of the follicular capsule, weakening the wall enabling further swelling of the entire follicle; degeneration of the stigma; and growth of new vessels into the follicle wall with prostaglandins (causing vasodilation) secreted into the follicular tissue. The combination of follicular swelling and stigma degeneration causes the follicle to rupture and discharge of the ovum.

Corpus luteum. Following ovulation, the remaining granulosa and theca interna cells rapidly become lutein cells, which proliferate, enlarge, secrete and then degenerate over about 12 days; during enlargement, they become filled with lipid inclusions giving them a yellowish appearance. The granulosa cells produce large amounts of progesterone and oestrogen, while the theca cells produce androgens (androstenedione, testosterone); they also secrete small amounts of inhibin which inhibits secretion of FSH by the adenohypophysis. Low concentrations of both FSH and LH cause the corpus luteum to degenerate completely (involution), being replaced by connective tissue and then absorbed. The cessation of oestrogen, progesterone and inhibin secretion removes the feedback inhibition of the adenohypophysis allowing it to once again begin secreting FSH and LH, which

initiates the growth of new follicles and the start of a new cycle. The paucity of oestrogen and progesterone secretion leads to menstruation (page 546).

Oestrogens. Within plasma, oestrogen is present in three forms (β-oestradiol, oestrone and oestriol), with the quantity and potency of β-oestradiol being more than that of oestrone and oestriol. Oestrogen is transported mainly by albumin, with some by globulin; the binding is loose so that the hormones are easily released into the tissues.

Effects. During puberty the secretion of oestrogens markedly increases, leading to cellular proliferation and tissue growth of the sex organs (ovaries, Fallopian tubes, uterus, vagina) and external genitalia (mons pubis, labia major and minor). There is a change in vaginal epithelium from cuboidal to stratified, making it more resistant to trauma and infection. In addition to an increase in the size of the uterus, there are important changes in the endometrium, with oestrogens causing a marked proliferation of the endometrial stroma and development of the endometrial glands, which later provide nutrition to the implanted ovum.

Oestrogen is also responsible for the development of secondary sexual characteristics in females: development of hair over the pubis (usually triangular in shape) and axilla, scalp hair grows profusely but body hair growth is less; the skin becomes soft and smooth, with its vascularity increasing; the shoulders narrow while the hips broaden, the thighs converge and arms diverge; fat deposition increases in the breasts and buttocks; the pelvis broadens increasing the transverse diameter, becoming round or oval rather than heart-shaped as in males; the larynx remains prepubertal.

In addition to increased fat deposits in the breast, oestrogen also causes development of stromal tissue, lobules and alveoli, and growth of an extensive duct system. These changes prepare the breast for lactation; however, progesterone is also required to complete breast growth, as well as prolactin for lactation.

Oestrogen increases osteoblast activity, with growth increasing rapidly at puberty; however, it also causes early fusion of the shaft and epiphysis of long bones, the effect being more pronounced in females than the effect of testosterone in males; growth in females usually stops earlier than in males. In older ages, oestrogen secretion becomes scanty (or ceases) and can lead to osteoporosis leaving the bones weak, fragile and susceptible to fracture.

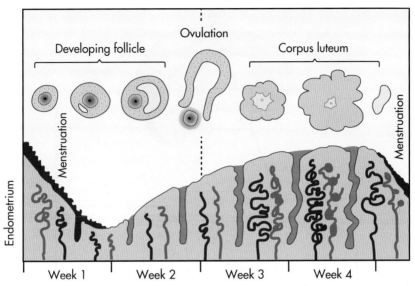

Fig. 4.109 Uterine changes during the menstrual cycle.

Oestrogen induces anabolism of proteins increasing total body protein; causes deposition of fat in the subcutaneous tissues (breast, buttocks, thighs); and increases sodium and water retention by the renal tubules, being more significant during pregnancy.

Regulation of secretion. By FSH released by the adenohypophysis, which in turn is stimulated by GnRH secreted by the hypothalamus. There is a negative feedback mechanism whereby oestrogen inhibits the secretion of both FSH and GnRH; granulosa cells in the ovaries also inhibit oestrogen secretion.

Progesterone. Progesterone is secreted by theca interna cells during the follicular stage (1st half) of the menstrual cycle, with large amounts being secreted during the secretory stage (2nd half) of the menstrual cycle; small amounts are also secreted by the adrenal cortex. During pregnancy the corpus luteum secretes large amounts during the 1st trimester; the placenta does the same during the 2nd and 3rd trimesters. It is transported in blood by albumin and globulin. Within a few minutes of being secreted, progesterone is degraded by the liver into other steroids, with the main end product being pregnanediol, which is conjugated with glucuronic acid and excreted in urine.

Effects. Progesterone is mainly associated with the final preparation of the uterus for pregnancy and of the breasts for lactation. It promotes secretory activities of the Fallopian tubes to provide nutrition for the ovum prior to implantation, and for the uterine endometrium. Specifically, it increases the thickness of the endometrium by increasing the size and number of cells; the size of uterine glands, which become more tortuous, and secretory activity of its epithelial cells; deposition of lipids and glycogen in endometrial stromal cells; blood supply to the endometrium by increasing the size of the vessels and vasodilation (Fig. 4.109); and the thickness of the cervical mucosa inhibiting the transport of sperm into the uterus. Progesterone decreases the frequency of uterine contractions during pregnancy preventing expulsion of the implanted ovum, and inhibits release of LH from the hypothalamus via a feedback mechanism.

Other effects include promoting development of lobules and alveoli in the breasts, causing the breasts to enlarge by increasing their secretory activity and fluid accumulation in the subcutaneous tissue; increasing body temperature following ovulation; increasing respiration during the luteal phase of the menstrual cycle and pregnancy by decreasing the partial pressure of carbon dioxide in the alveoli; and increasing the reabsorption of sodium and water from the renal tubules.

Regulation of secretion. By LH from the adenohypophysis activating the corpus luteum, which in turn is influenced by GnRH secreted by the hypothalamus; the release of LH is inhibited by negative feedback (Fig. 4.110).

Puberty, menarche and menopause. The onset of adult sexual life begins with puberty, with menarche signalling the start of menstrual cycles; menopause usually occurs between ages 40 and 50 and signals irregular cycles with ovulation often failing to occur. Puberty is caused by a gradual increase in gonadotropic hormone

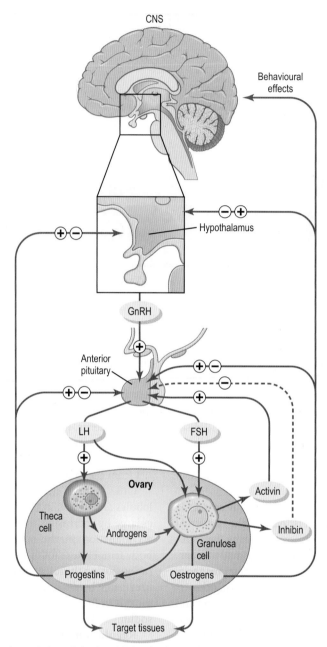

Fig. 4.110 Feedback regulation of the hypothalamic-pituitary-ovarian axis in females. *CNS,* Central nervous system; *FSH,* Follicle-stimulating hormone; *GnRH,* gonadotropin-releasing hormone; *LH,* luteinising hormone.

secretion by the adenohypophysis, beginning around 8 years of age (Fig. 4.111) and culminating in the onset of puberty, with menstruation beginning between ages 11 and 16 (average, 13 years).

Between ages 40 and 50 the sexual cycle becomes irregular with ovulation failing to occur, with the cycle ceasing completely within a few months/years; this period is the menopause caused by a decrease in the production of oestrogens by the ovaries as the number of primordial follicles approaches zero. When oestrogen production falls below a critical level they are unable to inhibit the production of FSH and LH, so that their secretion is continuous and in large quantities (Fig. 4.111). The loss of oestrogen often causes marked physiological changes: 'hot flushes'

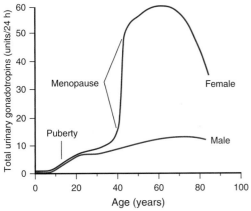

Fig. 4.111 The rates of secretion of gonadotropic hormones in males and females at different ages, showing an abrupt increase in females at menopause in females.

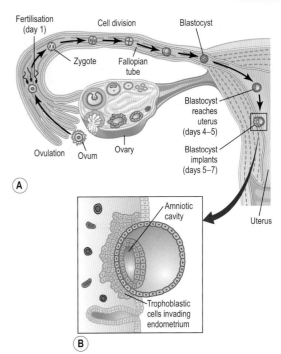

Fig. 4.112 (A) Ovulation and fertilisation of the ovum followed by implantation in the endometrial lining of the uterus. (B) Action of the trophoblast cells in implantation.

characterised by extreme flushing; psychic sensations of dyspnoea; irritability; fatigue; anxiety; and decreased strength and calcification of bones throughout the body.

Menstrual cycle. The menstrual cycle (average, 28 days; range 20–40 days) is characterised by a series of simultaneous changes in the ovaries, uterus, vagina and cervix; details of these changes, together with ovulation, can be found on pages 358 and 359. Details of the hormonal levels during the menstrual cycle can be found on page 357.

Common menstrual symptoms are abdominal pain, dysmenorrhea (menstrual pain), occasional nausea and vomiting, irritability, depression and migraine. Premenstrual syndrome (premenstrual stress syndrome, premenstrual stress, premenstrual tension) relates to the stress that appears before the onset of menstruation; it is caused by salt and water retention caused by oestrogen. Common features are mood swings, anxiety, irritability, emotional instability, headache, depression, constipation, abdominal cramps and abdominal swelling (bloating).

Menstruation without ovulation is common during puberty and a few years before menopause (perimenopause); it can lead to infertility. Common causes are hormonal imbalance; prolonged strenuous exercise; eating disorders; hypothalamic dysfunction; pituitary, ovarian or adrenal gland tumours; and long-term drug use (steroidal oral contraceptives).

Hypogonadism. Reduced secretion can be the result of poorly formed (or lack of) ovaries or genetically abnormal ovaries secreting the wrong hormones due to missing enzymes in the secretory cells. Absent or non-functional ovaries prior to puberty lead to female eunuchism, in which the secondary sexual characteristics fail to appear and the sexual organs remain infantile.

Removal of the ovaries in adults leads to regression of the uterus, a decrease in the size of the vagina with thin easily damaged epithelium and breast atrophy; the same changes occur after menopause.

Irregular menses and amenorrhea can occur due to low levels of oestrogen; a critical level is needed for rhythmical menstrual cycles. Prolonged ovarian cycles are usually associated with failure of ovulation, possibly due to insufficient secretion of LH at the time of the pre-ovulatory surge.

Hypergonadism. This is rare because excessive secretion by the ovaries automatically decreases gonadotropin production limiting the production of ovarian hormones; clinically it is only recognised in the presence of a feminising tumour. Granulosa cell tumours can develop (more often after menopause), which secrete large amounts of oestrogen leading to hypertrophy of the endometrium and irregular bleeding; bleeding may be the 1st and only indication of a tumour.

Pregnancy, Parturition and Lactation

Pregnancy

Fertilisation, cleavage and implantation. Once the ovum has been fertilised by a sperm, a series of events are set in motion; fertilisation occurs within the Fallopi-

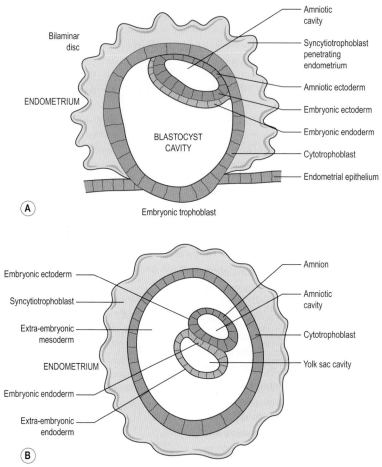

Fig. 4.113 (A) Implantation of the fertilised egg. (B) Appearance of the yolk sac.

an tube. Within 12 hours, the male and female pronuclei have fused forming a zygote, within another 12 hours cleavage occurs consisting of repeated mitotic divisions forming increasing numbers of cells (blastomeres) without an increase in total cytoplasmic mass; the 16-cell mass is a morula. After 4–5 days, the zygote reaches the uterus where it remains free before becoming implanted in the endometrium (Fig. 4.112); prior to implantation, the blastocyst obtains its nutrients from endometrial secretions (uterine milk). Just before implantation a layer of spherical cells (trophoblasts) releases proteolytic enzymes over the surface of the endometrium, digesting and liquefying it, allowing the morula to become implanted.

The morula takes in uterine fluid through the zona pellucida forming a blastocyst cavity (Fig. 4.113A) separating the inner cell mass from the trophoblast, except near the polar trophoblast overlying the inner cell mass; during blastocyst formation, the zona pellucida thins and is eventually shed.

During the early stages of implantation (6–8 days), the inner cell mass differentiates eventually forming the complete embryo. Cells facing the blastocyst cavity form a single layer of primary embryonic endoderm, with the remaining cells forming another layer (embryonic ectoderm), which also gives rise to the embryonic mesoderm (Fig. 4.113B). The amniotic cavity appears between these cells and an overlaying layer of cells (amniotic ectoderm) derived from the deep aspect of the polar trophoblast (Fig. 4.113B). Surrounding the blastocyst cavity, the trophoblast forms the cytotrophoblast and the syncytiotrophoblast, which penetrates the endometrial lining of the uterus (Fig. 4.113B). The inner cell mass gives rise to all future cells of the embryo, being no more than a bilaminar disc: the remaining blastocyst forms the foetal membranes.

As the amniotic cavity is formed, the blastocyst cavity becomes lined by extra-embryonic endoderm cells so that the blastocyst wall consists of three layers

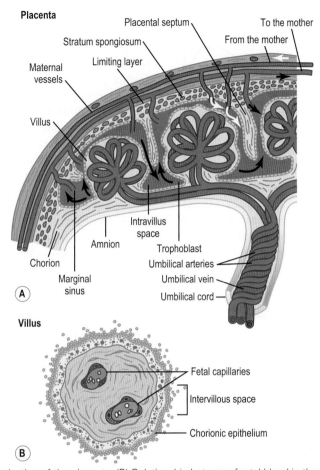

Placenta

Placental septum

To the mother

From the mother

Stratum spongiosum

Maternal vessels

Limiting layer

Villus

Intravillus space

Amnion

Trophoblast

Chorion

Umbilical arteries

Marginal sinus

Umbilical vein

Umbilical cord

(A)

Villus

Fetal capillaries

Intervillous space

Chorionic epithelium

(B)

Fig. 4.114 (A) Organisation of the placenta. (B) Relationship between foetal blood in the villus capillaries and maternal blood in the intervillous spaces.

comprising an outer trophoblast layer (extra-embryonic ectoderm, comprising cytotrophoblast and syncytiotrophoblast), middle loose reticular layer (extra-embryonic mesoderm) and inner layer (extra-embryonic endoderm); the remaining space is the yolk sac (Fig. 4.113B).

As the trophoblast cells in the morula develop into cords, they attach to the endometrium; blood capillaries grow into the cords from the vascular system of the newly forming embryo. Some 21 days following fertilisation, blood begins to be pumped by the developing foetal heart; at the same time, blood sinuses supplied with maternal blood develop around the outsides of the trophoblastic cords. The trophoblast cells send out more and more projections, which become placental villi into which the foetal capillaries grow forming the placenta (Fig. 4.114).

Placenta. The placenta functions to provide diffusion of oxygen and nutrients from maternal to foetal blood, and dif-

fusion of excretory products from foetal to maternal blood. As pregnancy progresses, permeability increases due to thinning of the membrane diffusion layers and expansion of the surface area through which diffusion occurs (Fig. 4.115). Further details of the placenta can be found on page 548.

Dissolved oxygen in the large maternal sinuses passes into foetal blood by simple diffusion, driven by an oxygen pressure gradient from maternal to foetal blood. The foetus is able to obtain sufficient oxygen because; foetal haemoglobin has a greater affinity for oxygen than adult haemoglobin (Fig. 4.116); haemoglobin concentration in foetal blood is 50% greater than that of the mother; and haemoglobin can carry more oxygen at low P_{CO_2} than at high P_{CO_2} (Bohr effect).

Hormonal factors during pregnancy. The placenta forms large quantities of human chorionic gonadotropins, oestrogens, progesterone and human

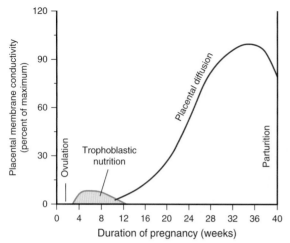

Fig. 4.115 Foetal nutrition during pregnancy.

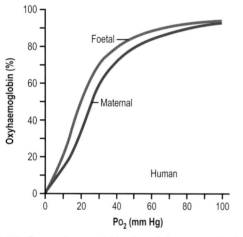

Fig. 4.116 Oxygen-haemoglobin dissociation curves for foetal and maternal blood. (Data from Metcalfe J, Moll W, Bartels H: Gas exchange across the placenta. Fed Proc 23:775, 1964.)

chorionic somatomammotropin throughout pregnancy (Fig. 4.117). Human chorionic gonadotropin is secreted by the syncytial trophoblast cells into the mother's fluid; it prevents involution of the corpus luteum causing it to secrete large quantities of oestrogens and progesterone preventing menstruation, as well as causing the endometrium to continue growing and storing nutrients. The decidua-like cells that develop during a normal cycle become swollen and nutritious decidual cells at the time of implantation.

Oestrogens secreted by the placenta are not synthesised from basic substrates; they are formed almost entirely from androgenic steroid compounds (DHEA, 16-

hydroxydehydroepiandrosterone) formed in the mother's adrenal glands and those of the foetus. Foetal adrenal glands are extremely large, with 80% constituting a 'foetal zone' with the primary function of secreting DHEA. During pregnancy large quantities of oestrogen cause enlargement of the uterus, external genitalia and breasts, together with growth of the breast ductal structure. It also relaxes pelvic ligaments and softens the symphysis pubis making it more elastic; these changes facilitate the passage of the foetus through the birth canal.

Progesterone is secreted in large quantities by the placenta during the later stages of pregnancy (Fig. 4.117); it causes the decidual cells to develop in the endometrium; decreases the contractility of the pregnant uterus; contributes to the development of the zygote prior to implantation, specifically increasing secretions from the Fallopian tubes; and during pregnancy help oestrogen prepare the breasts for lactation.

Human chorionic somatomammotropin secretion by the placenta starts in the 5th week of pregnancy, increasing rapidly for the remainder of the pregnancy. It results in some breast development, having a similar action to GH, causes decreased insulin sensitivity and decreased utilisation of glucose in the mother making large quantities of glucose available for the foetus, promotes the release of free fatty acids from the mother's fat stores providing an alternative maternal energy source during pregnancy.

Because of the increased metabolic load on the mother, most other non-sexual endocrine glands react to pregnancy; the pituitary enlarges and increases its production of corticotropin, thyrotropin and prolactin; the thyroid gland enlarges increasing its thyroxine production; the parathyroid glands enlarge causing calcium absorption from the mother's bones to maintain calcium ion concentration in the maternal extracellular fluid, during lactation the secretion of parathormone is intensified. The secretion of relaxin, a hormone secreted by the corpus luteum and placental tissues, is increased by the stimulating effect of human chorionic gonadotropin at the same time as increased secretion of oestrogens and progesterone; it is thought to cause relaxation of the pelvic ligaments, inhibit uterine contractions during pregnancy and possibly softens the cervix at the time of parturition.

Maternal responses to pregnancy. Under the influence of excessive hormones, the maternal sexual organs increase in size; there are also marked changes in appearance. There is weight gain, mostly during the 2nd and 3rd trimesters, accompanied by an increased desire for food; basal metabolic rate increases by about 15%, especially in the latter half of

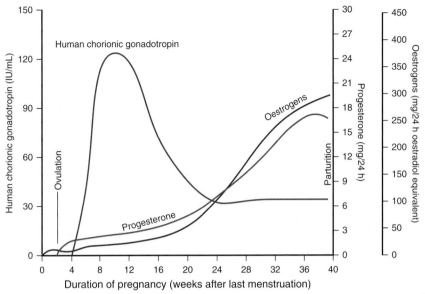

Fig. 4.117 Rate of secretion of oestrogens and progesterone, together with the concentration of human chorionic gonadotropin at different stages of pregnancy.

pregnancy; cardiac output increases up to the 27th week of pregnancy then returns to just above normal; blood volume increases during the latter half of pregnancy due to increased fluid retention by the kidneys; bone marrow becomes increasingly active producing extra red blood cells accompanying the excess fluid; respiratory and ventilation rates both increase; urine production is slightly increased, with increased resorptive capacity by the renal tubules for sodium, chloride and water, accompanied by increased blood flow and glomerular filtration rates due to renal vasodilation.

> **CLINICAL PHYSIOLOGY:** Lack of sufficient iron in the diet can lead to hypochromic anaemia.

> **CLINICAL PHYSIOLOGY:** Some mothers experience a rapid rise in arterial blood pressure to hypertensive levels, being associated with leakage of large amounts of protein into the urine (preeclampsia/toxaemia). It is characterised by excess salt and water retention by the kidneys, weight gain, oedema and hypertension; there is also impaired vascular endothelium functioning, with arterial spasm occurring in many parts of the body (kidneys, brain, liver). Preeclampsia may be initiated by insufficient blood supply to the placenta. Eclampsia (an extreme form of preeclampsia) is characterised by vascular spasm throughout the body; clonic seizures, sometimes followed by coma; liver malfunction; and a generalised toxic condition of the body. It occurs shortly before birth: without treatment (the administration of rapidly acting vasodilating drugs and/or inducing birth) it can be fatal.

Parturition (childbirth). Weak, irregular, short, usually painless (Braxton Hicks) contractions occur from the 6th week of pregnancy; they can be triggered by touching the abdomen, movement of the foetus in the uterus, physical activity, sexual intercourse and dehydration. Towards the end of pregnancy, the contractions become more intense as the uterus becomes progressively more excitable; strong rhythmical contractions eventually occur which help expel the baby. During pregnancy, progesterone inhibits uterine contractility, while oestrogens tend to increase contractility; from the 7th month, oestrogen secretion continues to increase while progesterone secretion remains constant (or decreases slightly). Oxytocin also increases uterine contractions; the myometrium increases its oxytocin receptors increasing its responsiveness; oxytocin secretion by the neurohypophysis increases at the time of labour; and cervical stretching causes a neurogenic reflex via the hypothalamic paraventricular and supraoptic nuclei causing the neurohypophysis to secrete more oxytocin. In addition, foetal adrenal glands secrete large amounts of cortisol and foetal membranes release high concentrations of prostaglandins during labour; both can increase the intensity of uterine contractions.

Stages of labour. In the 1st stage, contractions start at the fundus of the uterus (page 543) and move downwards pushing the foetal head against the cervix, dilating it and stimulating cervical muscles, resulting in reflex contractions of the uterus. Once started uterine contractions become stronger and stronger via a positive feedback mechanism, producing more uterine contractions of increasing intensity. The 1st stage is a period of progressive cervical dilation, usually lasting between 8 and 24 hours for the 1st pregnancy, but considerably less in subsequent pregnancies. In addition, there is also intense contraction of the abdominal muscles.

Prior to the 2nd stage, once the cervix is fully dilated the foetal membranes usually rupture with the loss of amniotic fluid. The foetal head moves through the dilated cervix and the vaginal canal until the completion of delivery; this stage generally lasts about 30 minutes for the 1st pregnancy and less for subsequent pregnancies.

With each contraction, the mother experiences considerable pain, with the cramping pain of early labour being caused by hypoxia of the myometrium due to compression of the blood vessels. During the 2nd stage of labour, the pain increases in severity being caused by cervical and perineal stretching, as well as stretching or tearing of structures in the vaginal canal. The pain is conducted by somatic nerves instead of visceral sensory nerves.

In the 3rd stage, for 10–45 minutes after birth uterine contractions continue with the uterus becoming smaller and smaller, causing a shearing effect between the uterine walls and placenta, separating the placenta from its implantation site. This opens the placental sinuses causing bleeding, uterine contraction following delivery constricts the vessels that previously supplied blood to the placenta; prostaglandins formed at placental separation cause additional blood vessel spasms.

Mechanics of parturition. The head is usually expelled first; however, in breech births (5% of births) the buttocks or feet appear first. The head acts as a wedge opening the birth canal as the foetus is pushed downwards during delivery; once the head has emerged the shoulders and rest of the body soon follow.

Uterine involution. The uterus involutes in the 4–5 weeks following parturition, becoming less than half its immediate postpartum weight within 1 week and by 4 weeks may become as small as it was before pregnancy, especially if the mother is breastfeeding: lactation suppresses gonadotropin and ovarian oestrogens secretion. During early involution the placental site on the endometrial surface autolyses leading to a vaginal discharge (lochia) lasting about 10 days; initially, it is bloody becoming serous. The endometrial surface then becomes re-epithelialised ready for the next cycle.

Lactation

Breast (mammary gland). At birth the breast (mammary gland) is rudimentary, developing during puberty under the direct stimulation of oestrogens during the menstrual cycle, with growth increasing during pregnancy when the glandular tissues become fully developed in readiness for the production of milk; there is also fat deposition (Fig. 4.118A). Oestrogen secreted by the placenta causes the ductal system to grow and branch; GH, prolactin, adrenal glucocorticoids and insulin all increase protein metabolism during breast development. The final development into a milk-secreting organ requires progesterone, which acts with oestrogen causing additional growth of breast lobules (Fig. 4.118B), with the budding of alveoli and development of secretory characteristics in the alveolar cells.

Prolactin. While oestrogens and progesterone are essential for breast development, they both inhibit milk secretion; in contrast, prolactin promotes milk secretion, with its concentration in maternal blood rising steadily from the 5th week (Fig. 4.119). The placenta also secretes large amounts of human chorionic somatomammotropin supporting the effect of prolactin. Prior to the birth, only small amounts of fluid are secreted daily due to the suppressive effects of oestrogens and progesterone. Colostrum is the fluid secreted for a few days before and after parturition; it has similar concentrations of proteins and lactose as milk, but almost no fat.

Milk secretion. This occurs in two phases: the initiation of secretion (lactogenesis) by prolactin; and the maintenance of secretion (galactopoiesis) by the secretion of GH, thyroxine and cortisol, which are responsible for the continuous supply of glucose, amino acids, fatty acids, calcium and other substances necessary for milk production.

Suckling by the infant is responsible for continuous milk production; impulses from the nipple stimulate the hypothalamus which releases prolactin-releasing factors resulting in prolactin secretion from the adenohypophysis, with the prolactin acting on glandular tissues to maintain the functional activity of the breast.

Milk ejection. Although milk is continuously secreted in the alveoli, it does not readily flow into the ductal system; it must be ejected from the alveoli into the ducts by combined neurogenic and hormonal reflexes involving oxytocin. Sensory impulses from the nipples pass to the hypothalamus promoting oxytocin release, which is carried in the blood to the breasts where it causes

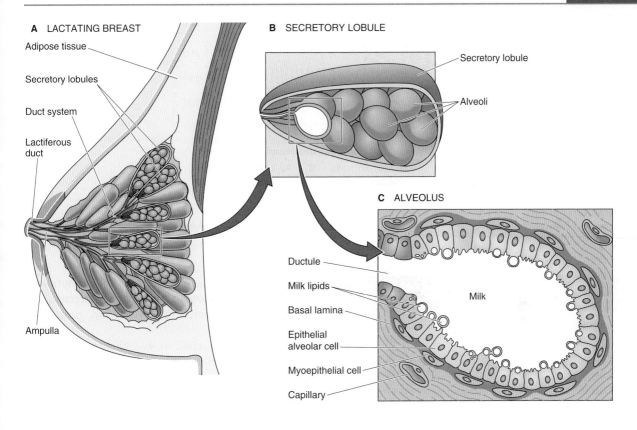

A LACTATING BREAST

Adipose tissue

Secretory lobules

Duct system

Lactiferous duct

Ampulla

B SECRETORY LOBULE

Secretory lobule

Alveoli

C ALVEOLUS

Ductule

Milk lipids

Basal lamina

Epithelial alveolar cell

Myoepithelial cell

Capillary

Milk

Fig. 4.118 (A) The breast showing the secretory lobules, alveoli and lactiferous ducts. (B) Enlargement of a lobule. (C) Milk-secreting cells within an alveolus.

myoepithelial cells (Fig. 4.118C) to contract expressing milk from the alveoli into the ducts (milk ejection reflex, milk let-down reflex).

> **APPLIED PHYSIOLOGY:** Suckling on one breast causes milk to flow in both breasts. When the mother fondles the baby or hears it cry, this emotional signal can trigger the hypothalamus to cause milk ejection.

Composition of breast milk. At the height of lactation, the mother can eject 1.5 L of milk per day, draining large amounts of energy from the mother; between 650 and 750 kilocalories are required per litre produced. The constituents of breast milk are shown in Table 4.13, although the composition and caloric content depend on the mother's diet and other factors (e.g., fullness of the breasts). About 50 g of fat enters milk each day, as well as 100 g of lactose, which is derived from the mother's glucose; 2–3 g of calcium phosphate may be lost by the mother each day therefore an adequate intake of milk and vitamin D is required.

> **APPLIED PHYSIOLOGY:** Maternal bone decalcification is not usually an issue during pregnancy but may become so during lactation.

Milk also provides the baby with protection against infection; many types of antibodies and other anti-infectious agents are secreted in milk alongside the nutrients, as well as neutrophils and macrophages, some of which are lethal to bacteria that could cause deadly infections in the newborn.

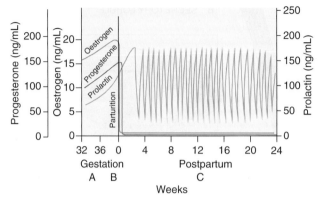

Fig. 4.119 The secretion of oestrogens, progesterone and prolactin before and after parturition in nursing mothers.

TABLE 4.13	The Composition of Breast Milk
Constituent	**Percentage Content**
Water	88.4
Fat	3.3
Lactose	6.8
Casein	0.9
Lactalbumin and other proteins	0.4
Calcium, iron, vitamins A and D, minerals	0.2

Pineal Gland

A small gland located in the diencephalon above the hypothalamus. It has two types of cells (large epithelial (parenchymal) and neuroglial). The main function of the gland is the secretion of melatonin by the parenchymal cells; melatonin production is stimulated by darkness and is important in modulating sleep patterns during the circadian cycle. Internal secretions of the gland inhibit development of the gonads thus inhibiting the onset of puberty; when damaged in children development of the gonads and skeleton are accelerated.

> **APPLIED PHYSIOLOGY:** In adults, the gland is calcified; however, the parenchymal cells still secrete melatonin.

Kidneys

Details of the gross anatomy of the kidneys can be found on page 509. As well as its role in excretion the kidney also has an endocrine function secreting five hormonal substances (erythropoietin, thrombopoietin, renin, 1,25 dihydroxycholecalciferol (calcitriol) and prostaglandins).

Erythropoietin is secreted by endothelial cells of peritubular capillaries, with the stimulus for secretion being hypoxia; it stimulates the bone marrow causing erythropoiesis.

Thrombopoietin secretion by the kidney (and liver) stimulates the production of platelets.

Renin is secreted by the granular cells of the juxtaglomerular apparatus; when released into the blood it acts on α-2 globulin (angiotensinogen/renin substrate). It converts angiotensinogen into angiotensin I, which in turn is converted into angiotensin II; further details can be found on page 516.

Calcitriol is activated by parathormone. It has an important role in the maintenance of blood calcium levels by acting on the intestinal epithelium to enhance the absorption of calcium from the gastrointestinal tract into the blood.

Prostaglandins secreted by the kidney are PGA_2 and PGE_2, which act on the juxtaglomerular cells and type I interstitial cells in the kidney medulla; they decrease blood pressure by systemic vasodilation, diuresis and natriuresis.

Heart

Details of the gross anatomy and function of the heart can be found on page 118. The atrial muscle secretes *atrial natriuretic peptide* when it is overstretched (e.g., increased blood volume); it increases the excretion of sodium (increased glomerular filtration rate, inhibition of sodium resorption from the distal convoluted tubules, increased sodium secretion into the renal tubules) and decreases blood pressure (vasodilation, inhibition of renin secretion, inhibition of the vasoconstriction effects of angiotensin II and catecholamines).

Brain natriuretic peptide is secreted by cardiac muscle; it has similar actions as atrial natriuretic peptide.

Thymus

Details of the thymus and its functions can be found on page 163. In in addition to its lymphoid function, it also has an endocrine function. The gland secretes thymosin, which accelerates lymphopoiesis and the proliferation of T lymphocytes, and thymin (thymopoietin), which suppresses neuromuscular activity by inhibiting acetylcholine release.

Hypothalamus

Details of the hypothalamus, as well as its endocrine function, can be found on page 255.

Local Hormones

These are hormones which act in the area of their secretion; they are usually released in an inactive form and activated by some condition or substance. They can be classified as hormones synthesised either in tissues (prostaglandins and related substances, other local hormones) or in the blood (serotonin, angiotensin, kinins).

Local Hormones Produced in Tissues

Prostaglandins and related hormones. Prostaglandins (PGA_2, PGD_2, PGE_2, PGF_2), thromboxanes (thromboxane A_2, thromboxane B_2), prostacyclin, leukotrienes and lipoxins (lipoxin A, lipoxin B) are derived from arachidonic acid; collectively they are eicosanoids.

Prostaglandins have a variety of physiological actions in the body: on blood, they accelerate the capacity of red blood cells to pass through capillaries; on blood vessels, PGE_2 causes vasodilation; on the gastrointestinal tract, they reduce gastric secretion; on the respiratory system, PGE_2 causes bronchodilation; on lipids, they inhibit the release of free fatty acids from adipose tissue; in the brain, they control or alter the actions of neurotransmitters; on reproduction, they regulate the reproductive cycle, with PGE_2 having an important role during parturition by increasing the force of uterine contraction;

and on the kidney, by stimulating the juxtaglomerular apparatus enhancing the secretion of renin, diuresis and natriuresis.

Thromboxane A_2 is secreted in platelets causing vasoconstriction, acceleration of platelet aggregation and clot formation; thromboxane B_2 is the metabolite of thromboxane A_2.

Prostacyclin is produced in the endothelial and smooth muscle cells of blood vessels; it causes vasodilation, as well as inhibiting platelet aggregation.

Leukotrienes promote inflammatory reactions, being the mediators of allergic responses; they are released when some allergic agents combine with antibodies (e.g., IgE). They cause bronchiolar and arteriolar constriction, vascular permeability and attract neutrophils and eosinophils to the site of inflammation.

Lipoxin A causes vasodilation of capillary vessels, while both lipoxin A and B inhibit the cytotoxic effects of killer T cells.

Other local hormones. *Acetylcholine* is the cholinergic neurotransmitter at the neuromuscular junction; it is secreted by nerve endings (presynaptic terminals), preganglionic and postganglionic parasympathetic nerves, preganglionic sympathetic nerves, postganglionic sympathetic nerves supplying eccrine sweat glands, sympathetic vasodilator nerves in skeletal muscle, and nerves in amacrine cells of the retina and other cells (mast cells, gastric mucosa, lungs, many regions of the brain). It produces the excitatory function of synapses by opening sodium channels, activates smooth muscle in the gastrointestinal and urinary tracts and causes vasodilation. Acetylcholine acts extremely quickly but is immediately destroyed after acting by acetylcholinesterase present in the synaptic cleft.

Serotonin (5-hydroxytryptamine) is secreted by the hypothalamus, limbic system, cerebellum, spinal cord, retina, gastrointestinal tract, lungs and platelets; it inhibits pain sensations, causes vasoconstriction, mood depression and induces sleep.

Histamine is secreted by nerve endings in the hypothalamus, limbic cortex and other parts of the cerebral cortex and spinal cord, as well as being released from tissues in allergic conditions, inflammation and damage. It is an excitatory substance increasing the motility of the gastrointestinal tract; when released from tissues it causes vasodilation, enhanced capillary permeability to fluid and plasma proteins from blood to the affected tissue producing oedema.

Substance P is secreted by nerve endings in the spinal cord and retina, and by the gastrointestinal tract (in the presence of chyme); it is a neurotransmitter for pain, as well as a neurotransmitter in the gastrointestinal tract increasing mixing and propulsive movements of the small intestine.

Heparin is secreted by mast cells and basophils; it acts as a natural anticoagulant.

Leptin is secreted by adipocytes in adipose tissue; it plays an important role in controlling adipose tissue and fat intake by acting on the hypothalamus and inhibiting the feeding centre, at the same time stimulating the metabolic reactions involved in the utilisation of fat stored in adipose tissue.

Details of *gastrointestinal hormones* can be found throughout the digestive physiology section (page 485).

Local Hormones Produced in Blood

Serotonin see above.

Angiotensinogen See page 516.

Kinins (bradykinin, kallidin) are biologically active hormones circulating in blood belonging to the kinin (kinin-kallikrein) system. Bradykinin dilates blood vessels and decreases blood pressure, increasing blood flow throughout the body and the permeability of capillaries during inflammatory conditions resulting in oedema; it also stimulates pain receptors and causes contraction of extravascular smooth muscle, especially in the intestines. Kallidin is a vasodilator.

SELF-TEST QUESTIONS

1. Concerning the skull, which of the following statements is NOT correct?
   a. Diploic veins communicate with the intracranial venous sinuses.
   b. The bregma is the region between the parietal and occipital bones.
   c. The frontal bone may show a metopic suture.
   d. The pterion is the junction between the frontal, parietal, temporal and sphenoid bones.
   e. The shape and size of the skull are determined by intracranial pressure.

2. Concerning the scalp, which of the following statements is correct?
   a. Its blood supply is by numerous branches.
   b. Lacerations to the scalp rarely bleed.
   c. It comprises three layers of tissue.
   d. The whole of the scalp is innervated by cervical nerves.
   e. The pericranium forms the inner surface of the skull vault.

3. Which of the following structures is NOT associated with the foramen ovale?
   a. Mandibular nerve
   b. Lesser petrosal nerve
   c. Middle meningeal artery
   d. Emissary vein
   e. Otic ganglion

4. Which of the following structures is NOT located in the infratemporal fossa?
   a. Medial pterygoid
   b. Maxillary artery
   c. Inferior alveolar nerve
   d. Chorda tympani
   e. Facial nerve

5. Which of the following nerves is NOT sensory to the skin on the face?
   a. Supratrochlear
   b. Infraorbital
   c. Mental
   d. Lesser occipital
   e. Greater auricular

6. Which of the following foramen is NOT located on the base of the skull?
   a. Carotid canal
   b. Jugular foramen
   c. Anterior condylar canal
   d. Pterygopalatine canal
   e. Foramen spinosum

7. Concerning the cranial fossae, which of the following statements is NOT correct?
   a. The falx cerebri is attached to the crista galli.
   b. The frontal lobes of the cerebral hemispheres sit on the orbital part of the frontal bone.
   c. The optic canal communicates with the anterior cranial fossa.
   d. The lateral part of the middle cranial fossa contains the temporal lobe of the brain.
   e. The posterior cranial fossa is covered by the tentorium cerebelli.

8. Which of the following structures does NOT pass through the jugular foramen?
   a. Superior petrosal sinus
   b. Vagus nerve
   c. Sigmoid sinus
   d. Accessory nerve
   e. Glossopharyngeal nerve
9. Concerning the brain, which of the following statements is NOT correct?
   a. Glial cells make up half the total volume of the brain.
   b. Collections of cell bodies with a similar function form a ganglion.
   c. The brainstem consists of the midbrain, pons and medulla oblongata.
   d. The cortex of the cerebellum is grey matter.
   e. A tract is a collection of axons with different functions.
10. Concerning the medulla oblongata, which of the following statements is correct?
   a. It is continuous inferiorly with the pons.
   b. The medial lemniscus carries proprioceptive fibres and tactile impulses.
   c. The glossopharyngeal nerve emerges from its dorsal surface.
   d. Its ventral surface forms part of the floor of the 4th ventricle.
   e. The superior cerebellar peduncle connects it to the cerebellum.
11. Concerning the pons, which of the following statements is NOT correct?
   a. It lies anterior to the cerebellum.
   b. It has large ventral and small dorsal parts.
   c. It is grooved anteriorly by the basilar artery.
   d. Lesions of the lateral segment of the lower pons lead to spastic hemiplegia.
   e. The dorsal part contains cranial nerve nuclei.
12. Concerning the midbrain, which of the following statements is NOT correct?
   a. It passes through the gap in the tentorium cerebelli.
   b. Cerebral peduncles extend from its upper border.
   c. The red nucleus sends efferent fibres to the frontal cortex.
   d. The colliculi are four rounded projections from the dorsal surface.
   e. The inferior colliculus is the reflex centre for hearing.

13. Concerning the cerebellum, which of the following statements is correct?
   a. Each cerebellar hemisphere controls the same side of the body.
   b. It is the largest part of the forebrain.
   c. Each hemisphere is divided into two lobes.
   d. The flocculonodular lobe is responsible for maintaining muscle tone.
   e. Inferior cerebellar peduncles pass superiorly into the medulla oblongata.
14. Concerning the cerebellum, which of the following statements is NOT correct?
   a. It has an inner medulla of white matter.
   b. It is involved in the coordination of muscle activity during movement.
   c. Bilateral dysfunction leads to a staggering unsteady gait.
   d. Two pairs of peduncles connect the cerebellum to the brainstem.
   e. The neocerebellum regulates fine body movements.
15. Concerning the thalamus, which of the following statements is NOT correct?
   a. It is the largest part of the diencephalon.
   b. The right and left thalamus are separated by the 4th ventricle.
   c. Each is an oval mass of grey matter surrounded by white matter.
   d. It is a higher centre for pain and extremes of temperature.
   e. The metathalamus receives afferent fibres concerned with vision.
16. Concerning the thalamus, which of the following statements is correct?
   a. The hypothalamus hangs from its ventrodorsal surface.
   b. The epithalamus is part of the limbic system.
   c. The medial geniculate body is concerned with auditory sensation.
   d. The hypothalamus has neural and vascular connections with the pineal gland.
   e. All sensory inputs relay directly in the thalamus.
17. Concerning the cerebrum, which of the following statements is NOT correct?
   a. The two hemispheres communicate via the corpus callosum.
   b. The occipital lobe is concerned with vision.

c. The frontal lobe is associated with motor functions, intellect and personality.

d. The postcentral gyrus is the primary somatosensory cortex.

e. The parietal lobe is separated from the temporal lobe by the calcarine sulcus.

18. Which of the following is NOT a descending motor tract?
    a. Rubrospinal
    b. Medial reticulospinal
    c. Olivospinal
    d. Ventral spinocerebellar
    e. Tectospinal

19. Concerning the corpus striatum, which of the following statements is NOT correct?
    a. Lesions lead to loss of automatic associative movement.
    b. It regulates muscle tone.
    c. The putamen is an efferent nucleus.
    d. The globus pallidus sends fibres to the hypothalamus.
    e. It influences the precentral motor cortex to control extrapyramidal activity.

20. Concerning the basal ganglia, which of the following statements is NOT correct?
    a. They are part of the pyramidal system.
    b. It includes the corpus striatum.
    c. The amygdaloid body is part of the limbic system.
    d. They are areas of grey matter.
    e. The lentiform nucleus is divided into larger lateral and smaller medial parts.

21. Concerning the ventricular system, which of the following statements is correct?
    a. It is not continuous with the central canal of the spinal cord.
    b. Tela choroidea are double-layered folds of arachnoid mater.
    c. Each lateral ventricle communicates directly with the 4th ventricle.
    d. The lateral ventricles are located mainly in the temporal lobes.
    e. The choroid plexuses produce cerebrospinal fluid.

22. Concerning cerebrospinal fluid, which of the following statements is NOT correct?
    a. It functions to regulate intracranial pressure.
    b. It occupies the subdural space.
    c. It is a modified tissue fluid.

d. It regulates the composition of electrolytes.

e. Its biochemical analysis can be used as a diagnostic tool.

23. Concerning the motor system, which of the following statements is NOT correct?
    a. The extrapyramidal system directly innervates lower motor neurons.
    b. The corticospinal tract starts in the precentral gyrus.
    c. Fibres in the corticospinal tract terminate at different levels in the anterior horn of the spinal grey matter.
    d. Extrapyramidal tracts are not modulated by the central nervous system.
    e. Peripheral nerves carry impulses to skeletal muscles.

24. Which of the following are NOT linked to interactions of the limbic system.
    a. Encephalopathy
    b. Autonomic regulation
    c. Visual processing
    d. Epilepsy
    e. Olfaction

25. Which of the following sinuses is NOT situated between layers of dura mater?
    a. Transverse sinus
    b. Superior sagittal sinus
    c. Sigmoid sinus
    d. Inferior sagittal sinus
    e. Sphenoid sinus

26. Concerning the meninges, which of the following statements is NOT correct?
    a. Arachnoid villi are projections of pia mater.
    b. The diaphragma sellae is a fold of dura covering the pituitary fossa.
    c. At the foramen magnum, the dura mater is continuous with the endosteum lining the vertebral canal.
    d. The arachnoid mater lines the dura mater.
    e. The pia mater follows every convolution of the brain.

27. Concerning the blood supply to the brain, which of the following statements is NOT correct?
    a. The basilar artery supplies the occipital lobe.
    b. The auditory and speech areas are supplied by the middle cerebral artery.
    c. The anterior cerebral artery supplies the visual cortex.

d. Central branches of the middle cerebral artery are the most susceptible to rupture.

e. The anterior cerebral artery supplies the motor and sensory areas of the lower limb.

28. Concerning cranial nerves, which of the following statements is NOT correct?
a. Olfactory nerve fibres pass through the cribriform plate of the ethmoid.
b. The abducens nerve innervates superior oblique.
c. Lesion of an optic nerve gives rise to monocular blindness.
d. The trochlear nerve arises from the dorsal aspect of the midbrain.
e. The mandibular division of the trigeminal nerve contains motor fibres.

29. Concerning cranial nerves, which of the following statements is correct?
a. The superior alveolar nerves are branches of the maxillary nerve.
b. The facial nerve arises from four nuclei.
c. The glossopharyngeal nerve innervates the muscles of the pharynx.
d. The accessory nerve arises entirely from the spinal cord.
e. The vagus lies outside the carotid sheath.

30. Concerning mastication, which of the following statements is NOT correct?
a. The temporomandibular joint has two compartments.
b. In opening and closing the mouth the mandible rotates about an axis through the lingulae.
c. In forward dislocation of the mandible the head of the mandible moves beyond the articular eminence.
d. Protraction of the mandible is produced by lateral pterygoid.
e. Side-to-side movements of the mandible are produced by masseter and temporalis.

31. The infratemporal fossa does NOT communicate with the:
a. orbit
b. pterygomaxillary fossa
c. temporal fossa
d. nasal cavity
e. middle cranial fossa

32. Concerning the face, which of the following statements is NOT correct?
a. It is supplied by the facial artery.

b. The facial vein communicates with intracranial venous sinuses.
c. The main function of the facial muscles is to facilitate facial expressions.
d. All lymph drains into the deep cervical nodes.
e. The skin is innervated by branches of the trigeminal nerve.

33. Concerning the orbit and its contents, which of the following statements is correct?
a. The roof of the orbit is formed by the greater wing of the sphenoid.
b. Orbital fascia encloses the orbital contents.
c. The superior orbital fissure communicates with the anterior cranial fossa.
d. All extraocular muscles are innervated by the oculomotor nerve.
e. The central artery of the retina is a direct branch of the anterior cerebral artery.

34. Concerning the eyeball, which of the following statements is NOT correct?
a. It is supported inferiorly by the suspensory ligament.
b. The outer layer is vascular.
c. The middle layer comprises the choroid, ciliary body and iris.
d. The inner layer is light-sensitive.
e. The visual axis passes between the centre of the cornea and fovea centralis.

35. Concerning orbital contents, which of the following statements is correct?
a. The lacrimal gland is located in the superomedial aspect of the orbit.
b. Lacrimal fluid contains antimicrobial agents.
c. Parasympathetic stimulation regulates blood flow through the lacrimal gland.
d. The ophthalmic artery enters the orbit via the superior orbital fissure.
e. Short ciliary nerves innervate dilator pupillae.

36. Concerning the nasal cavity, which of the following statements is NOT correct?
a. The superior and middle conchae are part of the ethmoid.
b. The nasolacrimal duct opens into the inferior meatus.
c. It communicates posteriorly with the nasopharynx.
d. Epistaxis occurs most frequently in the anterior part of nasal septum.
e. Parasympathetic secretomotor innervation is by the maxillary division of the trigeminal nerve.

37. Concerning the oral cavity, which of the following statements is NOT correct?
    a. The vestibule lies between the lips and cheeks externally and the teeth internally.
    b. The lips help to keep saliva and food within the mouth.
    c. The arterial supply to the lips does not anastomose across the midline.
    d. There are 16 permanent teeth in each jaw.
    e. The mucous membrane covering the tongue contains taste buds.

38. Concerning salivary glands, which of the following statements is correct?
    a. The secretions of the parotid gland are mainly serous.
    b. The submandibular gland is entirely superficial.
    c. The sublingual gland lies in the sublingual fossa on the lateral surface of the body of the mandible.
    d. Parasympathetic secretomotor innervation to the submandibular gland is by the glossopharyngeal nerve.
    e. The parotid duct opens opposite the lower 2nd molar.

39. Concerning the ear, which of the following statements is NOT correct?
    a. The middle ear contains the malleus, incus and stapes.
    b. Middle ear infections can result in a dulling or loss of taste.
    c. The external ear directs sound waves towards the tympanic membrane.
    d. Tensor tympani dampens down movements of the stapes in response to loud noises.
    e. Displacement of perilymph in the inner ear is facilitated by movement of the round window.

40. Concerning the neck, which of the following statements is NOT correct?
    a. The brachial plexus emerges between scalenus anterior and scalenus medius.
    b. Bony support is provided by eight cervical vertebrae.
    c. The accessory nerve passes obliquely across the floor of the posterior triangle on levator scapulae.
    d. The subclavian artery crosses the 1st rib posterior to the scalene tubercle.
    e. The prevertebral fascia splits to enclose trapezius.

41. Concerning the neck, which of the following statements is NOT correct?
    a. The carotid sheath contains the internal jugular vein.
    b. The sympathetic chain lies posteromedial to the carotid sheath.
    c. Pretracheal fascia surrounds the larynx, thyroid gland and trachea.
    d. The retropharyngeal space extends from the base of the skull to the posterior mediastinum.
    e. The investing layer of fascia extends into the axilla as the axillary sheath.

42. Concerning the pharynx and larynx, which of the following statements is correct?
    a. The muscles of the larynx are innervated by the external laryngeal nerve.
    b. The vocal cords lie lateral to the vestibular folds.
    c. The pharynx extends from the base of the skull to the level of the 6th cervical vertebra.
    d. The larynx does not move during swallowing.
    e. Mucous membrane lining the oropharynx is innervated by the vagus.

43. Concerning the thyroid gland, which of the following statements is NOT correct?
    a. It lies deep to the infrahyoid muscles.
    b. Hyperthyroidism is characterised by weight loss.
    c. The isthmus lies opposite the 2nd to 4th tracheal cartilages.
    d. Thyroid secretion is controlled by the neurohypophysis.
    e. Thyroid follicles are the functional units of the gland.

44. Concerning the root of the neck, which of the following statements is NOT correct?
    a. The apex of the lung projects above the middle one-third of the clavicle.
    b. The subclavian vein crosses the 1st rib posterior to scalenus anterior.
    c. The thoracic duct drains into the junction of the internal jugular and subclavian veins on the left.
    d. The phrenic nerve passes across scalenus anterior from lateral to medial.
    e. The vagus nerves enter the thorax anterior to the subclavian artery.

45. Concerning the endocrine system, which of the following statements is correct?
    a. Cell-to-cell signalling involves hormones.
    b. Steroid hormones are secreted by the adrenal cortex.

c. Dopamine is a neurotransmitter.

d. Protein hormones are secreted by the adrenal medulla.

e. Hormones bind with receptors on the cell membrane.

46. Concerning endocrine glands, which of the following statements is correct?

a. They coordinate and regulate body functions.

b. The thyroid gland only secretes thyroxine.

c. Acromegaly is caused by excess secretion of growth hormone before puberty.

d. The pituitary gland is connected to the thalamus by the infundibulum.

e. The pineal gland controls the function of many other endocrine glands.

47. Concerning hormones, which of the following statements is NOT correct?

a. Prolactin stimulates the breasts to produce milk.

b. Adrenocorticotrophic hormone stimulates the adrenal gland to produce cortisol.

c. In males, follicle-stimulating hormone is known as interstitial cell stimulating hormone.

d. Oxytocin affects uterine contractions during pregnancy.

e. Growth hormone stimulates growth and repair.

48. Which of the following is NOT a disorder associated with the adenohypophysis?

a. Gigantism

b. Cushing's disease

c. Simmonds' disease

d. Dwarfism

e. Diabetes insipidus

49. Concerning the thyroid and parathyroid glands, which of the following statements is NOT correct?

a. Calcitonin is secreted by parafollicular cells.

b. Cretinism occurs due to congenital absence of the parathyroid glands.

c. The parathyroid glands are embedded in the posterior surface of the lobes of the thyroid gland.

d. Hyperparathyroidism can cause bone pain.

e. Hypersecretion of thyroxine causes muscle weakness.

50. Concerning the adrenal glands, which of the following statements is NOT correct?

a. Disruption of the adrenal cortex causes fluid and electrolyte disruption.

b. The adrenal cortex and medulla do not function independently.

c. The zona glomerulosa secrete aldosterone.

d. The zona reticularis secretes androgens.

e. Cortisol promotes amino acid mobilisation from muscle.

51. Concerning the islets of Langerhans, which of the following statements is NOT correct?

a. Each islet is associated with several small blood capillaries.

b. They are located in the pancreas.

c. Carbohydrates increase insulin secretion.

d. Insulin promotes fatty acid synthesis.

e. Severe diabetes mellitus can lead to extreme muscle weakness.

52. Concerning diabetes, which of the following statements is correct?

a. Symptoms of type II diabetes appear rapidly.

b. Autoimmune disorders increase insulin production.

c. Type II diabetes is associated with increased plasma insulin concentrations.

d. Type II diabetes is due to a lack of insulin.

e. When blood glucose levels decrease it exerts large osmotic pressures in the extracellular fluid.

53. Concerning the gonads, which of the following statements is NOT correct?

a. Testosterone is responsible for the development of male sexual characteristics.

b. Sertoli cells support and nourish spermatogenic cells.

c. Decreased thyroxin secretion inhibits fertility.

d. Testosterone is formed by Leydig cells.

e. There are rhythmical changes in the rates of secretion of female hormones.

54. Concerning the gonads, which of the following statements is NOT correct?

a. Ovarian changes are dependent on gonadotropic hormones secreted by the adenohypophysis.

b. Oestrogen is responsible for the development of secondary sexual characteristics in females.

c. Progesterone is associated with preparation of the uterus for pregnancy.

d. Menstruation without ovulation can occur during puberty.

e. Sexual function is controlled by the release of hormones by the pituitary.

55. Which of the following is NOT associated with menstrual symptoms?
   a. Nausea and vomiting
   b. Oligomenorrhea
   c. Irritability
   d. Abdominal pain
   e. Depression and migraine

56. Concerning pregnancy and parturition, which of the following statements is NOT correct?
   a. Fertilisation occurs in the uterus.
   b. The placenta allows diffusion of oxygen and nutrients from maternal to foetal blood.
   c. During the later stages of pregnancy progesterone is secreted in large amounts by the placenta.
   d. Iron deficiency can lead to hypochromic anaemia.
   e. Braxton Hicks contractions occur from the 6th week of pregnancy.

57. Concerning parturition and labour, which of the following statements is correct?
   a. During labour contractions, start at the cervix.
   b. The foetal head acts as a wedge opening the birth canal.
   c. Pain in the 2nd stage of labour is due to cervical and perineal stretching.
   d. Foetal membranes release large amounts of cortisol.
   e. Towards the end of pregnancy the uterine contractions become less intense.

58. Which of the following is NOT a local hormone?
   a. Serotonin
   b. Substance P
   c. Dopamine
   d. Prostacyclin
   e. Heparin

59. Concerning the intracranial venous sinuses, which of the following statements is NOT correct?
   a. The internal carotid artery runs through the cavernous sinus.
   b. The transverse sinus passes around the posterolateral walls of the posterior cranial fossa.
   c. They lack the adventitial and muscular layers of veins.
   d. The inferior sagittal sinus is enclosed in the free edge of the falx cerebri.
   e. The superior petrosal sinus and transverse sinus form the internal jugular vein.

60. Concerning the thalamus, which of the following statements is correct?
   a. Anterior nuclei send efferent fibres to the mammillothalamic tract.
   b. Posterior nuclei receive afferent fibres from other thalamic nuclei.
   c. It receives its arterial supply from branches of the posterior cerebral artery.
   d. Anterior nuclei have no role in autonomic visceral activities.
   e. The subthalamus lies between the medulla oblongata and thalamus.

Upper Limb

CONTENTS

Key Concepts, 378
Learning Outcomes, 378
Overview, 378
Introduction, 378
Pectoral Region, 379
  Clavicle, 379
  Sternoclavicular Joint, 381
    Movements, 382
  Scapula, 383
  Acromioclavicular Joint, 384
    Movements, 384
  Movements of the Pectoral Girdle, 384
    Protraction and retraction, 385
    Elevation and depression, 385
    Lateral and medial rotation, 385
  Muscles, 386
Arm, 387
  Humerus, 387
  Shoulder Joint, 391
    Movements, 393
    Relations, 396
  Axilla, 398
    Axillary Artery, 398
    Axillary Vein, 398
    Brachial Plexus, 398
    Lymph Nodes, 400
  Compartments of the Arm, 402
    Anterior Compartment, 402
    Posterior Compartment, 404
    Muscles, 404
Forearm, 404
  Radius, 404
  Elbow Joint, 407

    Movements, 408
  Cubital Fossa, 411
  Radioulnar Joints, 412
    Movements, 412
  Compartments of the Forearm, 414
    Anterior Compartment, 414
    Posterior Compartment, 418
Wrist, 418
  Carpus, 420
  Wrist Joint, 420
    Movements, 420
Hand, 424
  Metacarpals and Phalanges, 425
  Carpometacarpal Joints, 426
    Movements, 427
  Metacarpophalangeal Joints, 427
    Movements, 428
  Interphalangeal Joints, 430
    Movements, 430
  Function of the Hand, 432
    Precision Grips, 435
    Power Grips, 435
  Blood Supply and Lymphatic Drainage, 435
    Arterial Supply, 435
    Venous Drainage, 435
    Lymphatic Drainage, 435
Summary of Nerves and Muscles, 435
  Major Nerves of the Upper Limb and the Muscles
    They Innervate, 435
    Axillary Nerve, 435
    Radial Nerve, 436
    Musculocutaneous Nerve, 436
    Ulnar Nerve, 436

Median Nerve, 438
Muscles Supplied by Each Root of the Brachial
    Plexus, 441
Movements in Each Region of the Upper Limb, the
    Muscles Responsible and Their Innervation, 442
    Pectoral Girdle, 442

Shoulder Joint, 442
Elbow Joint, 442
Radioulnar Joints, 443
Wrist Joint, 443
Joints of the Fingers, 443
Joints of the Thumb, 443

KEY CONCEPTS

- The upper limb enables the hand to function irrespective of its position in space.
- Joint stability is through articular surface shape, ligaments and muscle activity.
- Muscles function to stabilise joints: producing movement is secondary.
- Muscles crossing several joints promote coordinated movement and function.
- A wide range of movements is achieved by combinations of muscle actions.

- Muscles of the anterior arm are innervated by the musculocutaneous nerve; the anterior forearm by the median nerve (with exceptions); the posterior arm and forearm by the radial nerve; and the hand by the ulnar nerve (with exceptions).
- Skin of the lateral arm is innervated by C5/C6; the lateral forearm by C7; the hand by C8; the medial forearm by T1 and the medial arm by T2.
- The hand's rich nerve and blood supply make it a tactile and manipulative organ.

LEARNING OUTCOMES

By the end of this chapter you should be able to:
- Identify, palpate and examine the scapula, clavicle, humerus, radius, ulna, carpus, metacarpals and phalanges.
- Examine and assess movements of the pectoral girdle, the shoulder, elbow, radioulnar and wrist joints and joints of the hand and digits.
- Appreciate the influence of pathology and/or trauma on the function of the pectoral girdle, the shoulder, elbow, radioulnar and wrist joints and joints of the hand and digits.
- Locate, palpate and examine muscles associated with the pectoral girdle, arm, forearm and hand.
- Appreciate the influence of pathology and/or trauma on the muscles of the upper limb.
- Describe the location of the axilla and the significance of its contents.

- Appreciate the influence of pathology and/or trauma to the axilla and its contents.
- Describe the location of the cubital fossa and the significance of its contents.
- Appreciate the influence of pathology and/or trauma to the cubital fossa and its contents.
- Describe the formation, course and distribution of the brachial plexus and its branches.
- Appreciate the influence of pathology and/or trauma to the brachial plexus and its branches.
- Describe the origin, course and distribution of the major blood vessels of the upper limb.
- Assess the brachial, radial and ulnar pulse.
- Describe the lymphatic drainage of the upper limb, including the regions which drain into specific lymph nodes in the axilla.

OVERVIEW

This chapter considers the upper limb and is organised into five sections (pectoral girdle, arm, forearm, wrist, hand); within each section, the anatomy, function, and relevant applied and clinical anatomy are considered. At the end of the chapter is a summary of the major nerves arising from the brachial plexus and the muscles supplied by each; the muscles supplied by each nerve root of the brachial plexus; and the movements possible in each region (pectoral girdle, shoulder, elbow, forearm, hand), the muscles producing them together with their innervation.

INTRODUCTION

The upper limb has almost no locomotor function, being used primarily for grasping (prehension) and manipulation; nevertheless, it retains the ability to act as a locomotor prop as when pulling the trunk towards the hand by grasping an immobile object, as well as being used in conjunction with a walking aid during gait (walking) or other activity. Due to this loss of locomotor function the bones of the upper limb are not as robust as their counterparts in the lower limb.

The upper limb is attached to the trunk by the pectoral girdle (scapula, clavicle) with the only point of articulation being the sternoclavicular joint; the pectoral girdle connects the upper limb to the head, neck and thorax. Between the trunk and hand are a series of joints which enable the hand to be brought to any point in space and held there steadily and securely while performing tasks.

The upper limit of the upper limb can be considered as the superior surface of the clavicle anteriorly and the superior border of the scapula posteriorly. The arm lies between the shoulder and elbow joints, the forearm between the elbow and wrist joints and the hand beyond the wrist; the hand has anterior (palmar) and posterior (dorsal) surfaces (Fig. 5.1).

> **DEVELOPMENT:** The upper limb develops as a swelling of the body wall projecting at right angles to the surface opposite the lower cervical and 1st thoracic segments. It has ventral and dorsal surfaces and cephalic (preaxial, marked by the thumb) and caudal (postaxial, marked by the little finger) borders (Figs 5.2 and 5.3(i)). As the limb grows in length (Fig. 5.3(ii)), it becomes segmented (arm, forearm, hand) and folded ventrally so that the ventral surface becomes medial (Fig. 5.3(iii)), with the convexity of the elbow directed laterally (Fig. 5.3(iv)). At a later stage, the upper limb undergoes a process of adduction and rotation so that the preaxial border becomes lateral and the postaxial border medial, with the convexity of the elbow lying on the posterior aspect of the limb (Fig. 5.3(v)). As a result, the flexor surface of the upper limb comes to lie anterior and the extensor surface posterior.

The upper limb is surrounded by superficial fascia, like a sleeve, but shows regional differences between the shoulder and hand. In the shoulder and arm it contains a variable amount of fat; at the elbow there is a subcutaneous bursa between the skin and olecranon (page 406), which may become enlarged in individuals who habitually lean on their elbows (student's elbow); in the hand, there are a number of specialisations which tend to enhance its tactile and/or prehensile functions (page 424).

> **APPLIED ANATOMY:** In females, as a secondary sexual characteristic there is an increased deposition of fat in the superficial fascia around the shoulder and arm, which tends to increase after middle age.

The deep fascia of the upper limb is continuous with that of the upper back and hence to the superior nuchal line on the occipital bone (page 234), the ligamentum nuchae in the cervical region (page 199) and supra and interspinous ligaments in the thorax (page 199).

PECTORAL REGION

The bones of the pectoral (shoulder) girdle are the scapula and clavicle. The scapula sits against the posterior thoracic cage separated from it by muscles, whereas the clavicle acts as a strut between the upper limb, via the acromioclavicular joint, and trunk (thoracic cage), via the sternoclavicular joint (Fig. 5.4), steadying and bracing the pectoral girdle during movements of the upper limb.

Although movements of the pectoral girdle accompany nearly all movements of the shoulder joint, the shoulder joint is not part of the pectoral girdle. Nevertheless, it is the sum of movements of the mutually independent but interrelated acromioclavicular, sternoclavicular and shoulder joints which give the upper limb its freedom of movement. The mobility of the pectoral girdle-shoulder joint complex has implications for stabilisation of the upper limb during activities. Stability is due to the powerful muscles attaching the pectoral girdle to the thorax, vertebral column, head and neck; these same muscles act as shock absorbers when body weight is received by the upper limbs.

Clavicle

> **DEVELOPMENT:** The clavicle ossifies in membrane, being the first bone in the body to begin ossifying and the last to completely fuse. Two primary centres appear in the shaft during the 5th week *in utero* spreading towards each end of the bone; a secondary centre appears in the medial end between 14 and 18 years, which fuses with the shaft between age 18 and 20 in females and 23 and 25 in males.

A long curved subcutaneous bone (Fig. 5.5) between the sternum and acromion of the scapula (page 383) which acts as a strut holding the scapula laterally, facilitating a wide range of movement of the upper limb. The medial two-thirds (triangular in cross-section) is convex forwards and the flattened lateral one-third is concave forwards. Its anterior and posterior surfaces are smooth, the superior surface is rough in its medial part and the inferior surface is marked centrally by a groove for subclavius, with roughened areas medially for the costoclavicular ligament and laterally for the coracoclavicular ligament. The large quadrangular medial (sternal) end has a large facet

REGIONS   BONES   JOINTS

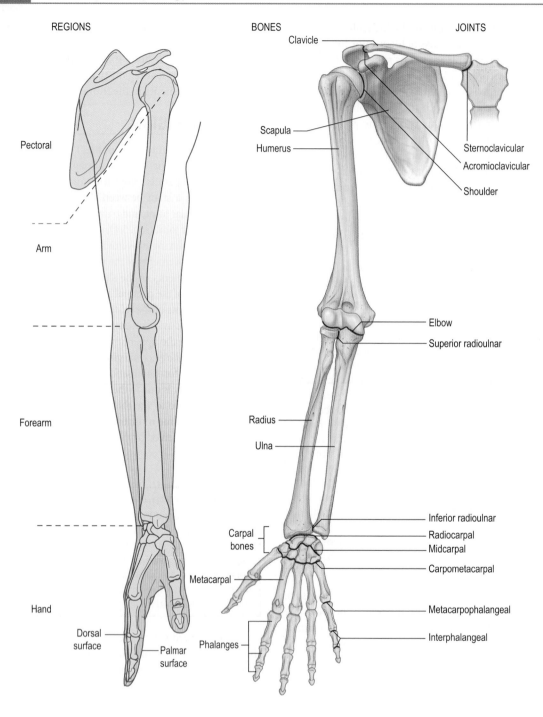

Pectoral

Arm

Forearm

Hand

Clavicle

Scapula
Humerus

Sternoclavicular
Acromioclavicular

Shoulder

Elbow
Superior radioulnar

Radius
Ulna

Inferior radioulnar
Radiocarpal
Midcarpal

Carpometacarpal

Metacarpophalangeal

Interphalangeal

Carpal bones

Metacarpal

Phalanges

Dorsal surface
Palmar surface

Fig. 5.1 Regions, bones and joints of the upper limb.

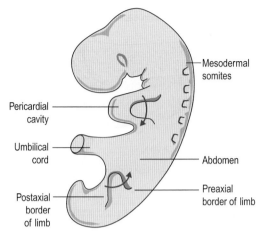

Fig. 5.2 Development of the upper and lower limb buds and their direction of rotation.

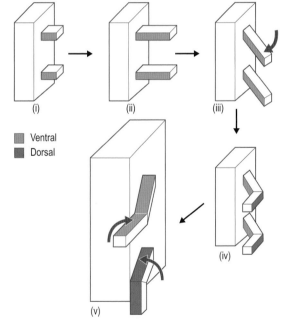

Fig. 5.3 Rotation of the upper and lower limb buds during development.

for articulation with the manubrium (page 68) at the sternoclavicular joint; the flattened lateral (acromial) end has a flat oval facet for articulation with the acromion at the acromioclavicular joint.

APPLIED ANATOMY: In slender individuals, the whole length of the clavicle can often be seen and palpated directly under the skin. The line of the sternoclavicular joint medially and acromioclavicular joint laterally can also be identified.

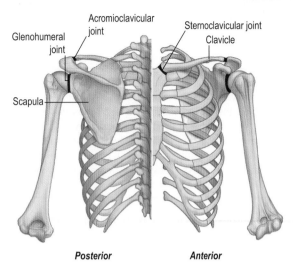

Fig. 5.4 Relationship between the pectoral girdle and thorax.

CLINICAL ANATOMY: Compressive forces along the length of the clavicle (as in falling on an outstretched hand or elbow) are transmitted via the coracoclavicular and costoclavicular ligaments and not the acromioclavicular and sternoclavicular joints and can cause fracture at the junction of the medial two-thirds and lateral one-third. The lateral fragment is depressed and adducted by the weight of the limb, while the medial fragment is raised by the action of the neck muscles. Excessive tensile stresses tend to cause joint dislocation rather than a fracture, while excessive rotational stresses tend to result in damage to the acromioclavicular (and sternoclavicular) joint and their associated ligaments rather than fracturing the bone.

Although not part of the thoracic inlet, the clavicle can, nevertheless, be considered as a boundary of the root of the neck (page 331) as structures from the neck and thorax pass deep to the clavicle between it and the 1st rib to enter the upper limb.

Sternoclavicular Joint

A synovial joint providing the only point of articulation between the upper limb and trunk (Fig. 5.6). Functionally it acts as a ball-and-socket joint, even though it does not have the form of one. Although the articular surfaces are reciprocally concavoconvex, they are not particularly congruent. Congruence is improved by the presence of a fibrocartilaginous intra-articular disc, which completely divides the joint into two separate cavities.

> **APPLIED ANATOMY:** In addition to improving congruence between the articular surfaces of the sternoclavicular joint, the intra-articular disc also holds the medial end of the clavicle against the manubrium preventing the clavicle moving superomedially when strong thrusting forces are transmitted from the upper limb or when the lateral end of the clavicle is depressed, as when carrying a heavy weight in the hand.

The fibrous joint capsule is strengthened by anterior and posterior sternoclavicular and interclavicular ligaments (Fig. 5.6A), while the strong extracapsular costoclavicular ligament (Fig. 5.6B) limits elevation of the medial end of the clavicle, as well as preventing excessive anterior and posterior movement.

The joint is reinforced anteriorly and posteriorly by muscle attachments, which posteriorly separate it from the brachiocephalic vein and common carotid artery on the left and brachiocephalic trunk on the right (Fig. 5.7). The superior vena cava lies just below the right sternoclavicular joint at the lower border of the 1st costal cartilage. The phrenic and vagus nerves also pass close to the posterior aspect of each joint.

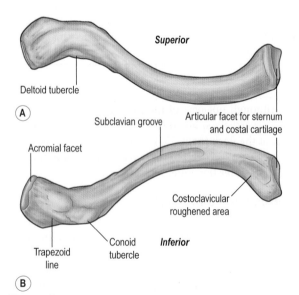

Fig. 5.5 Superior (A) and inferior (B) aspects of the right clavicle.

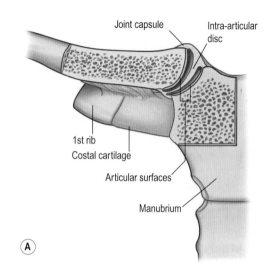

(A)

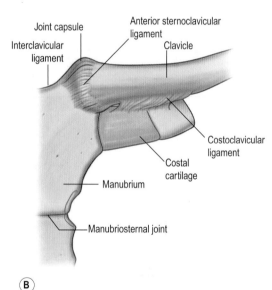

(B)

Fig. 5.6 (A) Section through the right sternoclavicular joint showing the articular surfaces and intra-articular disc; (B) ligaments associated with the left sternoclavicular joint.

Movements

The medial end of the clavicle can be elevated and depressed, protracted and retracted and undergo axial rotation (Fig. 5.8), with the movements (except axial rotation) taking place with the costoclavicular ligament as the fulcrum. Elevation, depression, protraction and retraction involve gliding between the clavicle and intra-articular disc, as well as between the disc and sternum. The axis of axial rotation passes through the centre of

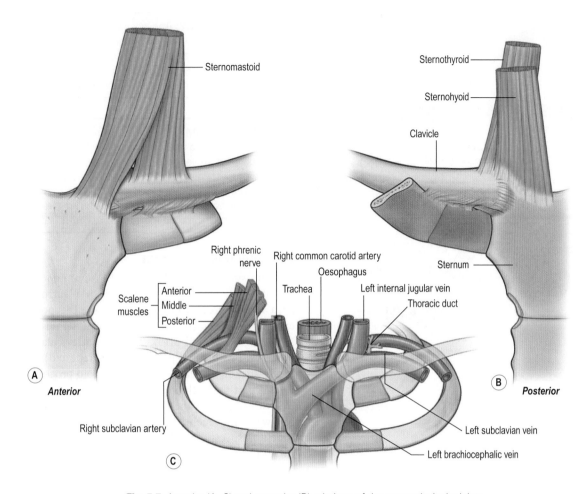

Fig. 5.7 Anterior (A, C) and posterior (B) relations of the sternoclavicular joints.

the articular surfaces of the sternoclavicular and acromioclavicular joints.

Scapula

> **DEVELOPMENT:** A primary centre appears in the body by the 8th week *in utero*. Secondary centres (2) appear in the coracoid process during the 1st year (fusing with the body between 12 and 14 years), and in the acromion (2), glenoid fossa, medial border and inferior angle between ages 12 and 14 (fusing with the body between 20 and 25 years).

A large, flat, triangular bone overlying the 2nd to 7th ribs on the posterolateral aspect of the thorax (Fig. 5.4), it has three borders (thin superior border between the superior and lateral angles; long thin medial border between the superior and inferior angles; thick lateral border between the inferior angle and glenoid fossa), three angles (superior, lateral, inferior) and two surfaces (costal, dorsal). It has three bony processes (coracoid, acromion, spine). The spine divides the dorsal surface into smaller supraspinous and larger infraspinous fossae (Fig. 5.9).

The lateral angle forms the shallow pear-shaped glenoid fossa, being broader below, which faces anterolaterally and articulates with the head of the humerus forming the shoulder joint (page 391). The large, quadrilateral acromion is the expanded lateral end of the spine and projects forwards at right angles to the spine. The lower border of the crest of the spine

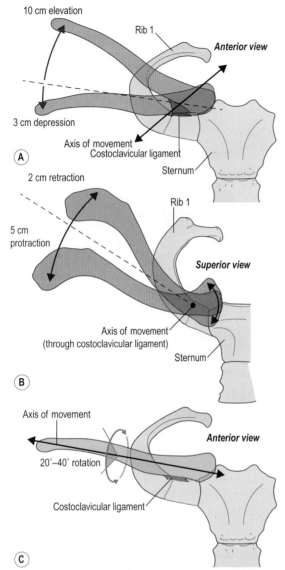

Fig. 5.8 Movements of the clavicle at the sternoclavicular joint during (A) elevation and depression, (B) protraction and retraction (viewed from above) and (C) axial rotation.

> **APPLIED ANATOMY:** The position of the scapula on the chest wall is determined by the tone in muscles attaching it to the thorax, humerus, head and neck. These same muscles produce movements of the scapula as an adjunct to movements of the upper limb.

> **APPLIED ANATOMY:** There is an important arterial anastomosis around the scapula involving branches from the subclavian, axillary and posterior intercostal arteries from the descending aorta (Fig. 5.10). On the left side this anastomosis enables blood to reach the descending aorta (reversed blood flow) in coarctation of the aorta (page 136), in which case the vessels become dilated.

Acromioclavicular Joint

A plane synovial joint between the acromion of the scapula and lateral end of the clavicle surrounded by a loose fibrous capsule (Fig. 5.11). The powerful extracapsular coracoclavicular ligament stabilises the joint (Figs. 5.11 and 5.15). The coracoclavicular ligament has two distinct parts (conoid, trapezoid) which firmly anchor the clavicle to the coracoid process. The conoid part limits the forward movement of the scapula with respect to the clavicle and the trapezoid part backward movement. The anterosuperior and posterosuperior aspects of the joint are covered by deltoid and trapezius, providing additional stability.

> **CLINICAL ANATOMY:** Due to the slope of the joint surfaces, in dislocations the lateral end of the clavicle tends to override the acromion resulting in downwards displacement of the acromion under the clavicle.

Movements

Movements at the acromioclavicular joint are entirely passive being caused by movement of the scapula against the clavicle. Protraction and retraction occur about a vertical axis and elevation and depression about a sagittal axis, both through the joint, and axial rotation about a longitudinal axis associated with medial and lateral rotation of the scapula (Fig. 5.12).

Movements of the Pectoral Girdle

The pectoral girdle is the link between the upper limb and the axial skeleton. It increases the range of movement of the shoulder joint (page 393) by changing the relative position of the glenoid fossa with respect to the chest wall. In all

continues as the lateral border of the acromion, with the junction being the acromial angle; the upper border of the crest is continuous with the medial border of the acromion and has a facet for articulation with the clavicle at the acromioclavicular joint. The hook-like coracoid process is directed anterosuperiorly, with its horizontal part projecting anterolaterally and tip lying below the junction of the middle and lateral one-third of the clavicle.

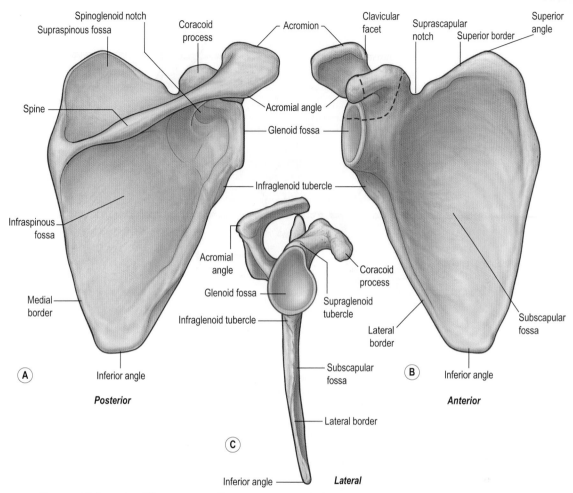

Fig. 5.9 (A) Posterior, (B) anterior and (C) lateral aspects of the right scapula: the *dashed red lines* represent the lines of fusion between the parts of the scapula.

movements, the clavicle acts as a strut holding the shoulder away from the trunk, providing greater freedom of movement of the upper limb. Most movements of the shoulder joint are accompanied by movements of the pectoral girdle.

Protraction and retraction

In protraction, the scapula moves forwards around the chest wall (rounding the shoulders); there may be some associated lateral rotation. While in retraction the medial border of the scapula moves towards the vertebral column (bracing the shoulders) (Fig. 5.13A and B)). Between the extremes of movement, the scapula forms a solid angle of 40 to 45 degrees, with the angle between the clavicle and scapula decreasing to 60 degrees in protraction and increasing to 70

degrees in retraction. The linear range of movement of the scapula around the chest wall is about 15 cm.

Elevation and depression

Elevation (shrugging the shoulders) and depression have a linear range of movement of 10–12 cm; it is usually accompanied by a small degree of rotation (Fig. 5.13C).

Lateral and medial rotation

Lateral (forward) rotation involves lateral movement of the inferior angle of the scapula around the chest wall accompanied by an upward movement so that the glenoid fossa is turned increasingly upwards. Medial

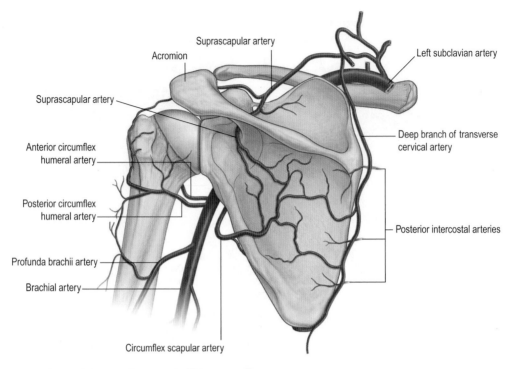

Fig. 5.10 Posterior aspect of the scapula and humerus showing the vessels involved in supplying the shoulder region, as well as the scapular collateral anastomosis.

rotation returns the scapula to its resting position (Fig. 5.13D). Scapula rotation occurs about an axis perpendicular to the plane of the scapula close to the root of the spine; it has a total range of 60 degrees (Fig. 5.13D).

> **APPLIED ANATOMY:** After some 30 degrees abduction and/or flexion of the arm the scapula begins to laterally rotate. After 30 degrees of scapula rotation the coracoclavicular ligament becomes taut causing the clavicle to rotate about its long axis (the superior surface becomes increasingly directed posteriorly), enabling the scapula to continue rotating a further 30 degrees.

Muscles

The clavicle and especially the scapula give attachment to many muscles, some of which anchor the pectoral girdle to the thorax, while others control the position of the upper limb. Muscles producing movements of the pectoral girdle, together with their attachments, actions

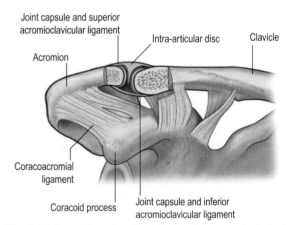

Fig. 5.11 Coronal section through the right acromioclavicular joint.

and innervation are given in Table 5.1: their position in relation to the pectoral girdle and shoulder region are shown in Fig. 5.18.

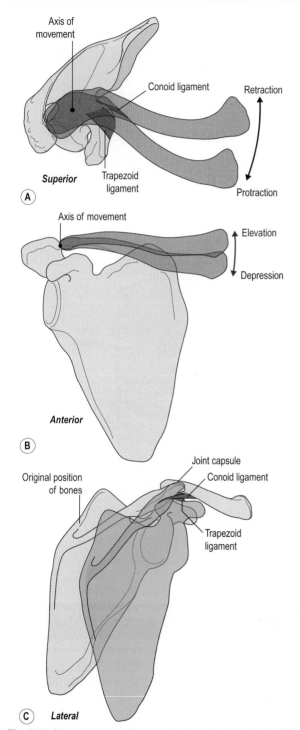

Fig. 5.12 Movements at the acromioclavicular joint during (A) protraction and retraction about a vertical axis; (B) elevation and depression about a sagittal axis and (C) axial rotation of the scapula.

THORACIC OUTLET SYNDROME: A variety of neurovascular syndromes resulting from compression of the subclavian artery, the trunks of the brachial plexus or less commonly the axillary or subclavian veins, caused by a drooping pectoral girdle, a cervical rib or fibrous band, or an abnormal 1st rib. Nerve compression causes atrophy and weakness of the muscles of the hand and, in advanced cases the forearm, with pain and sensory disturbance in the arm. Arterial compression leads to ischaemia, paraesthesia, numbness and weakness of the affected arm. Venous obstruction may result in thrombus formation in the axillary vein following exercise, with the symptoms being pain, oedema and skin discoloration. The syndromes tend to occur more frequently in females and in those aged 20 to 40.

ARM

The arm extends between the shoulder (articulation of the humerus with the scapula) and the elbow (articulation of the humerus with the radius and ulna) joints. It has anterior (flexor) and posterior (extensor) compartments separated by medial and lateral intermuscular septa. The deep fascia around the shoulder is extremely strong, with that attached to the clavicle being traced into the neck superiorly. It is continuous with that of the anterior abdominal wall. Medial to the shoulder is the clavipectoral fascia which attaches to the floor of the axilla (suspensory ligament of the axilla). It is also connected to the axillary sheath surrounding the axillary vessels and brachial plexus (page 398). In the arm, the deep fascia forms an investing layer around the muscles, attaching to the medial and lateral epicondyles of the humerus and olecranon process (page 406), becoming continuous with the deep fascia of the forearm.

Humerus

DEVELOPMENT: A primary centre appears in the shaft during the 8th week *in utero*. At the proximal end secondary centres appear in the head, greater and lesser tubercles during the 1st, 3rd and 5th years, which join together to form a single cap of bone between ages 6 and 8. This fuses with the shaft between ages 18 and 20 in females and 20 and 22 in males. At the distal end secondary centres appear in the capitulum, trochlea and lateral epicondyle during the 2nd, 9th/10th and 12th to 14th years, which join together by age 14 and then fuse with the shaft at age 15 in females and 18 in males. A separate centre (outside the joint capsule) appears in the medial epicondyle between ages 6 and 8, fusing with the shaft between ages 15 and 18. Most growth in length of the humerus occurs at its proximal end.

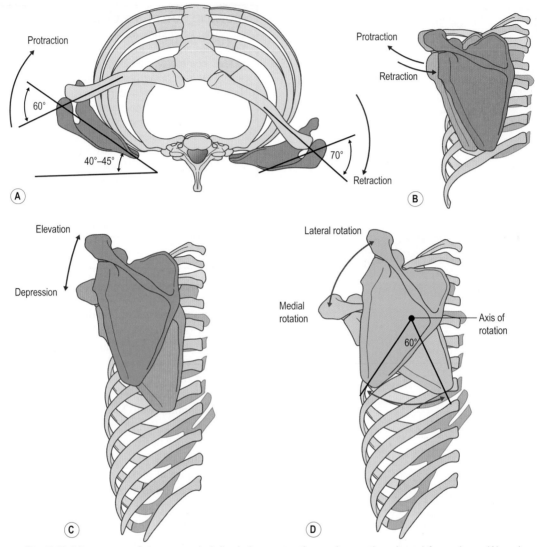

Fig. 5.13 Movements of the pectoral girdle during protraction and retraction viewed from above (A) and behind (B), elevation and depression (C) and axial rotation (D).

TABLE 5.1	Muscles Producing Movements of the Pectoral Girdle, Together With Their Attachments, Actions and Innervation		
Muscle	**Attachments**	**Action**	**Innervation (Root Value)**
Subclavius	From the 1st rib near its junction with the costal cartilage to the inferior surface (subclavian groove) of the clavicle	Steadies the clavicle against the sternum during movements of the pectoral girdle	Nerve to subclavius (C5, C6)
Rhomboid major	From the spinous processes of T2–T5 and intervening supraspinous ligament to the medial scapular border below the root of the spine	Retraction and medial rotation: important stabiliser when other muscle groups are active	Dorsal scapular nerve (C5)

TABLE 5.1   Muscles Producing Movements of the Pectoral Girdle, Together With Their Attachments, Actions and Innervation (cont'd)

Muscle	Attachments	Action	Innervation (Root Value)
Rhomboid minor	From the spinous processes of C7 and T1, and ligamentum nuchae to the medial scapular border near the root of the spine	Retraction and medial rotation: important stabiliser when other muscle groups are active	Dorsal scapular nerve (C5)
Trapezius	From the superior nuchal line and external occipital protuberance, ligamentum nuchae and spinous processes of C7 to T12 to the posterior border of the lateral third of the clavicle (upper fibres), medial border of the acromion and upper border of the crest of the spine of the scapula (middle fibres), and the inferior edge of the medial end of the spine of the scapula (lower fibres)	Stabilises the scapula during movements of the upper limb: the upper fibres elevate the pectoral girdle to maintain the level of the shoulders against the effects of gravity or when carrying a weight, they can also laterally flex the neck and together with the lower fibres produce lateral rotation of the scapula; the middle fibres retract the pectoral girdle and may be aided by both the upper and lower fibres; the lower fibres pull down the medial part of the scapula, especially against resistance	Motor, spinal part of the accessory nerve (XI): sensory, C3 and C4
Serratus anterior	By fleshy digitations from the outer surfaces of the upper eight or nine ribs and intervening fascia to the costal surface of the medial border of the scapula	Stabilises the scapula during movements of the upper limb by holding the medial border against the chest wall; protraction of the pectoral girdle, being involved in all thrusting, pushing and punching movements; in conjunction with the upper fibres of trapezius the lower digitations rotate the scapula laterally	Long thoracic nerve (C5–C7)
Pectoralis minor	From the outer surfaces of the 3rd, 4th and 5th ribs to the coracoid process	Pulls the coracoid process (and scapula) forwards and downwards; helps transfer the weight of the trunk to the upper limbs when leaning on the hands; with the scapula fixed it can act as an accessory muscle of respiration	Medial pectoral nerve (C6–C8)
Levator scapulae	From the transverse processes of C1 to C3/C4 to the medial border of the scapula above the root of the spine	Elevation and retraction of the pectoral girdle; it also resists downward movement when carrying a load; with trapezius both sides extend the neck	Dorsal scapular nerve (C5) and directly from C3 and C4

CLINICAL ANATOMY: Paralysis of *trapezius* (especially its upper part) results in the scapula moving forwards around the chest wall, with the inferior angle moving medially. The smooth curve of its upper border may become markedly angular. Paralysis of *serratus anterior* results in 'winging' of the scapula in which the medial border stands away from the chest wall severely affecting the function and mobility of the upper limb. The upper limb cannot be abducted more than 90 degrees.

A typical long bone with a shaft and proximal and distal ends. The proximal end carries the rounded head, neck and greater and lesser tubercles with the intervening intertubercular (bicipital) groove; the expanded distal end has medial and lateral supracondylar ridges leading to the medial and lateral epicondyles, the rounded capitulum and pulley-like trochlea (Fig. 5.14) for articulation with the head of the radius and the trochlear notch of the ulna, respectively.

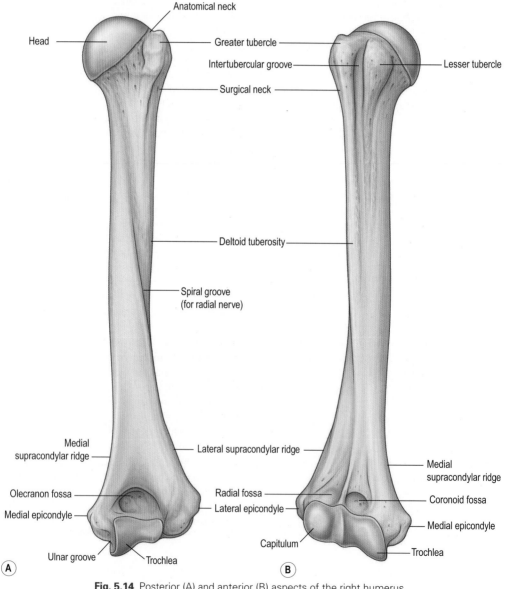

Fig. 5.14 Posterior (A) and anterior (B) aspects of the right humerus.

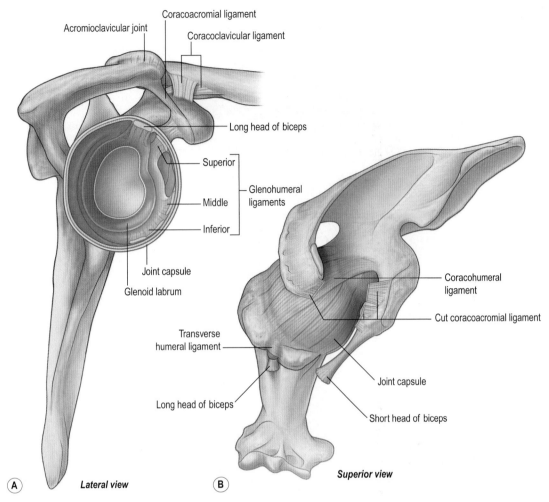

Coracoacromial ligament

Acromioclavicular joint

Coracoclavicular ligament

Long head of biceps

Superior

Glenohumeral
ligaments

Middle

Inferior

Joint capsule

Glenoid labrum

Transverse
humeral ligament

Long head of biceps

Coracohumeral
ligament

Cut coracoacromial ligament

Joint capsule

Short head of biceps

Superior view

A   *Lateral view*   **B**

Fig. 5.15 (A) Lateral aspect of the shoulder joint with the humeral head removed; (B) anterolateral aspect of the shoulder joint showing the joint capsule and transverse, coracohumeral, coracoacromial and coracoclavicular ligaments.

CLINICAL ANATOMY: Below the tubercles is the surgical neck. It can fracture due to a fall on the outstretched arm, occurring more frequently in the elderly and is often impacted (page 34). Displaced fractures are potentially more serious as they can damage vessels or nerves in the axilla. Bone metastases are common here and can lead to pathological fracture.

The upper half of the shaft is cylindrical and lower half triangular. It has three surfaces (anteromedial, anterolateral, posterior), with the deltoid tubercle on its posterior surface and spiral (radial) groove spiralling around the lateral aspect of the shaft (Fig. 5.14). Anteriorly at the distal end are the lateral radial and medial coronoid fossae for the head of the radius and coronoid process of the ulna in elbow joint flexion, respectively;

posteriorly is the olecranon fossa for the olecranon process of the ulna in elbow joint extension.

APPLIED ANATOMY: Distally, the lateral and medial epicondyles can be felt, together with the medial supracondylar ridge. Behind the medial epicondyle the ulnar nerve can be rolled against the bone giving tingling sensations in the fingers ('funny bone').

CLINICAL ANATOMY: The medial epicondyle is liable to fracture due to it being subcutaneous and prominent; fracture may compromise the ulnar nerve.

Shoulder Joint

A synovial ball-and-socket joint between the shallow pear-shaped glenoid fossa of the scapula (page 383), which is

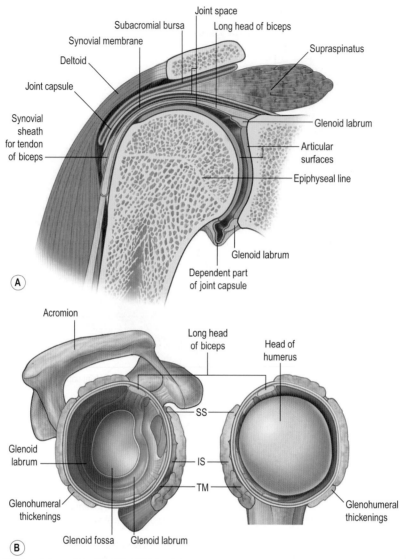

Fig. 5.16 (A) Coronal section through the shoulder joint showing the reflection of the synovial membrane around the long head of biceps; (B) the joint opened showing blending of the rotator cuff muscles with the joint capsule. *IS*, Infraspinatus; *SS*, supraspinatus; *TM*, teres minor.

deepened by the fibrocartilaginous glenoid labrum (Figs 5.15A and 5.16A), and the rounded head of the humerus. Because of the shape of its articular surfaces, the joint has little inherent stability. A loose, cylindrical fibrous capsule connects the two bones with the majority of fibres passing horizontally between the scapula and humerus (Fig. 5.15B); some fibres pass obliquely and transversely.

The anterior part of the capsule is thickened and strengthened by three glenohumeral ligaments (Figs 5.15A and (5.16A). As the tendons of the 'rotator cuff' muscles (Table 5.2) approach the humerus they spread out over the joint capsule, strengthening and supporting it by acting as

variable length ligaments (Figs 5.16B and 5.17). There are two openings within the capsule, one at the upper end of the intertubercular groove allowing the long head of biceps to pass into the arm (Fig. 5.16A), and the other between the superior and middle glenohumeral ligaments.

Although not directly associated with the joint capsule, the coracoacromial ligament, together with the coracoid process and acromion, form a fibro-osseous arch above the head of the humerus (Fig. 5.15A). The arch increases the surface area upon which the humeral head is supported when forces are transmitted upwards along the humerus.

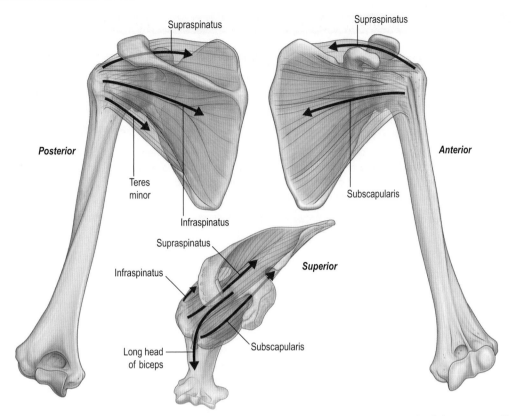

Fig. 5.17 Posterior, anterior and superior aspects of the shoulder region showing the role of the rotator cuff muscles in stabilising the shoulder joint.

CLINICAL ANATOMY: Anterior dislocation is the most common disruption of the shoulder joint, resulting from the humeral head slipping anteriorly out of the glenoid fossa when the arm is forcibly abducted and laterally rotated. It damages the joint capsule, as well as muscles attached to it, destabilising the joint. In recurrent cases, surgical intervention includes repair of the capsule and/or shortening the tendon of subscapularis. Subluxation of the shoulder joint is where the rotator cuff muscles fail to maintain the normal alignment of the joint surfaces following trauma or stroke (paralysis), making the joint painful.

CLINICAL ANATOMY: Frozen shoulder is a condition of unknown origin where the soft tissues surrounding the joint become inflamed and painful, restricting movement in most directions.

Movements

The shoulder joint has a greater range of movement than any other joint, with movement being possible about an infinite number of axes passing through the centre of the humeral head. The movements possible are flexion/extension, abduction/adduction and medial/lateral rotation. However, the axes about which movements occur have to be carefully defined as the plane of the glenoid fossa is inclined 45 degrees to both the sagittal and coronal planes. Two sets of axes about which movement occurs can be defined, one with respect to the cardinal planes of the body (Fig. 5.18A) and another with respect to the plane of the glenoid fossa (Fig. 5.18B).

APPLIED ANATOMY: All movements, except axial rotation, are a combination of gliding and rolling of the articular surfaces against each other.

APPLIED ANATOMY: The association of shoulder and pectoral girdle movements increases the range and power of movements of the upper limb. In patients with fixed or fused shoulders, a large degree of upper limb mobility with respect to the trunk can still be achieved due to pectoral girdle movements.

TABLE 5.2   The Attachments, Action and Innervation of Muscles Acting at the Shoulder Joint

Muscle	Attachments	Action	Innervation (Root Value)
Pectoralis major[a]	From the medial half of the anterior surface of the clavicle, anterior surface of the sternum and upper six costal cartilages to the lateral lip of the intertubercular groove of the humerus	Powerful adductor and medial rotator of the arm at the shoulder joint	Medial (C8, T1) and lateral (C5–C7) pectoral nerves
Deltoid[a]	From the anterior border of the lateral third of the clavicle (anterior fibres), lower border of the crest of the spine of the scapula (posterior fibres) and lateral margin of the acromion by four tendinous slips (middle fibres) to the deltoid tuberosity of the humerus	Involved in all movements of the arm at the shoulder joint except adduction	Axillary nerve (C5, C6)
Biceps brachii[a] (see Table 5.4)			
Coracobrachialis	From the coracoid process of the scapula to the medial side of the shaft of the humerus	Adductor and weak flexor of the arm at the shoulder joint	Musculocutaneous nerve (C6, C7)
Latissimus dorsi[a]	From the thoracolumbar fascia and spinous processes of T7 to S5, outer lip of the iliac crest, outer surfaces of the lower three or four ribs, and inferior angle of the scapula (via fascia) to the floor of the intertubercular groove of the humerus	Strong adductor and medial rotator of the arm at the shoulder joint; strong extensor of the flexed arm; with the scapula fixed it retracts the pectoral girdle	Thoracodorsal nerve (C6–C8)
Teres major[a]	From the dorsal surface of the scapula near the inferior angle to the medial lip of the intertubercular groove on the humerus	Adduction and medial rotation of the arm at the shoulder joint; it can help extend the flexed arm	Lower subscapular nerve (C6, C7)
Triceps brachii[a] (see Table 5.4)			Radial nerve (C6–C8)
Supraspinatus[b]	From the medial two-thirds of the supraspinous fossa of the scapula to the upper facet on the greater tubercle of the humerus	Initiates abduction of the arm at the shoulder joint	Suprascapular nerve (C5, C6)
Subscapularis[b]	From the medial two-thirds of the subscapular fossa of the scapula to the lesser tubercle of the humerus	Strong medial rotator of the arm at the shoulder joint; also assists adduction	Upper and lower subscapular nerves (C5–C7)
Teres minor[a,b]	From the upper two-thirds of the lateral border of the scapula to the lower facet on the greater tubercle of the humerus	Lateral rotator of the arm at the shoulder joint; also adducts the abducted arm	Axillary nerve (C5, C6)
Infraspinatus[a,b]	From the medial two-thirds of the infraspinous fossa of the scapula to the middle facet on the greater tubercle of the humerus	Lateral rotation of the arm at the shoulder joint	Suprascapular nerve (C5, C6)

[a]Shown in Fig. 5.20.
[b]'Rotator cuff' muscles.

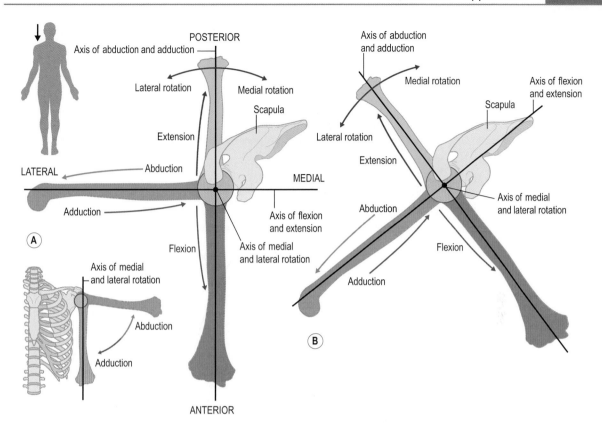

Fig. 5.18 Axes of movement at the shoulder joint with respect to (A) the cardinal planes of the body and (B) the plane of the glenoid fossa.

CLINICAL ANATOMY: The importance of the axes with respect to the plane of the glenoid fossa is in the treatment of some shoulder injuries. When the joint is abducted to 90 degrees in the plane of the glenoid fossa there is no asymmetric tension in the joint capsule and/or surrounding muscles.

The movements discussed below are with respect to the plane of the glenoid fossa. Details of the muscles producing each movement are given in Table 5.2.

Flexion and extension. In flexion, the arm moves forwards and medially across the chest wall and in extension the arm is carried backwards and laterally (Fig. 5.19A). Flexion has a range of 110 degrees and extension 70 degrees, being limited by the greater tubercle of the humerus making contact with the coracoacromial arch. The range of flexion can be increased to 180 degrees and extension to greater than 90 degrees by movements of the pectoral girdle.

Flexion is produced by pectoralis major, anterior fibres of deltoid, long head of biceps brachii and coracobrachialis; extension by latissimus dorsi, teres major, posterior fibres of deltoid and the long head of triceps.

Abduction and adduction. In abduction, the arm moves anterolaterally away from the trunk (Fig. 5.19B). It has a range of 120 degrees, of which only the first 25 degrees occur without concomitant rotation of the scapula; between 30 and 180 degrees scapular rotation augments shoulder abduction in the ratio of 1:2. Adduction beyond the neutral position is not possible due to the presence of the trunk.

Abduction is produced by supraspinatus and deltoid; adduction by coracobrachialis, pectoralis major, latissimus dorsi and teres major.

CLINICAL ANATOMY: Where the tendon of supraspinatus passes over the humeral head below the acromion it may become inflamed. Pain is experienced during abduction, most commonly between 60 and 120 degrees ('painful arc' syndrome). The tendon can also rupture without inflammation, making initiation of abduction difficult.

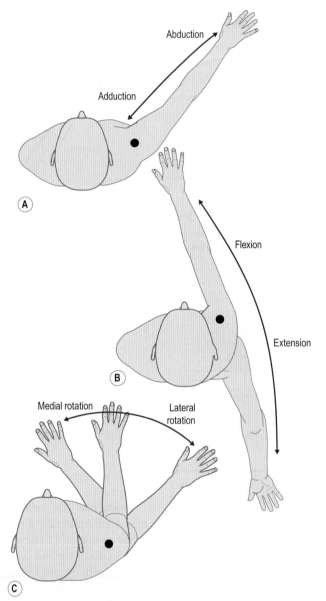

Fig. 5.19 (A) Abduction and adduction, (B) flexion and extension and (C) medial and lateral rotation of the arm at the shoulder joint.

Medial and lateral rotation. In medial rotation, the anterior surface of the arm is turned medially, while in lateral rotation it is turned laterally (Fig. 5.19C). The maximum ranges of medial and lateral rotation are 90 and 80 degrees, respectively. The combined range of rotation is greatest with the arm hanging by the side, being 90 degrees with the arm horizontal and negligible with the arm vertical.

Medial rotation is produced by subscapularis, teres major, latissimus dorsi, pectoralis major and anterior fibres of deltoid; lateral rotation by teres minor, infraspinatus and posterior fibres of deltoid.

Relations

The shoulder joint is completely surrounded by muscles passing between either the pectoral girdle or thorax and humerus (Fig. 5.20). These contribute to its stability, as well as producing movement; they also help protect the joint and suspend the upper limb from the pectoral girdle.

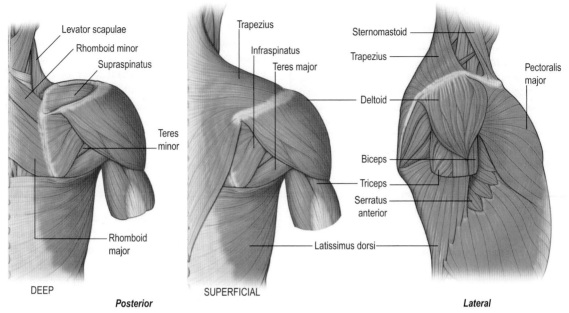

Fig. 5.20 Muscles of the shoulder region.

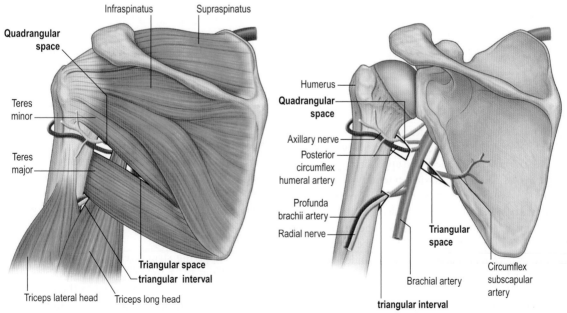

Fig. 5.21 Posterior aspect of the shoulder region showing the position of the quadrangular and triangular spaces and triangular interval, together with their contents.

Below and medial to the shoulder joint are 'spaces' which transmit important structures. The boundaries of each space and the structures each transmits are shown in Fig. 5.21.

> **CLINICAL ANATOMY:** Downwards dislocation of the head of the humerus or prolonged upward pressure (e.g., falling asleep with the arm hanging over the back of a chair) may cause temporary or permanent damage to the axillary nerve, with loss of function of deltoid and teres minor.

> **CLINICAL ANATOMY:** Fractures of the shaft of the humerus or pressure from the axillary pad of an incorrectly used crutch may compress the radial nerve, leading to radial nerve palsy (wrist drop), which will affect the functional use of the hand (Fig. 5.22).

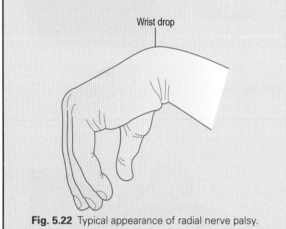

Fig. 5.22 Typical appearance of radial nerve palsy.

Axilla

A pyramidal-shaped space inferomedial to the shoulder joint between the arm and thorax enables vessels and nerves to pass between the neck and upper limb (Fig. 5.23). The apex is formed by the clavicle anteriorly and scapula posteriorly, with the outer border of the 1st rib medially; the concave base (floor) is formed by deep fascia extending over serratus anterior to the deep fascia of the arm attached to the anterior and posterior axillary folds; the anterior wall is formed by pectoralis major (the lower rounded border is formed by twisting of its muscle fibres), posterior wall by subclavius and teres major, medial wall by serratus anterior and lateral wall by the intertubercular groove (Fig. 5.23).

> **APPLIED ANATOMY:** With the arm fully abducted the axillary folds disappear, the axillary hollow may be replaced by a bulge.

The principal contents of the axilla are blood vessels (axillary artery and its branches, axillary vein and its tributaries) and nerves (brachial plexus and its branches) and lymph nodes (Fig. 5.23). The major blood vessels and nerve trunks are enclosed within an extension of the prevertebral layer of cervical fascia (axillary sheath), adherent to the clavipectoral fascia behind pectoralis minor, which blends with the tunica adventitia of the vessels beyond the 2nd part of the axillary artery.

Axillary Artery

Continuation of the subclavian artery at the lateral border of the 1st rib becoming the brachial artery at the lower border of teres major. It is divided into three parts by pectoralis minor, with the 1st part giving one branch (superior thoracic artery), the 2nd part two branches (thoracoacromial and lateral thoracic arteries) and 3rd part three branches (subscapular, anterior and posterior circumflex humeral arteries).

> **APPLIED ANATOMY:** The axillary artery describes a curve from the midpoint of the clavicle passing immediately below the coracoid process to the intertubercular groove of the humerus posterior to coracobrachialis. Its pulse can be felt in the lateral wall of the axilla behind coracobrachialis, a useful pressure point to control distal bleeding, although paraesthesia can result from pressure on the median, ulnar and radial nerves as they are closely related to the artery at this point.

Axillary Vein

The continuation of the superficial basilic vein at the lower border of teres major after it has pierced the deep fascia opposite the humeral attachment of coracobrachialis and travelled along the medial side of the brachial vessels.

Brachial Plexus

Nerves supplying structures in the upper limb are all derived from the brachial plexus, a complex of intermingling nerve roots originating in the neck from the ventral rami of the lower four cervical and 1st thoracic spinal cord segments (C5 to T1). There may be contributions from C4, T2 or both; these are the roots of the brachial plexus (Fig. 5.24). Each nerve receives an autonomic sympathetic contribution: C5 and C6 receive grey rami from the middle cervical ganglion,

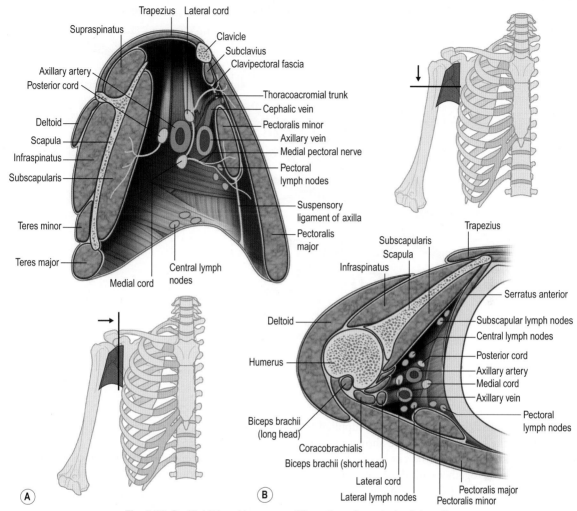

Fig. 5.23 Sagittal (A) and transverse (B) sections through the right axilla.

and C7, C8 and T1 from the inferior or stellate ganglion.

The upper two roots (C5, C6) usually unite to form the upper trunk, C7 continues as the middle trunk and the lower two roots (C8, T1) form the lower trunk (Fig. 5.24). The trunks are found between the scalene muscles and upper border of the clavicle in the posterior triangle of the neck (page 319). The lower trunk may groove the upper surface of the 1st rib behind the subclavian artery. The T1 root is always in contact with the rib.

Just above the clavicle each trunk divides into anterior and posterior divisions, which supply the flexor and extensor compartments of the upper limb, respectively. All posterior divisions unite to form the posterior cord, the upper two anterior divisions form the lateral cord, while the lower anterior division continues as the medial cord (Fig. 5.24). The cords pass into the axilla initially posterolateral to the axillary artery and then in their named positions with respect to the 2nd part of the axillary artery behind pectoralis minor. The cords and axillary artery are bound together in the axillary sheath. A number of branches arise from the roots, trunks and cords (Fig. 5.24), the major nerves being the axillary and radial nerves from the posterior cord, the musculocutaneous and lateral head of the median nerve from the lateral cord, and the ulnar and medial head of the median nerve from the medial cord

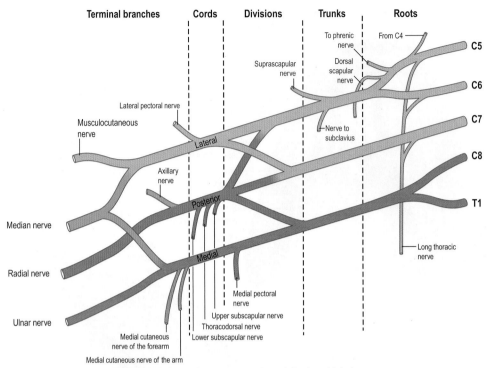

| Terminal branches | Cords | Divisions | Trunks | Roots |

Fig. 5.24 Schematic representation of the brachial plexus.

(Fig. 5.24). The muscles of the upper limb supplied by branches from the brachial plexus are shown in Table 5.3, while the distribution of the cutaneous branches of the major nerves, together with the dermatome supplied by each nerve root, are shown in Fig. 5.25.

> **CLINICAL ANATOMY:** Erb's palsy results from damage to the C5 and C6 roots of the brachial plexus. The axillary nerve is affected with the individual usually being unable to abduct or externally rotate the shoulder joint. It commonly occurs when there is an excessive increase in the angle between the neck and shoulder stretching, rupturing or tearing (avulsion) the nerve roots. It is the most common (48%) birth-related neuropraxia.

Lymph Nodes

The axillary lymph nodes are distributed in the axillary fat throughout the axilla, but can be considered as being in five groups, of which four lie below pectoralis minor (central, posterior/subscapular, lateral/humeral, anterior/pectoral) and one above (apical) (Fig. 5.26).

The central group of nodes lie above the floor of the axilla receiving lymph from all areas of the upper limb; however, the main upper limb drainage is to the lateral nodes. The pectoral nodes receive drainage from the breast and anterior chest wall (Fig. 5.27), while the scapular region and upper back drain to the subscapular nodes. Efferent vessels from these groups pass to central and then apical nodes, the latter also receiving efferent vessels from the superficial infraclavicular nodes (Fig. 5.27).

All lymph from the upper limb passes through the apical group where efferent vessels condense to form the subclavian lymph trunk. On the right, the trunk drains directly into the right lymphatic duct, while on the left it joins the thoracic duct.

> **APPLIED ANATOMY:** Infection and/or inflammation of the upper limb and posterior and anterior chest wall (including the breast) usually results in enlargement of the lymph nodes in the axilla. With careful palpation the site of infection/inflammation may be able to be determined.

Nerve	Muscles Supplied
Dorsal scapular nerve	Rhomboid major and minor
Suprascapular nerve	Supraspinatus and infraspinatus
Medial pectoral nerve	Pectoralis major and minor
Lateral pectoral nerve	Pectoralis major
Upper subscapular nerve	Subscapularis
Lower subscapular nerve	Subscapularis, teres major
Thoracodorsal nerve	Latissimus dorsi
Axillary nerve	Deltoid, teres minor
Musculocutaneous nerve	Coracobrachialis, biceps brachii, brachialis (medial two-thirds)
Median nerve	*In the forearm:* pronator teres, flexor carpi radialis, flexor digitorum superficialis, flexor pollicis longus, flexor digitorum profundus (lateral half), pronator quadratus *In the hand:* abductor, flexor and opponens pollicis, lateral two lumbricals
Radial nerve	Triceps brachii, anconeus, brachialis (lateral third), brachioradialis, extensors carpi radialis longus and brevis, supinator, extensor digitorum, extensor digiti minimi, extensor carpi ulnaris, extensors pollicis longus and brevis, extensor indicis, abductor pollicis longus
Ulnar nerve	*In the forearm:* flexor carpi ulnaris, flexor digitorum profundus (medial half) *In the hand:* palmaris brevis, abductor, flexor and opponens digit minimi, medial two lumbricals, palmar and dorsal interossei, adductor pollicis

TABLE 5.3   Muscles of the Upper Limb Supplied by Branches of the Brachial Plexus

Major branches are in bold.

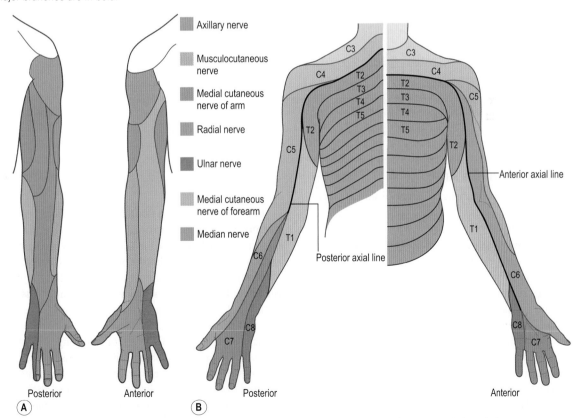

Fig. 5.25 (A) Cutaneous innervation of the upper limb; (B) dermatomes of the upper limb and thorax.

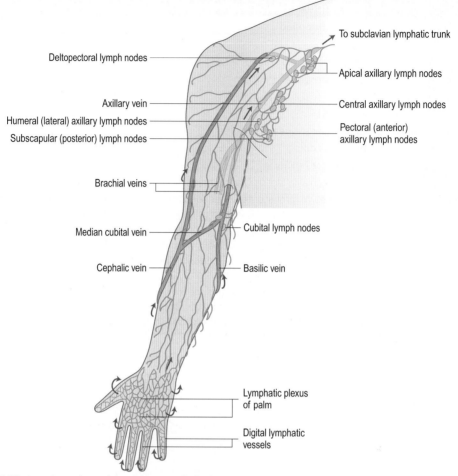

Fig. 5.26 Anterior surface of the right upper limb showing its lymphatic drainage and major groups of nodes.

Compartments of the Arm

The arm has two compartments: anterior and posterior.

Anterior Compartment

The anterior compartment contains the flexor muscles (coracobrachialis, biceps brachii, brachialis), the musculocutaneous, median and ulnar nerves, and the brachial artery surrounded by its vena comitantes, and the basilic and cephalic veins (Fig. 5.28).

Cephalic vein. From the elbow the cephalic vein passes along the lateral side of the biceps tendon to enter the groove anterior to the shoulder joint between deltoid and pectoralis major (deltopectoral groove). At the level of the coracoid process of the scapula it turns medially between pectoralis major and minor, piercing

the clavipectoral fascia to drain into the axillary vein (see Fig. 5.65).

Basilic vein. From the elbow the basilic vein passes along the medial side of the proximal arm, then pierces the deep fascia to ascend alongside the brachial vessels becoming the axillary vein at the lower border of teres major (see Fig. 5.65).

Brachial artery. Continuation of the axillary artery at the lower border of teres major, terminating at the level of the neck of the radius in the cubital fossa (page 411), where it divides into radial (lateral) and ulnar (medial) branches (see Fig. 5.64). It lies on the long and medial heads of triceps, coracobrachialis and brachialis, being covered anteriorly by biceps brachii. In the arm it gives the profunda brachii artery. Branches of the brachial artery and profunda brachii anastomose around the elbow joint.

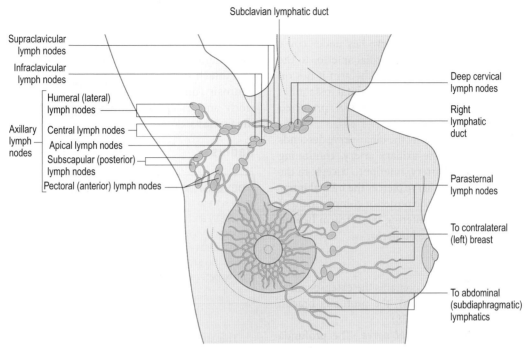

Fig. 5.27 Lymphatic drainage of the right anterior chest wall and breast.

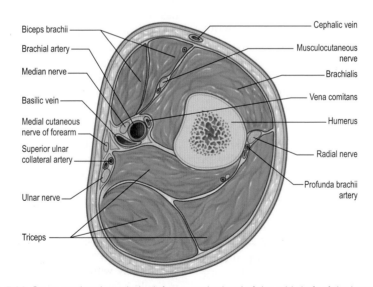

Fig. 5.28 Cross-section through the left arm at the level of the mid-shaft of the humerus.

APPLIED ANATOMY: The brachial pulse can be felt along its whole length by compressing the artery against the humerus; the pulse is best felt at the level of the medial epicondyle. It is at this level where Korotkoff sounds can be heard when measuring blood pressure.

Musculocutaneous nerve. Initially lateral to the axillary artery, the musculocutaneous nerve descends between the artery and coracobrachialis and then between biceps and brachialis to reach the lateral side of the arm (see Fig. 5.68A). At the elbow it pierces the deep fascia between biceps and brachioradialis as the lateral cutaneous nerve of the forearm (see Fig. 5.68A).

Median nerve. The median nerve lies under cover of biceps crossing from lateral to medial anterior to the brachial artery. In the lower part of the arm it lies on brachialis (see Fig. 5.70A) and in the cubital fossa it lies medial to the brachial artery (see Fig. 5.38A) protected by the bicipital aponeurosis.

Ulnar nerve. From the axilla the ulnar nerve descends on the medial side of the axillary artery, continuing medially to the brachial artery, anterior to triceps. In the distal half of the arm, the nerve pierces the medial intermuscular septum to enter the posterior compartment of the arm (see Fig. 5.69A), entering the forearm behind the medial epicondyle of the humerus.

Posterior Compartment

The posterior compartment contains the extensor muscles (triceps brachii, anconeus), the profunda brachii artery and radial nerve (Fig. 5.28).

Profunda brachii and radial nerve. The profunda brachii (branch of the brachial artery) and radial nerve (branch of the posterior cord of the brachial plexus) pass through the triangular interval and into the spiral (radial) groove of the humerus to enter the posterior compartment of the arm.

Muscles

The main action of muscles in the arm is to produce flexion (biceps brachii, brachialis, pronator teres) or extension (triceps, anconeus) of the forearm at the elbow joint, with biceps also being a strong supinator (page 412) of the forearm. Details of the attachments, action and innervation of the arm muscles are given in Table 5.4.

FOREARM

The forearm extends between the elbow (articulation of the radius and ulna with the humerus) and the wrist (articulation of the radius and ulna, via an intra-articular disc, with the proximal row of carpal bones) joints; it has anterior (flexor) and posterior (extensor) compartments separated by an interosseous membrane (see Fig. 5.44). Joints between the proximal and distal ends of the radius and ulna permit supination and pronation of the forearm about its length (page 412).

The deep fascia around the elbow is strong because many muscles arise from either the common flexor (anterior aspect of the medial epicondyle) or extensor (lateral surface of the lateral epicondyle) origins also attach to the overlying fascia: the bicipital aponeurosis (medial expansion of biceps brachii) anteriorly and triceps attachment posteriorly strengthen the fascia.

Radius

> **DEVELOPMENT:** A primary centre appears in the shaft during the 8th week *in utero*. At birth the head, radial tuberosity and distal end are cartilaginous. Secondary centres appear in the distal end during the 1st year, fusing with the shaft between 20 and 22 years; the head at age 6, fusing with the shaft between 15 and 17 years and radial tuberosity between 14 and 15 years, which soon fuses with the shaft.

The shorter lateral bone of the forearm (Fig. 5.29). It has a proximal head, shaft and distal expanded end with distinct articular surfaces. The disc-shaped head has a concave upper surface with a flattened outer surface, below which is a constricted neck. The neck slopes medially as it approaches the shaft. Where the shaft joins the neck it is round, becoming triangular lower down. In its upper quarter the shaft has a slight medial convexity continuous with the lateral convexity lower down. Anteromedially on the upper part of the shaft at its maximum convexity is the radial tuberosity (Fig. 5.29B). The shaft has three borders (rounded anterior and posterior, sharp medial interosseous) and three surfaces (convex posterior and lateral, concave anterior).

Proximally, the radius articulates with the capitulum of the humerus at the elbow joint (page 407), and distally with the scaphoid and lunate at the wrist (radiocarpal) joint (page 418). It also articulates proximally and distally with the ulna at the superior and inferior radioulnar joints (page 412).

> **APPLIED ANATOMY:** The head of the radius can be felt on the posterolateral aspect of the elbow, especially in elbow extension. It can be felt rotating during pronation and supination.

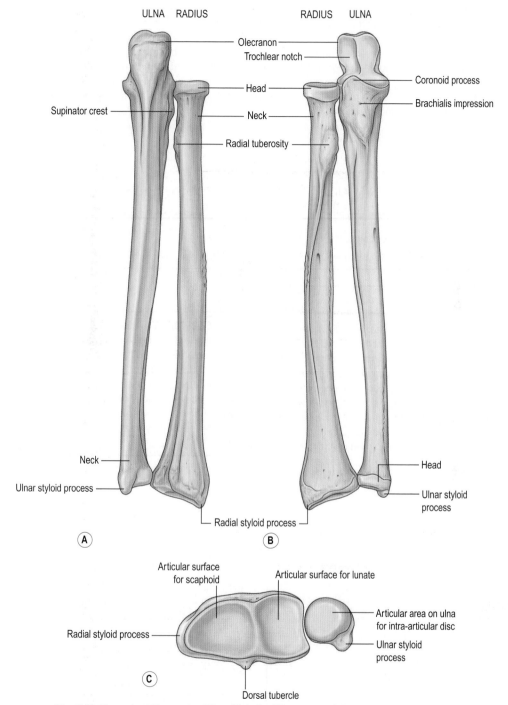

ULNA RADIUS   RADIUS ULNA

Olecranon

Trochlear notch

Coronoid process

Head

Brachialis impression

Supinator crest

Neck

Radial tuberosity

Neck

Head

Ulnar styloid process

Ulnar styloid process

Radial styloid process

(A)

(B)

Articular surface for scaphoid

Articular surface for lunate

Articular area on ulna for intra-articular disc

Radial styloid process

Ulnar styloid process

(C)

Dorsal tubercle

Fig. 5.29 Posterior (A), anterior (B) and inferior (C) aspects of the right radius and ulna.

CLINICAL ANATOMY: A *Colles' fracture* (transverse fracture in the lower 2–3 cm of the radius with the fragment displaced posteriorly (Fig. 5.30)) can result from a fall on the outstretched hand with the wrist extended; the hand is displaced laterally and dorsally. The ulna is not usually involved; however, its styloid process may be torn off. Alternatively, the fall can result in dislocation at the radiocarpal, but not the inferior radioulnar joint. A *Smith's fracture* (transverse fracture of the radius with the fragment displaced anteriorly (Fig. 5.30)) can result from a fall on the outstretched arm with the wrist flexed, a direct blow to the dorsal forearm or more commonly a palmar fall with the wrist slightly dorsiflexed. There may be more than one fragment and may/may not involve the radiocarpal joint.

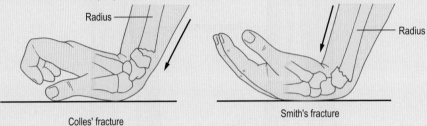

Radius   Radius

Colles' fracture   Smith's fracture

Fig. 5.30 Colles' and Smith's fractures of the radius showing displacement of the fracture fragment.

CLINICAL ANATOMY: Greenstick fractures occur in long bones, usually in children, due to their flexibility and present as an incomplete break with associated arm displacement. In the radius (or ulna) they can occur at three sites (proximal, medial, distal end of the bone). Greenstick fractures are of three types: a transverse fracture around the cortex extending to the middle of the bone (Fig. 5.31), a torus (buckling) fracture caused by impaction, and a bow fracture when the bone is curved along its longitudinal axis. Intense pain, swelling of the affected area, the presence of an abnormally bent or twisted limb, slight bruising and guarding of the affected area, and/or decreased range of movement of the injured part usually accompany the fracture. In some cases, there may be no associated symptoms.

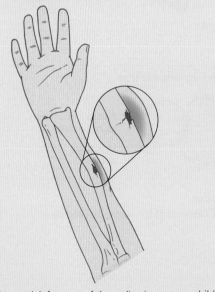

Fig. 5.31 Greenstick fracture of the radius in a young child.

Ulna

DEVELOPMENT: A primary centre appears in the shaft during the 8th week *in utero*, with the shaft, coronoid process and most of the olecranon ossifying from this centre. Secondary centres appear in the head during the 5th year, fusing with the shaft between 20 and 22 years; and remainder of the olecranon at age 11, fusing with the shaft between 16 and 19 years. There may be several secondary centres associated with the olecranon.

The longer medial bone of the forearm (Fig. 5.29). It has a large proximal end presenting as a hook-like projection, a shaft and a small rounded distal end. The proximal end has two projecting processes (olecranon posteriorly, coronoid anteriorly) enclosing a concave articular surface (trochlear notch). Medially below the notch is another articular surface (radial notch) separated from the trochlear notch by a sharp border. The distal end has a narrow neck which expands into a rounded head; the styloid process projects posteromedially. The shaft has three borders (rounded anterior and posterior, sharp lateral interosseous) and three surfaces (convex posterior and medial, concave anterior).

Proximally, the ulna articulates with the trochlea of the humerus at the elbow joint (page 407), and distally with the articular disc separating it from the wrist (radiocarpal) joint (page 418). It also articulates proximally and distally with the radius at the superior and inferior radioulnar joints (page 412).

APPLIED ANATOMY: The olecranon and epicondyles of the humerus form an equilateral triangle in full elbow flexion and lie in a straight line in full elbow extension. Disruption of this triangle may indicate a fracture or dislocation.

APPLIED ANATOMY: The outline of the olecranon can be felt proximally. It forms the 'point' of the elbow in flexion. Distally, the neck, head and styloid process can be felt. When the forearm is fully pronated the head of the ulna becomes prominent on the back of the wrist.

CLINICAL ANATOMY: The olecranon can be fractured in direct falls onto the point of the elbow. An avulsion fracture of the olecranon can result from a sudden powerful pull of triceps on its attachment.

CLINICAL ANATOMY: Inflammation of the olecranon bursa (olecranon bursitis) near the point of the elbow can be due to trauma or infection. It is associated with inflammatory conditions such as rheumatoid arthritis and gout.

Elbow Joint

A synovial hinge joint between the capitulum and trochlea of the humerus proximally and head of the radius and trochlear notch of the ulna distally. When viewed laterally the distal end of the humerus projects anteroinferiorly at about 45 degrees and the trochlear notch projects anterosuperiorly at about 45 degrees (Fig. 5.32A). This arrangement promotes a large range of flexion at the joint by delaying contact between the humerus and ulna. When viewed anteriorly the ulna deviates laterally forming the carrying angle (Fig. 5.32B).

APPLIED ANATOMY: The carrying angle is less in males (10–15 degrees) than in females (20–25 degrees).

The transverse axis of the elbow joint passes from inferior, posterior and medial to superior, anterior and lateral (Fig. 5.32B). Although the axis of movement may change slightly during flexion and extension, the joint behaves as a hinge joint. The joint is completely surrounded by a fibrous capsule, which includes the superior radioulnar joint, and is strengthened at the sides by strong lateral (radial) and medial (ulnar) collateral ligaments (Fig. 5.33).

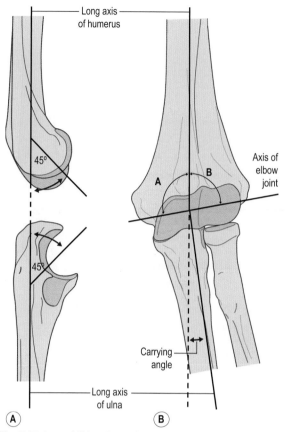

Fig. 5.32 Lateral (A) and anterior (B) aspects of the elbow joint.

The collateral ligaments cross the axis of movement and are therefore relatively tense in all joint positions.

CLINICAL ANATOMY: Supracondylar fractures are common in children falling on an outstretched arm. They are often comminuted (page 34) and may be complex to treat with vascular (brachial artery) and nerve (median) complications.

CLINICAL ANATOMY: Forceful abduction applied to the forearm may rupture the ulnar collateral ligament or more commonly result in avulsion of the medial epicondyle, with potential damage to the ulnar nerve. If the fracture does not unite or the ligament heal, the forearm becomes increasingly abducted, with stretching of the ulnar nerve leading to sensory disturbances and muscle weakness or paralysis.

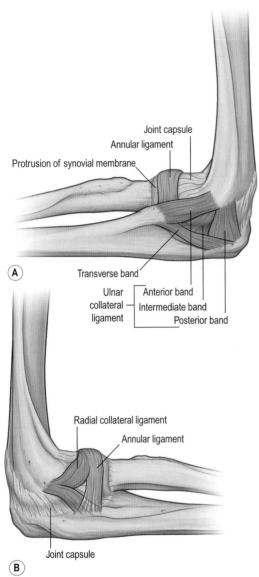

Fig. 5.33 Medial (A) and lateral (B) collateral ligaments of the elbow joint.

CLINICAL ANATOMY: In young children the head of the radius can be dislocated when traction forces are applied to the forearm and hand, because it is relatively small compared to the annular ligament. In older individuals a fall on the hand with the forearm extended can tear the annular ligament with a consequent anterior dislocation of the radial head (Fig. 5.34A); extreme pronation can also tear the annular ligament. The majority of elbow dislocations involve backward movement of the ulna through the relatively weak posterior capsule, often accompanied with coronoid process fracture (Fig. 5.34B). Both the radius and ulna may be involved because of the connections at the superior radioulnar joint. Backward dislocation can produce pressure on the brachial artery causing it to go into spasm reducing the blood supply to the forearm and hand. Pressure on the artery can also occur in supracondylar fractures as the lower fragment moves forwards. There may also be injury to the median nerve with a consequent loss of pronation and reduced function of the hand; there is considerable swelling around the elbow joint.

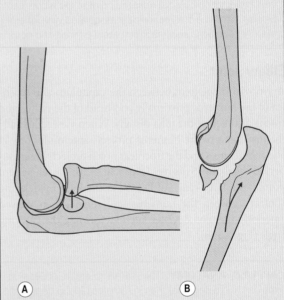

Fig. 5.34 (A) Dislocation of the radial head into the cubital fossa; (B) posterior dislocation of the ulna with coronoid process fracture.

Movements

The shape of the articular surfaces, together with the collateral ligaments, restricts movement at the joint to flexion and extension (Fig. 5.36). The active range of flexion is 145 degrees, while the passive range is 160 degrees. Extension is zero as this corresponds to the anatomical position; however, a small amount (5 degrees) of hyperextension may be possible. Except at the extremes of flexion and extension, movement at the joint is one of sliding rather than rolling.

When going from flexion to extension contact between the articular surfaces change. Contact between the trochlea and trochlear notch progressively increases

APPLIED ANATOMY: The alignment of the olecranon and humeral epicondyle can be used to assess the nature of the trauma in individuals with a swollen elbow. The alignment is unchanged (Fig. 5.35A) in supracondylar fractures but is changed in dislocations (Fig. 5.35B). If an apparently dislocated joint cannot be reduced fracture of the olecranon needs to be considered, especially if the joint is unstable.

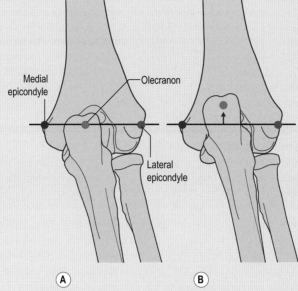

Fig. 5.35 Normal alignment (A) and malalignment (B) of the olecranon and humeral epicondyles.

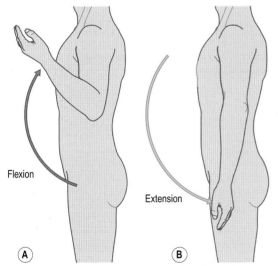

Fig. 5.36 Flexion (A) and extension (B) of the forearm at the elbow joint. (Adapted from Chao EY, Morrey BF. Three-dimensional rotation of the elbow. J Biomech 1978;11:57–74.)

(Fig. 5.37A), with the head of the radius only coming into contact with the capitulum after 90 degrees flexion (Fig. 5.37B).

The main muscles involved in flexing the forearm at the elbow joint are biceps brachii, brachialis, brachioradialis and pronator teres, although other muscles crossing anterior to the joint also contribute; similarly, the main muscles involved in extending the forearm at the elbow joint are triceps brachii and anconeus, although these are only active against resistance. Details of the attachments, action and innervation of the muscles crossing the elbow joint are given in Table 5.4.

CLINICAL ANATOMY: *Tennis elbow* is tenderness and pain caused by a tear in or near the common extensor attachment on the lateral epicondyle. It can be the result of sudden flexion of the wrist when the extensors are contracted but is more commonly the result of repeated gripping in everyday activities (cumulative trauma disorders). *Golfer's elbow* affects the common flexor attachment on the medial epicondyle. Pain and tenderness occur with repeated strain of the elbow flexors.

TABLE 5.4	The Attachments, Action and Innervation of Muscles Acting at the Elbow Joint		
Muscle	**Attachments**	**Action**	**Innervation**
Biceps brachii	From the supraglenoid tubercle above the glenoid fossa of the scapula (*long head*) and the cora-coid process of the scapula (*short head*) to the radial tuberosity of the radius	Its main action is flexion of the forearm at the elbow joint and supination of the forearm at the superior and inferior radioulnar joints: it is also a weak flexor of arm at the shoulder joint; if deltoid is paralysed biceps can be re-educated to abduct the arm at the shoulder when the arm is laterally rotated	Musculocuta-neous nerve (C5, C6)
Brachialis	From the distal two-thirds of the anterior surface of the shaft of the humerus and medial and lateral inter-muscular septa to the inferior part of the coronoid process of the ulna	Flexion of the forearm at the elbow joint	Musculocuta-neous nerve (C5, C6)
Brachioradialis	From the upper two-thirds of the lateral supracondylar ridge of the humerus to the lateral surface of the radius above the styloid process	Flexion of the forearm at the elbow joint, especially when the forearm is in mid pronation/supination; helps return forearm to this mid position from the extremes of either pronation or supination	Radial nerve (C5, C6)
Pronator teres[a]			
Flexor carpi radialis[b]			
Flexor carpi ulnaris[b]			
Flexor digitorum superficialis[c]			
Palmaris longus[b]			
Triceps brachii	From the infraglenoid tubercle below the glenoid fossa of the scapula (*long head*), above and lateral to the spiral groove of the humerus (*lateral head*) and posterior surface of the humerus below and medial to the spiral groove (*medial head*) to the posterior aspect of the proximal surface of the olecranon of the ulna and deep fascia of the forearm; all heads unite	The main action is extension of the forearm at the elbow joint: it also adducts and extends the flexed arm at the shoulder joint	Radial nerve (C6–C8)
Anconeus	From the lateral epicondyle of the humerus to the olecranon and upper quarter of the posterior surface of the ulna	Assists extension of the forearm at the elbow joint	Radial nerve (C7, C8)
Extensor carpi radialis longus[b]			
Extensor carpi radialis brevis[b]			
Extensor carpi ulnaris[b]			
Extensor digitorum[b]			
Extensor digiti minimi[b]			

[a]See Table 5.5 for details.
[b]Although these muscles contribute to flexion or extension of the forearm at the elbow joint, their main action is either at the wrist (a) or in the digits (b); details are given in Tables 5.6 and 5.7, respectively.

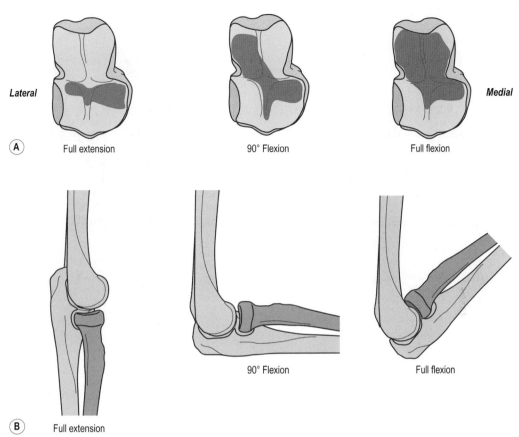

Fig. 5.37 (A) Contact areas between the trochlea of the humerus and trochlear notch of the ulna; (B) contact between the head of the radius and capitulum.

Cubital Fossa

A triangular space bounded above by an imaginary line between the medial and lateral epicondyles, laterally by the medial border of brachioradialis and medially by the lateral border of pronator teres (Fig. 5.38A). The floor is mainly formed by brachialis with supinator infero-laterally and the roof by the deep fascia of the forearm, reinforced medially by the bicipital aponeurosis (Fig. 5.38A). The deep fascia separates the superficial veins from the deeper structures (Fig. 5.38B).

> **CLINICAL ANATOMY:** This is an important area as the large superficial veins are used for venepuncture, whereas the deeper brachial artery is used for determining blood pressure.

Within the fossa deep to the deep fascia are, from medial to lateral, the median nerve, brachial artery and tendon of biceps. The median nerve passes between the two heads of pronator teres to enter the forearm. The brachial artery divides into radial and ulnar arteries at the level of the neck of the radius, with the radial artery passing inferolaterally over the biceps tendon deep to brachioradialis and the ulnar artery inferomedially deep to pronator teres. Both arteries are involved in an extensive anastomosis around the elbow region together with branches from the brachial artery and profunda brachii (Fig. 5.39). The tendon of biceps passes to attach to the radial tuberosity.

The ulnar nerve passes behind the medial epicondyle of the humerus on the ulnar collateral ligament. It does not pass through the cubital fossa.

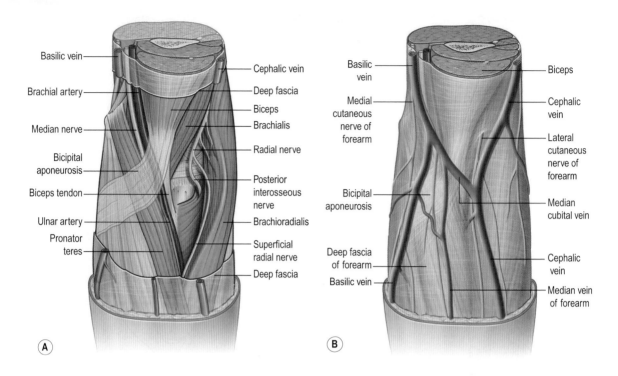

Fig. 5.38 Anterior aspect of the left cubital fossa showing the deep (A) and superficial (B) structures.

CLINICAL ANATOMY: Compression of the ulnar nerve can occur as it passes through a fibrous tunnel behind the medial epicondyle. Compression can be due to an abnormal valgus angle caused by an earlier fracture or by joint deformity/trauma due to rheumatoid arthritis or osteoarthritis.

Radioulnar Joints

The superior radioulnar joint is between the head of the radius and the radial notch of the ulna and annular ligament (Fig. 5.40). The inferior radioulnar joint is between the head of the ulna and ulnar notch on the distal end of the radius (Fig. 5.41). The superior joint is continuous with the elbow joint, while the inferior joint is separated from the wrist (radiocarpal) joint by an articular disc between the radius and ulna.

Movements

Combined movements at the superior and inferior radioulnar joints permit pronation and supination of the forearm. In supination the radius and ulna lie parallel to each other, while in pronation the radius moves anterolaterally across the ulna (Fig. 5.42).

During pronation the head of the radius rotates within the fibro-osseous ring formed by the radial notch and annular ligament (Fig. 5.43A), at the same time the ulna moves into slight extension and medial displacement. The ulna does not rotate but describes an arc of movement while remaining parallel to itself (Fig. 5.43B). The total range of pronation and supination is almost 180 degrees.

APPLIED ANATOMY: Below the lateral epicondyle the head of the radius can be felt rotating within the fibro-osseous ring formed by the radial notch of the ulna and annular ligament.

Muscles producing pronation are pronators teres and quadratus and supination are biceps brachii and supinator (Table 5.5).

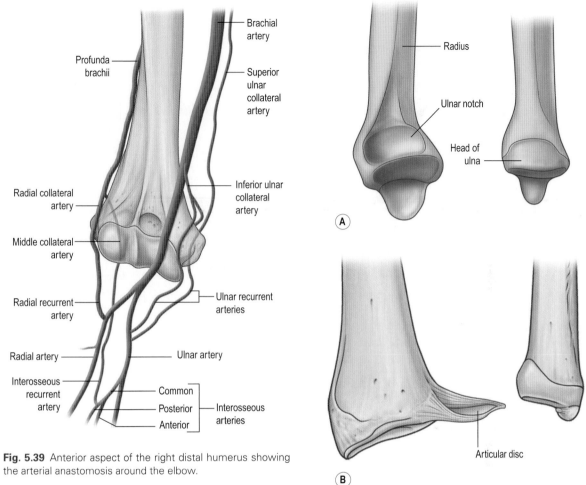

Fig. 5.39 Anterior aspect of the right distal humerus showing the arterial anastomosis around the elbow.

Fig. 5.41 The medial (A) and inferior (B) aspects of the inferior radioulnar joint.

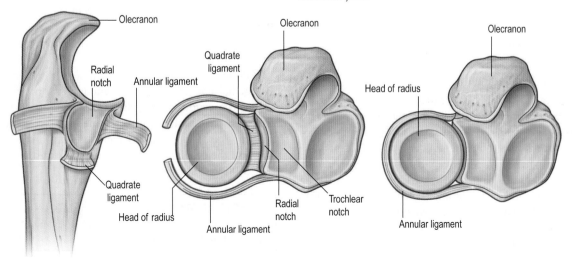

Fig. 5.40 The superior radioulnar joint.

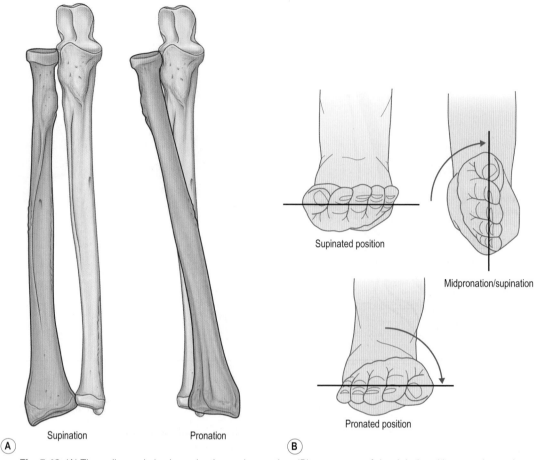

Fig. 5.42 (A) The radius and ulna in supination and pronation; (B) movement of the right hand in pronation and supination with the elbow flexed at 90 degrees.

Compartments of the Forearm

The forearm has two compartments separated by an interosseous membrane attached to the adjacent interosseous borders of the radius and ulna (Fig. 5.44).

Anterior Compartment

The anterior (flexor) compartment contains brachioradialis, the flexor muscles of the wrist (flexors carpi radialis and ulnaris, palmaris longus) and digits (flexors digitorum superficialis and profundus, and pollicis longus), the median, anterior interosseous and ulnar nerves, the radial, ulnar and anterior interosseous arteries with their vena comitantes, and the basilic and cephalic veins (Fig. 5.45).

Cephalic vein. The cephalic vein is a continuation of the lateral end of the dorsal venous network/arch of the hand ascending on the anterolateral aspect of the forearm

as far as the elbow, where it communicates with the basilic vein via the median cubital vein (Fig. 5.38B, see also Fig. 5.65). The median cubital vein (or occasionally the cephalic vein) receives the anterior vein of the forearm (antebrachial vein).

Basilic vein. The basilic vein is a continuation of the medial end of the dorsal venous network/arch of the hand ascending along the medial side of the forearm then passing anterior to the medial epicondyle of the humerus. It is joined by tributaries from the forearm and the median cubital vein anterior to the elbow (Fig. 5.38B, see also Fig. 5.65).

CLINICAL ANATOMY: The large superficial veins near the elbow (cephalic, basilic, median cubital, median vein of the forearm) are frequently used for venepuncture.

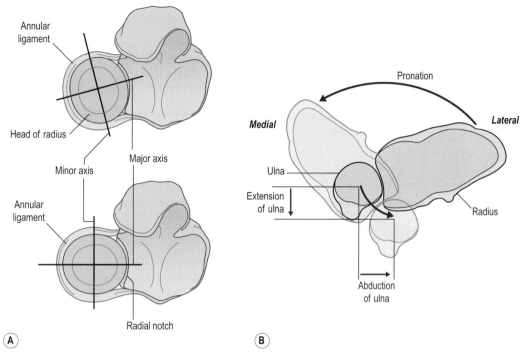

Fig. 5.43 (A) Rotation of the radial head within the fibro-osseous ring; (B) movement of the radius and ulna at the right inferior radioulnar joint during pronation.

TABLE 5.5 **The Attachments, Action and Innervation of Muscles Involved in Pronation and Supination of the Forearm**

Muscle	Attachments	Action	Innervation (Root Value)
Pronator teres	From the lower part of the medial supracondylar ridge (*upper head*) and medial epicondyle of the humerus (*lower head*) to the pronator ridge on the ulna	Pronates the forearm at the radioulnar joints: it is also a weak flexor of the forearm at the elbow joint	Median nerve (C6, C7)
Pronator quadratus	Fibres pass transversely between the lower quarter of the anterior surfaces of the ulna and radius	Initiates pronation of the forearm at the superior and inferior radioulnar joints	Anterior interosseous branch of median nerve (C8, T1)
Biceps brachii[a]			
Supinator	From the inferior aspect of the lateral epicondyle of the humerus, lateral collateral and annular ligaments (*upper head*) and supinator crest and fossa of the ulna (*lower head*) to the posterior, lateral and anterior aspects of the radius between the neck of the radius and attachment of pronator teres	Supinates the forearm at the radioulnar joints; is most powerful with the elbow flexed to 120 degrees	Posterior interosseous branch of the radial nerve (C5, C6)
Brachioradialis[a]			

[a]See Table 5.4.

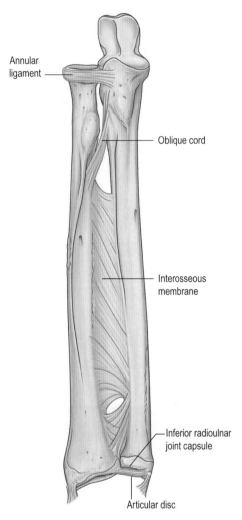

Annular ligament

Oblique cord

Interosseous membrane

Inferior radioulnar joint capsule

Articular disc

Fig. 5.44 Anterior aspect of the forearm showing the interosseous membrane between the radius and ulna.

Radial artery. The radial artery arises from the brachial artery in the cubital fossa level with the neck of the radius and passes inferolaterally over the tendon of biceps brachii deep to brachioradialis, where it continues on the lateral aspect of the forearm medial to the tendon of brachioradialis as far as the wrist (see Fig. 5.64). During its course the radial artery is joined on its lateral side by the superficial branch of the radial nerve. In the distal forearm the artery lies lateral to the tendon of flexor carpi radialis. The radial artery leaves the forearm by coursing around the lateral side of the wrist to enter the hand by passing through the two heads of the 1st dorsal

interosseous and of adductor pollicis and the bases of the 1st and 2nd metacarpals.

> **APPLIED ANATOMY:** The radial artery may pass from medial to lateral just deep to the deep fascia of the forearm superficial to the muscles of the anterior compartment.

> **APPLIED ANATOMY:** With the forearm in midpronation the course of the radial artery is indicated by a slightly convex line from the tendon of biceps in the cubital fossa down the medial side of brachioradialis to the anterior aspect of the radial styloid process.

> **CLINICAL ANATOMY:** The radial pulse can be felt against the distal end of the radius lateral to the tendon of flexor carpi radialis.

Ulnar artery. Ulnar artery is the other terminal branch of the brachial artery. In the cubital fossa it gives the common interosseous artery which immediately divides into anterior and posterior interosseous arteries which run either side of the interosseous membrane (see Fig. 5.64). The ulnar artery passes inferomedially deep to pronator teres, then courses medially lying on flexor digitorum profundus under cover of flexor carpi ulnaris as far as the wrist. The artery is joined on its medial side by the ulnar nerve.

> **APPLIED ANATOMY:** The course of the ulnar artery is represented by a medially convex line from the biceps tendon in the cubital fossa to the pisiform and hook of the hamate at the wrist, where it divides into deep and superficial branches.

> **CLINICAL ANATOMY:** As both the radial and ulnar arteries are relatively superficial, they can be lacerated, for example, when the hand passes through a window. If only one artery is involved, it can be ligated to stem the flow of blood. Because of the contribution of both vessels to the deep and superficial palmar arches (page 435) the blood supply to the hand is preserved.

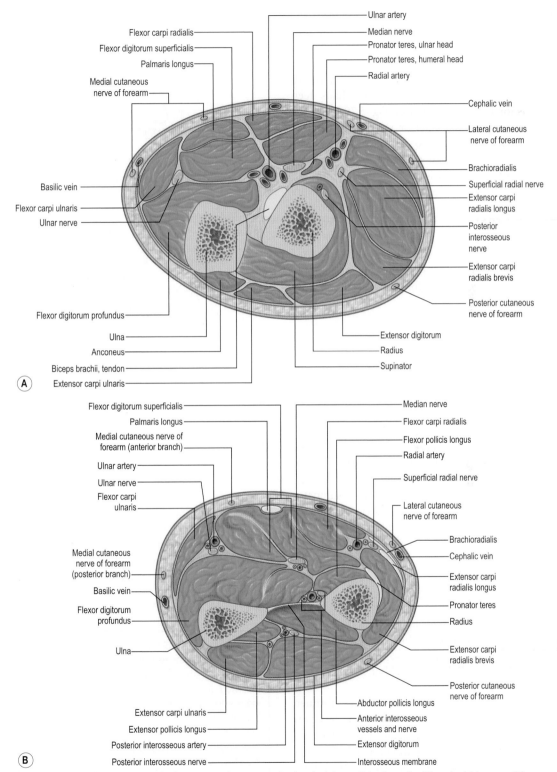

Ulnar artery
Median nerve
Pronator teres, ulnar head
Pronator teres, humeral head
Radial artery
Flexor carpi radialis
Flexor digitorum superficialis
Palmaris longus
Medial cutaneous nerve of forearm
Cephalic vein
Lateral cutaneous nerve of forearm
Brachioradialis
Superficial radial nerve
Extensor carpi radialis longus
Basilic vein
Flexor carpi ulnaris
Ulnar nerve
Posterior interosseous nerve
Extensor carpi radialis brevis
Posterior cutaneous nerve of forearm
Flexor digitorum profundus
Ulna
Anconeus
Biceps brachii, tendon
Extensor carpi ulnaris
Extensor digitorum
Radius
Supinator

A

Flexor digitorum superficialis
Palmaris longus
Medial cutaneous nerve of forearm (anterior branch)
Ulnar artery
Ulnar nerve
Flexor carpi ulnaris
Median nerve
Flexor carpi radialis
Flexor pollicis longus
Radial artery
Superficial radial nerve
Lateral cutaneous nerve of forearm
Brachioradialis
Cephalic vein
Extensor carpi radialis longus
Pronator teres
Radius
Extensor carpi radialis brevis
Medial cutaneous nerve of forearm (posterior branch)
Basilic vein
Flexor digitorum profundus
Ulna
Posterior cutaneous nerve of forearm
Extensor carpi ulnaris
Extensor pollicis longus
Posterior interosseous artery
Posterior interosseous nerve
Abductor pollicis longus
Anterior interosseous vessels and nerve
Extensor digitorum
Interosseous membrane

B

Fig. 5.45 Transverse sections through the forearm at the level of the radial tuberosity (A) and mid-forearm (B).

Median nerve. It enters the forearm between the two heads of pronator teres, then runs below the tendinous arch connecting the heads of flexor digitorum superficialis, being closely bound to its deep surface. It becomes superficial at the wrist between the tendons of flexors digitorum superficialis and carpi radialis deep to palmaris longus (if present) (see Fig. 5.70A). In the cubital fossa it gives the anterior interosseous nerve, which descends on the anterior aspect of the interosseous membrane with the anterior interosseous artery.

Ulnar nerve. It enters the forearm by passing through the two heads of flexor carpi ulnaris to descend on the medial side of the forearm on flexor digitorum profundus (see Fig. 5.69A) lateral to the ulnar artery. Proximal to the wrist it pierces the deep fascia to lie lateral to the tendon of flexor carpi ulnaris and then passes anterior to the flexor retinaculum, with the ulnar artery, lateral to the pisiform, where it divides into superficial and deep branches.

Posterior Compartment

The posterior (extensor) compartment contains the extensor muscles of the wrist (extensors carpi radialis longus and brevis, extensor carpi ulnaris) and digits (extensors digitorum, indicis, digiti minimi and pollicis brevis), abductor pollicis longus, and the posterior interosseous nerve and artery (Fig. 5.45).

Posterior interosseous nerve. The deep branch of the radial nerve arising anterior to the lateral epicondyle of the humerus entering the posterior compartment of the forearm by passing through the two heads of supinator (see Fig. 5.67A). It then runs on the posterior surface of the interosseous membrane with the posterior interosseous artery.

WRIST

The wrist connects the hand to the forearm (Fig. 5.46). It is not a single joint but comprises the articulation with the forearm (radiocarpal joint), that between the proximal and distal rows of carpal bones (midcarpal joint), and those between individual carpal bones (intercarpal joints) (Fig. 5.47).

At the wrist the deep fascia becomes thinner, although thickenings of transverse fibres form the flexor and extensor retinacula. The retinacula hold the tendons crossing the wrist in place preventing them 'bowstringing'. On the front of the wrist the flexor retinaculum

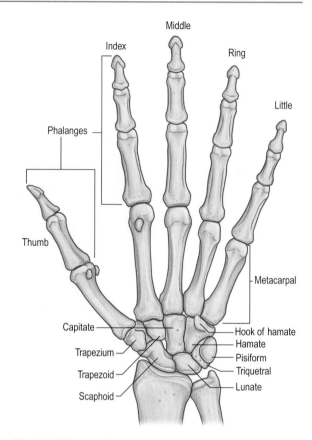

Fig. 5.46 The anterior aspect of the left distal radius and ulna, wrist and hand.

acts as a strong band converting the carpal sulcus into a tunnel transmitting the tendons of flexor pollicis longus, and digitorum superficialis and profundus, as well as the median nerve: the tendon of flexor carpi radialis passes in a tunnel through the flexor retinaculum. The median nerve lies anterior to the tendons of flexor digitorum superficialis (Fig. 5.48).

CLINICAL ANATOMY: As the median nerve passes deep to the flexor retinaculum it can be compressed if the synovial sheaths surrounding the muscles become inflamed, as well as during some wrist movements, giving rise to 'carpal tunnel (median nerve) syndrome'. There is loss of sensation over the lateral 3½ digits, weakness of the grip involving the thumb and atrophy of the thenar muscles (flexor and abductor pollicis brevis, opponens pollicis) (Fig. 5.49).

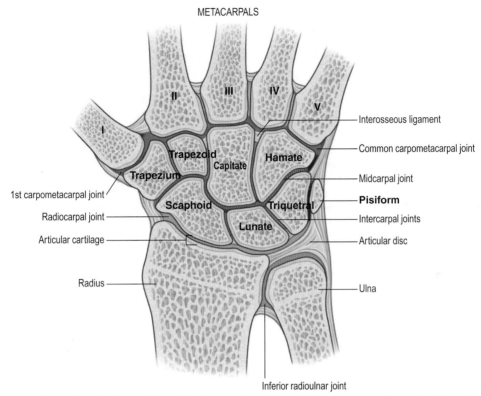

Fig. 5.47 Coronal section through the wrist showing the relationship between the radiocarpal, midcarpal and intercarpal joints.

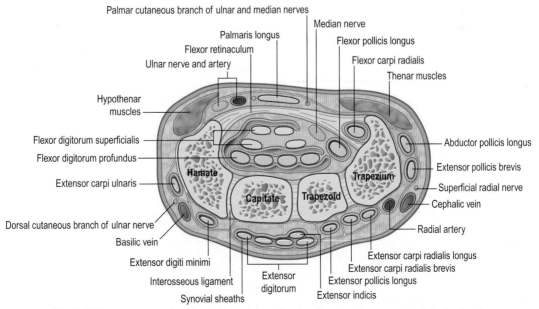

Fig. 5.48 Transverse section through the right wrist showing structures passing into the hand.

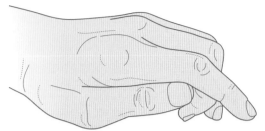

Fig. 5.49 Typical median nerve deformity of the hand.

CLINICAL ANATOMY: The ulnar nerve and artery pass superficial to the flexor retinaculum (Fig. 5.48) in a semirigid canal (Guyon's canal/tunnel) between the pisiform medially and hook of hamate laterally, where the nerve can become compressed, leading to a typical ulnar nerve deformity of the hand, with 'clawing' of the little and ring fingers due to paralysis/weakness of the interossei and lumbricals (Fig. 5.50).

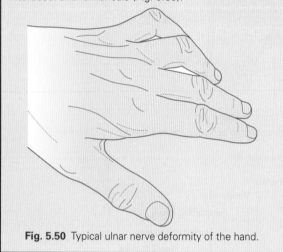

Fig. 5.50 Typical ulnar nerve deformity of the hand.

On the back of the wrist is the extensor retinaculum. Septa pass from its deep surface to the distal ends of the radius and ulna converting the grooves on the dorsum of the wrist into six compartments, each lined by a synovial sheath (Fig. 5.48).

Carpus

DEVELOPMENT: Each carpal bone ossifies from a single centre, except the scaphoid which may have two centres and the hamate (one for the hook of the hamate). During the 1st year centres for the capitate and hamate appear, followed by those for the triquetral between 2 and 4 years, lunate between 3 and 5 years, scaphoid, trapezium and trapezoid between 4 and 6 years, and pisiform between 9 and 11 years. Ossification is not complete until between 20 and 25 years.

CLINICAL ANATOMY: In the majority (>70%) of individuals the blood supply to the scaphoid is from distal to proximal. Following scaphoid fracture it is, therefore, important that the fragments are properly aligned. Non-union can lead to avascular necrosis of the proximal fragment accompanied by pain and swelling over the 'anatomical snuffbox' (page 424).

The wrist (carpus) consists of eight separate bones arranged around the capitate, but are usually considered as being in two rows. From lateral to medial, the proximal row comprises the scaphoid, lunate, triquetral and pisiform, and distal row the trapezium, trapezoid, capitate and hamate (Figs. 5.46 and 5.47). A strong fibrous capsule, reinforced by dorsal, palmar and collateral ligaments, surrounds the wrist.

APPLIED ANATOMY: The position of the radiocarpal joint is given by a slightly convex line proximally between the radial styloid process and head of the ulna.

Wrist Joint
Movements
Movements at the radiocarpal and midcarpal joints take place simultaneously, with the combined axis of movement being through the head of the capitate (Fig. 5.52). Because of the functional interdependence of the wrist and hand, all movements of the hand tend to be accompanied by movements at the wrist.

The line of action of the muscles at the wrist is oblique to the axes of movement (Fig. 5.53). The carpal flexors and extensors fix the wrist during flexion and extension of the fingers to prevent the digital muscles from losing power and efficiency.

APPLIED ANATOMY: During movements at the wrist, the extrinsic finger flexor tendons press and move against the walls of carpal tunnel. In flexion they are supported by the flexor retinaculum and in extension the carpal bones. Compression of the flexor tendons, as well as of their surrounding synovial sheaths, may compress the median nerve and be an important factor in carpal tunnel (median nerve) syndrome.

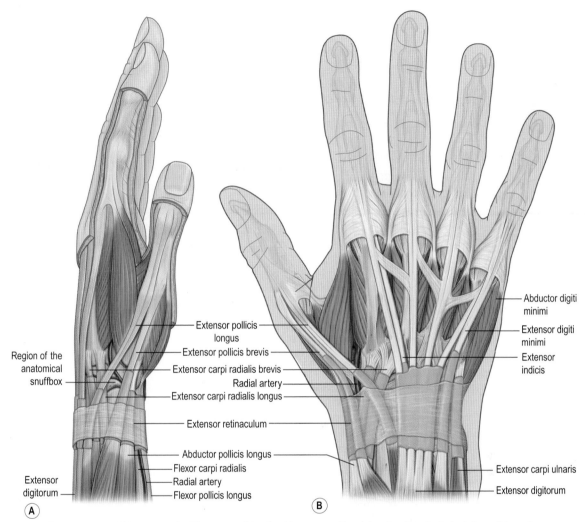

Region of the
anatomical
snuffbox

Extensor pollicis
longus

Extensor pollicis brevis

Extensor carpi radialis brevis

Radial artery

Extensor carpi radialis longus

Extensor retinaculum

Abductor pollicis longus

Flexor carpi radialis

Radial artery

Flexor pollicis longus

Extensor
digitorum

Abductor digiti
minimi

Extensor digiti
minimi

Extensor
indicis

Extensor carpi ulnaris

Extensor digitorum

(A)   (B)

Fig. 5.51 Lateral (A) and posterior (B) aspects of the distal forearm and hand showing the principal relations of the wrist.

CLINICAL ANATOMY: Tinel's test (Hoffmann-Tinel sign) is used to test for compression neuropathy. It is commonly used in diagnosing carpal tunnel (median nerve) syndrome. Tapping (percussion) over the median nerve at the wrist eliciting a tingling ('pins and needles') sensation in the distribution of the nerve at or distal to the site of the lesion is taken as a positive sign, indicating nerve compression. A positive sign can also indicate nerve regeneration.

Flexion and extension. In flexion the palmar aspect of the hand moves towards the anterior surface of the forearm, while in extension the dorsal aspect moves towards the posterior surface of the forearm. The range of each movement is approximately 85 degrees (Fig. 5.52), which tends to decrease with increasing age, with females having a greater range than males. Movement occurs about a transverse axis through the head of the capitate (Fig. 5.52). Flexion is limited by tension in the extensor tendons and is greatly reduced if the fingers are fully flexed.

The main muscles producing flexion are flexors carpi radialis and ulnaris, and palmaris longus (Table 5.6), with contributions from flexors digitorum superficialis and profundus and flexor pollicis longus. The main muscles producing extension are extensors carpi radialis longus and brevis and extensor carpi

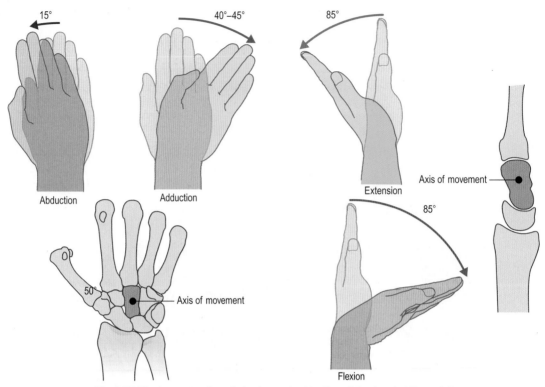

Fig. 5.52 Flexion, extension, abduction and adduction of the hand at the wrist.

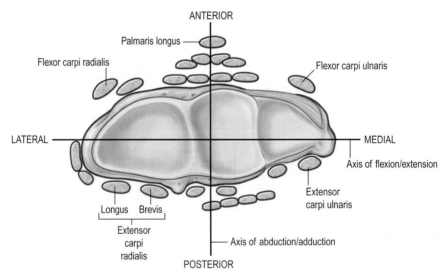

Fig. 5.53 Inferior surface of the right radius and intra-articular disc of the radiocarpal joint showing the relationship of the tendons producing movement at the wrist to the axes of flexion/extension and abduction/adduction.

ulnaris (Table 5.6), with contributions from extensors digitorum, indicis, digiti minimi, pollicis longus and brevis.

Abduction (radial deviation) and adduction (ulnar deviation). In abduction the tips of the fingers move laterally and in adduction they move medially (Fig. 5.52).

	TABLE 5.6 The Attachments, Action and Innervation of Muscles Involved in Movements of the Wrist		
Muscle	**Attachments**	**Action**	**Innervation (Root Value)**
Flexor carpi radialis	From the medial epicondyle of the humerus via the common flexor origin to the palmar surfaces of the bases of the 2nd and 3rd metacarpals	Flexion and abduction of the hand at the wrist joint	Median nerve (C6, C7)
Flexor carpi ulnaris	From the medial epicondyle of the humerus via the common flexor origin (*humeral head*) and upper two-thirds of the posterior border of the ulna (*ulnar head*) to the hook of the hamate and base of the 5th metacarpal; it also attaches to and invests the pisiform	Flexion and adduction of the hand at the wrist joint	Ulnar nerve (C7, C8)
Palmaris longus	From the medial epicondyle of the humerus via the common flexor origin to the superficial surface of the flexor retinaculum and apex of the palmar aponeurosis	Flexion of the hand at the wrist joint: by tightening the palmar fascia it may also cause slight flexion at the metacarpophalangeal joints	Median nerve (C8)
Flexor digitorum superficialis[a] (see Table 5.7)			
Flexor digitorum profundus[a] (see Table 5.7)			
Flexor pollicis longus[a] (see Table 5.7)			
Extensor carpi radialis longus	From the lower third of the lateral supracondylar ridge to the posterior surface of the base of the 2nd metacarpal	Extension and abduction of the hand at the wrist joint	Radial nerve (C6, C7)
Extensor carpi radialis brevis	From the lateral epicondyle of the humerus via the common extensor tendon and lateral collateral ligament to the posterior surface of the base of the 3rd metacarpal	Extension and abduction of the hand at the wrist joint	Posterior interosseous branch of the radial nerve (C6, C7)
Extensor carpi ulnaris	From the lateral epicondyle of the humerus via the common extensor tendon and posterior border of the ulna to the tubercle on the medial side of the base of the 5th metacarpal	Extension and adduction of the hand at the wrist joint	Posterior interosseous branch of the radial nerve (C7, C8)
Extensor digitorum[a] (see Table 5.7)			
Extensor indicis[a] (see Table 5.7)			

Continued

TABLE 5.6 The Attachments, Action and Innervation of Muscles Involved in Movements of the Wrist—cont'd

Muscle	Attachments	Action	Innervation (Root Value)
Extensor digit minimi[a] (see Table 5.7)			
Extensor pollicis longus[a] (see Table 5.7)			
Extensor pollicis brevis[a] (see Table 5.7)			

[a]Although these muscles contribute to flexion or extension of the hand at the wrist, their main action is on the digits; details are given in Table 5.7.

The range of abduction is 15 degrees and adduction 40 to 45 degrees, with both decreasing with increasing age. Movement occurs about an anteroposterior axis through the head of the capitate (Fig. 5.52). Abduction is more limited than adduction due to the distal projection of the radial styloid process and closing of the lateral part of the midcarpal joint space.

Abduction is produced by flexor carpi radialis and extensor carpi radialis longus and brevis, and adduction by flexor and extensor carpi ulnaris (Table 5.6).

On the posterolateral aspect of the wrist, with the thumb extended a slight hollow can be seen between the tendons of abductor pollicis longus and extensor pollicis brevis within the same synovial sheath laterally and the tendon of extensor pollicis longus medially. This is the 'anatomical snuffbox' (Fig. 5.51A).

> **APPLIED ANATOMY:** From proximal to distal in the floor of the 'anatomical snuffbox', the tip of the radial styloid process, scaphoid, trapezium and base of the 1st metacarpal can be palpated.

> **APPLIED ANATOMY:** The radial pulse can be felt in the 'anatomical snuffbox' as it compressed against the scaphoid.

HAND

The hand is an extremely mobile structure endowed with fine sensory discrimination. It is used to grip and manipulate the environment, being capable of applying large gripping forces between the thumb and fingers, yet can also perform precision movements. It also relays information regarding texture and surface contour, warns against the extremes of hot and cold and prevents collisions, especially when sight cannot be used. These motor and sensory functions have considerable representation in the motor and sensory cortices of the brain (see Fig. 4.21). There are four fingers and a thumb (or five digits) in each hand, with the fingers being identified as index (2nd digit), middle (3rd digit), ring (4th digit) and little (5th digit).

On the dorsum of the hand the superficial fascia is loose and thin, while on the palm, as well as the palmar surfaces of the digits it is specialised. In the centre of the palm strong bands of connective tissue connect the skin to the palmar aponeurosis (thickening of deep fascia); overlying the thenar and hypothenar regions fixation of the skin to the deep fascia is less marked, nevertheless, the superficial fascia is thicker and less fibrous to facilitate gripping actions of the hand. The pads on the palmar surfaces of the distal phalanges are highly specialised with numerous tactile nerve endings. Here the skin is firmly attached to the distal two-thirds of the distal phalanx.

There are two layers of deep fascia: the deeper layer covers the interosseous muscles and encloses adductor pollicis; the superficial layer is the strong, dense, thick, triangular palmar aponeurosis bound to the superficial fascia. The palmar aponeurosis has its apex at the wrist and base at the webs of the fingers, from which four slips pass into the fingers to become continuous with the digital sheaths of the flexor tendons. Each slip further divides giving attachments to the deep transverse metacarpal ligament, capsule of the metacarpophalangeal (MCP) joint and sides of the proximal phalanx.

In some individuals, especially the elderly, the medial part of the palmar aponeurosis and fibrous flexor sheaths of the ring and little fingers can become shortened (contracted) leading to progressive flexion of the fingers at the MCP and proximal interphalangeal (PIP) joints, with an inability to extend the fingers even passively. In severe cases, the distal interphalangeal (DIP) joint may become hyperextended. This is a *Dupuytren contracture* (Fig. 5.54).

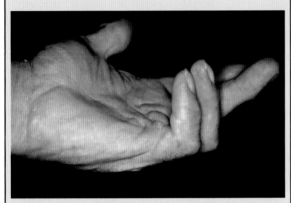

Fig. 5.54 The appearance of Dupuytren's contracture.

APPLIED ANATOMY: Septa pass down from the medial and lateral borders of the palmar aponeurosis fusing with the fascia covering the interossei, dividing the palm into three compartments: the lateral compartment contains the thenar muscle, the intermediate the long flexor tendons and lumbricals surrounded by loose connective tissue and the medial the hypothenar muscles. The intermediate compartment is divided into lateral and medial midpalmar spaces by an incomplete septum from the deep aspect of the connective tissue to the shaft of the 3rd metacarpal. These spaces communicate proximally with a potential space in front of pronator quadratus, while distally they are prolonged around each lumbrical into the web of the fingers, which in turn communicates with the subaponeurotic space on the dorsum of the hand deep to the extensor tendons.

CLINICAL ANATOMY: Accumulations of fluid in the midpalmar spaces following injury or infection of the hand can track back in the deep aspect of the flexor compartment or, via the web spaces of the fingers, up the posterior aspect of the forearm in the loose superficial fascia.

The synovial sheaths surrounding the tendons of the digital flexors at the wrist continue into the palm of the hand, with those to the thumb and little finger extending into the digit. Separate sheaths are present for the index, middle and ring fingers (Fig. 5.55A). In the fingers the tendons and their sheaths are held close to the phalanges by digital fibrous sheaths to prevent bowstringing of the tendons, ensuring that their pull produces movement at the MCP and interphalangeal (IP) joints. The fibro-osseous canals are formed by a shallow groove on the anterior surface of the phalanx and a fibrous sheath attached to the palmar edges of the phalanx (Fig. 5.55B), Most fibres of the sheath are arranged transversely, but at the IP joints they have a criss-cross arrangement allowing flexion to occur (Fig. 5.56).

CLINICAL ANATOMY: Infection of the synovial sheaths within the palm or of those in the thumb and little finger can track back and present as a swelling proximal to the wrist.

CLINICAL ANATOMY: 'Trigger finger' is a localised swelling of a flexor digitorum profundus tendon proximal to the tendon sheath and fibro-osseous canal. When the finger is flexed the swelling moves into the canal causing difficulty during extension. The same condition can affect the tendon of flexor pollicis longus in the thumb.

Metacarpals and Phalanges

DEVELOPMENT: Primary centres for each metacarpal appear in the shaft in the 9th week *in utero*, with secondary centres appearing in the heads of the 2nd to 5th metacarpals between 2 and 3 years and the base of the 1st metacarpal slightly later. Fusion of the epiphysis with the shaft occurs between ages 17 and 19. Primary centres for the shafts of the phalanges appear between the 8th and 12th week *in utero*, with secondary centres appearing in the bases during the 2nd and 3rd years. Fusion of the epiphysis and shaft occurs between ages 17 and 19.

The metacarpals, numbered M1 to M5 from lateral to medial, lie in the palm of the hand (Fig. 5.46), with each being a long bone with a proximal quadrilateral base, shaft with a slight longitudinally curved palmar concavity,

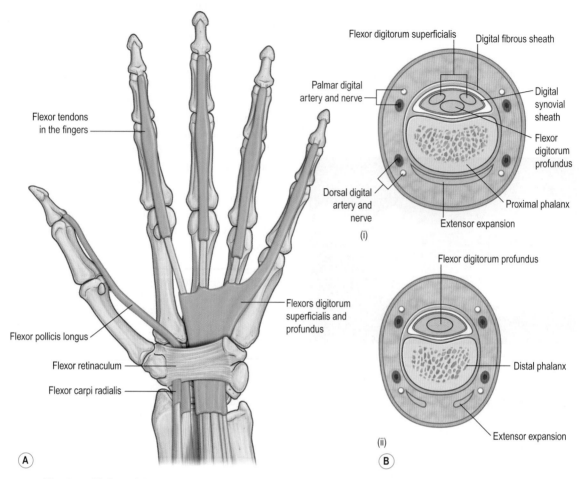

Fig. 5.55 (A) Synovial sheaths associated with the flexor tendons at the wrist and in the hand; (B) cross-section of a digit at the (i) proximal and (ii) distal phalanx showing the digital fibrous sheath and the arrangement of the tendons and synovial sheaths.

and distal rounded head. M1 is rotated approximately 90 degrees to the other metacarpals (Fig. 5.46). The bases of the metacarpals articulate with the distal row of carpal bones (M1 with the trapezium, M2 the trapezoid and capitate, M3 the capitate, M4 and M5 with the hamate) and heads with the proximal phalanges (Fig. 5.46). The relationship of the metacarpals to the surface creases of the wrist and palm is shown in Fig. 5.57.

Each hand contains 14 phalanges, three in each finger and two in the thumb (Fig. 5.46). Each phalanx has a large proximal end, a curved shaft convex dorsally and a rounded pulley-shaped distal head (in the distal phalanx the head is expanded to support the pulp pad of the digit).

> **APPLIED ANATOMY:** With the fingers flexed the metacarpal heads are the knuckles; the dorsal surface of the shaft and the line of the carpometacarpal joint (CMJ) can be felt. The heads of the proximal and middle phalanges can be felt on the dorsal surface with the fingers flexed, as can the proximal and DIP joints.

Carpometacarpal Joints

The bases of the medial four metacarpals and medial three carpal bones of the distal row form the plane synovial common carpometacarpal joint (CMJ), which has an irregular joint line (Fig. 5.47). The 1st metacarpal (M1)

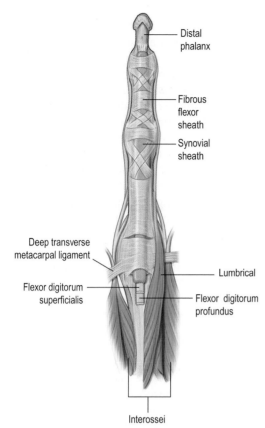

Fig. 5.56 Anterior aspect of a finger showing the organisation of the fibres in a digital fibrous sheath.

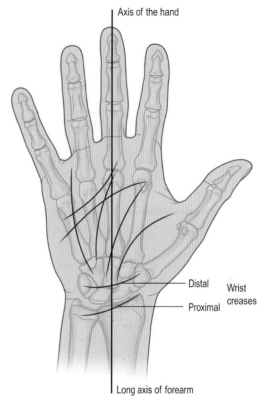

Fig. 5.57 Anterior aspect of the right hand showing the relationship of the surface creases of the wrist and palm to the underlying bones.

and trapezium form the synovial saddle-shaped 1st CMJ (Fig. 5.47). Each joint is surrounded by a fibrous capsule reinforced by ligaments. Dorsal and palmar carpometacarpal ligaments for the common CMJ; radial carpometacarpal and anterior and posterior oblique ligaments for the 1st CMJ. The common CMJ provides a firm base between the joints of the wrist and those of the hand. In contrast, the shape of the articular surfaces and loose joint capsule gives the 1st CMJ a large degree of mobility.

Movements

There is little or no movement at the common CMJ. The 2nd, 3rd and 4th metacarpals are essentially immobile; the 5th can undergo slight flexion in grasping and slight rotation during opposition (page 430) of the thumb to the little finger. In contrast, the 1st

CMJ is capable of flexion and extension, abduction and adduction, and axial rotation/opposition (Fig. 5.58). Details of the muscles involved in producing these movements of the thumb, together with other joints of the thumb at which they act are given in Table 5.7.

Metacarpophalangeal Joints

These are structurally and functionally similar in the fingers and thumb. The proximal articular surface is the rounded head of the metacarpal and the distal surface the base of the proximal phalanx (Fig. 5.59). The joints are surrounded by a loose fibrous capsule reinforced at the sides by collateral ligaments; those associated with the thumb contain sesamoid bones. The anterior and posterior aspects of the joint capsule are replaced by the palmar ligament and tendon of extensor digitorum in each finger, while the tendon of extensor pollicis longus either replaces or strengthens the posterior joint capsule in the thumb.

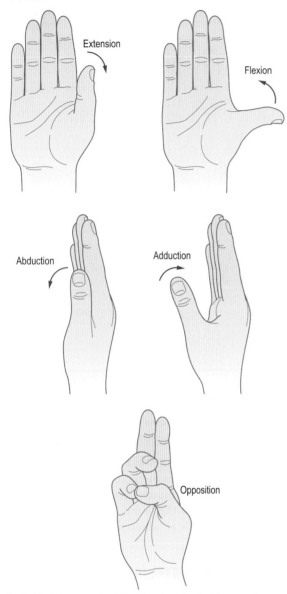

Fig. 5.58 Movements of the thumb at the 1st carpometacarpal joint.

> **CLINICAL ANATOMY:** A common deformity in rheumatoid arthritis, induced by synovitis of the MCP joint, leads to narrowing of the articular cartilage and attenuation of the collateral ligaments, with palmar subluxation of the proximal phalanx on the metacarpal head, creating laxity of the flexor complex. Under the pull of the flexor tendons there may be further subluxation of the proximal phalanx associated with an ulnar deviation, especially in the index and middle fingers.

Movements

The movements possible at the MCP joints are flexion and extension, abduction and adduction and axial rotation (Fig. 5.60). Axial rotation in the fingers is passive, while that in the thumb is active.

Flexion and extension. In the thumb, this occurs about an anteroposterior axis through the head of the metacarpal and about a transverse axis through the head of the metacarpal in each finger. In extension the anterior surface of the metacarpal head articulates with the palmar ligament, which moves past the metacarpal head turning upon itself to glide along the palmar surface of the shaft during flexion. The range of flexion is 60 degrees for the thumb, slightly less than 90 degrees for the index finger, progressively increasing towards the little finger. Flexion at one finger is limited by tension in the deep transverse metacarpal ligaments, being ultimately limited by the collateral ligaments. Extension in the thumb is zero but may reach 50 degrees in the fingers. Passive extension in the fingers can be as much as 90 degrees.

The main muscle producing flexion of the thumb at the MCP joint is flexor pollicis brevis aided by flexor pollicis longus, and of the fingers are the lumbricals (Table 5.8) aided by flexors digitorum superficialis and profundus. The main muscle producing extension of the thumb is extensor pollicis from the flexed position, while in the fingers it is extensor digitorum, aided by extensor indicis in the index finger and extensor digiti minimi in the little finger (Table 5.7).

Abduction and adduction. In the thumb abduction and adduction occur about a transverse axis and in the fingers about an anteroposterior axis through the metacarpal head. The fingers move away from or towards the long axis of the hand (middle finger) (Fig. 5.57). The range of abduction in the thumb is 15 degrees with negligible adduction, while in the fingers abduction and adduction, each has a range of 30 degrees. When the fingers are flexed to 90 degrees the collateral ligaments limit abduction and adduction to no more than 10 degrees.

Abduction and adduction in the thumb are produced by abductor pollicis brevis and adductor pollicis (Table 5.8), respectively. Abduction of the fingers is produced by the dorsal interossei (Table 5.8) for the index, middle and ring fingers and abductor digiti minimi (Table 5.8) for the little finger, aided by the 1st and 2nd lumbricals for the index and middle fingers.

TABLE 5.7   **Muscles of the Forearm Whose Action Is on the Digits: Attachments, Action and Innervation**

Muscle	Attachments	Action	Innervation (Root Value)
Flexor digitorum superficialis	From the medial epicondyle via the common flexor origin, ulnar collateral ligament and coronoid process of the ulna (*medal (humeroulnar) head*) and the upper two-thirds of the anterior surface of the radius (*lateral (radial) head*) to the palmar surface of the middle phalanx of the finger after splitting to allow the tendon of flexor digitorum profundus to pass through (Fig. 5.62)	Primarily flexes the metacarpophalangeal and proximal interphalangeal joints; assists flexion at the wrist joint	Median nerve (C7, C8, T1)
Flexor digitorum profundus	From the coronoid process, upper three-fourth of the anterior and medial surfaces of the ulna and adjacent anterior surface of the interosseous membrane to the base of the palmar surface of the distal phalanx after passing through the tendon of flexor digitorum superficialis (see Fig. 5.62)	Primarily flexes the distal interphalangeal joint; assists in flexing the proximal interphalangeal, metacarpophalangeal and wrist joints	Anterior interosseous branch of the median nerve (C7, C8, T1)
Lumbricals[a]			
Flexor digiti minimi brevis[a]			
Flexor pollicis longus	From the anterior surface of the radius and adjacent interosseous membrane to the palmar surface of the base of the distal phalanx of the thumb	Flexion of the interphalangeal joint of the thumb; assists in flexion of the metacarpophalangeal and wrist joints	Anterior interosseous branch of the median nerve (C8, T1)
Extensor digitorum	From the lateral epicondyle of the humerus via the common extensor tendon dividing into four tendons near the wrist, with each expanding over the posterior aspect of the metacarpophalangeal joint with the central tendon attaching to the dorsal surface of the base of the middle phalanx and the lateral tendons to the dorsal aspect of the base of the distal phalanx (see Fig. 5.62)	Extension of the metacarpophalangeal joint; assists extension of both interphalangeal joints of the fingers	Posterior interosseous branch of the radial nerve (C7, C8)
Extensor indicis	From the posterior surface of the ulna and adjacent interosseous membrane to the dorsal digital expansion of the index finger	Assists extensor digitorum in the index finger, enabling it to extend independently; also aids extension of the hand at the wrist	Posterior interosseous branch of the radial nerve (C7, C8)
Extensor digit minimi	From the lateral epicondyle of the humerus via the common extensor tendon to the dorsal digital expansion of the little finger	Assists extensor digitorum in the little finger, enabling it to extend independently; also aids extension of the hand at the wrist	Posterior interosseous branch of the radial nerve (C7, C8)
Dorsal interossei[a]			

Continued

TABLE 5.7   Muscles of the Forearm Whose Action Is on the Digits: Attachments, Action and Innervation—cont'd

Muscle	Attachments	Action	Innervation (Root Value)
Palmar interossei[a]			
Extensor pollicis longus	From the lateral part of the middle one-third of the posterior surface of the ulna and adjacent interosseous membrane to the dorsal surface of the base of the distal phalanx of the thumb	Extends all joints of the thumb; assists in extension and abduction of the hand at the wrist	Posterior interosseous branch of the radial nerve (C7, C8)
Extensor pollicis brevis	From the middle part of the posterior surface of the radius and adjacent interosseous membrane to the dorsal surface of the base of the proximal phalanx of the thumb	Extends the carpometacarpal and metacarpophalangeal joints of the thumb	Posterior interosseous branch of the radial nerve (C7, C8)
Abductor pollicis longus	From the upper part of the ulna and radius (distal to anconeus and supinator) and adjacent interosseous membrane to the base of the 1st metacarpal	Abducts and extends the carpometacarpal joint of the thumb	Posterior interosseous branch of the radial nerve (C7, C8)

[a]Details can be found with the other intrinsic muscles of the hand in Table 5.8.

Adduction is produced by the palmar interossei (Table 5.8), aided by the 3rd and 4th lumbricals for the ring and little fingers.

Axial rotation (opposition). Active axial rotation is possible in the thumb, being important during opposition (Fig. 5.60B). Active rotation is always directed medially, whereas passive rotation can be in either direction. Active rotation is initially produced by the combined action of flexor and abductor pollicis brevis, with opponens pollicis contributing once rotation has started (Table 5.8). Active rotation in the fingers is not possible; however, passive rotation is possible due to the laxity of the joint ligaments and shape of the joint surfaces. The range of rotation in each direction is 45 degrees.

Interphalangeal Joints

The IP joints (proximal, distal) of the fingers and thumb are similar, being between the head of the proximal phalanx and base of the distal phalanx. A loose fibrous capsule surrounds each joint strengthened laterally by collateral ligaments and partly replaced anteriorly and posteriorly by the palmar ligament and extensor tendon, respectively.

Movements

Flexion and extension about a transverse axis, which for the middle, ring and little fingers runs increasingly obliquely (Fig. 5.61). In the thumb flexion has a range in excess of 90 degrees, with approximately 10 degrees of extension, whereas at the PIP joints of the fingers flexion is 90 degrees increasing to 135 degrees in the little finger and at the DIP joint flexion is 90 degrees in the little finger gradually decreasing towards the index finger. Active extension in the fingers is no more than 5 degrees.

In the thumb, flexion and extension of the IP joint is produced by flexor and extensor pollicis longus (Table 5.7), respectively. In the fingers, flexion of the PIP joint is produced by flexor digitorum superficialis, aided by flexor digitorum profundus, with flexion of the DIP joint being produced by flexor digitorum profundus. Extension of the joints is produced by the lumbricals and interossei via the dorsal digital (extensor) expansion, aided by extensor digitorum in all fingers and extensors indicis and digiti minimi in the index and little fingers (Table 5.7), respectively.

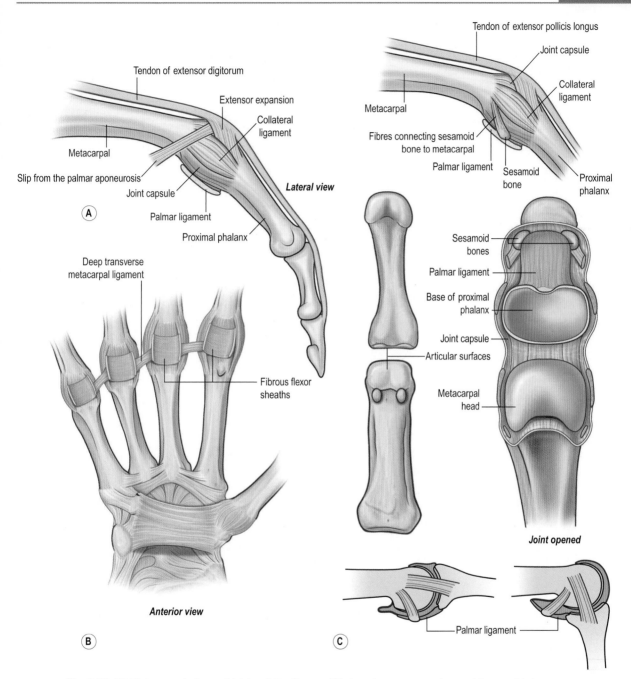

Fig. 5.59 (A) Metacarpophalangeal joints of the fingers; (B) deep transverse metacarpal ligament between the medial four metacarpal heads; (C) metacarpophalangeal joint of the thumb.

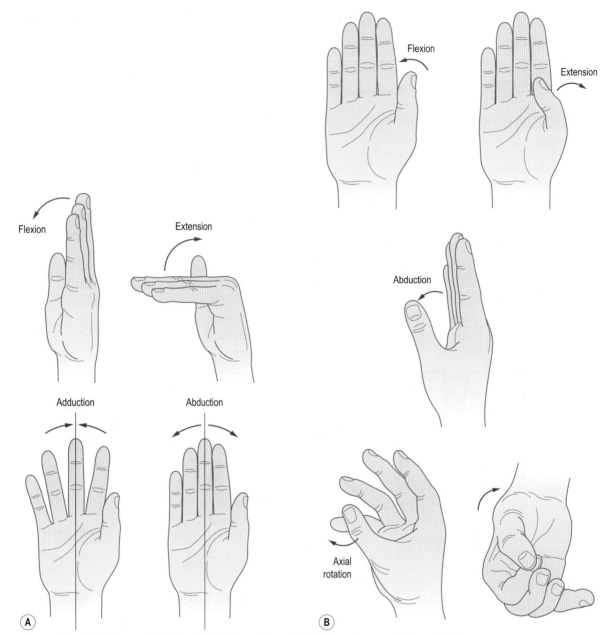

Fig. 5.60 Movements of the fingers (A) and thumb (B) at the metacarpophalangeal joints.

Function of the Hand

The skin over the pads of the digits is richly endowed with sensory receptors enabling sensing of the environment, including objects being manipulated; however, its major function is one of manipulation, as in gripping objects (prehension). There are two types of grip (precision, power) depending on the size, shape and weight of the object and the use to which it is put.

TABLE 5.8 Intrinsic Muscles of the Hand: Attachments, Action and Innervation

Muscle	Attachments	Action	Innervation (Root Value)
Flexor pollicis brevis[a]	From the distal border of the flexor retinaculum, trapezium, capitate and trapezoid to the base of the proximal phalanx of the thumb	Flexion of the thumb at the metacarpophalangeal and carpometacarpal joints: its continued action medially rotates the thumb	Median nerve (T1)
Abductor pollicis brevis[a]	From the flexor retinaculum, scaphoid and trapezium to the base of the proximal phalanx of the thumb	Abducts the thumb at the metacarpophalangeal and carpometacarpal joints	Median nerve (T1)
Opponens pollicis[a]	From the flexor retinaculum and trapezium to the lateral half of the anterior surface of the 1st metacarpal	Produces the complex mechanism of opposition of the thumb in which the thumb is pulled forwards and medially in an arc towards the fingers	Median nerve (T1)
Adductor pollicis	From the sheath of the tendon of flexor carpi radialis, bases of the 2nd, 3rd and 4th metacarpals, trapezoid and capitate (*transverse head*) and a longitudinal ridge on the anterior surface of the shaft of the 3rd metacarpal (*oblique head*) to the base of the proximal phalanx of the thumb	Adducts the thumb from a position of abduction	Deep branch of the ulnar nerve (T1)
Flexor digiti minimi brevis[b]	From the hook of the hamate and adjacent flexor retinaculum to the base of the proximal phalanx of the little finger	Flexion of the metacarpophalangeal joint of the little finger	Deep branch of the ulnar nerve (T1)
Abductor digiti minimi[b]	From the pisiform, pisohamate ligament and tendon of flexor carpi ulnaris to the dorsal digital expansion and ulnar side of the proximal phalanx of the little finger	Abducts the little finger away from the ring finger; aids extension of the interphalangeal joints	Deep branch of the ulnar nerve (T1)
Opponens digiti minimi[b]	From the hook of the hamate and adjacent flexor retinaculum to the medial half of the palmar surface of the 5th metacarpal	Pulls the little finger towards the palm at the same time rotating it laterally at the carpometacarpal joint	Deep branch of the ulnar nerve (T1)
Dorsal interossei	From the sides of adjacent metacarpals to the dorsal digital expansion and proximal phalanx: two attach to the middle finger and one each to the index and ring fingers (Fig. 5.62)	Abduct the index, middle and ring fingers away from the longitudinal axis of the hand; they also assist the lumbricals	Deep branch of the ulnar nerve (T1)
Palmar interossei	From the shaft of the metacarpal to the dorsal digital expansion and base of the proximal phalanx of the same digit (Fig. 5.62)	Adduction of the thumb, index, ring and little finger towards the middle finger: they also assist the lumbricals	Deep branch of the ulnar nerve (T1)
Lumbricals	From the lateral side of the tendon of flexor digitorum profundus to the lateral edge of the dorsal digital expansion (Fig. 5.62)	Flexion of the metacarpophalangeal and extension of the interphalangeal joints	Lateral two by the median nerve (T1), medial two by the ulnar nerve (T1)

[a]Muscles of the thenar eminence.
[b]Muscles of the hypothenar eminence.

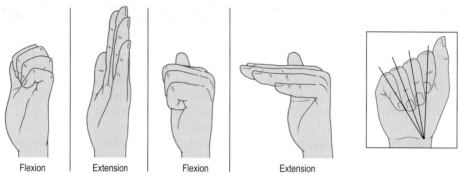

Flexion   Extension   Flexion   Extension

Fig. 5.61 Movements at the interphalangeal joints of the fingers.

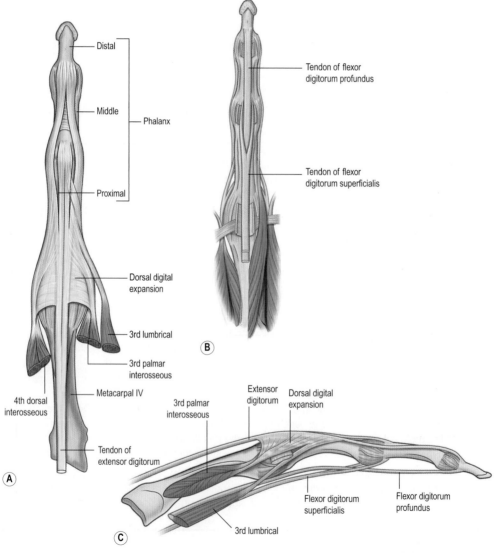

Fig. 5.62 Posterior (A), anterior (B) and lateral C) aspects of the left ring finger (4th digit) showing the relationship between flexors digitorum superficialis and profundus, the dorsal digital (extensor) expansion and its attachments.

Palmaris brevis, a small muscle arising from the medial border of the palmar aponeurosis and attaching into the skin on the medial border of the hand, assists the thumb in achieving a good grip.

Precision Grips

The object is usually small and may be fragile, being seized between the pads of the digits which spread around the object conforming to its shape. It involves rotation at the CM joint of the thumb and at the MCP joints of the thumb and finger(s) involved, using the intrinsic muscles of the hand and flexors digitorum superficialis, profundus and pollicis longus. Types of precision grip are pincer (terminal opposition), subterminal opposition (tripod), pinch and subtermino-lateral (key) (Fig. 5.63A–D).

> **CLINICAL ANATOMY:** Precision grips are disrupted by trauma involving the median and ulnar nerves.

Power Grips

These are used when considerable force is required and involve the hand as well as the fingers. The flexors and extensors of the wrist work strongly to stabilise the wrist, while the long finger flexors and intrinsic muscles of the hand grip the object. Types of power grip are oblique palmar, ball, span, cylinder and hook (Fig. 5.63E–I).

Blood Supply and Lymphatic Drainage
Arterial Supply

The radial artery enters the hand after passing across the floor of the anatomical snuffbox, through the two heads of the 1st dorsal interosseous and of adductor pollicis. The ulnar artery passes superficial to the flexor retinaculum. Both arteries give deep and superficial branches which contribute to the superficial and deep palmar arches in the hand. The radial artery also gives the princeps pollicis and radialis indicis branches (Fig. 5.64).

> **APPLIED ANATOMY:** Because the thumb is supplied by the large princeps pollicis artery, when assessing the pulse of an individual it should be done using the index and/or middle finger, otherwise the pulsations felt may be your own and not that of the individual.

> **APPLIED ANATOMY:** The *superficial palmar arch* lies deep to the palmar aponeurosis, with its distal convexity level with the flexor surface of the extended thumb. It gives four common palmar digital arteries, which each divide into proper digital arteries supplying the sides of the little, ring, middle and index fingers. The *deep palmar arch* lies deep to the long flexor tendons and their synovial sheaths on the metacarpal bases, with its distal convexity 2 cm distal to the distal wrist crease. It gives rise to the palmar metacarpal arteries.

Venous Drainage

The venous drainage of the hand, and upper limb as a whole, is by superficial vessels which lie in the superficial fascia and deep vessels which accompany the arteries. Both sets of vessels have valves promoting proximal drainage (Fig. 5.65). On the dorsal aspect of the hand is the variable dorsal venous network/arch. From its medial side the basilic vein arises and from its lateral side the cephalic vein.

Lymphatic Drainage

The lymphatic drainage of the hand, and upper limb as a whole, is by a superficial intermeshing network of vessels just below the skin and by deep lymphatic channels below the deep fascia (Fig. 5.26).

SUMMARY OF NERVES AND MUSCLES
Major Nerves of the Upper Limb and the Muscles They Innervate
Axillary Nerve

From the posterior cord (C5, C6) of the brachial plexus: it supplies deltoid (C5, C6) and teres minor (C5, C6) and gives the upper lateral cutaneous nerve of the arm (Figs. 5.25 and 5.66).

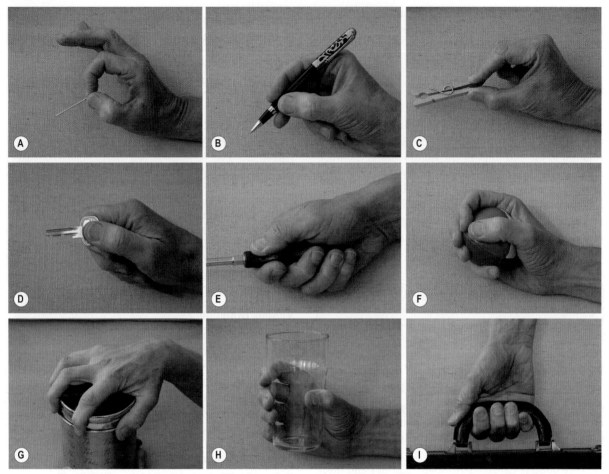

Fig. 5.63 Types of grip: (A) pincer; (B) subterminal opposition; (C) pinch; (D) subtermino-lateral; (E) oblique palmar; (F) ball; (G) span; (H) cylinder; (I) hook.

Radial Nerve

From the posterior cord (C5–C8, (T1)) of the brachial plexus: it supplies triceps (C6–C8), anconeus (C7, C8), lateral third of brachialis (C5, C6), brachioradialis (C5, C6), extensor carpi radialis longus (C6, C7) and from its posterior interosseous (deep) branch supinator (C5, C6), extensor carpi radialis brevis (C6, C7), extensor digitorum (C7, C8), extensor digiti minimi (C7, C8), extensor carpi ulnaris (C7, C8), extensor pollicis longus (C7, C8), extensor pollicis brevis (C7, C8), extensor indicis (C7, C8), abductor pollicis longus (C7, C8), and gives the posterior cutaneous nerve of the arm, the lower lateral cutaneous nerve of the arm, the posterior cutaneous nerve of the forearm and superficial radial branch (Figs 5.25 and 5.67).

Musculocutaneous Nerve

From the lateral cord (C5–C7) of the brachial plexus: it supplies coracobrachialis (C6, C7), biceps brachii (C5, C6) and medial two-thirds of brachialis (C5, C6) and gives the lateral cutaneous nerve of the forearm (Figs 5.25 and 5.68).

Ulnar Nerve

From the medial cord (C7, C8, T1) of the brachial plexus: it supplies flexor carpi ulnaris (C7, C8), medial half of flexor digitorum profundus (C7, C8, T1), palmaris brevis (T1) and from its deep branch abductor digit minimi (T1), flexor digiti minimi (T1), opponens digit minimi (T1), medial two lumbricals (T1), palmar interossei (T1), dorsal interossei (T1), adductor pollicis (C8, T1),

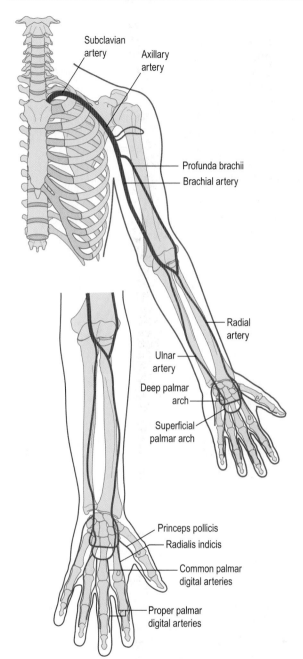

Fig. 5.64 Anterior aspect of the thorax, left upper limb and palmar aspect of the hand showing the position and course of the major arteries of the upper limb.

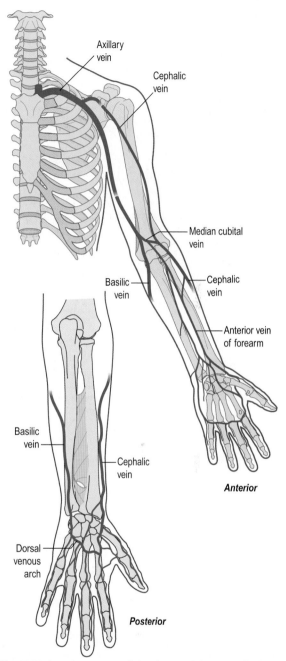

Fig. 5.65 Anterior aspect of the thorax, right upper limb and dorsum of the hand showing the position and course of the major veins of the upper limb.

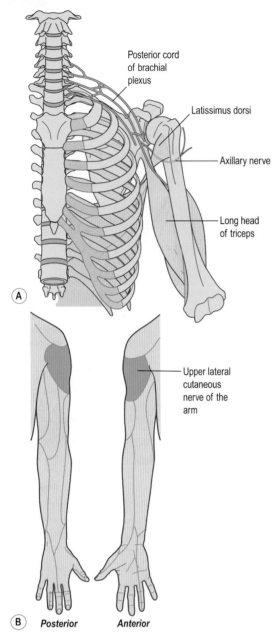

Fig. 5.66 (A) Anterior aspect of the thorax and right arm showing the course of the axillary nerve; (B) cutaneous distribution of the axillary nerve.

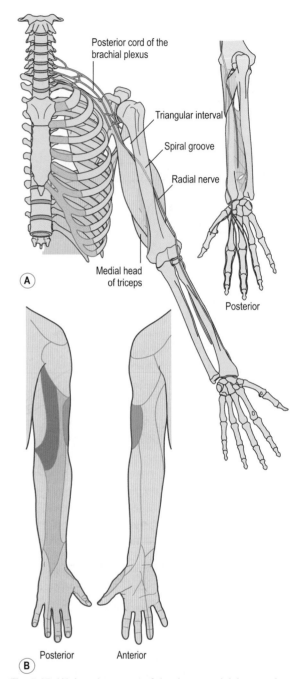

Fig. 5.67 (A) Anterior aspect of the thorax and right arm showing the course of the radial nerve; (B) cutaneous distribution of the radial nerve.

palmaris brevis (T1) and gives palmar, dorsal, superficial and digital cutaneous branches (Figs 5.25 and 5.69).

Median Nerve

From the lateral (C5–C7) and medial (C8, T1) cords of the brachial plexus: it supplies pronator teres (C6, C7),

flexor carpi radialis (C6, C7), palmaris longus (C8), flexor digitorum superficialis (C7, C8, T1), abductor pollicis longus (C7, C8), flexor pollicis brevis (T1), opponens pollicis (T1) and from its anterior interosseous branch

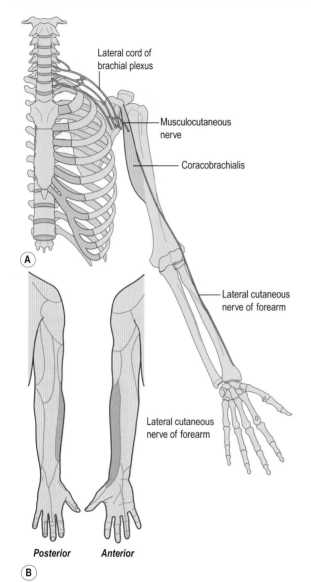

Lateral cord of
brachial plexus

Musculocutaneous
nerve

Coracobrachialis

Lateral cutaneous
nerve of forearm

Lateral cutaneous
nerve of forearm

Posterior   Anterior

Fig. 5.68 (A) Anterior aspect of the thorax and upper limb showing the course of the musculocutaneous nerve; (B) cutaneous distribution of the musculocutaneous nerve.

flexor pollicis longus (C8, T1), lateral half of flexor digitorum profundus (C7, C8, T1), pronator quadratus, lateral two lumbricals (T1) and gives palmar, lateral, medial and digital cutaneous branches (Figs 5.25 and 5.70).

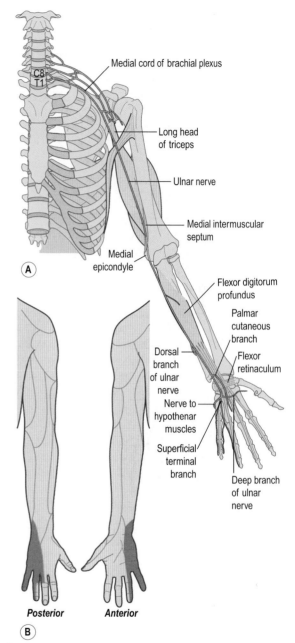

C8
T1

Medial cord of brachial plexus

Long head
of triceps

Ulnar nerve

Medial intermuscular
septum

Medial
epicondyle

Flexor digitorum
profundus

Palmar
cutaneous
branch

Flexor
retinaculum

Dorsal
branch
of ulnar
nerve

Nerve to
hypothenar
muscles

Superficial
terminal
branch

Deep branch
of ulnar
nerve

Posterior   Anterior

Fig. 5.69 (A) Anterior aspect of the thorax and right arm showing the course of the ulnar nerve; (B) cutaneous distribution of the ulnar nerve.

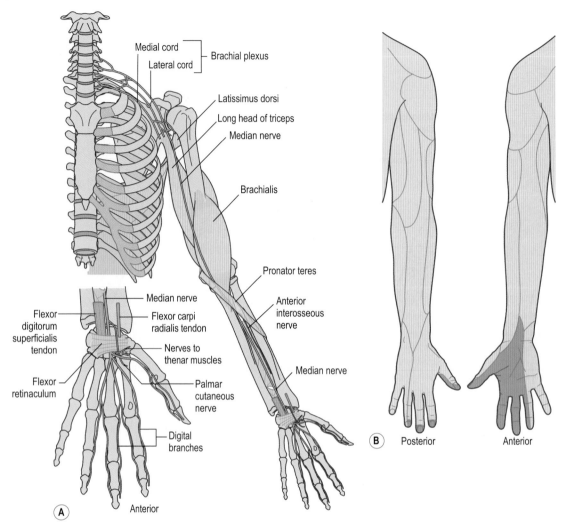

Fig. 5.70 (A) Anterior aspect of the thorax and right arm showing the course of the median nerve; (B) cutaneous distribution of the median nerve.

Muscles Supplied by Each Root of the Brachial Plexus

Root value				
C5	C6	C7	C8	T1
Levator scapulae[a]				
Rhomboid major				
Rhomboid minor				
Supraspinatus				
Deltoid				
Biceps brachii				
Teres minor				
Infraspinatus				
Brachialis				
Brachioradialis				
Supinator				
	Serratus anterior			
	Pectoralis minor			
	Subscapularis			
	Coracobrachialis			
	Extensor carpi	radialis longus		
	Extensor carpi	radialis brevis		
	Teres major			
	Pronator teres			
	Anconeus			
	Flexor carpi radialis			
		Triceps brachii		
		Latissimus dorsi		
		Pectoralis major		
		Flexor carpi ulnaris		
		Extensor carpi	ulnaris	
		Extensor digitorum		
		Extensor indicis		
		Extensor digiti	minimi	
		Extensor pollicis	longus	
		Extensor pollicis	brevis	
		Abductor pollicis	longus	
		Flexor digitorum	superficialis	
		Flexor digitorum	profundus	
			Palmaris longus	
			Adductor pollicis	
			Pronator	quadratus
				Flexor pollicis longus

Root value				
C5	**C6**	**C7**	**C8**	**T1**
				Flexor pollicis brevis
				Abductor pollicis brevis
				Opponens pollicis
				Abductor digiti minimi
				Opponens digiti minimi
				Dorsal interossei Palmar interossei
				Palmaris brevis

[a]Also innervated by C3 and C4 roots; trapezius is innervated by the accessory nerve (CN XI).

Movements in Each Region of the Upper Limb, the Muscles Responsible and Their Innervation

Pectoral Girdle

Movement	Muscles (root value of innervation)
Retraction	Rhomboid major (C5) Rhomboid minor (C5) Trapezius (CN XI)
Protraction	Serratus anterior (C5–C7) Pectoralis minor (C5–C7)
Elevation	Trapezius (upper fibres) (CN XI) Levator scapulae (C3–C5)
Depression	Pectoralis minor (C5–C7) Trapezius (lower fibres) (CN XI)
Lateral rotation	Trapezius (CN XI) Serratus anterior (C5–C7)
Medial rotation	Rhomboid major (C5) Rhomboid minor (C5) Levator scapulae (C3–C5) Pectoralis minor (C5–C7)

Shoulder Joint

Movement	Muscles (root value of innervation)
Abduction	Supraspinatus (C5, C6) Deltoid (C5, C6)
Adduction	Coracobrachialis (C6, C7) Pectoralis major (C5–C8, T1) Latissimus dorsi (C6–C8) Teres major (C6, C7)
Flexion	Pectoralis major (C5–C8, T1) Deltoid (anterior fibres) (C5, C6) Coracobrachialis (C6, C7) Biceps brachii (long head) (C5, C6)
Extension	Latissimus dorsi (C6–C8) Teres major (C6, C7) Pectoralis major (to midline) (C5–C8, T1) Deltoid (posterior fibres) (C5, C6) Triceps brachii (long head) (C6–C8)
Medial rotation	Subscapularis (C5–C7) Teres major (C6, C7) Latissimus dorsi (C6–C8) Pectoralis major (C5–C8, T1) Deltoid (anterior fibres) (C5, C6)
Lateral rotation	Teres minor (C5, C6) Infraspinatus (C5, C6) Deltoid (posterior fibres) (C5, C6)

Elbow Joint

Movement	Muscles (root value of innervation)
Flexion	Biceps brachii (C5, C6) Brachialis (C5, C6) Brachioradialis (C5, C6) Pronator teres (C6, C7) Superficial forearm flexors:

Flexor digitorum superficialis
(C7, C8, T1)
Flexor carpi radialis (C6, C7)
Flexor carpi ulnaris (C7, C8)
Palmaris longus (C8)

Extension	Triceps brachii (C6–C8) Anconeus (C7, C8) *Superficial forearm extensors:* *Extensor carpi radialis longus* *(C6, C7)* *Extensor carpi radialis brevis* *(C6, C7)* *Extensor carpi ulnaris (C7, C8)* *Extensor digitorum (C7, C8)* *Extensor digiti minimi (C7, C8)*

Radioulnar Joints

Movement	Muscles (root value of innervation)
Supination	Supinator (C5, C6) Biceps brachii (C5, C6) Brachioradialis (C5, C6)
Pronation	Pronator teres (C6, C7) Pronator quadratus (C8, T1) Brachioradialis (C6, C7)

Wrist Joint

Movement	Muscles (root value of innervation)
Flexion	Flexor carpi radialis (C6, C7) Flexor carpi ulnaris (C7, C8) Palmaris longus (C8) *Digital flexors:* *Flexor digitorum superficialis* *(C7, C8, T1)* *Flexor digitorum profundus* *(C7, C8, T1)* *Flexor pollicis longus (C8, T1)*
Extension	Extensor carpi radialis longus (C6, C7) Extensor carpi radialis brevis (C6, C7) *Digital extensors:* *Extensor digitorum (C7, C8)* *Extensor indicis (C7, C8)* *Extensor digiti minimi (C7, C8)* *Extensor pollicis longus (C7, C8)* *Extensor pollicis brevis (C7, C8)*
Abduction (radial deviation)	Flexor carpi radialis (C6, C7) Extensor carpi radialis longus (C6, C7)
	Extensor carpi radialis brevis (C6, C7)
Adduction (ulnar deviation)	Flexor carpi ulnaris (C7, C8) Extensor carpi ulnaris (C7, C8)

Joints of the Fingers

Each finger comprises three joints: MCP, PIP, DIP joints.

Movement	Muscles (root value of nerve supply)
Flexion	Flexor digitorum profundus at DIP, PIP and MCP (C7, C8, T1) Flexor digitorum superficialis at PIP and MCP (C7, C8, T1)
Extension	Extensor digitorum at DIP, PIP and MCP (C7, C8) Extensor indicis at DIP, PIP and MCP of index finger (C7, C8) Extensor digiti minimi at DIP, PIP and MCP of little finger (C7, C8)
Abduction	Dorsal interossei at MCP (T1) Abductor digiti minimi at MCP of little finger (T1)
Adduction	Palmar interossei at MCP (T1)
Opposition	Opponens digiti minimi at CMJ of little finger (T1)

Joints of the Thumb

The thumb comprises three joints: CMJ, MCP, IP joints.

Movement	Muscles (root value of nerve supply)
Flexion	Flexor pollicis longus at IP and MCP (T1) Flexor pollicis brevis at MCP (T1)
Extension	Extensor pollicis longus at IP and MCP (C7, C8) Extensor pollicis brevis at MCP (C7, C8)
Abduction	Abductor pollicis longus at CMJ (C7, C8) Abductor pollicis brevis at CMJ (T1)
Adduction	Adductor pollicis at CMJ (T1)
Opposition	Opponens pollicis at CMJ (T1)

Within the hand, many muscles of the digits cross several joints and are therefore involved in complex combined movements. Interaction of the extrinsic and intrinsic muscles of the fingers and thumb allows a wide range of complex grips and functions of the hand.

SELF-TEST QUESTIONS

1. Concerning muscles of the arm, which of the following statements is NOT correct?
   a. Triceps brachii crosses two joints.
   b. Brachialis is innervated by the musculocutaneous nerve.
   c. Brachioradialis extends the forearm at the elbow joint.
   d. Anconeus extends the elbow joint.
   e. Coracobrachialis adducts the arm at the shoulder joint.

2. Which of the following muscles is innervated directly by the radial nerve?
   a. Brachialis
   b. Brachioradialis
   c. Supinator
   d. Extensor carpi radialis brevis
   e. Coracobrachialis

3. Concerning deltoid, which of the following movements does it NOT contribute to?
   a. Flexion
   b. Medial rotation
   c. Extension
   d. Adduction
   e. Lateral rotation

4. Concerning the pectoral region, which of the following statements is NOT correct?
   a. It is the region where the upper limb meets the trunk.
   b. The shoulder joint is part of the pectoral girdle.
   c. The clavicle ossifies in membrane.
   d. The scapula does not articulate directly with the axial skeleton.
   e. Clavicular fractures occur at the junction of the medial two-thirds and lateral third.

5. Concerning movements of the scapula, which of the following statements is NOT correct?
   a. The sternoclavicular joint contains a complete intra-articular disc.
   b. Elevation is produced by trapezius.
   c. Elevation is usually accompanied by slight rotation.
   d. During abduction of the upper limb the clavicle undergoes rotation.
   e. In retraction, the scapula moves forwards around the chest wall.

6. Concerning the arm, which of the following statements is correct?
   a. It is the region between the pectoral girdle and elbow joint.
   b. The medial and lateral intermuscular septa give attachment to biceps brachii.
   c. The distal end of the humerus articulates with the head of the ulna.
   d. The medial and lateral epicondyles of the humerus can be palpated.
   e. The anatomical neck of the humerus is frequently fractured in falls on the outstretched arm.

7. Concerning the shoulder joint, which of the following statements is NOT correct?
   a. It is between the head of the humerus and glenoid fossa of the scapula.
   b. In subluxation the rotator cuff muscles fail to maintain normal joint alignment.
   c. It commonly dislocates posteriorly.
   d. The fibrous capsule surrounding the joint is loose.
   e. The tendon of the long head of biceps brachii passes through the joint.

8. Concerning movements at the shoulder joint, which of the following statements is correct?
   a. Combined flexion and extension has a range of 180 degrees.
   b. Movement of the pectoral girdle does not increase the range of movement of the upper limb.
   c. With respect to the plane of the scapula in flexion the arm moves in a parasagittal plane.
   d. Painful arc syndrome occurs between 60 and 120 degrees of extension.
   e. Pectoralis minor is a powerful adductor and medial rotator.

9. What is the root value of the musculocutaneous nerve?
   a. C5
   b. C5, C6

c. C5, C6, C7

d. C6, C7

e. C6, C7, C8

10. Which of the following muscles does NOT have a direct attachment to the scapula?

a. Teres minor

b. Trapezius

c. Pectoralis minor

d. Latissimus dorsi

e. Serratus anterior

11. Concerning the axilla, which of the following statements is NOT correct?

a. The anterior wall is formed by pectoralis major.

b. The axillary vein is a continuation of the cephalic vein.

c. The axillary artery passes posterior to pectoralis minor.

d. The trunks of the brachial plexus are enclosed within the axillary sheath.

e. It contains numerous lymph nodes.

12. Concerning the brachial plexus, which of the following muscles is NOT innervated by the median nerve?

a. Pronator teres

b. Pronator quadratus

c. Flexor carpi radialis

d. Flexor pollicis longus

e. Flexor carpi ulnaris

13. Which nerve innervates latissimus dorsi?

a. Dorsal scapular

b. Suprascapular

c. Thoracodorsal

d. Upper subscapular

e. Lower subscapular

14. Which of the following groups of lymph nodes receive drainage directly from the anterior chest wall and breast?

a. Central

b. Pectoral

c. Apical

d. Subscapular

e. Lateral

15. Concerning the anterior compartment of the arm, which of the following statements is NOT correct?

a. The brachial artery gives the profunda brachii.

b. The basilic vein pierces the deep fascia.

c. The brachial pulse can be felt by pressing the brachial artery against the humerus.

d. The musculocutaneous nerve becomes the lateral cutaneous nerve of the forearm at the elbow.

e. The median nerve lies on biceps brachii.

16. Concerning the forearm, which of the following statements is NOT correct?

a. The distal end of the radius moves medially over the ulna during pronation.

b. The ulnar articulates with the lunate.

c. A Colles' fracture involves the lower end of the radius.

d. The anterior compartment muscles are mainly innervated by the median nerve.

e. The olecranon forms the 'point' of the elbow in flexion.

17. Concerning the elbow joint, which of the following statements is correct?

a. It is a synovial pivot joint.

b. Brachialis is an extensor.

c. Contact between the articular surfaces remains constant during flexion and extension.

d. Supracondylar fractures are common in children.

e. The ulnar head is surrounded by the annular ligament.

18. Concerning the cubital fossa, which of the following statements is NOT correct?

a. The lateral border is the medial border of brachioradialis.

b. Brachialis forms the floor.

c. It contains, from medial to lateral, the tendon of biceps brachii, brachial artery and median nerve.

d. The deep fascia separates the superficial veins from deeper structures.

e. The brachial artery is used for determining blood pressure.

19. Concerning the forearm, which of the following statements is NOT correct?

a. An interosseous membrane divides it into anterior and posterior compartments.

b. The basilic vein is a continuation of the lateral end of the dorsal venous network.

c. The radial pulse can be felt lateral to the tendon of flexor carpi radialis.

d. The ulnar artery gives the common interosseous artery.

e. The median nerves pass between the two heads of pronator teres.

20. What is the root value of the innervation of biceps brachii?
    a. C5
    b. C5, C6
    c. C5, C6, C7
    d. C6, C7
    e. C6, C7, C8
21. Concerning the wrist, which of the following statements is NOT correct?
    a. In carpal tunnel syndrome there is sensory loss over the lateral 3½ digits.
    b. The ulnar nerve and artery pass superficial to the flexor retinaculum.
    c. There are six extensor compartments.
    d. The flexor retinaculum attaches to the hamate and scaphoid.
    e. The midcarpal joint is between the radius, scaphoid and lunate.
22. Concerning movements at the wrist, which of the following statements is NOT correct?
    a. Flexion and extension occur about a transverse axis through the lunate.
    b. Movements of the hand are accompanied by movements at the wrist.
    c. Tinel's test can be used to diagnose carpal tunnel syndrome.
    d. The range of adduction is greater than that of abduction.
    e. Palmaris longus flexes the wrist.
23. Which of the following does NOT form part of the floor of the anatomical snuffbox?
    a. Scaphoid
    b. Base of the 1st metacarpal
    c. Trapezoid
    d. Radial styloid process
    e. Trapezium
24. Concerning the hand, which of the following statements is NOT correct?
    a. Dupuytren's contracture affects the ring and little fingers.
    b. The intermediate compartment of the palm is divided into medial and lateral spaces.
    c. Infections of the midpalmar space can track back to the deep aspect of the forearm.
    d. Trigger finger is a localised swelling of a flexor digitorum superficialis tendon.
    e. The lateral compartment of the palm contains the thenar muscles.

25. Concerning the digits, which of the following statements is correct?
    a. Each has three phalanges.
    b. The medial side of the 4th digit is innervated by the median nerve.
    c. Rotation at the metacarpophalangeal joints of the fingers is passive.
    d. Abduction of the fingers is produced by the palmar interossei.
    e. In the thumb abduction and adduction occur in the plane of the palm.
26. Concerning the palm, which of the following statements is NOT correct?
    a. There is little movement at the common carpometacarpal joint.
    b. The tendons of flexor digitorum profundus lie superficial to those of flexor digitorum superficialis.
    c. Palmar subluxation of the proximal phalanx on the metacarpal head is due to thinning of the articular cartilage.
    d. Flexion of the metacarpophalangeal joints of the fingers is produced by the lumbricals.
    e. The deep palmar arch lies deep to the long flexor tendons.
27. Which of the following muscles is NOT innervated directly by the median nerve?
    a. Flexor digitorum profundus
    b. Pronator teres
    c. Abductor pollicis longus
    d. Opponens pollicis
    e. Flexor carpi radialis
28. Which of the following is NOT a precision grip?
    a. Terminal opposition
    b. Pinch
    c. Subterminal opposition
    d. Span
    e. Subtermino-lateral opposition
29. Concerning the blood supply to the hand, which of the following statements is NOT correct?
    a. The superficial palmar arch lies deep to the palmar aponeurosis.
    b. The dorsal venous network gives rise to the cephalic and basilic veins.
    c. The radial artery enters the hand between the two heads of adductor pollicis.
    d. The ulnar artery contributes to both the superficial and deep palmar arches.

e. The individual's pulse should always be taken with the thumb.

30. Which of the following muscles is NOT innervated by the C5 and C6 nerve root?
    a. Brachioradialis
    b. Supinator
    c. Rhomboid major
    d. Deltoid
    e. Supraspinatus

31. Which nerve root supplies the skin of the hand?
    a. C5
    b. C6
    c. C7
    d. C8
    e. T1

32. Which of the following muscles produces protraction of the pectoral girdle?
    a. Rhomboid major
    b. Serratus anterior
    c. Trapezius
    d. Pectoralis major
    e. Levator scapulae

33. Which of the following muscles does NOT produce adduction of the arm at the shoulder joint?
    a. Supraspinatus
    b. Coracobrachialis
    c. Pectoralis major
    d. Latissimus dorsi
    e. Teres major

34. Which of the following combinations of muscles produce abduction of the hand at the wrist?
    a. Extensor carpi ulnaris and extensor carpi radialis
    b. Extensor carpi ulnaris and flexor carpi ulnaris
    c. Flexor carpi radialis and extensor carpi radialis brevis
    d. Flexor carpi ulnaris and extensor carpi radialis longus
    e. Flexor carpi radialis and flexor pollicis longus

35. Concerning the forearm, which of the following statements is NOT correct?
    a. The ulnar nerve enters through the two heads of flexor carpi ulnaris.
    b. The posterior interosseous nerve enters through the two heads of supinator.
    c. Biceps brachii is a powerful pronator.
    d. Flexor pollicis longus is a deep muscle in the anterior compartment.
    e. Brachioradialis attaches to the radial styloid process.

Abdomen, Pelvis and Perineum

CONTENTS

Key Concepts, 449
Learning Outcomes, 450
Overview, 450
Abdomen and Pelvis, 450
  Anterior and Lateral Abdominal Walls, 453
    Inguinal Canal, 456
    Innervation of the Abdominal Wall, 458
  Pelvic Floor, 458
  Abdominal Regions, 459
Digestive System, 461
    Structure of the Digestive Tract, 463
  Digestive Tract, 464
    Stomach, 465
    Small Intestine, 468
    Large Intestine/Colon, 472
    Rectum and Anal Canal, 476
    Liver and Biliary System, 477
    Pancreas, 482
  Application, 484
    Spleen, 484
  Digestive Physiology, 485
    Regulation of Food Intake and Energy Storage, 485
    Mixing and Propulsion of Food Through the
      Digestive Tract, 488
    Nutrition, 497
Urinary System, 508
  Kidney, 509
    Renal Physiology, 513
    Urine Formation, 515
    Diuretics, 521
    Kidney Diseases, 522
  Ureter, 523
  Bladder, 523

    Bladder Filling, 527
  Urethra, 527
    Nerve Supply to the Bladder and Urethral
      Sphincters, 528
  Micturition, 528
    Facilitation or Inhibition by the Brain, 529
    Voluntary Urination, 529
    Abnormalities of Micturition, 529
Reproductive System, 530
  Sex Determination, 531
  Male Reproductive System, 532
    Testis, 532
    Excretory Genital Ducts, 534
    Accessory Glands, 535
    Semen, 537
    Penis, 538
  Female Reproductive System, 541
    Ovary, 541
    Uterine (Fallopian) Tubes, 542
  Uterus, 543
    Vagina, 549
Perineum, 550
  Urogenital Triangle, 550
    Female External Genitalia, 552
    Male External Genitalia, 555
    Superficial Fascia, 555
  Anal Triangle, 555
    External Anal Sphincter, 555
  Neurovascular Supply of the Perineum, 556
    Nerves, 556
    Arteries, 556
    Veins, 557
    Lymphatics, 557

KEY CONCEPTS

- The abdominal cavity comprises the abdomen and pelvis: the perineum is separated from the pelvis by the pelvic floor.
- The anterolateral abdominal walls are muscular.
- There is an oblique passage through the lower antero-lateral abdominal wall.
- The digestive, urinary and reproductive systems lie within the abdominal cavity.
- The digestive system comprises oesophagus, stomach, small intestine (duodenum, jejunum, ileum), colon (ascending, transverse, descending, sigmoid), rectum and anal canal.
- Ingested food consists of carbohydrates, fats and proteins.
- Vitamins and minerals are an essential part of a healthy diet.
- There are 10 essential amino acids (i.e., they cannot be produced in the body).
- An imbalance of energy intake and expenditure results in either obesity or weight loss.
- The urinary system comprises kidneys, ureter, bladder and urethra.
- The digestive and urinary systems work together to maintain essential body functions.
- The male reproductive system comprises testes, various ducts, prostate and penis.
- The female reproductive system comprises ovaries, uterine tubes, uterus and vagina.
- The uterus is responsible for protecting and nurturing the developing infant.

LEARNING OUTCOMES

At the end of this chapter, you should be able to:
- Describe and locate muscles of the anterolateral abdominal wall and understand their function.
- Understand the formation of the inguinal canal and spermatic cord.
- Describe and locate the nine regions and four quadrants of the abdomen and the contents of each.
- Describe the components of the digestive system and the function of each.
- Understand the role of different parts of the digestive system in absorbing nutrients and in the production and elimination of waste.
- Understand the role of enzymes in the breakdown of ingested food in different parts of the digestive tract.
- Appreciate the influence of pathology and/or trauma on the digestive system.
- Describe the components of the urinary system and the function of each.
- Understand the role of different parts of the urinary system in the production of urine.
- Appreciate the influence of pathology and/or trauma on the urinary system.
- Describe the components of the male and female reproductive systems and the function of each.
- Appreciate the influence of pathology and/or trauma on the male and female reproductive systems.

OVERVIEW

This chapter is divided into two major sections (abdomen and pelvis, perineum), with an outline of the anatomy of each region being considered, including the organs found in each region, before considering the physiology of the digestive/gastrointestinal, renal/urinary and reproductive systems. The abdomen and pelvis form the larger part of the trunk, lying below the thorax, being bounded posteriorly in the midline by the vertebral column and sacrum, posteriorly, laterally and anteriorly by the abdominal muscles (page 453), superiorly by the diaphragm (page 73) and inferiorly by the pelvic floor (page 458); the perineum lies below the pelvic floor. Because the diaphragm is concave superiorly, some organs (stomach, liver, kidneys) lie at thoracic levels. The abdominopelvic cavity comprises the abdominal and pelvic cavities (Fig. 6.1).

ABDOMEN AND PELVIS

The structural support of the abdomen is located posteriorly, being the lumbar part of the vertebral column (page 188), with the anterior and lateral aspects consisting of muscles attached to the thorax, pelvis and vertebral column.

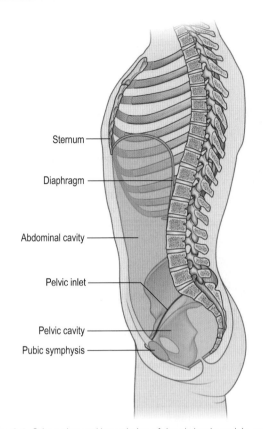

Sternum

Diaphragm

Abdominal cavity

Pelvic inlet

Pelvic cavity

Pubic symphysis

Fig. 6.1 Orientation and boundaries of the abdominopelvic cavity.

Over the back of the abdomen (trunk) the superficial fascia is thick and contains a large amount of fat held within a meshwork of fibres; at the front and sides there is a variable amount of fat. In the superficial fascia of the anterior abdominal wall fat is commonly deposited in middle age, in the upper part of the abdomen in males and lower part in females. As the superficial fascia passes downwards towards the thigh it divides into two layers (Fig. 6.2A and B), between which lie the superficial vessels and nerves; it is continuous with the superficial fascia of the thigh (page 565). The fatty superficial layer (Camper's fascia) is of variable thickness and is continuous over the inguinal ligament with the superficial fascia of the thigh and with a similar layer in the perineum. In males the superficial layer continues over the penis and, after losing its fat and fusing with the deeper layer, continues into the scrotum where it forms a specialised fascial layer containing smooth muscle fibres (dartos fascia). In females the superficial layer retains some fat and is a component of the labia majora.

The deeper layer (Scarpa's fascia) is a thin elastic membrane attached, in the lower part of the abdominal wall,

loosely to the external oblique aponeurosis and more firmly to the linea alba and symphysis pubis (page 569). In the lower abdomen this membranous layer replaces the deep fascia proper. It passes superficial to the inguinal ligament to attach to the fascia lata of the thigh 2 cm below and parallel to the inguinal ligament. In males, the extensions of the deep membranous layer firmly attach to the pubic symphysis and pass inferiorly onto the dorsum and sides of the penis (fundiform ligament of the penis) (Fig. 6.2C). In females, the membranous layer continues into the labia majora and anterior part of the perineum.

Over the anterior and lateral parts of the trunk, the deep fascia has no special features, being relatively thin and elastic to enable the abdomen to expand. It may be replaced by the external oblique aponeurosis and membranous layer of superficial fascia in the lower part of the abdomen. The back is covered by a layer of deep fascia of variable thickness attaching to the thoracic and lumbar vertebral spines, iliac crest and back of the sacrum. It is continuous with the deep fascia laterally. Deep to the superficial muscles of the back (page 203) in the lower thoracic, lumbar and sacral regions is an extremely strong layer of deep fascia (thoracolumbar fascia).

The thoracolumbar fascia comprises three separate layers (see Fig. 3.21): the posterior layer is superficial to erector spinae extending from the sacrum and iliac crest to the angles of the ribs (page 70); the middle layer is sandwiched between erector spinae and quadratus lumborum and extends from the 12th rib to the iliac crest; the thin anterior layer lies in front of quadratus lumborum, fusing with the middle layer at its lateral border, extending between the iliac crest and 12th rib and transverse process of L1, where it is thickened forming the lateral arcuate ligament (page 74). The single layer of fascia formed laterally gives attachment to transversus abdominis and internal oblique of the anterior and lateral abdominal wall. In the lumbar region it acts as a protective membrane filling the gap between the 12th rib and iliac crest.

Lining the abdominopelvic cavity is a serous membrane (peritoneum); some structures are surrounded by peritoneum (intraperitoneal) (Fig. 6.3A), while others are only partly covered (retroperitoneal) (Fig. 6.3B).

> **APPLIED ANATOMY:** Although structures may be intra or retroperitoneal none are contained within the intraperitoneal space. All lie outside it within the abdominal and pelvic cavities.

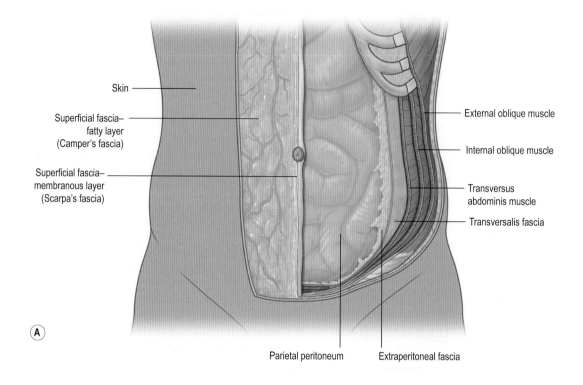

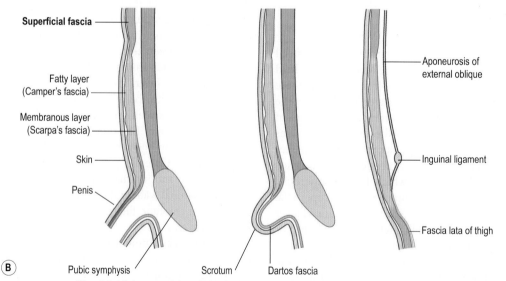

Fig. 6.2 (A) Layers of the abdominal wall; (B) arrangement of the superficial fascia.

As well as supporting many abdominal organs, the folds/reflections of peritoneum provide routes for the passage of blood vessels, lymphatics and nerves to and from the organs. The peritoneal cavity is sub-divided into the greater and lesser (omental bursa) sacs (Fig. 6.4, see also Fig. 6.13). The greater sac extends from the diaphragm superiorly to the pelvic cavity inferiorly, while the lesser sac lies behind the stomach and liver and is continuous with the greater sac at the epiploic/omental foramen.

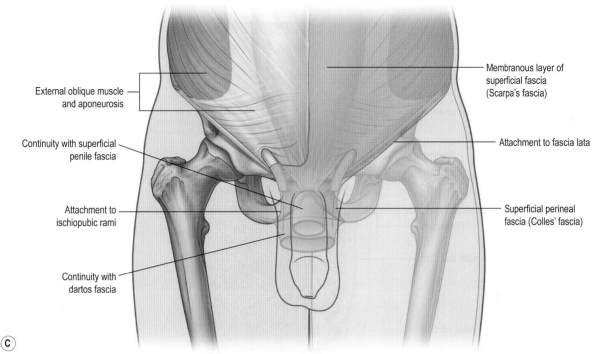

External oblique muscle and aponeurosis

Continuity with superficial penile fascia

Attachment to ischiopubic rami

Continuity with dartos fascia

Membranous layer of superficial fascia (Scarpa's fascia)

Attachment to fascia lata

Superficial perineal fascia (Colles' fascia)

Fig. 6.2, cont'd (C) continuity of the membranous layer of superficial fascia into other areas.

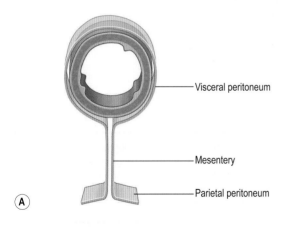

Visceral peritoneum

Mesentery

Parietal peritoneum

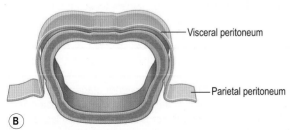

Visceral peritoneum

Parietal peritoneum

Fig. 6.3 The arrangement of the peritoneum in which some structures become intraperitoneal (A) while others remain retroperitoneal (B).

CLINICAL ANATOMY: Peritonitis is inflammation of the peritoneum, usually resulting from bacterial or fungal infection. There are two types of peritonitis: spontaneous bacterial peritonitis, which develops as a complication of liver (cirrhosis) or kidney disease, and secondary peritonitis, which is the result of rupture/perforation of the peritoneum or as a complication of other medical conditions. Peritonitis requires prompt medical attention to counteract the infection, as well as the underlying medical condition. If left untreated it can lead to severe, potentially life-threatening infection throughout the body.

Anterior and Lateral Abdominal Walls

There is no bony support for the anterior and lateral abdominal walls; they are muscular to allow expansion of the abdominal and pelvic contents, as well as being important in producing movements of the trunk (page 200). From superficial to deep the muscles are external oblique, internal oblique and transversus abdominis, with rectus abdominis anteriorly in the midline (Fig. 6.5). Anteriorly, the aponeuroses of the external and internal oblique and transversus abdominis form

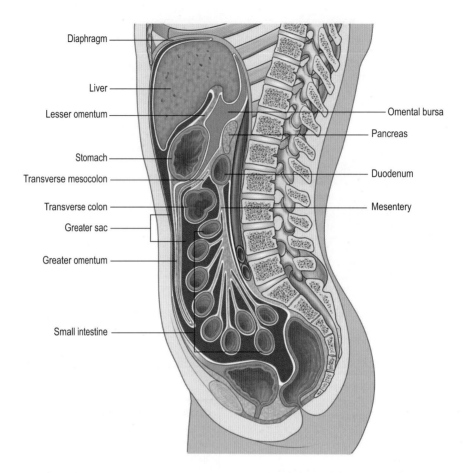

Fig. 6.4 The greater and lesser (omental bursa) sacs of the peritoneal cavity showing some peritoneal reflections (mesentery, transverse mesocolon, greater and lesser omentum).

the rectus sheath surrounding rectus abdominis (Fig. 6.2B). The sheaths fuse along their medial borders at the linea alba. Above the costal margin the sheath is only present anteriorly, being formed by external oblique; between the costal margin and midway between the umbilicus and symphysis pubis it is formed anteriorly by the aponeuroses of external and internal oblique and posteriorly by those of internal oblique and transversus abdominis (Fig. 6.5D (i)); below this all aponeuroses pass anteriorly so that the posterior wall is deficient (Fig. 6.5D (ii)). The lower border of the posterior wall has a crescentic border (arcuate line) below which rectus abdominis lies directly on the transversalis fascia, separating it from extraperitoneal fat and the peritoneum. A small muscle (pyramidalis) lies within the rectus sheath. It is attached to the pubic crest and linea alba.

APPLIED ANATOMY: Rectus abdominis has three tendinous intersections in the anterior part of the muscle which are attached to the rectus sheath, giving the appearance of a 'six-pack' in lean, muscular individuals.

APPLIED ANATOMY: Pyramidalis tenses the linea alba providing a stable attachment from which the abdominal muscles can work, particularly when the trunk is flexed.

CLINICAL ANATOMY: In the latter stages of pregnancy (page 361), the linea alba stretches increasing the distance between the rectus abdominis muscles (divarication/diastasis recti), with separation being as much as 5 cm; postpartum it returns to normal providing undue strains are avoided.

Details of the attachments, action and innervation of the muscles of the abdominal wall can be found in Table 6.1.

> **APPLIED ANATOMY:** Abdominal muscle contraction combined with appropriate sphincter relaxation increases pressure on the bladder aiding micturition, on the rectum assisting defaecation, and on the stomach it helps in vomiting. In the final stages of childbirth (parturition) it helps expel the foetus from the uterus. When the diaphragm is relaxed increased intra-abdominal pressure presses the abdominal viscera against its lower surface pushing it upwards so that, when the rima glottidis (glottis) (page 330) is opened, air is forced from the lungs in a violent explosive cough or sneeze.

> **APPLIED ANATOMY:** The combined action of the abdominal muscles and the diaphragm produces a muscular corset holding the abdominal viscera in place, with the effect being increased during lifting, creating a 'pneumatic' cushion in front of the lumbar spine; holding the breath to anchor the diaphragm often occurs when moving a heavy object.

> **CLINICAL ANATOMY:** Access to the abdomen is through incisions in the anterior abdominal wall at or around the region of interest. They are usually large to allow good access and visual inspection. A central craniocaudal incision from the xiphoid process to the symphysis pubis provides access to the whole of the abdominopelvic cavity enabling exploratory procedures to be undertaken (laparotomy).

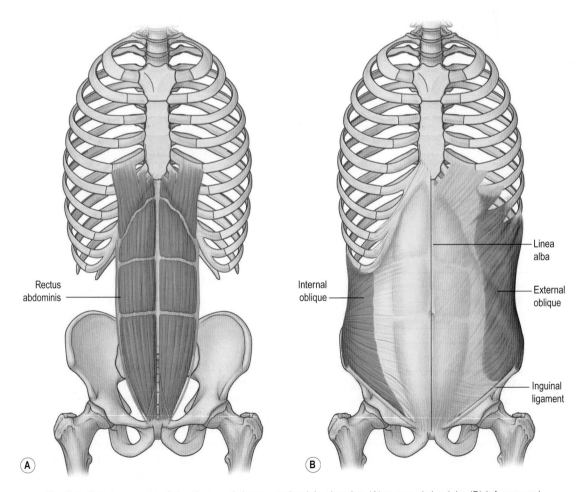

Fig. 6.5 Anterior aspect of the thorax, abdomen and pelvis showing (A) rectus abdominis; (B) left external oblique and right internal oblique;

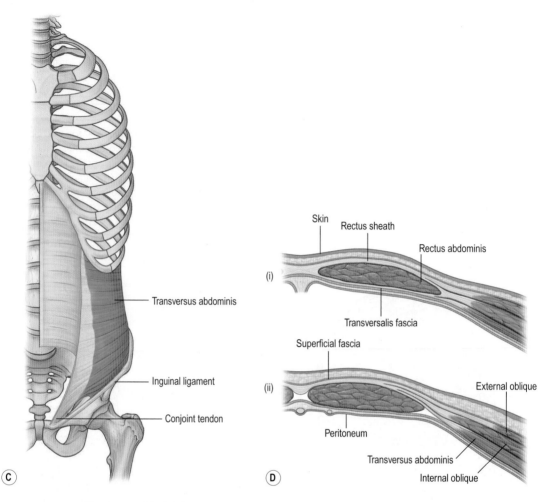

Skin
Rectus sheath
Rectus abdominis
(i)
Transversalis fascia

Superficial fascia
(ii)
External oblique
Peritoneum
Transversus abdominis
Internal oblique

Transversus abdominis

Inguinal ligament

Conjoint tendon

(C)

(D)

Fig. 6.5 cont'd (C) left transverse abdominis; (D) formation of the rectus sheath.

CLINICAL ANATOMY: Pain from surgical incisions of the abdominal muscles frequently causes their inhibition, making coughing difficult and painful; this can lead to infection.

CLINICAL ANATOMY: Laparoscopic/keyhole/minimally invasive surgery is performed through one or more small (1–2 cm) incisions. It results in smaller scars, is less painful for the patient and has shorter recovery times. To create sufficient space for operative procedures the abdominal wall is elevated by inflating the cavity with gas (carbon dioxide). Keyhole surgery can be used for appendectomy, cholecystectomy, hernia repair, and orthopaedic, urological and gynaecological procedures. Robot-assisted surgery is routinely used worldwide where it enhances the surgeon's dexterity; such surgery can also be performed remotely.

Inguinal Canal

An oblique passage through the anterior abdominal wall for the passage of the spermatic cord into the scrotum in males (page 555) and round ligament of the uterus into the labia majora in females (page 552), as well as the ilioinguinal nerve in both sexes (Fig. 6.6).

It begins as a round opening in the transversalis fascia (deep inguinal ring) 1.5 cm above the midpoint of the inguinal ligament and ends as a deficit in the aponeurosis of external oblique (superficial inguinal ring) above the pubic tubercle and medial end of the inguinal ligament. Throughout its course the floor is formed by the inguinal ligament; the anterior wall is formed by the aponeurosis of external oblique, reinforced

TABLE 6.1   The Attachments, Action and Innervation of the Muscles of the Abdominal Wall

Muscle	Attachments	Action	Nerve Supply (Root Value)
Rectus abdominis	From the symphysis pubis and pubic crest to the xiphoid process and costal cartilages of the 5th–7th ribs: it is enclosed within the rectus sheath	Both sides flex the trunk or with the thorax fixed lift the anterior part of the pelvis reducing lumbar lordosis; individually it laterally flexes the trunk	T5/T6–T12
External oblique	From the outer aspects of the lower eight ribs and their costal cartilages, the fibres run inferomedially to the anterior two-thirds of the iliac crest and rectus sheath: it has a free posterior border between the 12th rib and iliac crest with the lower free border forming the inguinal ligament	Both sides flex the trunk or with the thorax fixed lift the anterior part of the pelvis reducing lumbar lordosis; individually it laterally flexes and rotates the trunk	T7–T12
Internal oblique	From the lateral two-thirds of the inguinal ligament, anterior two-thirds of the iliac crest and thoracolumbar fascia, the fibres fan out running superolaterally to the lower four ribs posteriorly and the rectus sheath anteriorly: its lower part blends with the lower part of transversus abdominis forming the conjoint tendon, which attaches to the pubic crest	Both sides flex the trunk or with the thorax fixed lift the anterior part of the pelvis reducing lumbar lordosis; individually it laterally flexes and rotates the trunk	T7–T12, L1
Transversus abdominis	From the lateral one-third of the inguinal ligament, anterior two-thirds of the iliac crest and thoracolumbar fascia and lower six ribs the fibres run horizontally to the rectus sheath: the fibres arising from the inguinal ligament blend with the lower part of internal oblique forming the conjoint tendon, which attaches to the pubic crest	Helps to increase intra-abdominal pressure during expulsive acts; compresses the abdominal viscera	T7–T12, L1

in its lateral one-third by muscular fibres of internal oblique; the posterior wall is formed by the transversalis fascia reinforced in its medial one-third by the conjoint tendon; the roof is formed by the arching fibres of internal oblique and transversus abdominis passing from front to back as they form the conjoint tendon (Fig. 6.6).

APPLIED ANATOMY: In adults the reinforcements of the anterior and posterior walls of the inguinal canal lie opposite the deep and superficial inguinal rings, respectively.

APPLIED ANATOMY: In the foetus and young children, the deep and superficial rings lie opposite each other, facilitating the passage of structures from the abdomen into the groin (the testes and associated structures in males).

As the spermatic cord (or round ligament of the uterus) passes through the canal it receives three coverings: from the margins of the deep inguinal ring it receives the internal spermatic fascia from the transversalis fascia; from the lower border of internal oblique it receives the cremasteric fascia containing cremaster; and from the margins of the superficial ring it receives the external spermatic fascia from the external oblique aponeurosis.

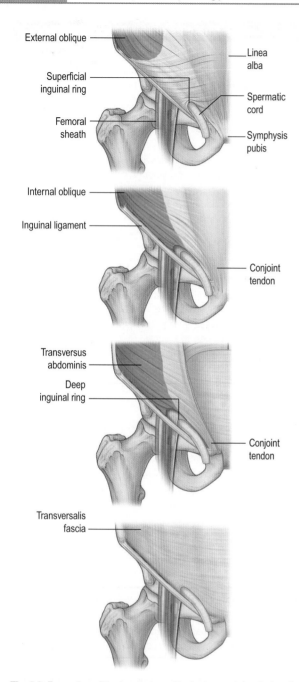

External oblique

Linea alba

Superficial inguinal ring

Spermatic cord

Femoral sheath

Symphysis pubis

Internal oblique

Inguinal ligament

Conjoint tendon

Transversus abdominis

Deep inguinal ring

Conjoint tendon

Transversalis fascia

Fig. 6.6 Formation of the inguinal canal in the lower abdominal wall.

CLINICAL ANATOMY: The inguinal canal is a weakness in the anterior abdominal wall. Contraction of the abdominal muscles may squeeze mobile abdominal viscera through the superficial inguinal ring (hernia); however, these same muscles, when contracting, also narrow the canal and reduce the size of the superficial and deep inguinal rings.

Herniae. An abdominal hernia is a protrusion of gut and the covering peritoneum through an opening into a space where it is not normally found. It can be internal (hiatus hernia, page 74) or external giving an obvious 'lump'. The commonest type (75%) of external hernia is inguinal hernia followed by femoral hernia; both need to be distinguished from other 'lumps in the groin'. Factors predisposing to external herniae include: sex (inguinal hernias are more common in males); raised intra-abdominal pressure (coughing, straining, lifting); a patent processus vaginalis (page 533); weak abdominal muscles.

CLINICAL ANATOMY: There is a danger of strangulation (twisting of the intestine and occlusion of its blood supply) with external hernias. Prompt surgical intervention is required to prevent gangrenous necrosis.

Inguinal hernia. Most inguinal hernias are indirect in which a loop of small intestine enters the deep inguinal ring and follows the course of the spermatic cord through the abdominal wall, with the bulge appearing above the inguinal ligament medial to the pubic tubercle; they tend to occur predominantly in males. Once through the superficial inguinal ring, the hernia enters the scrotum (or labia majora in females). In direct hernias, the protruding gut pushes through the posterior wall of the inguinal canal, usually deep to or just medial to the superficial ring: an indirect hernia passes along the inguinal canal.

Femoral hernia. These tend to be twice as common in females as in males, particularly in females who have had children. The loop of gut pushes through the femoral ring at the entrance to the femoral canal into the femoral sheath (page 579), appearing below the inguinal ligament lateral to the pubic tubercle. The hernia is limited by the fascia lata, except at the saphenous opening (page 588), through which it may progress.

Innervation of the Abdominal Wall

The skin of the anterior and lateral abdominal wall is innervated by the lower five intercostal (T7–T11), subcostal (T12), iliohypogastric (L1) and ilioinguinal (L1) nerves (Fig. 6.7).

Pelvic Floor

The right and left levator ani and coccygeus form a gutter-like floor across the lower part of the pelvis separating the pelvic cavity from the perineum (Fig. 6.8). Both muscles unite in the midline, but for most of their

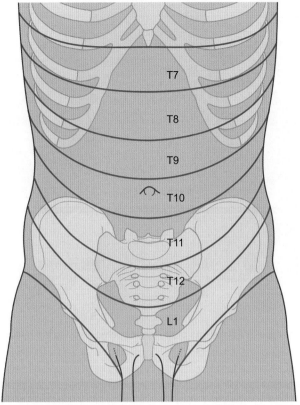

Fig. 6.7 Dermatomes of the anterolateral abdominal wall.

extent they are separated in males by the prostate anteriorly and anus posteriorly, and in females by the urethra and vagina anteriorly and anus posteriorly. Details of the attachments, action and innervation of the pelvic muscles can be found in Table 6.2.

CLINICAL ANATOMY: Levator ani is extremely important in supporting the uterus. It can become excessively stretched during childbirth or surgically traumatised by episiotomy. Stretching can adversely affect its action on the anus, and more commonly the urethra in females, leading to stress incontinence (leakage of urine and faeces when intra-abdominal pressure is raised). Stress incontinence is less common in males, but may occur following prostatectomy. In both males and females pelvic floor exercises may help restore levator ani function.

Details of the bony pelvis can be found on page 567. It is continuous with the abdomen superiorly and separated from the perineum inferiorly by the pelvic floor. It contains the terminal parts of the digestive, renal and reproductive systems, which pass into the perineum via openings in the pelvic floor.

Abdominal Regions

The abdomen can be divided into nine regions projected onto the anterior abdominal wall by the intersection of horizontal transpyloric and transtubercular planes and vertical right and left midclavicular planes (Fig. 6.9A). The transpyloric plane lies midway between the jugular notch (page 68) and upper border of the symphysis pubis (page 569); the transtubercular plane passes

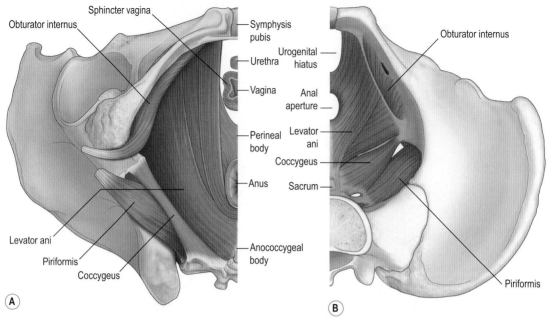

Fig. 6.8 Inferior (A) and superior (B) aspects of the female pelvis showing the muscles of the pelvic floor.

	TABLE 6.2	**The Attachments, Action and Innervation of Muscles of the Pelvic Floor**		
Muscle	Attachments	Action	Nerve Supply (Root Value)	
Levator ani	From the inner surface of the pubic body, obturator membrane and ischial spine the fibres run backwards, downwards and medially towards the midline, inserting into the perineal body, sides of the anal canal and anococcygeal raphe between the anal canal and coccyx: it usually consists of two distinct parts (iliococcygeus, pubococcygeus)	Supports the pelvic viscera, especially in females, having a constricting effect on openings in the pelvic floor, both reflexively and voluntarily	Ventral rami of S3, S4 and perineal branch of the pudendal nerve (S4)	
Coccygeus	From the spine of the ischium, sacrospinous ligament and lower two parts of the sacrum to the midline raphe	Assists levator ani in supporting the pelvic viscera and maintaining intra-abdominal pressure: it also pulls the coccyx forwards after defaecation and parturition	Ventral ramus of S4	

through the iliac tubercles (page 568). Alternatively, the abdomen can be divided into quadrants centred on the umbilicus (Fig. 6.9B).

CLINICAL ANATOMY: Even though the position of the umbilicus is variable, the quadrants are used extensively in clinical practice.

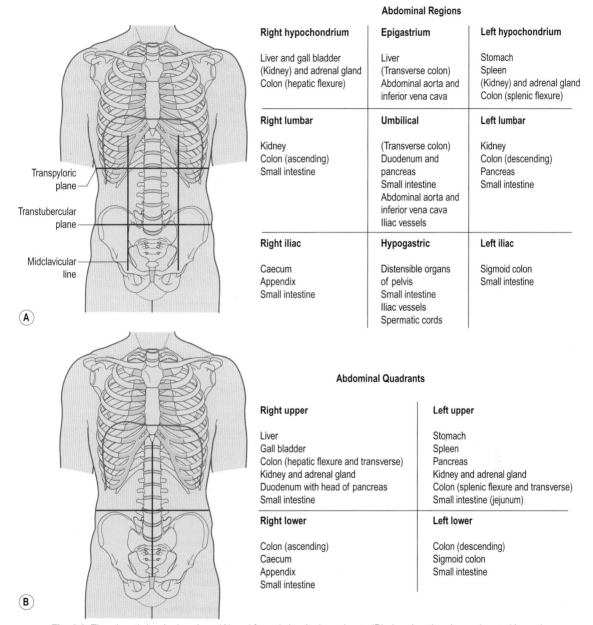

Abdominal Regions

Right hypochondrium	Epigastrium	Left hypochondrium
Liver and gall bladder (Kidney) and adrenal gland Colon (hepatic flexure)	Liver (Transverse colon) Abdominal aorta and inferior vena cava	Stomach Spleen (Kidney) and adrenal gland Colon (splenic flexure)
Right lumbar	**Umbilical**	**Left lumbar**
Kidney Colon (ascending) Small intestine	(Transverse colon) Duodenum and pancreas Small intestine Abdominal aorta and inferior vena cava Iliac vessels	Kidney Colon (descending) Pancreas Small intestine
Right iliac	**Hypogastric**	**Left iliac**
Caecum Appendix Small intestine	Distensible organs of pelvis Small intestine Iliac vessels Spermatic cords	Sigmoid colon Small intestine

Transpyloric plane

Transtubercular plane

Midclavicular line

(A)

Abdominal Quadrants

Right upper	Left upper
Liver Gall bladder Colon (hepatic flexure and transverse) Kidney and adrenal gland Duodenum with head of pancreas Small intestine	Stomach Spleen Pancreas Kidney and adrenal gland Colon (splenic flexure and transverse) Small intestine (jejunum)
Right lower	**Left lower**
Colon (ascending) Caecum Appendix Small intestine	Colon (descending) Sigmoid colon Small intestine

(B)

Fig. 6.9 The nine abdominal regions (A) and four abdominal quadrants (B) showing the viscera located in each region/quadrant.

Digestive System

DEVELOPMENT: The primitive gut (foregut, midgut, hindgut) forms during the 4th week from lateral folding of the embryo (Fig. 6.10) and incorporation of the dorsal part of the yolk sac; the rest of the yolk sac and allantois remain outside the embryo. Endoderm of the primitive gut gives rise to the epithelial lining of most of the digestive tract and its derivatives (biliary system, parenchyma of the liver and pancreas) except at the cranial and caudal extremities

Continued

where it is derived from ectoderm. The splanchnic mesoderm surrounding the primitive gut gives rise to the muscular and connective tissue (peritoneal) components. The foregut gives rise to the oesophagus, trachea and lung buds (see Fig. 2.27), stomach, proximal duodenum, liver and biliary system and pancreas; the midgut forms the primary intestinal loop, which because of the rapid growth of the liver and kidneys projects into the umbilical cord between the 6th and 10th weeks (see Fig. 6.30), it gives rise to the distal duodenum, jejunum, ileum, caecum, appendix, ascending and proximal transverse colon; the hindgut forms the distal transverse, descending and sigmoid colon, rectum and upper part of the anal canal (the lower part of the anal canal is derived from the proctodeum).

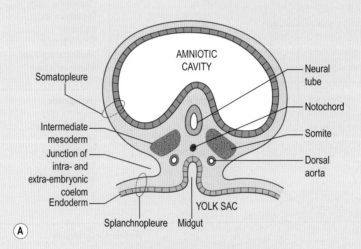

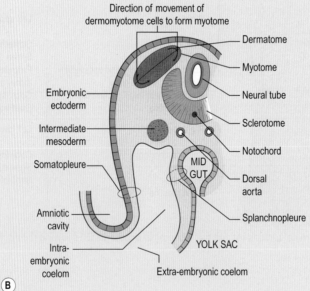

Fig. 6.10 Formation of the gut tube at 3 (A) and 4 (B) weeks.

CLINICAL ANATOMY: Failure of the midgut to return to the abdomen between the 10th and 12th weeks of development, with persistence of intestine or the presence of other abdominal viscera (stomach, liver) in the umbilical cord results in an omphalocele (exomphalos), which is caused by malrotation of the bowels when returning to the abdomen. Omphalocele occurs in 1 in 4000 births and is associated with high mortality (25%) and severe malformations (cardiac anomalies, 50%; neural tube defects, 40%). Some 15% of live born infants with omphalocele have chromosomal abnormalities and 30% have other congenital abnormalities.

Structure of the Digestive Tract

All parts of the digestive tract have a common structural organisation, being a hollow tube of variable diameter with the wall comprising four main layers: mucosa, submucosa, muscularis and serosa (Fig. 6.11).

The mucosa (mucous membrane) comprises an epithelial lining supported by the lamina propria of loose connective tissue, containing blood vessels, lymphatics, smooth muscle cells, and occasionally small glands. The muscularis mucosa separates the mucosa from the submucosa. The submucosa comprises denser connective tissue with larger blood and lymph vessels and Meissner's plexus of autonomic nerves. It may also contain glands and significant accumulations of lymphoid tissue. The muscularis layer (muscularis externa) consists of smooth muscle cells organised as two layers (inner circular and outer longitudinal) separated by connective tissue containing blood and lymph vessels and the myenteric (Auerbach) plexus of autonomic nerves organised into small ganglia connected by pre- and post-ganglionic nerve fibres. Contractions, generated and coordinated by the myenteric plexus, of the muscularis externa mix and propel the luminal contents along the digestive tract (peristalsis). The serosa is a thin layer of loose connective tissue rich in blood

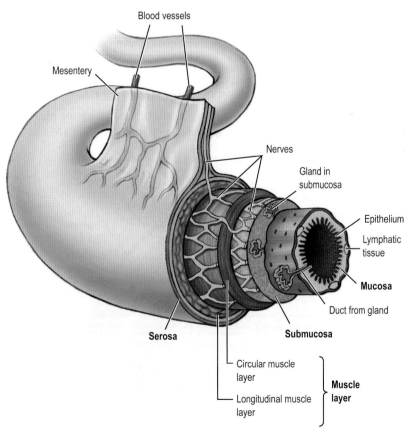

Fig. 6.11 The four main layers of the digestive tract.

vessels, lymphatics and adipose tissue, with a simple squamous epithelial covering (mesothelium). In the abdomen it is continuous with the peritoneum. Where the digestive tract is not suspended (retroperitoneal) the serosa is replaced by a thick connective tissue layer (adventitia) which merges with the surrounding tissues.

> **APPLIED ANATOMY:** Free immune cells and lymphoid nodules in the mucosa and submucosa are part of the mucosa-associated lymphoid/lymphatic tissue (MALT).

Enteric nervous system. The enteric nervous system comprises millions of neurons and enteric glial cells in the walls of the digestive tract. Ganglia, containing neuronal cell bodies, and glia are connected by bundles of axons forming myenteric (Auerbach) and submucosal (Meissner) plexuses (Fig. 6.12) extending from the oesophagus to the anal sphincters. The myenteric plexus mainly controls peristalsis and submucosal gut secretions, intestinal transport of water and electrolytes, and regulation of local blood flow. There are complex interactions between the enteric and autonomic nervous systems. The enteric system is capable of sustaining local reflex activity independent of the central nervous system (CNS). The enteric plexuses can function independent of the autonomic nervous system; however, parasympathetic stimulation increases its activity, while sympathetic stimulation decreases it.

More than a dozen neurotransmitters are released by nerve endings of different types of enteric neurons. As in the parasympathetic and sympathetic systems, the main neurotransmitters are acetylcholine and noradrenaline/norepinephrine, others being adenosine 5'-triphosphate, serotonin, dopamine, cholecystokinin (CCK), substance P, vasoactive intestinal polypeptide (VIP), somatostatin, leu-enkephalin, met-enkephalin and bombesin; the specific function (excitatory, inhibitory) of most of these is not well known. However, acetylcholine usually excites gastrointestinal activity and noradrenaline mostly inhibits it. Adrenaline reaching the digestive tract via blood following its secretion by the adrenal medulla (page 347) also tends to inhibit gastrointestinal activity.

> **CLINICAL ANATOMY:** In Hirschsprung disease (congenital aganglionic megacolon) or Chagas disease (trypanosomiasis infection), the enteric plexus is absent or severely injured, respectively; this disturbs digestive tract function and its motility, with dilations being produced in some areas.

Digestive Tract

Details of the oral cavity, pharynx and oesophagus can be found on pages 308, 326 and 87, respectively.

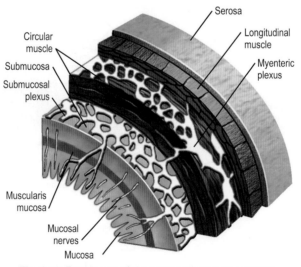

Fig. 6.12 Enteric part of the autonomic nervous system.

Stomach

DEVELOPMENT: The stomach appears as a dilation beyond the oesophagus in the 4th week. Due to differential growth, it rotates 90 degrees clockwise about its long axis acquiring greater and lesser curvatures, with the dorsal mesentery being carried to the left forming the lesser sac (omental bursa) behind the stomach (Fig. 6.13).

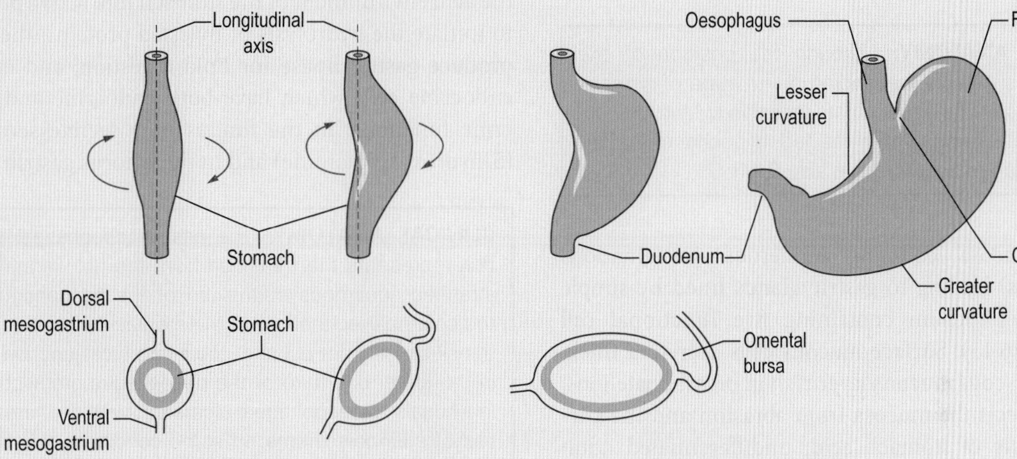

Fig. 6.13 Rotation of the stomach showing formation of the omental bursa.

The lesser omentum passes between the lesser curvature of the stomach and liver, while the greater omentum extends from the greater curvature draping over the transverse colon in front of the small intestine (Figs 6.4 and 6.14).

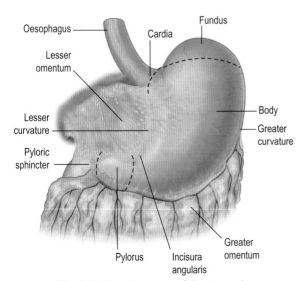

Fig. 6.14 Anterior aspect of the stomach.

CLINICAL ANATOMY: The greater omentum is referred to as the 'abdominal policeman' due to its ability to migrate to an inflamed area and wrap itself around the organ to seal off the inflammation. Inflamed bowel ceases peristalsis (paralytic ileus); however, the remainder continues to undergo peristalsis and 'massages' the greater omentum to the aperistaltic region, which then adheres to the inflamed/diseased area.

CLINICAL ANATOMY: The greater omentum is also an important site for metastatic tumour spread; direct transcoelomic omental spread is common in ovarian cancer. As the metastases develop the greater omentum becomes thickened, being referred to as an 'omental cake' on computed tomography (CTs) and during laparotomy.

The stomach lies free within the abdominal cavity, anchored only at its proximal and distal ends. It has greater and lesser curvatures and is divided into the fundus above the oesophageal opening, body below the fundus and pylorus separated from the body by the angular notch (Fig. 6.14); the pyloric antrum lies next to the body, with the thickened pyloric sphincter controlling the passage of gastric contents into the duodenum. In addition to the longitudinal and circular layers, the muscular wall contains an internal oblique layer. The interior is thrown into a series of longitudinal folds (rugae), which flatten when the stomach is stretched (full).

> **APPLIED ANATOMY:** Although the position of the stomach is variable, depending on its state of fullness and physique, its approximate position within the abdomen lies mainly within the left hypochondrium/left upper quadrant (Figs. 6.9 see also 6.24).

The mucosa contains numerous invaginations (gastric pits) leading to gastric glands lined by simple columnar epithelium containing five functional cell types (Fig. 6.15). Surface mucous cells secrete a thick, adherent viscous mucous layer rich in bicarbonate ions, which protects the mucosa from abrasion and the corrosive effects of stomach acid; undifferentiated adult stem cells (located in the isthmus) divide asymmetrically producing progenitor cells for all other epithelial cells; mucous neck cells; parietal (oxyntic) cells produce and secrete hydrochloric acid (HCl) and intrinsic factor (glycoprotein necessary for vitamin B_{12} uptake in the

small intestine), their activity is regulated by parasympathetic innervation and by the paracrine release of histamine and polypeptide gastrin from enteroendocrine cells; chief (zymogenic) cells contain secretory granules of inactive enzyme pepsinogens, which are converted in the acid environment of the stomach into active pepsins, to initiate the hydrolysis of ingested proteins: they also produce gastric lipase for lipid digestion; and enteroendocrine cells which have both endocrine and paracrine functions: in the fundus they secrete serotonin (5-hydroxytryptamine) and in the pylorus gastrin.

> **CLINICAL ANATOMY:** The gastro-oesophageal junction represents the transition from the non-keratinised stratified squamous epithelium of the oesophagus to the columnar epithelium of the stomach. However, the transition may not occur at the anatomical junction, but in the lower one-third of the oesophagus predisposing individuals to oesophageal ulceration with an increased risk of adenocarcinoma. In some conditions (oesophageal reflux) the stratified squamous oesophageal epithelium can undergo metaplasia and be replaced by columnar epithelium (Barrett's oesophagus), predisposing individuals to the development of oesophageal malignancy (adenocarcinoma).

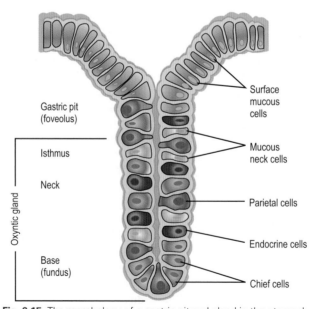

Fig. 6.15 The morphology of a gastric pit and gland in the stomach.

CLINICAL ANATOMY: Gastric and duodenal ulcers are painful lesions of the mucosa extending into deeper layers and can occur anywhere between the oesophagus and jejunum. They are the result of bacterial infection *(Helicobacter pylori)*, the effects of non-steroidal anti-inflammatory drugs, overproduction of HCl or pepsin, lowered production/secretion of mucous or bicarbonate.

CLINICAL ANATOMY: Achlorhydria (reduced hydrochloric acid production) is a chronic autoimmune disease destroying the gastric mucosa: the absence of parietal cells means that intrinsic factor is not secreted leading to pernicious anaemia. Lack of intrinsic factor is the most common cause of vitamin B_{12} deficiency; however, because the liver has extensive stores of B_{12} the disease may not be recognised until significant gastric mucosal changes have occurred. Symptoms include pain in the epigastrium; weight loss; heartburn; nausea; abdominal bloating; diarrhoea; acid regurgitation; feelings of fullness; vomiting; constipation and difficulty swallowing (dysphagia).

Innervation of the stomach. Parasympathetic innervation is from the vagus nerves by the anterior and posterior gastric nerves. The anterior gastric nerve is mainly a continuation of the left vagus and the posterior of the right vagus (page 92). The anterior gastric nerve runs on the anterosuperior surface of the stomach, while the posterior gastric nerve runs on the posteroinferior surface. The parasympathetic supply is motor to the musculature, inhibitory to the pyloric sphincter and secretomotor to the gastric glands. Sympathetic innervation is derived from the coeliac plexus, reaching the stomach through the sympathetic plexuses around the arteries. It is inhibitory to the musculature, motor to the pyloric sphincter, vasomotor to the vessels and also carries pain sensation from the stomach.

CLINICAL ANATOMY: Vagotomy (complete or partial section of the vagus nerves and/or its branches) is undertaken to reduce the rate of gastric secretions, as in treating peptic ulcers. The types of vagotomy are (i) truncal, (ii) selective and (iii) highly selective (Fig. 6.16).

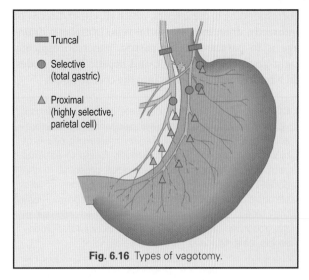

- ▬ Truncal
- ● Selective (total gastric)
- △ Proximal (highly selective, parietal cell)

Fig. 6.16 Types of vagotomy.

Arterial supply, venous and lymphatic drainage of the foregut. The arterial supply to the foregut (lower part of the oesophagus to the first part of the duodenum, pancreas, spleen and liver) is from the coeliac trunk, a branch of the abdominal aorta just below the diaphragm (Fig. 6.17). The venous drainage is by veins

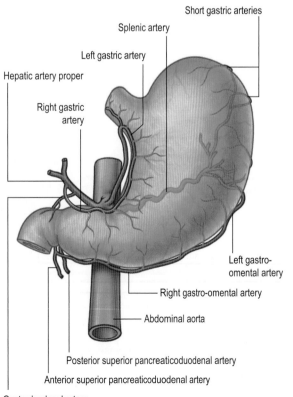

Short gastric arteries
Splenic artery
Left gastric artery
Hepatic artery proper
Right gastric artery
Left gastro-omental artery
Right gastro-omental artery
Abdominal aorta
Posterior superior pancreaticoduodenal artery
Anterior superior pancreaticoduodenal artery
Gastroduodenal artery

Fig. 6.17 Arterial supply to the foregut.

corresponding to the arteries, which all, either directly or indirectly, drain into the portal vein. Lymphatic drainage is to paracardial, left gastric, pancreaticosplenic, right gastroepiploic, pyloric and hepatic lymph nodes: all lymph eventually drains into the coeliac nodes.

> **CLINICAL ANATOMY:** Varices are dilated submucosal veins in the lining of the lower oesophagus and stomach (Fig. 6.18); they can be a life-threatening cause of bleeding. They are most commonly found in patients with portal hypertension or elevated pressure in the portal system resulting from the complications of liver cirrhosis. Varices tend not to show symptoms unless they bleed; however, individuals may experience pain in the abdomen, vomiting blood, black tarry and/or bloody stools, pale skin, dizziness and feeling faint.

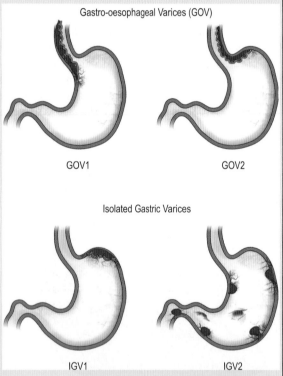

Fig. 6.18 Gastric and oesophageal varices: 1 and 2 refer to the location.

> **CLINICAL ANATOMY:** Chronic gastric inflammation (gastritis), pernicious anaemia and polyps predispose to stomach cancer. Because it is often not diagnosed until late in the course of the disease, survival rates are relatively low. Symptoms include vague epigastric pain, early fullness when eating, bleeding (leading to chronic anaemia) and obstruction.

Small Intestine

This comprises the duodenum, jejunum and ileum.

Duodenum. The C-shaped duodenum (Fig. 6.19) is retroperitoneal lying directly on the posterior abdominal wall overlying the vertebral column. It has thick muscular walls, with the interior thrown into regular circular folds (plicae circulares). The duodenum can be considered as being in four parts which surround the head of the pancreas: the first (superior) part is a continuation of the pylorus; the second (descending) part is crossed by the transverse colon and overlays the right kidney; the third (inferior) part crosses the inferior vena cava, aorta and vertebral column; the fourth (ascending) part terminates at the duodenojejunal junction. Secretions from the pancreas (pancreatic juice for the digestion of proteins, fats and carbohydrates) and liver (bile for the digestion of fats) drain into the second part of the duodenum, with the two ducts having a common site of entry (major duodenal papilla): at the terminal end of each duct a sphincter controls the flow of pancreatic secretions/bile into the duodenum.

> **CLINICAL ANATOMY:** The first part of the duodenum is clinically referred to as the ampulla or duodenal cap. It is the site of most duodenal ulcers.

Jejunum and ileum. The jejunum (proximal two-fifths) and ileum (distal three-fifths) are relatively mobile parts of the small intestine and fill the majority of the abdominopelvic cavity (Fig. 6.20). The jejunum is fixed to the posterior abdominal wall at the duodenojejunal junction and the ileum at the ileocaecal junction. The jejunum and ileum are suspended from the posterior abdominal wall by the mesentery (Fig. 6.4). They are the most common parts of the digestive tract associated with hernias.

The jejunum lies mostly in the left upper quadrant. It has thicker walls than the ileum with its inner mucosal lining characterised by numerous prominent circular folds (plica circulares); however, it has less prominent arterial arcades and longer vasa recta (straight arteries) (Fig. 6.21A). In contrast, the ileum lies mostly in the right lower quadrant. It has thinner walls, fewer and less prominent mucosal folds, shorter vas recta, more mesenteric fat and more arterial arcades (Fig. 6.21B). The ileum opens into the large intestine at the junction of the caecum and ascending colon (Fig. 6.22), with the opening surrounded by two ileocaecal folds. The folds

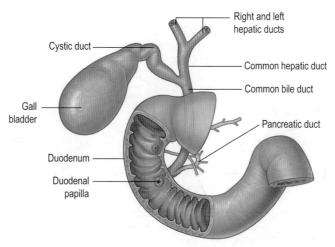

Fig. 6.19 Duodenum and its relationship to the bile and pancreatic ducts.

may prevent reflux from the caecum into the ileum, as well as regulating the passage of contents from the ileum into the caecum.

CLINICAL ANATOMY: Meckel's diverticulum (diverticulum ilei) is a common congenital disorder present in 2% of individuals. It is a small outpouching/bulge 5 cm long in the wall of the small intestine approximately 1 m proximal to the ileocaecal junction and usually contains tissue similar to that of the pancreas or stomach. It may be free within the abdomen or connected to the umbilicus by a fibrous cord. Symptoms include: gastrointestinal bleeding (blood in the stools); abdominal pain and cramping; bowel obstruction, which can cause pain, bloating, diarrhoea, constipation and vomiting; and diverticulitis (swelling of the intestinal wall). Bleeding is the most common symptom in children under 5, with bowel obstruction occurring more frequently in older children and adults. In children, diverticulitis may be misdiagnosed as appendicitis.

The mucosa and submucosa of the small intestine show a series of permanent circular or semicircular folds (plica circulares), which are best developed in the jejunum (Fig. 6.23A). Covering the entire mucosa and projecting into the lumen are short (0.5–1.5 mm) villi covered in a simple columnar epithelium of absorptive cells (enterocytes) interspersed with goblet cells (Fig. 6.23B). Each villus has a core of loose connective tissue extending from the lamina propria containing fibroblasts, smooth muscle fibres, lymphocytes, plasma cells, fenestrated capillaries and a central lymphatic (lacteal).

Between the villi are openings of short tubular glands or crypts (interstitial glands/crypts of Liebekühn). The epithelium of each villus is continuous with that of the glands/crypts and includes differentiating cells and pluripotent stem cells for all cell types in the small intestine and include: enterocytes (absorptive cells) having a brush border densely packed with microvilli, greatly increasing the surface area for nutrient absorption; goblet cells, interspersed among the enterocytes, secrete glycoprotein mucins which form mucous to protect and lubricate the intestinal lining; Paneth cells, located in the basal portion of the crypt below the stem cells, release lysozyme, phospholipase A and hydrophobic peptides (defensins), all of which bind and break down membranes of microorganisms and bacterial cell walls – they have an important role in innate immunity and in regulating the microenvironment of the crypts; enteroendocrine cells which secrete peptide hormones (somatostatin, serotonin, substance P, CCK, gastric inhibitory peptide (GIP), glucagon-like peptide (GLP-1), peptide YY, motilin, neurotensin, secretin); and M (microfold) cells, specialised epithelial cells in the ileal mucosa overlying Peyer patches (lymphoid tissue, part of MALT), selectively endocytose antigens transporting them to the underlying lymphocytes and dendritic cells, which then migrate to lymph nodes to elicit an appropriate immune response.

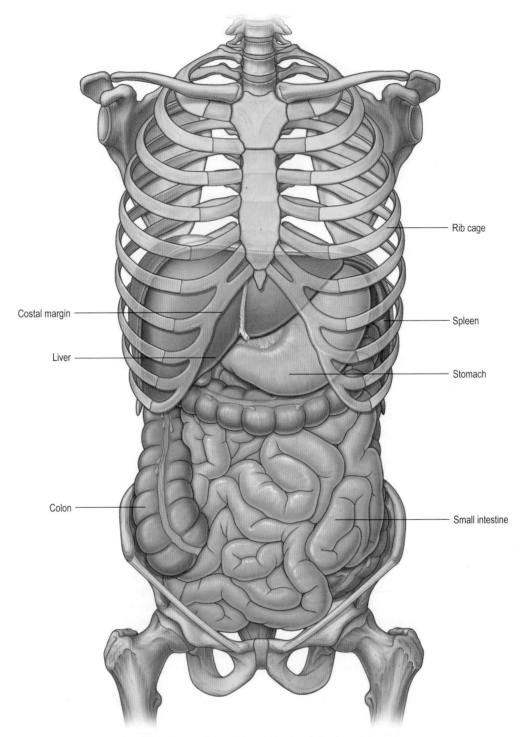

Fig. 6.20 The small intestine within the abdominopelvic cavity.

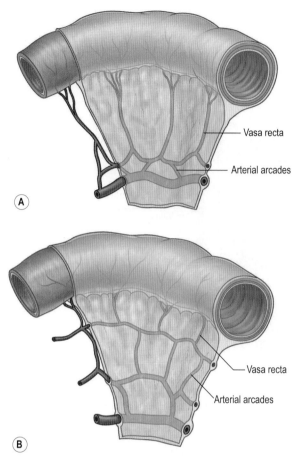

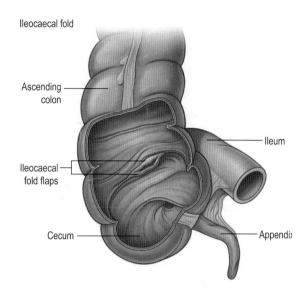

Fig. 6.22 The ileocaecal junction.

Mucous from these glands is alkaline to neutralise the chyme entering the duodenum from the pylorus, not only protecting the mucous membrane, but also bringing the pH of the chyme to an optimum level for pancreatic enzymes to act.

Fig. 6.21 Arterial supply to the jejunum (A) and ileum (B).

> **APPLIED ANATOMY:** The plica circulares increase the intestinal surface area 3-fold, the villi increase it a further 10-fold and the microvilli a further 20-fold, giving a total absorptive area of the small intestine in excess of 200 m².

Along the length of the small intestine are extensive blood and lymphatic vessels, nerve fibres, smooth muscle fibres and diffuse lymphoid tissue. The smooth muscle fibres produce rhythmic movements of the villi increasing their absorptive efficiency, as well as producing local movements of the plica circulares, helping to propel lymph from the lacteals into submucosal and mesenteric lymphatics. In the mucosa and submucosa of the proximal duodenum are large clusters of branched tubular mucous (duodenal/Brunner) glands with excretory ducts opening among the crypts.

> **CLINICAL ANATOMY:** Coeliac disease (coeliac sprue) is an immune reaction against gluten or other proteins in wheat, barley and rye. Gluten is also found in any food that contains these cereals (pasta, cakes, breakfast cereals, most types of bread, some sauces and ready meals, most beers). It affects the mucosa of the small intestine causing malabsorption and possible damage to or destruction of the villi, resulting in reduced nutrient absorption. Symptoms include diarrhoea, stomach aches, bloating and flatulence, indigestion, constipation and anaemia. More general symptoms include tiredness, unintentional weight loss, an itchy rash, infertility, peripheral neuropathy, ataxia and delayed puberty in children.

Arterial supply, venous and lymphatic drainage of the small intestine. The arterial supply is mainly by branches of the superior mesenteric artery, a branch of the abdominal aorta below the coeliac trunk. The superior mesenteric artery is the artery of the midgut (2nd part of the duodenum to two-thirds along the transverse

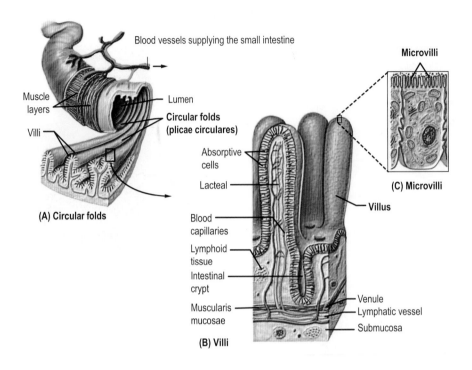

Fig. 6.23 (A) Layers of the small intestine. (B) Plica circulares covered in villi. (C) Schematic representation of a villus.

colon). The venous drainage is by veins corresponding to the arteries, which all, either directly or indirectly, drain into the portal vein. Lymphatic drainage is to pyloric, pancreaticoduodenal, hepatic, superior mesenteric and ileocolic nodes, with the lymph eventually reaching the coeliac nodes.

> **APPLIED ANATOMY:** The coeliac trunk and superior mesenteric artery may arise as a common trunk, which then divides.

Large Intestine/Colon

The large intestine comprises the caecum, appendix, colon (ascending, transverse, descending, sigmoid), rectum and anal canal. It is situated around the margins of the abdominopelvic cavity (Fig. 6.24). It has a larger internal diameter compared to the small intestine, peritoneal-covered accumulations of fat (appendices epiploicae/omental appendices), longitudinal muscles arranged in three narrow bands (taeniae coli, which converge to the base of the appendix) and is divided into sacculations (haustrations) along its length.

Caecum and appendix. The caecum is a blind ending sac lying below the ileocaecal opening in the right iliac fossa, being continuous above with the ascending colon. It is usually in contact with the anterior abdominal wall. Because of its mobility it is considered to be intraperitoneal, although its upper part lies directly on the posterior abdominal wall. Attached to its posteromedial wall is the appendix (Fig. 6.24), a narrow hollow blind-ended tube containing large aggregations of lymphoid tissue in its walls. It is suspended from the terminal ileum by the mesoappendix, which carries the appendicular vessels.

Duodenojejunal junction

Descending colon

Transverse colon

Ascending colon

Ileocaecal junction

Caecum

Appendix

Rectum

Bladder

Sigmoid colon

Fig. 6.24 The large intestine (colon) within the abdomen.

APPLIED ANATOMY: The base of the appendix lies at the junction of the lateral one-third and medial two-thirds of a line from the right anterior superior iliac spine to the umbilicus (McBurney's point). Although the base of the appendix is fixed, the position of the remainder is highly variable (Fig. 6.25). It can be retrocaecal (74%), pelvic (21%), subcaecal (3.5%), pre-ileal (1%) or posti-leal (0.5%).

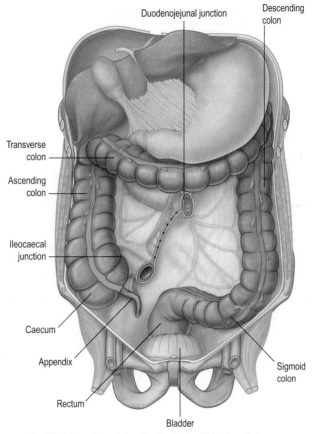

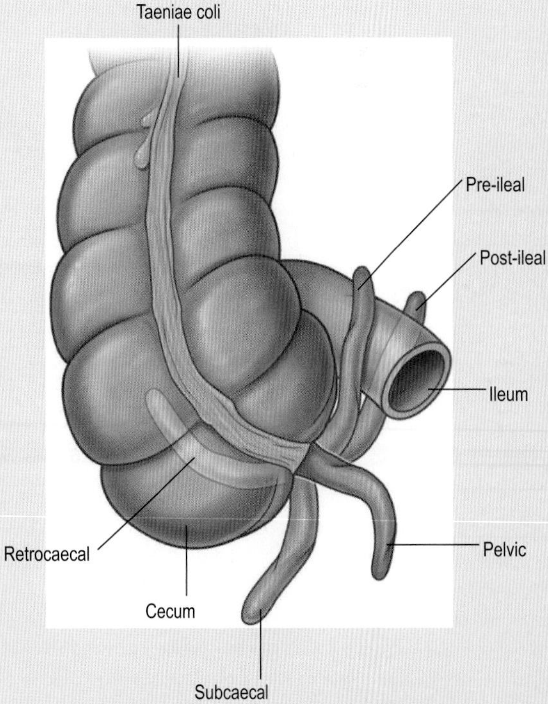

Taeniae coli

Pre-ileal

Post-ileal

Ileum

Retrocaecal

Cecum

Pelvic

Subcaecal

Fig. 6.25 Positions of the appendix.

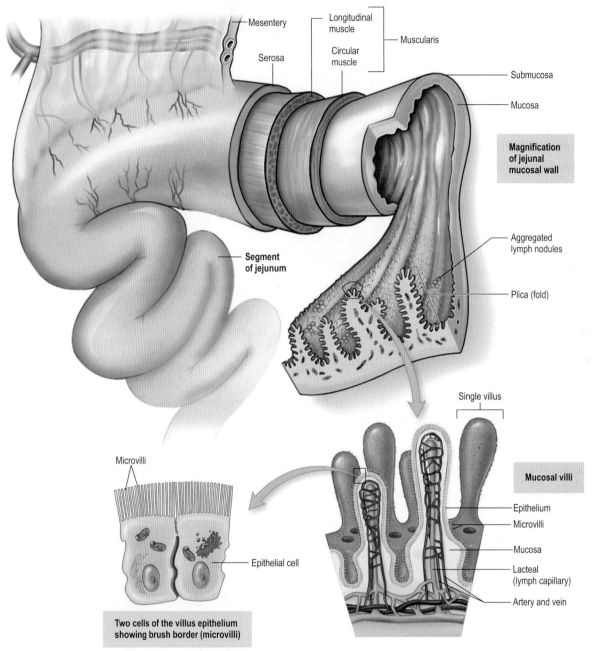

Mesentery

Longitudinal muscle

Muscularis

Circular muscle

Serosa

Submucosa

Mucosa

Magnification of jejunal mucosal wall

Segment of jejunum

Aggregated lymph nodules

Plica (fold)

Single villus

Microvilli

Mucosal villi

Epithelium

Microvilli

Mucosa

Epithelial cell

Lacteal (lymph capillary)

Artery and vein

Two cells of the villus epithelium showing brush border (microvilli)

Fig. 6.26 The wall of the large intestine.

CLINICAL ANATOMY: Acute appendicitis is an abdominal emergency, usually occurring when the appendix is obstructed by faecal matter or the lymphoid tissue has become enlarged. There is bacterial proliferation with invasion of the appendix wall, which becomes damaged by pressure necrosis. If unresolved it may lead to peritonitis. Initially, pain begins as a central, periumbilical, colicky pain, which tends to wax and wane, but after 6–10 hours it is constant and localised in the right iliac fossa. Individuals may develop a fever, nausea and vomiting.

Colon. The ascending and descending segments of the colon are retroperitoneal, while the transverse and sigmoid colon are intraperitoneal, suspended by the transverse and sigmoid mesocolon, respectively. At the junction of the ascending and transverse colon is the hepatic (right colic) flexure, just below the right lobe of the liver (page 478), and at the junction of the transverse and descending colon is the splenic (left colic) flexure, just below the spleen (pages 162 and 484). The splenic flexure is higher and more posterior than the hepatic flexure. The highly mobile transverse colon is suspended from the posterior abdominal wall by the transverse mesocolon, except where it lies directly on the duodenum and head of the pancreas.

The mucosa of the colon is penetrated throughout its length by tubular interstitial glands (Fig. 6.26), which together with the lumen are lined by goblet and absorptive cells (colonocytes), with a small number of enteroendocrine cells. The colonocytes have irregular microvilli and dilated intercellular spaces for active fluid absorption. Goblet cells become more numerous along the length of the colon and rectum. Epithelial stem cells are found in the lower one-third of each gland. The lamina propria is rich in lymphoid cells and nodules, which often extend into the submucosa. The richness in MALT is related to the large bacterial population of the colon. The appendix has little or no absorptive function but is a significant component of MALT.

CLINICAL ANATOMY: Herniation of the mucosa and submucosa of the colon can occur between the taeniae coli forming bulges (diverticula) leading to diverticulitis. It results from structural defects in the colon wall, high intraluminal pressure or constipation. Faecal material can become immobilised in the diverticula causing localised inflammation or diverticulitis.

CLINICAL ANATOMY: Crohn's disease is a chronic inflammatory bowel disorder occurring most commonly in the ileum or colon (Fig. 6.27), although it can occur anywhere along the digestive tract. It is an immune-related but not an autoimmune disease. It is considered to be the result of a combination of immune responses (excessive lymphocyte activity, inflammation), and environmental and genetic factors. Symptoms include abdominal pain, diarrhoea (which may be bloody if inflammation is severe), fever, abdominal distension and weight loss. Bowel obstruction can be a complication with chronic inflammation, with a greater risk of small bowel and colon cancer. Other symptoms include anaemia, skin rashes, arthritis and inflammation of the eye.

CLINICAL ANATOMY: Ulcerative colitis (colitis, proctitis) is an inflammatory bowel disease characterised by inflammation and ulceration of the wall of the large intestine, affecting the descending and sigmoid colon and rectum (Fig. 6.27). It can occur at any age, but is most common between 15 and 30 years. Symptoms include abdominal pain, diarrhoea with bloody stools, fatigue, loss of appetite and weight, eye inflammation, liver disease (hepatitis, cirrhosis), skin rashes and anaemia.

Arterial supply, venous and lymphatic drainage of the colon. The ascending and proximal two-thirds of the transverse colon are part of the midgut and are consequently supplied by branches of the superior mesenteric artery, while the distal one-third of the transverse colon, descending and sigmoid colon, rectum and upper part of the anal canal are supplied by branches of the inferior mesenteric artery (artery of the hindgut (Fig. 6.28)). The venous drainage is by veins corresponding to the arteries, which all, either directly or indirectly, drain into the portal vein. Lymphatic drainage is via epicolic nodes on the wall of the colon, paracolic nodes along the medial and lateral borders of the ascending and descending colon and mesenteric border of the transverse and sigmoid mesocolon, intermediate nodes along the right, ileocolic, middle and left colic vessels, and terminal colic nodes along the superior and inferior mesenteric arteries. Efferent vessels drain into the intestinal lymph trunk and then to the cisterna chyli.

Inflammatory bowel disease (IBD)

Crohn disease   Ulcerative colitis

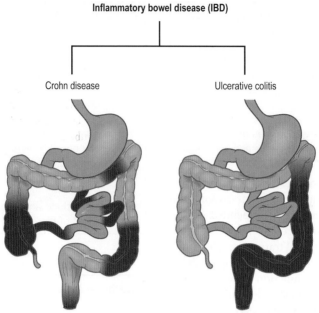

Fig. 6.27 Common isolated locations of Crohn disease and the more extensive colitis ulcerosa (ulcerative colitis).

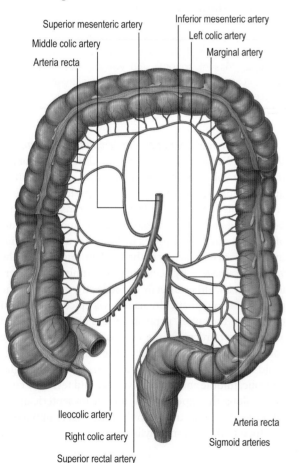

Superior mesenteric artery

Middle colic artery

Arteria recta

Inferior mesenteric artery

Left colic artery

Marginal artery

Ileocolic artery

Right colic artery

Superior rectal artery

Arteria recta

Sigmoid arteries

Fig. 6.28 Arterial supply to the large intestine.

> **CLINICAL ANATOMY:** Where the colon, liver and stomach lie directly against the diaphragm or posterior abdominal wall, veins from these organs communicate with veins of the posterior abdominal wall and are, therefore, potential sites of portosystemic anastomoses.

Rectum and Anal Canal

The retroperitoneal rectum is a continuation of the sigmoid colon, usually at the level of S3. The anal canal is a continuation of the large intestine below the rectum. The junction between the rectum and anal canal (anorectal junction) represents a marked change in direction as the puborectalis part of levator ani (page 458) surrounds and pulls the anorectal junction forwards. It is also the site of change from simple squamous epithelium with intestinal glands in the rectum to stratified squamous epithelium in the anal canal. It is the site most commonly affected by HPV (human papillomavirus), being where lesions are most likely to arise. A distinction is often made between anal canal/intra-anal and anal margin/perianal cancers.

The mucosa and submucosa of the anal canal are highly vascularised (venous sinuses) and thrown into a series of longitudinal folds (anal columns), with intervening anal sinuses. Faecal material accumulated in the rectum is eliminated by muscular contraction, with accompanying relaxation of the internal anal sphincter, continuous with the circular layer of the muscularis externa, and the external sphincter of skeletal muscle.

CLINICAL ANATOMY: The arterial supply to the rectum and anal canal is by branches from the inferior mesenteric (superior rectal artery), internal iliac (middle rectal artery) and internal pudendal arteries (inferior rectal artery) (Fig. 6.29). The lower one-third of the rectum and upper part of the anal canal is a site of a portosystemic anastomosis, which in cases of increased portal pressure can lead to haemorrhoids (piles), swellings containing enlarged veins (see Fig. 6.93); they can be internal or external: another site of portosystemic anastomosis is the lower one-third of the oesophagus. External piles appear as small bluish lumps under the skin around the anus and can be painful. Internal piles are not visible unless they protrude from the anus, with smaller piles returning spontaneously or can be pushed back into the anal canal; larger piles cannot. Symptoms include itching and pain around the anus, bleeding and discomfort during defaecation. Large internal piles can prevent the anal sphincter from closing properly resulting in the escape of faeces and intense itching around the anus.

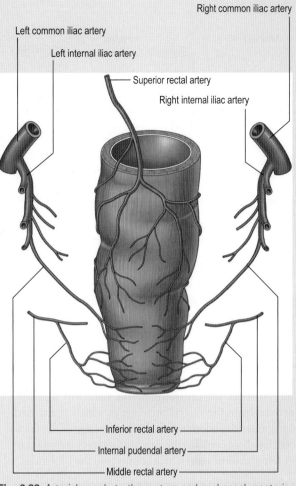

Fig. 6.29 Arterial supply to the rectum and anal canal, posterior aspect.

Labels in figure:
- Right common iliac artery
- Left common iliac artery
- Left internal iliac artery
- Superior rectal artery
- Right internal iliac artery
- Inferior rectal artery
- Internal pudendal artery
- Middle rectal artery

CLINICAL ANATOMY: Colorectal cancer is an adenocarcinoma which develops initially from benign adenomatous polyps in the mucosal epithelium. They usually occur in the rectum, sigmoid colon or distal colon. Polyps are more common in individuals with low-fibre diets, which reduces the bulk of faecal material prolonging contact of faecal toxins with the mucosa.

Liver and Biliary System

DEVELOPMENT: The liver, gall bladder and biliary system appear as an outgrowth (liver bud) from the proximal duodenum during the 4th week, which invaginates the septum transversum. The liver bud divides into two parts (pars cystica and pars hepatica) which enlarge and grow between the layers of the ventral mesentery (Fig. 6.30), giving rise to the gallbladder and cystic duct, and biliary system and terminal parts of the cords of the cells, respectively. The septum transversum gives rise to the fibrous stroma and capsule of the liver. The liver grows rapidly filling most of the abdominal cavity by the 9th week. Part of the liver (bare area) outgrows the ventral mesentery and comes to lie directly against the diaphragm (Fig. 6.30).

Continued

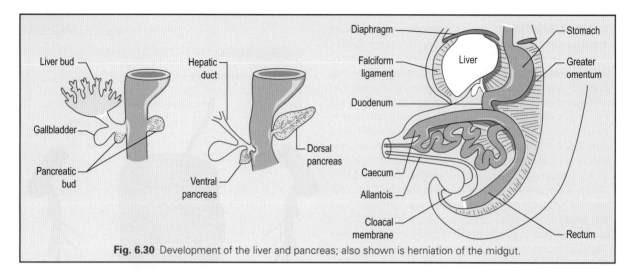

Fig. 6.30 Development of the liver and pancreas; also shown is herniation of the midgut.

Liver. The large, soft, reddish brown wedge-shaped liver lies in the right hypochondrium extending into the epigastrium and occasionally the left hypochondrium (upper right quadrant extending into the upper left quadrant). It has diaphragmatic (anterior, superior, posterior) and visceral (inferior) surfaces. It has a larger right and smaller left lobe, with smaller caudate and quadrate lobes, both functionally part of the left lobe (Fig. 6.31). The right and left lobes are separated by the falciform ligament (derived from the ventral mesentery), which is attached to the anterior abdominal wall. The free edge of the falciform ligament contains the ligamentum teres (remnant of the left umbilical vein) which connects to the umbilicus.

> **APPLIED ANATOMY:** The margins of the triangular bare area are continuous with the groove for the inferior vena cava, porta hepatis, fossa for the gallbladder and fissures for the ligamentum teres and venosum. The area outlined is devoid of a peritoneal covering (Fig. 6.31). The porta hepatis is the area where structures enter (portal vein, right and left hepatic arteries) or leave (hepatic ducts/bile duct) the liver; the ligamentum venosum is the obliterated ductus venosus, which shunted blood returning from the placenta, via the umbilical vein, to the inferior vena cava, thus bypassing the liver.

> **APPLIED ANATOMY:** Approximately 75% of blood entering the liver is via the portal vein, which receives nutrient-rich blood from the small and large intestines and spleen; however, it has a low oxygen content. The remaining 25% is via the hepatic artery, a branch of the coeliac trunk, with a normal arterial oxygen content.

> **APPLIED ANATOMY:** The portal venous system carries blood from the stomach, small and large intestines, spleen, pancreas and gallbladder. It is formed by the union of the superior mesenteric and splenic veins behind the neck of the pancreas (page 482). The inferior mesenteric vein (continuation of the superior rectal vein) drains into the splenic vein.

> **APPLIED ANATOMY:** The liver is held in place by peritoneal reflections; the two hepatic veins draining into the inferior vena cava; areolar connective tissue between it and the diaphragm and intra-abdominal pressure, which depends on the integrity of the abdominal wall muscles.

> **CLINICAL ANATOMY:** The anastomosis between the left branch of the portal vein and veins of the anterior abdominal wall via small paraumbilical veins passing along the ligamentum teres in the falciform ligament can, in the presence of high portal pressure, lead to the appearance of tortuous dilated veins radiating around the umbilicus (caput medusa).

The liver is the interface between the digestive system and blood, being the organ in which nutrients absorbed in the small intestine are processed before distribution throughout the body. The liver is organised into lobules arranged around a central vein (Fig. 6.32), onto which peripheral blood vessels converge (venule from the portal vein, arteriole from the hepatic artery) and bile ductule leave. The venule, arteriole and ductule constitute a portal triad, which

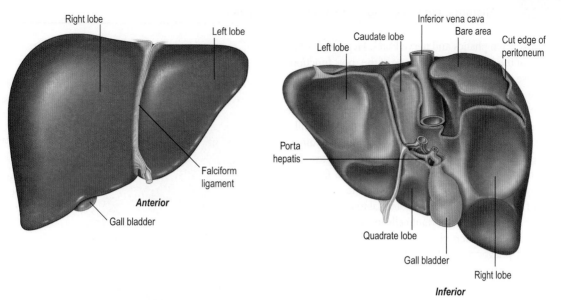

Right lobe

Left lobe

Falciform
ligament

Anterior

Gall bladder

Inferior vena cava

Bare area

Caudate lobe

Left lobe

Cut edge of
peritoneum

Porta
hepatis

Quadrate lobe

Gall bladder

Right lobe

Inferior

Fig. 6.31 Diaphragmatic and visceral surfaces of the liver.

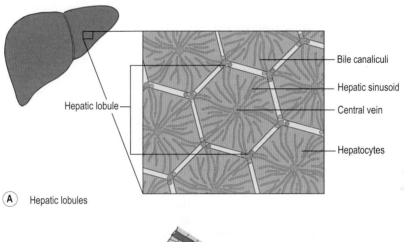

Hepatic lobule

Bile canaliculi

Hepatic sinusoid

Central vein

Hepatocytes

A Hepatic lobules

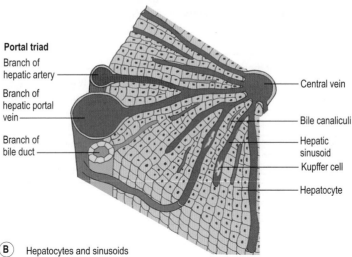

Portal triad

Branch of
hepatic artery

Branch of
hepatic portal
vein

Branch of
bile duct

Central vein

Bile canaliculi

Hepatic
sinusoid

Kupffer cell

Hepatocyte

B Hepatocytes and sinusoids

Fig. 6.32 (A) A hepatic lobule. (B) Blood vessels forming sinusoids as they pass between plates of hepatocytes draining into the central vein.

also contains lymphatics and nerve fibres. Hepatocytes line the walls of the sinusoids and are one of the most functionally diverse cells in the body. Between the plates of hepatocytes the anastomosing sinusoids have thin discontinuous linings of fenestrated endothelial cells surrounded by sparse basal lamina and reticular fibres, allowing plasma to fill a narrow perisinusoidal space (of Disse), bathing the numerous irregular villi projecting from the hepatocytes. The direct contact between hepatocytes and plasma facilitates most key hepatocyte functions involving the uptake and release of nutrients, proteins and potential toxins.

Other functionally important cells in the sinusoids are: specialised stellate macrophages (Kupffer cells), which recognise and phagocytose old erythrocytes releasing haem and iron for reuse and storage in ferritin complexes, they also remove bacteria and debris present in the portal blood; hepatic stellate cells (Ito cells) in the perisinusoidal space, which store vitamin A and other fat-soluble vitamins. Following injury to the liver they also produce extracellular matrix components, which become myofibroblasts, and cytokines, which help regulate Kupffer cell activity.

The apical surfaces of hepatocytes form bile canaliculi involved in the secretion of bile. They are elongated spaces with large surface areas due to the numerous short microvilli. The canaliculi form a complex anastomosing network of channels through the hepatocyte plates. They empty bile into the canals of Hering (Fig. 6.33), which are lined by cuboidal epithelial cells (cholangiocytes). The short bile canaliculi merge with the bile ductules, eventually forming the hepatic ducts.

Hepatocytes continually secrete bile, a mixture of bile acids (organic acids such as chloric acid), bile salts (deprotonated forms of bile acids), electrolytes, fatty acids, phospholipids, cholesterol and bilirubin.

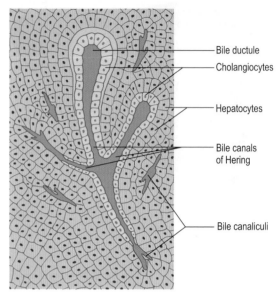

Fig. 6.33 Bile canaliculi and the canals of Hering.

The main digestive function of the liver is the production of bile, a complex substance for the emulsification, hydrolysis and uptake of fats in the small intestine. However, together with other liver cells they process the contents of blood, having many specific functions: synthesis and secretion of the major plasma proteins (albumin, fibrinogen, apolipoproteins, transferrin); conversion of amino acids to glucose (gluconeogenesis); breakdown (detoxification) and conjugation of ingested toxins, including some drugs; amino acid deamination producing urea, which is excreted by the kidneys; and storage of glucose in granules and triglycerides in small lipid droplets.

APPLIED ANATOMY: Bilirubin is a pigmented breakdown product of haem released mainly by splenic macrophages, but also by Kupffer cells. Released into the duodenum bilirubin is converted by intestinal bacteria into other pigmented products, some of which are absorbed by the intestinal mucosa to be processed and excreted again in the liver or excreted into urine by the kidneys. This is what gives faeces and urine their characteristic colour.

CLINICAL ANATOMY: Fatty liver disease is the abnormal accumulation of large lipid deposits containing triglycerides in hepatocytes (steatosis); it is reversible. It has multiple causes, but most commonly occurs in individuals with alcoholism or obesity. It can produce a progressive inflammation of the liver (hepatitis), usually referred to as steatohepatitis.

CLINICAL ANATOMY: Hepatitis is characterised by swelling and inadequate functioning of the liver. It can be acute or chronic, and when severe it can lead to liver failure and death. It can be the result of viral (hepatitis A and B, caused by contaminated water and food; sharing needles, or having unprotected sex with infected individuals; blood transfusions from infected individuals; inheritance from the mother during parturition) or bacterial (leptospirosis, Q fever) infection, excess alcohol consumption, excess administration of drugs (paracetamol), poisons (carbon tetrachloride, aflatoxin), Wilson's disease (a genetic disorder preventing the removal of excess copper, with it accumulating in the liver, brain and eyes), circulatory insufficiency, or inheritance from the mother during parturition. Symptoms include fever; nausea; vomiting, diarrhoea and weight loss; headache and weakness. Chronic hepatitis is characterised by stomach pain, pale skin, dark-coloured urine and pale stools, jaundice and changes in personality.

CLINICAL ANATOMY: Cirrhosis, often referred to as end-stage liver disease, results from long-term damage to the liver and can be due to a number of different causes: alcohol; viral infections (hepatitis B and C); non-alcohol related fatty liver disease (NAFLD); autoimmune hepatitis; primary biliary cholangitis (PBC) and other long-term diseases of the bile ducts (primary sclerosing cholangitis (PSC)) or biliary atresia (BA) in children; some inherited diseases (haemochromatosis, Wilson's disease); long-term contact with some drugs and poisons; and blood vessel disease (Budd-Chiari syndrome). The damage leads to scarring (fibrosis) with irregular nodules replacing the smooth liver tissue, resulting in the liver becoming harder. Cirrhosis is classified as compensated (the liver is coping with the damage and maintaining its important functions) and decompensated (the liver is not able to perform adequately all its functions). Individuals with decompensated liver disease often have serious symptoms and complications (portal hypertension, bleeding varices, ascites, hepatic encephalopathy). Early symptoms include generally feeling unwell and tired all the time; loss of appetite; loss of weight with muscle wasting; nausea and vomiting; tenderness/pain over the liver; spider-like small blood capillaries on the skin above the waist (spider angioma); blotchy red palms and sleep disturbances. Later symptoms as the liver is struggling to function include: intensely itchy skin; yellowing of the whites of the eyes and skin; white nails; clubbed fingers; hair loss; oedema of the legs, ankles and feet; swelling of the abdomen (ascites); dark urine; pale-coloured or dark/tarry stools; frequent nosebleeds and bleeding gums; easy bruising, with difficulty in stopping small bleeds; vomiting blood; frequent muscle cramps; right shoulder pain; enlarged breasts and shrunken testes in men; irregular or lack of menstrual cycle; impotence and loss of libido; dizziness and extreme fatigue (anaemia); shortness of breath; tachycardia; fevers with high temperatures and shivers; forgetfulness, memory loss, confusion and drowsiness; changes in personality; trembling hands, with small spidery writing; staggering gait; and increased sensitivity to drugs (medical, recreational) and alcohol. Red flag symptoms include fever with high temperature and shivers, often caused by infection; shortness of breath; vomiting blood; very dark or black/tarry stools and periods of mental confusion or drowsiness.

CLINICAL ANATOMY: The liver is capable of regeneration despite its slow rate of cell renewal. Hepatocyte loss due to toxins triggers mitosis in the remaining healthy hepatocytes (compensatory hyperplasia) to maintain the original tissue mass. Surgical removal of part of the liver elicits a similar response, with the regenerated liver being well organised replacing the functions of the destroyed/removed tissue. The regenerative capacity of the liver is important because a single donor liver can be divided and used in more than one recipient. Similarly, a liver lobe can be donated by a living relative for surgical transplantation with full liver function restored in both the donor and recipient.

CLINICAL ANATOMY: An important function of hepatocytes is the conjugation of water-insoluble yellow bilirubin by glucuronyl transferases to form water-soluble non-toxic bilirubin glucuronide. If not formed or excreted properly various diseases characterised by jaundice can result. Treatment of jaundice in the newborn is exposure to blue light from ordinary fluorescent tubes transforming unconjugated bilirubin into a water-soluble photoisomer which can be excreted by the kidneys.

CLINICAL ANATOMY: Most malignant tumours of the liver are derived from hepatocytes or cholangiocytes of the hepatic ducts. The pathogenesis of liver cancer is associated with a number of acquired disorders (chronic viral hepatitis (B or C), cirrhosis).

Biliary system. The right and left hepatic ducts, from the right and left lobes of the liver, unite forming the common hepatic duct, which in turn joins with the cystic duct to form the common bile duct (Fig. 6.19), which runs in the free margin of the lesser omentum. It then passes posterior to the 1st part of the duodenum behind the head of the pancreas to unite with the pancreatic duct before entering the second part of the duodenum (Fig. 6.19).

Gallbladder. An elongated pear-shaped structure situated on the inferior surface of the right lobe of the liver (Fig. 6.31); it has a fundus, body and neck. The neck is the twisted narrow part extending from the body. Its mucous membrane forms a spiral valve continuous with the cystic duct. The gallbladder stores and concentrates bile. To move stored bile into the duodenum, gallbladder contraction is induced by cholecystokin (CCK) released from enteroendocrine cells in the small intestine, with CCK being stimulated by the presence of ingested fats.

APPLIED ANATOMY: The fundus of the gallbladder is marked by a point at the tip of the right 9th costal cartilage (where the transpyloric plane crosses the linea semilunaris at the lateral side of the rectus sheath).

The mucous membrane lining the hepatic, cystic and common bile ducts is a simple columnar epithelium of cholangiocytes, with a relatively thin lamina propria and submucosa, which contains mucous glands in some regions of the cystic duct. The whole is surrounded by a thin muscularis, which becomes thicker near the duodenum and duodenal papilla, forming a sphincter regulating the flow of bile into the small intestine.

CLINICAL ANATOMY: A number of congenital anomalies are associated with the gallbladder: atresia, due to failure of the gallbladder and bile duct to canalise; absence, due to failure to develop as an outgrowth from the hepatic diverticulum; intrahepatic gallbladder, when it is partially or completely embedded in the liver; double gallbladder, due to division of the pars cystica (page 477) into two parts; and bifid gallbladder, in which the fundus and body are divided into two parts.

Pancreas

DEVELOPMENT: The pancreas develops from two buds (ventral and dorsal). The ventral bud arises from the hepatic bud (Fig. 6.30) and migrates to the right of the duodenum below the dorsal bud and forms the lower part of the head and uncinate process; the dorsal bud develops from the concavity of the duodenum (Fig. 6.30) and enlarges to form the tail, body and upper part of the head. The distal part of the duct of the dorsal bud and proximal part of the duct of the ventral bud join to form the main pancreatic duct, which in turn joins the common bile duct prior to opening into the 2nd part of the duodenum. Occasionally, the proximal part of the dorsal duct remains patent as an accessory pancreatic duct opening into the duodenum above the main pancreatic duct.

The pancreas is a mixed endocrine (insulin secretion) and exocrine (pancreatic juice secretion) gland lying obliquely across the posterior abdominal wall behind the lesser sac at the level of L1 (Fig. 6.34). It is divided into an uncinate process, head, narrow neck, body and tail, with the head lying within the C-shaped concavity of the duodenum and tail towards the hilum of the spleen; the uncinate process lies behind the superior mesenteric vessels.

CLINICAL ANATOMY: A number of congenital anomalies are associated with the pancreas: annular pancreas (pancreatic tissue surrounding the duodenum), due to an abnormal migration of the ventral pancreatic bud; accessory pancreas, a mass of pancreatic tissue in the submucosa of the pylorus of the stomach and cystic fibrosis of the pancreas, due to viscous secretions leading to obstruction of the pancreatic duct, followed by cystic formation and fibrosis of the pancreatic tissue.

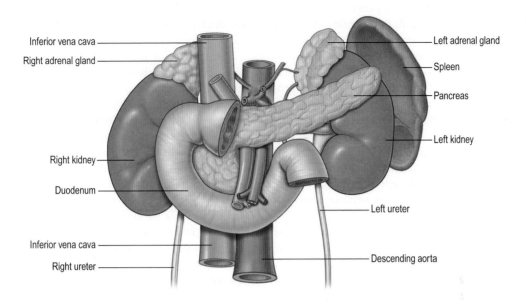

Fig. 6.34 Anterior aspect of the upper abdomen showing the relationship between the pancreas, duodenum, kidneys and spleen.

CLINICAL ANATOMY: Pancreatic cancer is usually associated with the duct cells and can arise anywhere in the gland, but occurs most frequently in the head near the duodenum. It is usually asymptomatic until growth and metastases are well advanced, with a subsequent high mortality. Nonspecific symptoms include upper abdominal pain, loss of appetite and weight loss. Most detected cancers have spread locally invading the portal vein, porta hepatis and superior mesenteric vessels; lymph node spread is also common. Surgical resection, if advised, is complex due the number of associated blood and lymphatic vessels. It involves resection of the region of the tumour, together with part of the duodenum, requiring a complex bypass procedure.

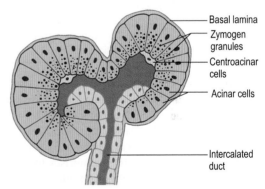

Fig. 6.35 A serous acinus in the pancreas.

The pancreas has a thin capsule of connective tissue with extended septa covering the larger vessels and ducts, separating the parenchyma into lobules containing serous acini (Fig. 6.35) surrounding isolated clusters of enteroendocrine cells (islets of Langerhans) (Fig. 6.36).

Cells of the serous acini produce digestive enzymes. Each acinus is drained by a short intercalated duct of simple squamous epithelium. Centroacinar and intercalated duct cells, under the influence of secretin, secrete large volumes of fluid rich in bicarbonate ions (HCO_3), which alkalinises, hydrates and transports the enzymes

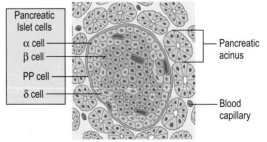

Fig. 6.36 An islet of Langerhans showing the four major types of cells.

produced in the acini. The alkaline pancreatic secretions are released into the duodenum to neutralise the acidic chyme entering from the stomach, creating an environment for optimal activity of pancreatic enzymes (proteases, α-amylase, lipases, nucleases (deoxyribonucleic acid (DNAase), ribonucleic acid (RNAase)). The proteases are secreted as inactive zymogens (trypsinogen, chymotrypsinogen, proelastase, kallikreinogen, procarboxypeptidase). The secretion of pancreatic enzymes is mainly regulated by the secretion of CCK, which stimulates secretion by the acinar cells, and secretin, which promotes water and HCO_3 secretion by the duct cells. Parasympathetic fibres also stimulate secretin from both acinar and duct cells.

Pancreatic tissue is protected against autodigestion by restricting protease activation to the duodenum; having a trypsin inhibitor co-packaged in the secretory granules with trypsin; and a low pH in the acini and duct system due to the presence of HCO_3.

> **CLINICAL ANATOMY:** In acute pancreatitis, the proenzymes may be activated and digest pancreatic tissue, which can lead to serious complications. Possible causes include infection, gallstones, alcoholism, drugs and trauma. Chronic pancreatitis can lead to progressive fibrosis and loss of pancreatic function.

The pancreatic islets (of Langerhans) are compact clusters of cells embedded within the acinar tissue. They are mainly located in the tail and constitute 1%–2% of pancreatic volume. A thin capsule surrounds each islet, with the cells arranged in cords separated by fenestrated capillaries (Fig. 6.36). Each islet comprises the following cell types: α (A) cells mainly secrete glucagon, which acts on several tissues to make energy stored in glycogen and fat available through glycogenolysis and lipolysis, increasing blood glucose content, they are usually found at the periphery; β (B) cells (the most numerous) produce insulin, which acts on several tissues to cause entry of glucose into cells promoting a decrease in blood glucose content; δ (D) cells secrete somatostatin, which inhibits release of other islet cell hormones through local paracrine action, it also inhibits the release of growth hormone (GH) and thyroid-stimulating hormone (TSH) from the anterior pituitary and HCl secretion by gastric parietal cells; and PP (pancreatic polypeptide) cells, more common in islets in the head, which secrete pancreatic polypeptide, stimulating activity in the gastric chief cells and inhibiting bile, pancreatic enzyme and bicarbonate secretion, as well as intestinal motility.

The activity of α and β cells is largely regulated by blood glucose levels above or below 70 mg/dL. Increased blood glucose levels stimulate β cells to release insulin and inhibit α cells from releasing glucagon, while decreased blood glucose levels stimulate α cells to release glucagon. Closely associated with 10% of islet cells are sympathetic and parasympathetic nerve fibres, which function as part of the control system for insulin and glucagon secretion. Sympathetic fibres increase glucagon secretion and inhibit insulin secretion, while parasympathetic fibres increase both glucagon and insulin secretion. It is the opposing action of these two hormones which helps to control precisely blood glucose concentrations, important in homeostasis.

The islets also normally contain some enterochromaffin cells similar to those in the digestive tract, which secrete hormones affecting the digestive system.

> **CLINICAL ANATOMY:** Diabetes mellitus is characterised by loss of the insulin effect and subsequent failure of cells to take up glucose, leading to increased blood sugar levels (hyperglycaemia). Type 1 (insulin-dependent) diabetes mellitus (IDDM) is caused by the loss of β cells due to autoimmune destruction. It is treated by regular injections of insulin. In Type 2 (non-insulin-dependent) diabetes mellitus (NIDDM) the β cells are present but fail to produce adequate levels of insulin in response to hyperglycaemia. The peripheral target cells also 'resist' or no longer respond to insulin. Type 2 diabetes is commonly associated with obesity, although multifactorial genetic components may be important in its onset.

Spleen

> **DEVELOPMENT:** The spleen arises during the 6th week from mesodermal cells in the dorsal mesogastrium. The cells form the parenchyma, stroma and capsule which become infiltrated by haematopoietic cells. It is supplied by the splenic artery, a branch of the coeliac trunk. The splenic vein joins the superior mesenteric vein to form the portal vein.

It is part of the reticuloendothelial system concerned with haematopoiesis in the foetus and the reutilisation of iron from haemoglobin of destroyed red blood cells. It is not part of the digestive system *per se.* The spleen has diaphragmatic and visceral surfaces, with the visceral surface having impressions for the stomach, left kidney, left colic (splenic) flexure and tail of the pancreas (Fig. 6.34).

APPLIED ANATOMY: The spleen lies in the left hypochondrium deep to the posterior parts of the 9th, 10th and 11th ribs, with its long axis aligned with the 10th rib. The medial end lies lateral to T10 and lateral end reaches the midaxillary line.

CLINICAL ANATOMY: Rupture of the spleen following a violent blow to the lower left ribs may produce massive intraperitoneal haemorrhage, which if left untreated or undiagnosed, can be fatal.

Digestive Physiology

Digestion is the process by which food is broken down into simpler chemical substances that can be absorbed into blood, distributed around the body and used as nutrients. The digestive process is achieved through the mechanical and enzymatic breakdown of food. The functions of the digestive system include the ingestion of food, breaking it into small particles, transporting these to different areas of the digestive tract; the secretion of enzymes and other substances necessary for digestion with the subsequent digestion and absorption of the food particles; and finally the removal of unwanted substances from the body in faeces and urine.

The amount of food ingested is mainly determined by the desire for food (hunger), with the type of food preferentially sought being determined by appetite. These mechanisms are important for maintaining an adequate nutritional supply for the body. The intake of carbohydrates, fats and proteins provides energy that can be used in various body functions or stored for use later. Energy intake and energy expenditure need to be balanced to ensure body weight and composition remain stable. When intake persistently exceeds expenditure, most of the excess is stored as fat, with body weight increasing. An insufficient energy intake to meet the body's metabolic demands leads to starvation and a loss of body mass.

Different foods contain different proportions of carbohydrates, fats, proteins, vitamins and minerals; therefore, an appropriate balance must be maintained between them to ensure that the body's metabolic needs are met. The mean energy available from each gram of carbohydrate as it is oxidised to carbon dioxide and water is 4 calories; from fat 9 calories; and from protein as it is oxidised to carbon dioxide, water and urea is 4 calories. However, the mean percentages absorbed in the digestive tract for carbohydrates is 98%, fat 95% and protein 92%. If the diet contains an abundance of carbohydrates and fats, almost all the body's energy requirements are derived from them, with little from protein; however, after the carbohydrate and fat stores have been depleted (as in starvation) the body's protein stores are rapidly consumed, sometimes at very high rates.

Regulation of Food Intake and Energy Storage

Approximately 27% of the energy ingested normally reaches the functional systems of the cells, much of which is converted to heat from protein metabolism, muscle activity and activities of the body's various organs and tissues. Excess energy is mainly stored as fat, while an energy intake deficit results in a loss of total body mass until energy intake is increased or death occurs.

Neural regulation of food intake. Centres in the hypothalamus (page 255) participate in the control of food intake. The lateral nuclei serve as a feeding centre, with stimulation leading to the need to eat; the ventromedial nuclei serve as the satiety centre, giving a sense of nutritional satisfaction inhibiting the feeding centre; the paraventricular and dorsomedial nuclei also have a role in regulating food intake, causing excessive eating and a depression of eating, respectively; the arcuate nuclei are regions where multiple hormones released from the digestive tract and adipose tissue converge to regulate food intake, as well as energy expenditure. Together these centres coordinate the processes controlling eating behaviour and the perception of satiety. At the same time these nuclei influence the secretion of several hormones important in regulating energy balance and metabolism, including those from the thyroid, adrenal glands and pancreatic islet cells.

The hypothalamus receives nerve impulses from the digestive tract giving sensory information about stomach filling (Fig. 6.37). Chemical signals from nutrients in the blood (glucose, amino acids, fatty acids) signal satiety; signals from the digestive hormones (peptide YY, CCK and insulin suppress further feeding; ghrelin

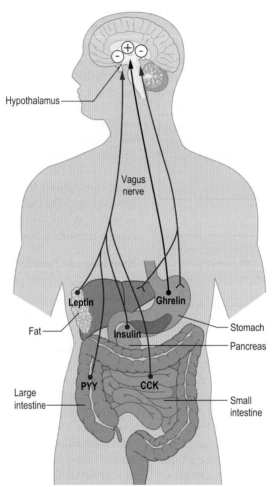

Fig. 6.37 Feedback mechanisms in the control of food intake: stretch receptors in the stomach activate sensory afferent pathways in the vagus and inhibit food intake. (See text for details.)

stimulates appetite; leptin inhibits food intake as fat cells increase in size); signals from the cerebral cortex (sight, smell, taste) influence feeding behaviour. Orexigenic substances (neuropeptide Y; agouti-related protein; melanin-concentrating hormone; orexins A and B; galanin; cortisol; ghrelin; endocannabinoids) stimulate feeding and anorexigenic substances (α-melanocyte-stimulating hormone; leptin; serotonin; noradrenaline/norepinephrine; corticotropin-releasing hormone (CRH); CCK; glucagon-like peptide; peptide YY) inhibit feeding.

Factors regulating food intake. Regulation can be considered as either short-term, preventing overeating at each meal, or intermediate and long-term, maintenance of energy stores within the body.

Short-term regulation. A number of rapid feedback signals are important in determining that the amount of food eaten meets nutritional needs. Stretch inhibitory signals from the distended stomach and duodenum, transmitted mainly by the vagus, suppress the feeding centre reducing the desire for food. In addition, hormonal factors also suppress feeding. CCK activates receptors on local sensory nerves in the duodenum contributing to satiation; its effects are short-lived and probably function to prevent overeating during meals. Peptide YY is released some 1–2 hours after eating, being stimulated by the calorific intake and composition of the food, especially the intake of fat. Glucagon-like peptide release is stimulated by the presence of food in the intestine, its release in turn enhances insulin secretion, both of which act to suppress appetite. Ghrelin blood levels rise during fasting, peaking just before eating, then rapidly fall after a meal.

Short-term regulation serves two other functions: firstly, it tends to make individuals eat smaller amounts of food at each meal, allowing the food to pass through the digestive tract at a steadier pace so that its digestive and absorptive mechanisms can work at optimal rates; secondly, it helps prevent individuals from eating excessive amounts that would be too much for the metabolic storage systems once the food has been absorbed.

Intermediate and long-term regulation. Decreases in blood glucose, amino acid and lipid levels increase the desire for food to return blood metabolite concentrations to normal. A rise in blood glucose level increases activity in the glucoreceptor neurons of the satiety centre in the ventromedial and paraventricular nuclei of the hypothalamus, as well as a decrease in the glucosensitive neurons in the hunger centre of the lateral hypothalamus. In addition, some amino acids and lipids also affect the firing of these same or closely related neurons.

Most stored energy comprises fat. The hypothalamus senses this energy storage through the action of leptin, which is released from adipocytes when adipose tissue increases. Stimulation of leptin receptors in the hypothalamic nuclei decreases the production of appetite stimulators (neuropeptide Y, agouti-related protein); increases the production of α-melanocyte-stimulating hormone, with activation of melanocortin receptors; increases production of CRH to decrease food intake; increases sympathetic activity increasing metabolic rate and energy expenditure; and decreases insulin production to decrease energy storage. However, social and cultural factors can result in continued excess food intake, even in the presence of high leptin levels.

Long-term regulation helps to maintain more or less constant stores of nutrients in the tissues.

Obesity. This is defined as an excess of body fat, with body mass index – BMI: weight (kg)/height (m^2) – often being used as a determinant of obesity, even though it is not a direct estimate of adiposity. An individual with a BMI of 25–29 is considered to be overweight and one with a BMI greater than 30 is considered to be obese; however, some individuals may have a high BMI due to a large muscle mass (muscle tissue weighs more than fat). It is preferable to define obesity in terms of the actual percentage of body fat, with obesity defined in males as having more than 25% total body fat and females more than 35%; however, specific methods (skinfold thicknesses, underwater weighing,

bioelectrical impedance) have to be used to assess total body fat; it is easier and more common to use BMI.

When more energy is consumed than expended body weight increases. The excess is stored as fat in the subcutaneous tissues and abdominal cavity, with the liver often accumulating significant amounts of fat in obese individuals.

Inanition, anorexia and cachexia

Inanition. The opposite of obesity, characterised by extreme weight loss due to either insufficient energy intake or pathophysiological conditions (psychogenic disturbances, hypothalamic abnormalities) that decreases the desire for food. In individuals with cancer the reduced desire for food may be associated with increased energy expenditure leading to weight loss.

Anorexia. The reduction in food intake caused mainly by diminished appetite, thus emphasising the role of central neural mechanisms in its pathophysiology in some diseases (cancer), when other conditions (pain, nausea) may cause a lowered intake of food. Anorexia nervosa (erroneously referred to as anorexia) is an eating disorder characterised by low weight, food restriction, body image disturbance, fear of gaining weight and an overpowering desire to be thin.

Cachexia. A metabolic disorder of increased energy expenditure leading to weight loss greater than that caused by reduced food intake. It is more common in individuals with lung cancer or cancers in the digestive system. The main symptoms are severe weight loss (including fat and muscle), loss of appetite, anaemia, weakness and fatigue. Cachexia and anorexia often occur together in individuals with acquired immunodeficiency disease (AIDS) and chronic inflammatory disorders. Central neural and peripheral factors contribute to cancer-induced anorexia and cachexia, with some inflammatory cytokines (tumour necrosis factor-α, interleukin-6, interleukin-1β, proteolysis-inducing factor) causing anorexia and cachexia.

Starvation. The major effect of starvation is the progressive depletion of tissue fat and protein as only small amounts of carbohydrate are stored in the body (glycogen in the liver and muscles). The rate of fat depletion continues until most fat stores are gone, even when protein is being utilised (Fig. 6.38).

Initially, protein undergoes rapid depletion as the easily mobilised protein is used directly for metabolism or is converted to glucose. Once the easily accessed protein has been depleted during the early phase of starvation, the rate of gluconeogenesis decreases with an accompanying decrease in the rate of protein depletion. The decreased

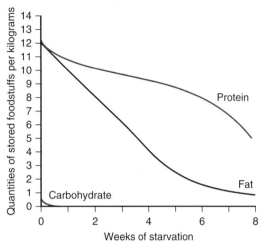

Fig. 6.38 Effect of starvation on the body's food stores.

availability of glucose initiates a series of events leading to the excessive utilisation and conversion of some of the fat breakdown products to ketone bodies, leading to the state of ketosis. Ketone bodies, like glucose, can cross the blood-brain barrier enabling brain cells to use them for energy; this process leads to a partial preservation of protein stores in the body. When the fat stores are almost completely depleted, protein stores again undergo rapid depletion. Because proteins are essential for cellular function, death usually occurs when the body's proteins have been depleted to half their normal level.

The stores of some vitamins, especially the water-soluble vitamins (B group, C), do not last long during starvation. After a week of starvation, mild vitamin deficiencies begin to appear, with severe deficiencies being present after several weeks. The deficiencies add to the debility, leading to death.

Mixing and Propulsion of Food Through the Digestive Tract

Chewing (mastication) and swallowing. Details of the muscles involved in chewing can be found on page 288 and of swallowing on page 328.

Secretion. Throughout the digestive tract secretory glands have two primary functions: firstly, digestive enzymes are secreted in most areas of the tract; and secondly, mucous glands provide mucous for lubrication and protection. Most digestive secretions occur in the presence of food, with the amount secreted being proportionate to that needed for proper digestion. In some parts of the tract the types of enzymes and other constituents of the secretions vary according to the type of food present. It is the

presence of food coming into contact with the epithelium that stimulates secretion. Part of this local effect, especially the secretion of mucous, is the result of direct contact stimulation of the surface glandular cells. Local epithelial stimulation (tactile, chemical irritation, distension) activates the enteric nervous system (page 464) within the gut wall, resulting in reflexes stimulating mucous glands on the epithelial surface and deep glands in the gut wall to increase their secretion. Parasympathetic stimulation increases the rate of secretion, while sympathetic stimulation results in a slight/moderate increase in secretion and vasoconstriction of vessels supplying the glands.

> **CLINICAL PHYSIOLOGY:** If parasympathetic and/or hormonal stimulation is already causing copious glandular secretions, sympathetic stimulation reduces the secretion, mainly through its vasoconstrictive action.

Mucous is a thick secretion comprising mainly water, electrolytes and glycoproteins. It differs slightly in different parts of the digestive tract. It has important properties: it adheres tightly to food or other particles spreading a thin film over their surfaces; it coats the gut wall, preventing contact between most food particles and the mucosa; it has a low resistance to slippage, enabling particles to slide along the epithelial surface; it causes faecal particles to adhere together to form faeces that are expelled during defaecation; it is strongly resistant to digestion by the digestive enzymes; and mucous glycoproteins are capable of buffering small amounts of either acids (it contains moderate amounts of bicarbonate ions) or alkalies, giving it amphoteric properties.

In the stomach and intestine, gastrointestinal hormones (polypeptides, polypeptide derivatives) are released by the presence of food entering the blood and carried to the glands, where they stimulate secretion. They help regulate the volume and nature of the secretions, particularly of gastric and pancreatic juices when food enters the stomach or duodenum.

The mixing of food begins in the mouth once food has been ingested. Chewing breaks it down into smaller segments by the grinding action of the teeth. In the mouth the chemical breakdown of the food begins as it is mixed with saliva secreted by the salivary glands (page 312).

Saliva. Mainly composed of water (99.5%) and containing enzymes (amylase (ptyalin), maltase, lingual lipase, lysozyme, phosphatase, carbonic anhydrase, kallikrein) and other organic substances (mucin, albumin, proline-rich proteins, lactoferrin, IgA, blood group antigens, free amino acids, non-protein nitrogenous substances (urea, uric acid, creatinine, xanthine, hypoxanthine)), with a small amount (0.5%) of solids containing inorganic substances (sodium, calcium, potassium, bicarbonate, bromide, chloride, fluoride, phosphate) and gases (oxygen, carbon dioxide, nitrogen).

> **CLINICAL PHYSIOLOGY:** Glucose is normally absent in saliva; however, it tends to be present in individuals with diabetes mellitus.

Saliva moistens and dissolves the ingested food, with mucin lubricating the bolus facilitating swallowing. The dissolved substances in food stimulate taste buds. The digestive enzymes initiate the breakdown of food: amylase acts on cooked or boiled starch converting it into dextrin and maltose, although the major part of this process occurs in the stomach; maltase converts maltose to glucose; and lingual lipase digests pre-emulsified fats and hydrolyses triglycerides of milk fat into fatty acids (diacylglycerol). The constant secretion of saliva keeps the mouth and teeth rinsed and free of food debris, and sheds epithelial cells and foreign particles, preventing bacterial growth (lysozyme kills staphylococcus, streptococcus and brucella); proline-rich proteins and lactoferrin have antimicrobial properties, with both stimulating tooth enamel formation. Proline-rich proteins also neutralise tannins; IgA has antimicrobial and antiviral actions.

Many organic and inorganic substances (mercury, potassium iodide, lead, thiocyanate) are excreted in saliva, along with some viruses (those causing rabies and mumps).

> **CLINICAL PHYSIOLOGY:** Excess urea is excreted in saliva nephritis and excess calcium in hyperparathyroidism.

> **APPLIED PHYSIOLOGY:** Substances which increase salivary secretion include sympathomimetic drugs (adrenaline, ephedrine), parasympathomimetic drugs (acetylcholine, pilocarpine, muscarine, physostigmine), histamine and anaesthetics (chloroform, ether), although deep anaesthesia decreases secretion due to central inhibition. Substances which decrease salivary secretion include: sympathetic (ergotamine, dibenamine) and parasympathetic (atropine, scopolamine) depressants.

> **CLINICAL PHYSIOLOGY:** A reduction in secretion (hyposalivation) can be temporary, due to emotional conditions (fear), fever or dehydration, or permanent, due to sialolithiasis (salivary duct obstruction), congenital absence or hypoplasia of the salivary glands, or Bell's palsy (damage to or paralysis of the facial nerve (page 276)). Excess secretion (hypersalivation) can occur during pregnancy or be the result of pathology (ptyalism, sialorrhea, sialism, sialosis); tooth decay or neoplasm in the mouth or tongue due to continuous irritation of the nerve endings; pathology of the oesophagus, stomach or small intestine; neurological disorders (cerebral palsy, mental retardation, cerebral stroke, parkinsonism) and nausea and vomiting.

In addition to hypo and hypersalivation, salivary secretion can be affected in the following:

Xerostomia (dry mouth) caused by dehydration or renal failure; Sjögren syndrome; radiotherapy; salivary gland or duct trauma; the side effects of antihistamines, antidepressants, monoamine oxidase inhibitors, antiparkinsonian drugs and antimuscarinic drugs; shock; after smoking marijuana. It gives rise to difficulties in mastication, swallowing and speech, and causes halitosis.

Drooling (ptyalism) occurs due to excess saliva production, often associated with an inability to retain saliva within the mouth. It occurs during the eruption of teeth in children; upper respiratory tract infection or nasal allergies in children; difficulty in swallowing; tonsillitis and peritonsillar abscess.

Chorda tympani syndrome, characterised by sweating while eating, can occur following trauma or surgical procedures which sever some parasympathetic fibres to the salivary glands. During nerve regeneration some fibres may deviate joining fibres innervating sweat glands.

Mumps (an acute viral infection affecting the parotid glands) is associated with puffiness of the cheeks (due to swelling of the parotid glands), fever, sore throat and weakness. It can also affect the meninges (page 264), gonads and pancreas.

Sjögren syndrome is an autoimmune disorder in which immune cells destroy exocrine glands (lacrimal, salivary). Symptoms include dry mouth, persistent cough, dryness of the eyes, skin, nose and vagina; in severe cases the kidneys, lungs, liver, pancreas, thyroid (page 331), blood vessels and brain may be affected.

Mixing. On leaving the mouth the food bolus enters the oesophagus where it is propelled towards the stomach by primary and secondary peristalsis. Primary peristalsis

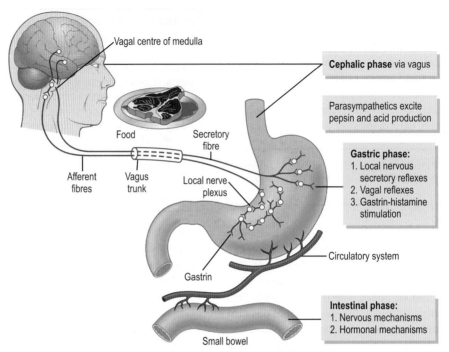

Fig. 6.39 Phases of gastric secretion and their regulation.

is a continuation of the wave that begins in the pharynx spreading into the oesophagus; secondary peristalsis results from distension of the oesophagus itself continuing until all food has emptied into the stomach, which relaxes, together with the duodenum, to receive the food bolus. At the lower end of the oesophagus is the lower oesophageal (gastro-oesophageal, cardiac) sphincter. As the peristaltic wave passes down the oesophagus it relaxes, allowing propulsion of food into the stomach.

into the remainder of the digestive tract; mixing of food with gastric secretions until it forms a semifluid mixture (chyme); and slow release of chyme into the small intestine for its proper digestion and absorption. As long as there is food in the stomach weak peristaltic (mixing) waves continue to move chyme towards the antrum. The stomach also has digestive, protective, haemopoietic and excretory functions, all of which are related to the secretion of substances by cells of the gastric pits. The regulation of gastric secretion is summarised in Fig. 6.39.

CLINICAL ANATOMY: Gastro-oesophageal reflux disease (GORD) is caused by weakness or abnormal relaxation of the gastro-oesophageal sphincter, allowing acid to flow back into the oesophagus, causing heartburn (acid indigestion). Symptoms include chest pain behind the sternum moving upwards into the neck and throat; a bitter or acid taste; difficulty in swallowing (dysphagia); persistent dry cough; hoarseness or sore throat; regurgitation of food or sour liquid (acid reflux) and sensation of a lump in the throat. It is common in the 1st few weeks and months of life as the sphincter has not matured sufficiently. Many babies with reflux gradually improve as they grow, particularly when they start to eat more solid foods and feed in an upright position.

APPLIED PHYSIOLOGY: When the stomach has been empty for several hours, hunger contractions (rhythmic peristaltic contractions in the body of the stomach) can occur, lasting for 2–3 minutes. They are most intense in young healthy individuals, being enhanced by low blood sugar levels. Hunger pangs refers to pain in the pit of the stomach. They do not usually begin until 12–24 hours after the last meal; however, in starvation they reach their greatest intensity after 3–4 days, gradually weakening in the following days.

The motor functions of the stomach are storage of large quantities of food so that it can be processed ready for passage

Stomach emptying is controlled by the degree of filling and the effects of gastrin on stomach peristalsis. Increased pressure in the stomach elicits local myenteric reflexes causing increased emptying and relaxation of the duodenum, and the presence of digestive products of proteins elicits the release of gastrin, causing the secretion of highly acidic gastric juice, which enhances emptying. More important, however, are the inhibitory feedback signals from the duodenum, including both enterogastric inhibitory nervous feedback reflexes and hormonal feedback via CCK. These work together to slow the rate of emptying when too much chyme is already in the small intestine or it is excessively acidic, contains too much unprocessed protein or fat, is hypotonic/hypertonic, or is irritating to the mucosa.

> **CLINICAL PHYSIOLOGY:** Acute gastritis (inflammation of the superficial layers of mucous membrane and infiltration with leucocytes, mainly neutrophils) is caused by *Helicobacter pylori* infection, excess alcohol consumption, excess use of non-steroidal anti-inflammatory drugs (NSAIDs) or trauma from nasogastric tubes. Chronic gastritis (inflammation of the deeper layers, with infiltration of more leucocytes) is caused by chronic *Helicobacter pylori* infection, long-term alcohol abuse and use of NSAIDs or autoimmune disease. There is atrophy of the gastric mucosa with loss of chief and parietal cells from the glands, decreasing the secretion. Symptoms of both acute and chronic gastritis include abdominal discomfort, nausea, vomiting, anorexia, indigestion, feeling of fullness and belching.

> **CLINICAL PHYSIOLOGY:** In gastric atrophy the stomach muscles shrink and become weak; there is also shrinking of the gastric glands, resulting in decreased secretion. It is caused by chronic gastritis (chronic atrophic gastritis), with atrophy of the gastric mucosa and loss of gastric glands. Autoimmune atrophic gastritis also causes gastric atrophy. Generally, there are no noticeable features; however, it can lead to achlorhydria (absence of hydrochloric acid in the gastric secretions) and pernicious anaemia. Some individuals may develop gastric cancer.

> **CLINICAL PHYSIOLOGY:** Peptic ulcer (gastric ulcer in the stomach, duodenal ulcer in the duodenum) involves erosion of the surface as a result of shedding or sloughing of inflamed necrotic tissue lining the organ. It is caused by: increased peptic activity due to excessive secretion of pepsin; hyperacidity of gastric secretions; reduced alkalinity of duodenal content; decreased mucin content in gastric secretions or decreased protective activity; constant emotional or physical stress; excessively spiced or smoked foods (classical causes); long-term use of NSAIDs (aspirin, ibuprofen, naproxen) and chronic *Helicobacter pylori* infection. Common symptoms include pain while eating or drinking (stomach ulcer) or 1–2 hours after eating and during the night (duodenal ulcer); nausea; vomiting; haematemesis (vomiting blood); heartburn (due to acid regurgitation); anorexia and weight loss.

> **CLINICAL PHYSIOLOGY:** Zollinger-Ellison syndrome is characterised by excess hydrochloric acid secretion, caused by a pancreatic tumour producing excess gastrin. Symptoms include abdominal pain; frequent and watery diarrhoea; difficulty eating and occasional haematemesis.

The pancreatic secretions empty into the duodenum, together with bile from the liver. Like saliva, it comprises 99.5% water and 0.5% solids, which are either organic or inorganic substances. The organic substances are mainly proteolytic (trypsin, chymotrypsin, carboxypeptidases, nuclease, elastase, collagenase, pancreatic amylase (an amylolytic enzyme)) or lipolytic (pancreatic lipase, cholesterol ester hydrolase, phospholipase A and B, colipase, bile-salt activated lipase) enzymes, together with albumin and globulin; the inorganic substances are sodium, calcium, potassium, magnesium, bicarbonate, chloride, phosphate and sulphate.

Pancreatic secretion is regulated: by unconditioned (food entering the mouth) and conditioned (acquired/learned) reflexes; following food entering the stomach and the release of gastrin transported to the pancreas in blood; when chyme enters the small intestine releasing many hormones, some of which stimulate secretion (secretin, CCK) and others inhibit secretion (pancreatic polypeptide, somatostatin, peptide YY, peptides (ghrelin, leptin)).

The regulation of pancreatic secretions is summarised in Fig. 6.40.

> **CLINICAL PHYSIOLOGY:** Inflammation of the pancreatic acini (pancreatitis) is rare but dangerous. Acute pancreatitis is more severe, being caused by excess alcohol intake or gallstones, and presents as severe upper abdominal pain, nausea and vomiting, loss of appetite, weight loss, fever and shock. Chronic pancreatitis develops from: repeated acute inflammation or chronic pancreatic damage; obstruction of the duodenal papilla; congenital anomalies of the pancreatic duct; cystic fibrosis; malnutrition; as well as being idiopathic. It can lead to complete destruction of the pancreas; absence of pancreatic enzymes; severe pain in the upper abdomen, radiating to the back; fever, nausea and vomiting; a tender and swollen abdomen and weight loss.

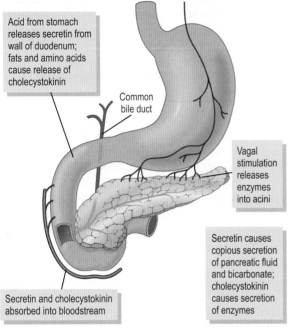

Acid from stomach releases secretin from wall of duodenum; fats and amino acids cause release of cholecystokinin

Common bile duct

Vagal stimulation releases enzymes into acini

Secretin causes copious secretion of pancreatic fluid and bicarbonate; cholecystokinin causes secretion of enzymes

Secretin and cholecystokinin absorbed into bloodstream

Fig. 6.40 Regulation of pancreatic secretion.

CLINICAL PHYSIOLOGY: Steatorrhea is the formation of bulky, foul smelling, frothy clay-coloured stools with large amounts of undigested fat due to impaired digestion and absorption. Causes include lack of pancreatic lipase; liver disease affecting bile secretion; coeliac disease and cystic fibrosis.

Bile is secreted by hepatocytes (page 480) and released into the duodenum together with secretions of the pancreas. It comprises 97.6% water and 2.4% solids, of which some are organic (bile salts, bile pigments, cholesterol, fatty acids, lecithin, mucin) and some inorganic (sodium, calcium, potassium, chloride, bicarbonate) substances. When stored in the gallbladder (page 482) its volume decreases due to the absorption of water and electrolytes (except calcium and potassium). The regulation of liver secretion and gallbladder emptying is summarised in Fig. 6.41.

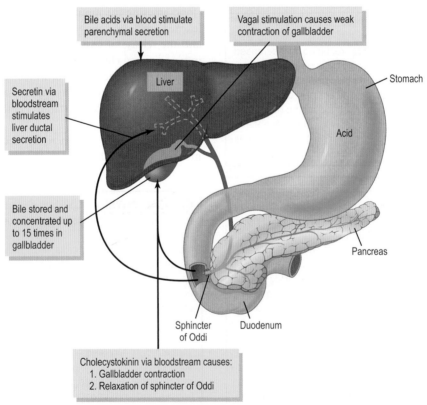

Bile acids via blood stimulate parenchymal secretion

Vagal stimulation causes weak contraction of gallbladder

Secretin via bloodstream stimulates liver ductal secretion

Liver

Stomach

Acid

Bile stored and concentrated up to 15 times in gallbladder

Pancreas

Sphincter of Oddi

Duodenum

Cholecystokinin via bloodstream causes:
1. Gallbladder contraction
2. Relaxation of sphincter of Oddi

Fig. 6.41 Liver secretion and gallbladder emptying.

APPLIED PHYSIOLOGY: Bile has a number of functions: digestive and absorptive, through the action of bile salts; excretory, through bile pigments (the major excretory products of bile), with heavy metals (copper, iron), some bacteria (typhoid bacteria), some toxins, cholesterol, lecithin and alkaline phosphatase also being excreted in bile; laxative action, through the action of bile salts; antiseptic action, by inhibiting the growth of certain bacteria by its natural detergent action; choleretic action, whereby bile salts stimulate bile secretion from the liver; the maintenance of a normal gut pH; prevention of gallstone formation, through the action of bile salts; lubrication, via mucin and gallbladder contraction (cholagogue action), by stimulating CCK secretion.

Secretions from the small intestine (succus entericus), as elsewhere in the digestive tract, comprise 99.5% water and 0.5% solids, which are either organic or inorganic substances. The organic substances are proteolytic enzymes (amino peptidase, dipeptidase, tripeptidase), enterokinase, amylolytic enzymes (sucrose, maltase, lactase, dextrinase, trehalase), lipolytic enzymes (lipase), mucous, intrinsic factor, and defensins; the inorganic substances are sodium, calcium, potassium, bicarbonate, chloride, phosphate and sulphate. The small intestine is responsible for the continued breakdown of the partially digested food and the absorption of carbohydrates, fats, proteins, vitamins, minerals and water. From the lumen these substances pass through the lacteals in the villi, cross the mucosa and

CLINICAL PHYSIOLOGY: The formation of gallstones (cholelithiasis) in the gallbladder or biliary ducts is associated with reabsorption of water from bile. It often originates with bile containing excessive amounts of normal bile components (Fig. 6.42). Saturation with cholesterol can lead to cholesterol stones (most common form); brown or black pigmented stones form when bile contains excessive amounts of unconjugated bilirubin, which can result from chronic haemolysis, as in sickle cell anaemia. Gallstones can lead to biliary obstruction or, more commonly, inflammation in acute or chronic cholecystitis. Removal of the gallbladder due to obstruction or chronic inflammation appears to have few major consequences on digestion.

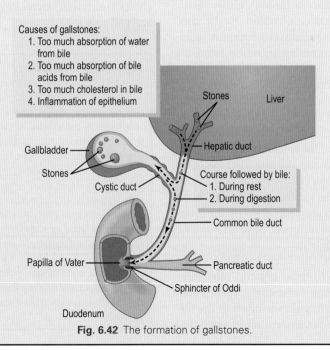

Causes of gallstones:
1. Too much absorption of water from bile
2. Too much absorption of bile acids from bile
3. Too much cholesterol in bile
4. Inflammation of epithelium

Stones

Liver

Gallbladder

Stones

Cystic duct

Hepatic duct

Course followed by bile:
1. During rest
2. During digestion

Common bile duct

Papilla of Vater

Pancreatic duct

Sphincter of Oddi

Duodenum

Fig. 6.42 The formation of gallstones.

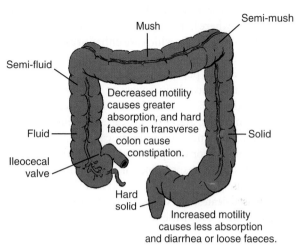

Fig. 6.43 Absorptive and storage functions of the large intestine.

either enter the blood directly or via the lymphatics. The regulation of succus entericus is by both nervous and hormonal mechanisms. Parasympathetic stimulation causes vasodilation and increased secretion, while sympathetic stimulation has the opposite effect: local nervous reflexes, initiated by chyme entering the small intestine, stimulate the mucosa through either tactile stimuli or irritation to increase secretion. At the same time the intestinal mucosa secretes enterocrinin, secretin and CCK, further promoting secretion from the intestinal glands.

As in the small intestine, secretions from the large intestine comprise 99.5% water and 0.5% solids; however, the composition of the solids differs markedly, there being no digestive enzymes while the concentration of bicarbonate is high. The solids consist of organic (albumin, globulin, mucin, urea, debris from epithelial cells) and inorganic (sodium, calcium, potassium, bicarbonate, chloride, phosphate, sulphate) substances. Acids formed by bacterial action are neutralised by the bicarbonate, while the presence of mucin helps to lubricate movement of the bowel contents.

The main function of the large intestine is the absorption of water, electrolytes, organic substances (glucose), alcohol and drugs (anaesthetic agents, sedatives, steroids); however, it is also involved in the formation of faeces through the absorption of water and other unwanted substances (mercury, lead, bismuth, arsenic). It also has a synthetic function in which bacterial flora synthesise vitamins B_{12} and K, which contribute to erythropoietic activity and blood clotting. The proximal half of the large intestine is concerned principally with absorption and the distal half with storage (Fig. 6.43).

Dietary fibre/roughage. A group of food particles which reach the large intestine without being digested. Sources are fruit, vegetables, cereals, bread and wheat grain. It provides a substrate for the microflora of the large intestine and increases bacterial mass. Anaerobic bacteria degrade the fermentable components, with some being absorbed and others excreted in faeces. The major components of dietary fibre are cellulose, hemicellulose, D-glucans, pectin, lignin and gums, of which cellulose, hemicellulose and pectin are partially digestible. Dietary fibre also contains minerals, antioxidants and other chemicals useful for health.

A diet with a high fibre content have health benefits as it delays stomach emptying; increase the formation of bulky soft faeces, which eases defaecation and contain antioxidants and other beneficial substances. Such diets tend to be low in energy and may be useful in weight reduction, with some components also reducing blood cholesterol levels, decreasing the risk of heart disease and gallstones.

APPLIED PHYSIOLOGY: Loose, fluid discharge of intestinal contents (diarrhoea) occurs due to increased movement of food through the digestive tract, with reduced water absorption in the large intestine. Acute diarrhoea is temporary, often due to infections, while chronic diarrhoea can be the result of disorders of the intestinal mucosa. Causes include: dietary factors (contaminated food or water, artificial sweeteners, spicy food); food intolerance (lactose, milk products); infection (bacteria (*Escherichia coli, salmonella, shigella*), viruses (rotavirus, hepatitis virus) and parasites (entamoeba, histolytica, *giardia lamblia*); reaction to medicines (antibiotics, antihypertensive drugs, antacids containing magnesium, laxatives) and intestinal diseases. Severe diarrhoea results in loss of water and electrolytes leading to dehydration and electrolyte imbalance. Chronic diarrhoea can result in hypokalaemia and metabolic acidosis.

APPLIED PHYSIOLOGY: Failure to void faeces (constipation) is due to the lack of intestinal movements, with faeces remaining in the colon for a long time where fluid is continually absorbed resulting in hard dry faeces. It produces discomfort. Causes include: diet (lack of fibre or liquid); irregular bowel habits, due to inhibition of normal defaecation reflexes; spasm of the sigmoid colon (spastic colon) preventing motility; disease; dysfunction of the myenteric plexus in the large intestine (megacolon) and drugs (diuretics, pain relievers/narcotics, antihypertensive drugs such as calcium channel blockers, antiparkinson drugs, antidepressants, anticonvulsants).

Movement of food through the digestive tract

Small intestine. Movements of the small intestine are a mixture of mixing and/or propulsive contractions: when a portion of the small intestine becomes distended, stretching of its wall elicits localised concentric contractions causing segmentation (Fig. 6.44). As one set of contractions relaxes, a new set often begins at a new point dividing the chyme into segments, promoting its mixing with the succus entericus. The frequency of contractions is normally 2–4 per minute, although with intense stimulation it can reach 12 per minute in the duodenum and proximal jejunum and 8–9 per minute in the ileum. Segmentation contractions are weaker when excitatory activity of the enteric nervous system is blocked by atropine.

Chyme is propelled through the small intestine by peristaltic waves (Fig. 6.44) moving it towards the anus. They are usually weak and die out after travelling 3–5 cm. Peristaltic activity increases after eating via the gastroenteric reflex initiated in the stomach and conducted mainly through the myenteric plexus along the wall of the small intestine. In addition, gastrin, motilin and serotonin all enhance motility, while secretin and glucagon inhibit it. In addition to moving chyme forwards, peristalsis also spreads it out along the intestinal mucosa.

APPLIED PHYSIOLOGY: The muscularis interna cause short folds to appear in the mucosa increasing the surface area for absorption. Individual muscle fibres extend into the villi, with their contraction and relaxation resulting in lymph flowing freely from the central lacteals of the villi into the lymphatic system. These contractions of the mucosa and villi are mainly initiated by local nerve reflexes in the submucosal plexus in response to the presence of chyme in the small intestine.

Ileocaecal valve. Its main function is the prevention of backflow into the small intestine. The ileocaecal sphincter remains slightly constricted controlling the slow emptying of ileal contents into the caecum. Following eating, peristalsis in the ileum intensifies and emptying of ileal contents into the caecum starts. Any resistance to emptying facilitates absorption. The regulation of the passage of chyme through the ileocaecal valve is shown in Fig. 6.45.

APPLIED PHYSIOLOGY: Inflammation of the appendix can cause intense spasm of the ileocaecal sphincter and partial paralysis of the ileum, which together can block emptying of the ileum into the caecum. These reflexes are mediated by the myenteric plexus and prevertebral sympathetic ganglia.

Stimulus by stretching of intestinal wall

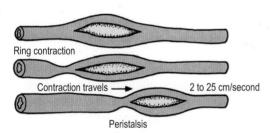

Ring contraction

Contraction travels →   2 to 25 cm/second

Peristalsis

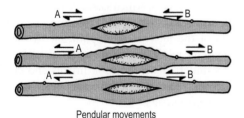

Pendular movements

Inactive state

Alternating contractions

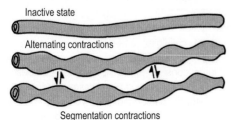

Segmentation contractions

Fig. 6.44 Movements of the small intestine.

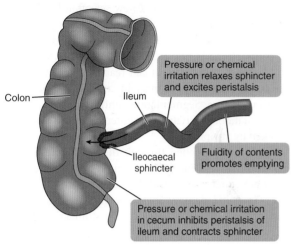

Colon

Ileum

Pressure or chemical irritation relaxes sphincter and excites peristalsis

Ileocaecal sphincter

Fluidity of contents promotes emptying

Pressure or chemical irritation in cecum inhibits peristalsis of ileum and contracts sphincter

Fig. 6.45 Emptying at the ileocaecal valve.

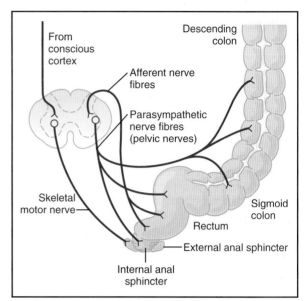

From conscious cortex

Descending colon

Afferent nerve fibres

Parasympathetic nerve fibres (pelvic nerves)

Skeletal motor nerve

Sigmoid colon

Rectum

External anal sphincter

Internal anal sphincter

Fig. 6.46 The defaecation reflex. Afferent and efferent fibres pass through pelvic parasympathetic nerves; voluntary control is mediated by the pudendal nerve; the defaecation centre is located in sacral spinal cord segments.

Large intestine. Because intense movements of the wall of the large intestine are not required, its movements tend to be sluggish; nevertheless, they have similar characteristics to those of the small intestine, having both mixing and propulsive actions. Large circular constrictions occur, occasionally almost occluding the lumen, which together with contraction of the longitudinal muscle causes unstimulated parts of the large intestine to bulge outwards into sacs (haustrations). With each contraction faecal material is rolled over so that it all comes into contact with the mucosa, promoting fluid and dissolved substances to be progressively absorbed.

Between the caecum and sigmoid colon mass movements, lasting many minutes, take over the propulsive role. They usually only occur one to three times a day. If a mass movement forces faeces into the rectum, the desire to defecate occurs immediately.

APPLIED PHYSIOLOGY: Irritation of the colon can initiate intense mass movements. Individuals with ulcerative colitis (page 475) frequently have mass movements which persist most of the time.

Defaecation. Most of the time the rectum is empty, but when faecal material enters it the desire to defecate is immediate. The continuous dribble of faecal matter through the anus is prevented by tonic constriction of the internal (smooth muscle) and external (skeletal muscle) anal sphincters. The external anal sphincter (page 555) is innervated by the pudendal nerve (page 580), part of the somatic nervous system and therefore under

voluntary control: it is usually kept continuously constricted, unless voluntary signals inhibit its constriction.

The deafecation reflex (Fig. 6.46) is initiated by distension of the rectum stimulating sensory nerve endings, with the impulses transmitted by afferent fibres to the defaecation centre in sacral segments of the spinal cord. The centre then sends motor impulses via efferent fibres of pelvic nerves, which cause strong contraction of the descending colon, sigmoid colon and rectum and relaxation of the internal anal sphincter. At the same time, voluntary relaxation of the external anal sphincter occurs under cortical control. Infants and children develop the defaecation reflex to enable them to control their bowel movements.

APPLIED ANATOMY: Flatulence is the production and release of a mixture of intestinal gases (flatus) from bacterial action on undigested sugars and polysaccharides (starch, cellulose), and digestion of flatulence food (cheese, yeast in bread, oats, onion, beans, cabbage, milk). Flatus consists of swallowed non-odorous gases (nitrogen, oxygen); non-odorous gases produced by microbes (methane, carbon dioxide, hydrogen) and odorous materials (low molecular weight fatty acids (butyric acid), reduced sulphur compounds (hydrogen sulphide, carbonyl sulphide)).

TABLE 6.3   Carbohydrate Digestion in Different Regions of the Digestive Tract

Region	Secretion	Enzyme	Substrate	End Product
Mouth	Saliva	Salivary amylase	Polysaccharides (cooked starch)	Disaccharides (dextrin, maltose)
Stomach	Gastric juice	Gastric amylase	Weak amylase	Negligible action
Small intestine	Pancreatic juice	Pancreatic amylase	Polysaccharides	Disaccharides (dextrin, maltose, maltotriose)
	Succus entericus	Sucrase	Sucrose	Glucose, fructose
		Maltase	Maltose and maltotriose	Glucose
		Lactase	Lactose	Glucose, galactose
		Dextrinase	Dextrin, maltose, maltotriose	Glucose
		Trehalase	Trehalose	Glucose

Nutrition

The biochemical and physiological process by which food is used to support life. It includes ingestion, digestion, absorption, assimilation, biosynthesis, catabolism and excretion. All ingested food is a combination of carbohydrate, fat and protein, with traces of vitamins and minerals. The aim of most chemical reactions in cells is to make the energy in food available to the numerous physiological systems of the cell.

All foods can be oxidised in cells, releasing large amounts of energy; however to provide this energy the chemical reactions need to be coupled with the system responsible for these physiological functions. Adenosine triphosphate (ATP) is an essential link between the energy-utilising and energy-producing functions; it can be gained and spent repeatedly. Energy from the oxidation of carbohydrates, fats and proteins is used to convert adenosine diphosphate (ADP) to ATP. This conversion is necessary for the active transport of molecules across cell membranes, muscle contraction and the performance of work, synthetic reactions which create hormones, cell membranes and other essential molecules of the body, conduction of nerve impulses, cell division and growth, and other physiological functions necessary to maintain life.

Carbohydrates. The human diet contains three types of carbohydrate: polysaccharides, with large polysaccharides (glycogen, amylose, amylopectin) in the form of starch (glucose polymers), glycogen is available in non-vegetarian diets, while amylose and amylopectin are available in vegetarian diets; disaccharides, in the form of sucrose (glucose and fructose) and lactose (glucose

and galactose) and monosaccharides, mostly as glucose and fructose, with other carbohydrates in the diet (alcohol, lactic acid, pyruvic acid, pectins, dextrins, carbohydrates in meat).

Digestion of carbohydrates. This occurs in the mouth, stomach and small intestine (Table 6.3). The final products of carbohydrate digestion are glucose, fructose and galactose, of which 80% is glucose.

Before glucose can be used by cells it must be transported through the cell membrane into the cellular cytoplasm. It does this by facilitated diffusion by which the glucose binds with protein carrier molecules in the cell membrane.

Absorption of carbohydrates. Carbohydrates are absorbed from the small intestine mainly as monosaccharides (glucose, galactose, fructose). Glucose is transported from the gut lumen into the epithelial cells in the mucous membrane by sodium cotransport. The energy for this is obtained by binding sodium ions and glucose molecules to a carrier protein. After absorption from the digestive tract much of the fructose and almost all of the galactose is rapidly converted to glucose in the liver. Glucose is, therefore, the final common pathway for the transport of almost all carbohydrates to the tissue cells.

Metabolism of carbohydrates. The release of energy from carbohydrates is mainly by oxidation (catabolism), with part of the energy used by cells and tissues for physiological actions, and the remainder stored as rich energy phosphate bonds, protein, carbohydrates and fats in the tissues (anabolism).

Following absorption into the cell, glucose can be immediately released for energy to the cell or stored as

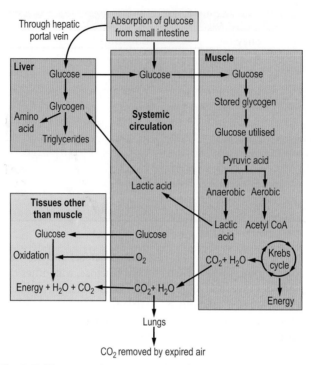

Fig. 6.47 Diagrammatic representation of carbohydrate metabolism.

glycogen. Liver and muscle cells can store large amounts of glycogen without significantly changing the osmotic pressure of the intracellular fluids. The breakdown of stored glycogen (glycogenolysis) is by the process of phosphorylation, catalysed by the enzyme phosphorylase, when stimulated by epinephrine/adrenaline or glucagon. Epinephrine is released by the adrenal medulla (page 347) under sympathetic stimulation. This stimulates liver and muscle cells to increase the availability of glucose for rapid energy metabolism. Glucagon is secreted by α cells in the pancreas when blood glucose levels fall too low and promotes the conversion of liver glycogen into glucose and its release into the blood. The rate of glucose transport is increased by insulin. The amount of glucose that can diffuse into cells, except those of the liver and brain, in the absence of insulin is insufficient to supply the amount required for its metabolism.

A diagrammatic representation of carbohydrate metabolism is given in Fig. 6.47; however, the associated biochemical processes are outside the scope of this text.

The reader is, therefore, referred to an appropriate textbook of physiology and/or biochemistry.

Fats/lipids. Fats/lipids are mostly consumed as neutral fats (triglycerides), being the major constituent of animal products and much less in plant products. In addition, the diet usually contains small amounts of cholesterol and cholesterol esters. Dietary fats are either saturated fats, triglycerides from only saturated fatty acids, or unsaturated, formed by dehydrogenation of saturated fatty acids. Unsaturated fats are mono-unsaturated, polyunsaturated (essential fatty acids of two types (Omega-3 and Omega-6)) or trans fats. The sources and functions of different dietary fats are shown in Table 6.4.

Digestion of fats/lipids. Fats are digested by lipolytic enzymes secreted in the mouth (lingual lipase), stomach (gastric lipase) and small intestine, with most fats being digested in the small intestine due to the presence of bile salts, pancreatic lipolytic enzymes and intestinal lipase (Table 6.5). The end products of fat digestion are fatty acids, cholesterol and monoglycerides.

TABLE 6.4 Sources and Functions of Dietary Fats

Type	Sources	Functions
Saturated fats	Full-fat milk, cream, cheese, butter; deep fried fast food; coconut and palm oil; fatty meat; commercially baked biscuits and pastries	Increases blood cholesterol, with the risk of atherosclerosis and coronary heart disease
Monounsaturated fats	Oils (canola, olive, peanut); nuts (cashews, almonds, hazelnuts, peanuts); margarine	Decreases blood cholesterol decreasing the risk of coronary heart disease
Polyunsaturated fats	Fruit and vegetables; vegetable oils (corn, soy, sunflower); walnuts; flax seeds; lean meat; fish and seafood; eggs	Decreases blood cholesterol and triglycerides reducing blood pressure, the risk of coronary heart disease, obesity, platelet aggregation. Increases disease-countering actions in the body
Trans fats	Milk; cheese; lamb and beef	Increases low-density lipoproteins (LPLs) increasing the risk of atherosclerosis and coronary heart disease

TABLE 6.5 Digestion of Lipids

Region	Secretion	Enzyme	Substrate	End Product
Mouth	Saliva	Lingual lipase	Triglycerides	Fatty acid 1, 2 diacylglycerol
Stomach	Gastric juice	Gastric lipase (weak)	Triglycerides	Fatty acids; glycerol
Small intestine	Pancreatic juice	Pancreatic lipase	Triglycerides	Monoglycerides; fatty acids
		Cholesterol ester lipase	Cholesterol ester	Free cholesterol; fatty acids
		Phospholipase A	Phospholipids	Lysophospholipids
		Phospholipase B	Lysophospholipids	Phosphoryl choline; free fatty acids
		Colipase	Facilitates action of pancreatic lipase	
		Bile-salt-activated lipase	Phospholipids Cholesterol esters	Lysophospholipids
	Succus entericus	Intestinal lipase	Triglycerides	Fatty acids; glycerol (weak action)

Absorption of fats/lipids. Monoglycerides, cholesterol and fatty acids enter cells of the intestinal mucosa by simple diffusion, from where further transport occurs. In the mucosal cells most monoglycerides are converted to triglycerides, which, together with cholesterol esters, are coated with a layer of protein, cholesterol and phospholipids forming chylomicrons. Because of their large size chylomicrons enter the lymph vessels and are then transferred to blood vessels. From the mucosal cells fatty acids enter the portal blood (transported as free or unesterified fatty acids). The presence of bile salts is essential for fat absorption. Most fats are absorbed in the upper part of the small intestine.

Fats are stored in adipose tissue (neutral/tissue fat) and the liver. As chylomicrons pass through the capillaries of adipose tissue or the liver the triglycerides are hydrolysed by lipoprotein lipase into free fatty acids and glycerol, which enter the fat cells (adipocytes/lipocytes) of the adipose tissue or liver, where they are again converted to triglycerides and stored. The other components of the chylomicron (cholesterol, phospholipids) are released into the bloodstream, where they combine with proteins to form lipoproteins. When energy is required by other tissues the stored triglycerides are hydrolysed into free fatty acids and glycerol, with the free fatty acid transported to the tissues in the bloodstream in combination with albumin.

Phospholipids have a number of functions: they are an important constituent of lipoproteins in blood, being essential for their formation, their absence results in abnormalities in the transport of cholesterol and other lipids; thromboplastin is necessary to initiate the clotting process; sphingomyelin acts as an electrical insulator in the myelin sheath around nerves; they donate phosphate radicals for different chemical reactions in tissues; and participate in the formation of structural elements, mainly membranes, in cells.

Cholesterol is slowly absorbed from the digestive tract into intestinal lymph. Being highly soluble in fat, but only slightly soluble in water, it is capable of forming esters with fatty acids. Plasma cholesterol concentration depends on: daily cholesterol intake; a highly saturated fat diet increases concentration, especially when associated with excess weight gain and obesity; unsaturated fatty acids decrease concentration; lack of insulin or growth hormone increase concentrations; and genetic disorders (mutations of the low-density lipoprotein (LDL) receptor gene) of cholesterol metabolism can increase concentrations.

Cholesterol is used by the: liver to form cholic acid (about 80%); adrenal glands to form adrenocortical hormones; testes to form testosterone; and ovaries to form progesterone and oestrogen. It is precipitated in the skin, together with other lipids, making it highly resistant to water-soluble substances and the action of many chemical agents. Cholesterol also helps prevent water evaporation from the skin.

Lipoproteins are small particles containing cholesterol, phospholipids, triglycerides and proteins (β globulins/apoproteins). They are classified into four types depending on their density:

Very-low-density lipoproteins (VLDL) contain high concentrations of triglycerides and moderate concentrations of cholesterol and phospholipids. They carry cholesterol from the liver to organs and tissues and are associated with atherosclerosis and heart disease.

Intermediate-density lipoproteins (IDL) are derived from VLDL by the removal of most of the triglycerides. They contain high concentrations of cholesterol and phospholipids due to the removal of triglycerides, and transport triglycerides, cholesterol and phospholipids from the liver to peripheral tissues.

Low-density lipoproteins (LDLs) are formed from IDL by the complete removal of triglycerides and only contain cholesterol and phospholipids. They carry cholesterol and phospholipids from the liver to different areas of the body (muscle, heart) and are responsible for the deposition of cholesterol on arterial walls (atherosclerosis), as well as increasing the risk of heart disease.

High-density lipoproteins (HDLs) contain high concentrations of proteins with low concentrations of cholesterol and phospholipids. They carry cholesterol and phospholipids from tissues and organs back to the liver for degradation and elimination, preventing the deposition of cholesterol on arterial walls.

LDL is often referred as 'bad cholesterol' as it takes cholesterol from the liver to different areas of the body, while HDL is often referred to 'good cholesterol' because it reduces blood cholesterol levels. HDL also helps in the normal functioning of some hormones and tissues of the body, as well as being used in the formation of bile. A high level of HDL is a good indicator of a healthy heart. Details of adipose tissue can be found on pages 27 and 502.

CLINICAL PHYSIOLOGY: Atherosclerosis is a disease of large and intermediate-sized arteries in which fatty lesions (atheromatous plaques) develop on the internal surfaces of arteries. It can be caused by damage to the vascular endothelium, which increases the expression of adhesion molecules on endothelial cells. Following damage circulating monocytes and lipids (mainly LDLs) accumulate at the site of injury. Monocytes cross the endothelium and enter the intima of the vessel wall and become macrophages, which ingest and oxidise the accumulated lipoproteins (macrophage foam cells) to form fatty streaks on the vessel wall (Fig. 6.48A). Over time the fatty streaks enlarge and coalesce, with the surrounding fibrous and smooth muscle tissues proliferating, forming larger and larger plaques (Fig. 6.48B) which can obliterate the vessel lumen. Atherosclerotic arteries become hardened due to the deposition of extensive amounts of dense connective tissue losing most of their distensibility; they are also easily ruptured. Where plaques protrude into the blood flow their rough surfaces can cause blood clots to develop, resulting in thrombus or embolus formation and sudden blockage of all blood flow in the artery. Risk factors, other than LDLs, include physical inactivity and/or obesity; diabetes mellitus; hypertension, increasing the risk of coronary artery disease; hyperlipidaemia and smoking.

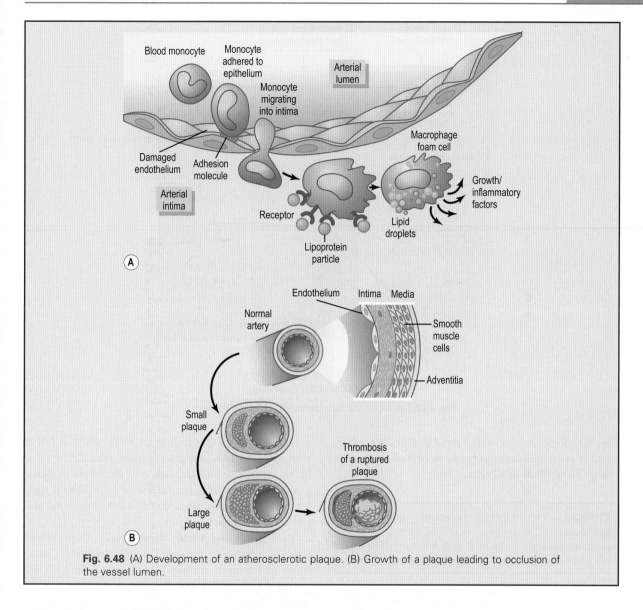

Fig. 6.48 (A) Development of an atherosclerotic plaque. (B) Growth of a plaque leading to occlusion of the vessel lumen.

Metabolism of fats/lipids. The initial stage in using triglycerides for energy is their hydrolysis into fatty acids and glycerol, which are both transported in the blood to active tissues where they are oxidised to release energy. Glycerol is immediately changed by intracellular enzymes into glycerol-3-phosphate, which enters the glycolytic pathway for glucose breakdown and is stored as energy. The fatty acids are degraded and oxidised in the mitochondria.

Carbohydrate utilisation, when excess quantities of carbohydrates are present, is preferred to that of fat. However, when carbohydrates are not available fat is mobilised from adipose tissue and used for energy. A number of hormonal changes occur to promote fatty acid mobilisation, among them being a decrease in insulin secretion (reducing the rate of glucose utilisation) and decreased fat storage. Epinephrine (adrenaline) and norepinephrine (noradrenaline), released from the adrenal medulla (page 347) by sympathetic stimulation, activate hormone-sensitive triglyceride lipase resulting in the rapid breakdown of triglycerides and mobilisation of fatty acids. During stress, corticotropin is released by the anterior pituitary (page 335) causing the adrenal cortex (page 343) to secrete glucocorticoids; both activate the same hormone-sensitive triglyceride lipase. Growth hormone can have a similar, but milder, effect.

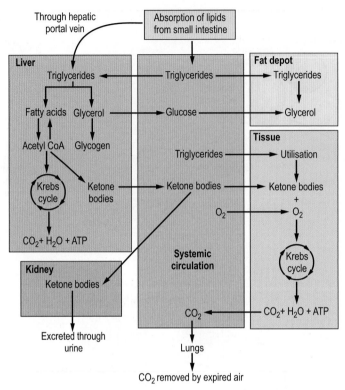

Fig. 6.49 Diagrammatic representation of fat metabolism.

Thyroid hormone also causes a rapid mobilisation of fat, possibly as an indirect response to an overall increase in energy metabolism in all cells.

> **CLINICAL PHYSIOLOGY:** Excessive corticotropin and glucocorticoid secretion over long periods of time occur in Cushing's syndrome, with fats frequently mobilised to such an extent that ketosis develops.

A diagrammatic representation of fat/lipid metabolism is given in Fig. 6.49; however, the associated biochemical processes are outside the scope of this text. The reader is, therefore, referred to an appropriate textbook of physiology and/or biochemistry.

Adipose tissue. A loose connective tissue consisting of adipocytes (fat cells, lipocytes), which is the storage site of fat in the form of triglycerides. It is of two types.

White adipose tissue (white fat) is distributed throughout the body deep to the skin (subcutaneous fat) and surrounds internal organs; the cells are unilocular having one large vacuole filled with fat. It has three functions: energy storage regulated by hormones, especially insulin, depending on blood glucose levels, with increases in blood glucose levels stimulating insulin to synthesise and store fat and decreases in blood glucose levels causing the release of fat, which is used for energy; heat insulation due to subcutaneous fat and protection of internal organs.

Brown adipose tissue (brown fat), a specialised form of adipose tissue, present only in certain areas (back of the neck, intrascapular region); the cells are multilocular, with each cell having many small vacuoles filled with fat. It does not store fat but utilises fat in the tissue releasing energy directly as heat. In this way it has an important role in regulating body temperature, especially in infants. The mitochondria contain an uncoupling protein (mitochondrial uncoupling protein 1/thermogenin), which allows the controlled entry of protons, without ATP synthesis, in order to generate heat.

> **APPLIED PHYSIOLOGY:** Brown fat is abundant in infants, forming 5% of total body fat. After infancy it gradually disappears, being only 1% in adults.

Proteins. Structural proteins, enzymes, nucleoproteins, proteins that transport oxygen, proteins in muscle causing contraction and many others performing specific intracellular and extracellular functions constitute 75% of the body solids. The principal constituents of proteins are amino acids. Proteins present in meat include collagen, albumin, myosin; in eggs include albumin, vitellin; in milk include casein, lactalbumin, albumin, myosin and in wheat include gluten (glutenin and gliadin).

Digestion of proteins. Proteins are digested by proteolytic enzymes secreted in the stomach (pepsin) and small intestine, with most proteins being digested in the duodenum and jejunum by the proteolytic enzymes of the pancreas (trypsin, chymotrypsin, carboxypeptidases) and the succus entericus (dipeptidases, tripeptidases, aminopeptidases). The final products of protein digestion are amino acids (Table 6.6).

Absorption of proteins. The products of digestion and absorption of proteins are almost entirely amino acids; only rarely are polypeptides and whole protein molecules absorbed from the digestive tract into the blood. Protein digestion and absorption extends over 2–3 hours, allowing only small quantities of amino acids to be absorbed at a time. After entering the blood excess amino acids are absorbed within 5–10 minutes by cells throughout the body, especially the liver, with the result that large concentrations of amino acids almost never accumulate in the blood and tissue fluids; nevertheless, the turnover of amino acids is very rapid. Amino acid molecules are too large to diffuse through cell membranes, consequently they move in and out of cells by either facilitated or active transport using carrier mechanisms. In the kidneys some amino acids are actively reabsorbed through the proximal tubular epithelium, removing them from the glomerular filtrate returning them to the blood.

Immediately after entering tissue cells the amino acids combine forming cellular proteins, which can be stored; however, many intracellular proteins can be rapidly decomposed into amino acids by intracellular lysosomal digestive enzymes and transported back into the blood. Exceptions are proteins in the nuclear chromosomes and structural proteins (collagen, muscle contractile proteins), which do not participate significantly in the reverse digestion and transport back out of cells. Growth hormone and insulin increase the formation of tissue proteins, whereas adrenocortical glucocorticoid hormones increase the concentration of plasma amino acids. There is a constant exchange of amino acids between tissue cells and blood. A tissue requiring proteins can synthesise them from amino acids in the blood, which are replenished by degradation of proteins from other cells, especially the liver.

TABLE 6.6 Digestion of Proteins

Region	Secretion	Enzyme	Substrate	End Product
Mouth	Saliva	No proteolytic enzymes		
Stomach	Gastric juice	Pepsin	Proteins	Proteases, peptones, large polypeptides
Small intestine	Pancreatic juice	Trypsin	Proteoses	Dipeptides, tripeptides, polypeptides
		Chymotrypsin	Peptones	
		Carboxypeptidases A and B	Dipeptides, tripeptides, polypeptides	Amino acids
	Succus entericus	Dipeptidases	Dipeptides	Amino acids
		Tripeptidases	Tripeptides	
		Amino peptidases	Large polypeptides	

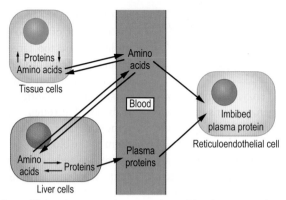

Fig. 6.50 Reversible equilibrium between plasma amino acids, plasma proteins and tissue proteins.

Plasma proteins. The major types of protein in plasma are: albumin, which provides colloid osmotic pressure in the plasma preventing its loss from capillaries; globulin, which performs enzymatic functions in the plasma, as well as being principally responsible for the body's natural and acquired immunity against invading organisms; and fibrinogen, which is important in forming blood clots that help repair leaks in the circulatory system. When tissues are depleted of proteins, the plasma proteins act as a source of rapid replenishment, being imbibed by tissue macrophages through pinocytosis and then split into amino acids, which are then transported back into blood for use throughout the body. There is a constant state of equilibrium between plasma proteins, amino acids in the plasma and tissue proteins (Fig. 6.50).

> **APPLIED PHYSIOLOGY:** An effective therapy for severe, acute whole-body protein deficiency is intravenous plasma protein transfusion. Within hours/days the amino acids of the infused proteins are forming new proteins in cells throughout the body.

Essential and non-essential amino acids. Ten amino acids (threonine, lysine, methionine, arginine, valine, phenylalanine, leucine, tryptophan, isoleucine and histidine), normally present in animal proteins, can be synthesised in cells. Because they can be synthesised, they are referred to as being non-essential amino acids. However, the remaining 10 amino acids (glycine, proline,

alanine, serine, cysteine, aspartic acid, glutamic acid, asparagine, glutamine and tyrosine) cannot be synthesised, or not in sufficient amounts for the body's needs, and are, therefore, referred to essential amino acids.

> **APPLIED PHYSIOLOGY:** The synthesis of non-essential amino acids requires derivatives of vitamin B_6 (pyridoxine), without which amino acids are poorly synthesised and protein formation cannot proceed normally.

Metabolism of proteins. Once cells are replete with protein, additional amino acids in body fluids are degraded and used for energy or stored mainly as fat or secondarily as glycogen. The degradation occurs almost entirely in the liver by the process of deamination (removal of amino groups from the amino acids). The ammonia released during deamination is removed from blood by conversion into urea, which diffuses from liver cells into the body fluids and is excreted by the kidneys. A diagrammatic representation of protein metabolism is given in Fig. 6.51; however, the associated biochemical processes are outside the scope of this text. The reader is, therefore, referred to an appropriate textbook of physiology and/or biochemistry.

> **APPLIED PHYSIOLOGY:** Of the 20 amino acids, 18 can be converted to glucose (gluconeogenesis) and 19 can be converted into keto or fatty acids (ketogenesis).

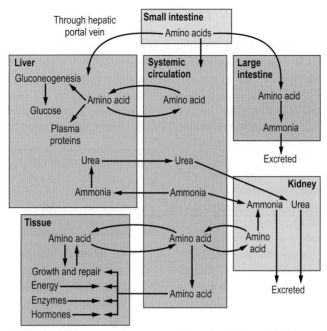

Fig. 6.51 Diagrammatic representation of protein metabolism.

CLINICAL PHYSIOLOGY: In serious liver disease ammonia accumulates in the blood. This is extremely toxic, especially to the brain, and can lead to hepatic coma.

When an individual eats no protein, a certain proportion of body protein is degraded into amino acids and then deaminated and oxidised. This is the obligatory degradation/loss of protein.

APPLIED PHYSIOLOGY: Except for the obligatory degradation of protein, during starvation the body uses carbohydrates and fats (protein sparers) for energy as long as they are available. When these begin to run out, usually after several weeks, the amino acids in blood are rapidly deaminated and oxidised for energy, with a rapid loss of tissue proteins, resulting in the deterioration of cellular function.

Vitamins. Small quantities of vitamins (organic compounds) are needed for normal metabolism, which cannot be produced in the body's cells. Important vitamins needed on a daily basis are:

Vitamin A (occurring in tissues as retinol) is needed to form the visual pigments to prevent 'night blindness'. It is also necessary for normal growth of most cells, especially for growth and differentiation of epithelial cells. Lack of vitamin A leads to: epithelium becoming stratified and keratinised, presenting as scaliness of the skin and acne; failure of growth in the young, including the arrest of skeletal growth; failure of reproduction, associated with atrophy of testicular germinal epithelium and occasionally interruption of the female menstrual cycle; and corneal keratinisation leading to blindness. The damaged epithelial structures may become infected (conjunctivitis, lining of the urinary and reproductive tracts).

Vitamin B$_1$ (thiamine) is needed for the final metabolism of carbohydrates and many amino acids. Thiamine deficiency (beriberi) results in decreased utilisation of pyruvic acid and some amino acids by tissues and increased utilisation of fats; chromatolysis and swelling of neuronal cells in the CNS, disrupting communication between them; degeneration of myelin sheaths in the central and peripheral nervous systems, with the peripheral nerves becoming extremely irritable, characterised by pain radiating along the course of one or several peripheral nerves; fibres/tracts within the spinal cord can degenerate leading to muscle weakness, atrophy and occasionally paralysis; peripheral vasodilation increasing venous return, with cardiac failure due to weakened cardiac muscle accompanied by peripheral oedema and ascites; and gastrointestinal deficiencies (indigestion, severe constipation, anorexia, gastric atony, hypochlorhydria).

Vitamin B$_2$ (riboflavin) combines in tissues forming flavin mononucleotide (FMN) and flavin adenine dinucleotide (FAD). These are hydrogen carriers in the oxidative systems of mitochondria. Riboflavin deficiency usually causes mild symptoms (digestive disturbances, burning sensations of the skin and eyes, skin cracking at the corners of the mouth, headaches, mental depression, forgetfulness). It may occur with deficiencies in thiamine or niacin, or both, leading to a number of deficiency syndromes (pellagra, beriberi, sprue, kwashiorkor).

Vitamin B$_6$ (pyridoxine) functions as a coenzyme for many chemical reactions related to amino acid and protein metabolism. In children, pyridoxine can cause seizures, dermatitis and digestive disturbances (nausea, vomiting).

Vitamin B$_{12}$ has several metabolic functions, including promoting growth and red blood cell formation and maturation. Its deficiency leads to pernicious anaemia; demyelination of nerve fibres, especially in the dorsal, and occasionally lateral, columns of the spinal cord, leading to loss of peripheral sensation and occasionally paralysis.

Vitamin C (ascorbic acid) is essential for the growth and strength of fibres in the subcutaneous tissue, cartilage, bone and teeth; without it the collagen fibres formed are defective and weak. In vitamin C deficiency (scurvy): after 20–30 weeks wounds can take months rather than weeks to heal, due to the failure of cells to deposit collagen fibrils and intercellular cement; bone growth also ceases, even though the epiphyses continue to proliferate no new collagen is laid down between the cells; bone fractures easily as osteoblasts cannot form new bone matrix and fails to heal; and blood vessel walls become fragile due to failure (i) of endothelial cells to be cemented together properly, and (ii) to form collagen fibrils normally present in vessel walls. Capillaries are likely to rupture leading to numerous small petechial haemorrhages, with those beneath the skin causing purpuric blotches.

> **CLINICAL PHYSIOLOGY:** In extreme scurvy muscle cells can fragment; lesions of the gums occur, accompanied by loosening of the teeth; mouth infections develop and vomiting of blood, bloody stools and cerebral haemorrhage occurs. A high fever usually develops before death occurs.

Vitamin D increases calcium absorption from the digestive tract and also helps control calcium deposition in bone.

Vitamin E has a protective role in the prevention of oxidation of unsaturated fats. In vitamin E deficiency the quantity of unsaturated fats in cells becomes diminished resulting in abnormal structure and function of cellular organelles (mitochondria, lysosomes) and even the cell membrane.

Vitamin K is important in blood coagulation; its deficiency results in poor/delayed blood clotting.

> **APPLIED PHYSIOLOGY:** It is rare for an individual to have a bleeding deficiency due to vitamin K in the diet; however, when colon bacteria are destroyed by large amounts of antibiotics it can rapidly occur because of a paucity in the normal diet.

Folic (pteroylglutamic) acid is required for growth and the maturation of red blood cells, being more potent than vitamin B$_{12}$. Folic acid deficiency leads to macrocytic anaemia, which is almost identical to pernicious anaemia, but can be effectively treated by folic acid alone.

Niacin (nicotinic acid) functions in the body as a coenzyme which combines with hydrogen as it is removed from food substrates by dehydrogenases. In niacin deficiency the normal rate of dehydrogenation cannot be maintained, so that the oxidative delivery of energy from food to cells cannot occur at normal rates. In the early stages there is muscle weakness and poor glandular secretion; however, with severe deficiency tissue death occurs, with pathological lesions appearing in many parts of the CNS, permanent dementia and/or psychoses. Skin exposed to mechanical or sun irritation develops a cracked, pigmented, scaly appearance; there is intense irritation and inflammation of the mucous membrane of the mouth and other parts of the digestive tract, which can lead to gastrointestinal haemorrhage.

> **APPLIED PHYSIOLOGY:** Niacin deficiency (pellagra) is exacerbated in individuals who eat a corn-based diet due to the lack of the amino acid tryptophan.

Pantothenic acid is mainly incorporated into the body as coenzyme A (CoA), which has many metabolic roles. Its deficiency can lead to depressed metabolism of carbohydrates and fats.

Mineral metabolism. As well as carbohydrates, fats, proteins and vitamins the body also requires minerals, some in extremely small amounts (trace elements), to function normally.

Magnesium acts as a catalyst for enzymatic reactions related to carbohydrate metabolism. Low concentrations cause increased irritability of the nervous system, peripheral vasodilation and cardiac arrhythmias, especially following acute myocardial infarction.

Calcium is present in bone and extracellular fluid. Excess levels in extracellular fluid can cause the heart to stop in systole and also be a mental depressant; low levels can cause spontaneous discharge of nerve fibres (tetany).

Phosphorus Phosphate is the major anion in intracellular fluid and is important for many metabolic processes.

Iron is essential for the transport of oxygen to the tissues and the operation of oxidative systems within cells; without iron life would cease in seconds. Two-thirds of iron in the body is in the form of haemoglobin (page 109).

Iodine is essential for the formation of thyroxine and triiodothyronine (page 340), which are responsible for the maintenance of normal metabolic rates in all cells.

Zinc is essential for the performance of many reactions associated with carbon dioxide metabolism, an integral part of many enzymes (including carbonic anhydrase). Carbonic anhydrase is responsible for the rapid combination of carbon dioxide with water in red blood cells of peripheral capillary blood and for the rapid release of carbon dioxide from pulmonary capillary blood into the alveoli. Carbonic anhydrase is also present in the digestive tract, kidney tubules and epithelial cells of many glands. Zinc is also important for the interconversions between pyruvic and lactic acid, and for the digestion of proteins in the digestive tract.

Fluorine does not appear to be necessary for metabolism, but its presence when teeth are being formed helps protect against caries. Excess fluorine intake (fluorosis) causes mottled teeth and, in more severe cases, enlarged bones.

Sodium is found mainly in body fluids helping to maintain blood volume and blood pressure by attracting and holding water. It is important in cellular osmotic processes (passage of fluids into and out of cells) and plays a key role in normal nerve and muscle function. The kidneys (page 509) maintain a consistent level of sodium in the body by adjusting the amount secreted in urine.

Potassium is the most abundant cation in the body. It is present in all body tissues, being required for normal cell function because of its role in maintaining intracellular fluid volume and transmembrane electrochemical gradients. It has a strong relationship with sodium in maintaining extracellular fluid volume, including plasma volume. It enters cells more readily than sodium instigating the brief sodium-potassium exchange across cell membranes. In nerve cells this electrical potential aids the conduction of nerve impulses; in muscle it helps generate muscle contractions and regulates the heartbeat. It also helps prevent the swelling of cells by pumping sodium out. If sodium is not pumped out water accumulates within the cell causing it to swell and eventually burst. It participates in the synthesis of protein from amino acids; functions in carbohydrate metabolism; is active in glycogen and glucose metabolism, converting glucose to glycogen for storage in the liver; and is important for normal growth and building muscle. While sodium is conserved by the body, there is no effective potassium conservation. When there is a potassium shortage the kidneys continue to excrete it.

Chloride is important in helping maintain acid-base fluid balance. It also helps muscles to contract and nerve cells to transmit impulses; aids digestion and prevents the growth of unwanted microbes in the stomach; and helps red blood cells exchange oxygen and carbon dioxide in the lungs and other parts of the body.

> **CLINICAL PHYSIOLOGY:** Cystic fibrosis is caused by a mutation in a protein that transports chloride ions out of cells. Signs and symptoms include salty skin; poor digestion and absorption, leading to poor growth; sticky mucous accumulation in the lungs, leading to increased susceptibility of respiratory infections; liver damage and infertility.

Cobalt is an essential component required for the normal functioning of the pancreas. It: helps absorb and process vitamin B_{12}; is used to treat illnesses, such as anaemia and some infectious diseases; aids in the repair of myelin; and helps in the formation of haemoglobin. It may be used in place of zinc.

Copper is crucial for brain and nervous system development; it also plays a role in the production and maintenance of myelin. It is a cofactor for several enzymes (cuproenzymes) involved in energy production, iron metabolism, neuropeptide activation, connective tissue and neurotransmitter synthesis. Copper is also involved in many physiologic processes (angiogenesis, neurohormone homeostasis, regulation of gene expression, brain development, pigmentation, immune system functioning), as well as acting as a defence against oxidative damage, which depends mainly on dismutases.

Manganese helps activate powerful antioxidant enzymes; converts fats and proteins into energy; supports cartilage and bone formation; protects mitochondria from free-radical damage and plays an important role in blood clotting and haemostasis in conjunction with vitamin K. Manganese deficiency is rare; symptoms include loss of bone mass and stunted growth in children.

Metabolic functions of the liver. The liver is a large chemically active pool of cells with a high metabolic rate. The cells share substrates and energy from one system to another, processing and synthesising multiple substances which are transported to other areas of the body.

Carbohydrate metabolism. The liver: stores large amounts of glycogen; converts galactose and fructose to glucose; is involved in gluconeogenesis and forms many chemical compounds from intermediate products of carbohydrate metabolism. It is important for maintaining normal blood glucose concentrations, with the storage of glycogen enabling it to remove excess glucose from blood, store it and then return it to blood when required. This is the glucose buffer function of the liver. Gluconeogenesis in the liver is also important in maintaining blood glucose concentration because it occurs significantly only when glucose levels fall below normal. Large amounts of amino acids and glycerol from triglycerides are then converted into glucose, helping to maintain blood glucose levels.

> **APPLIED PHYSIOLOGY:** In individuals with poor liver function, blood glucose concentration following a meal rich in carbohydrates can increase two to threefold compared to an individual with normal liver function.

Fat/lipid metabolism. Although most cells metabolise fat, specific aspects occur mainly in the liver: oxidation of fatty acids supplying energy for other body functions; synthesis of large amounts of cholesterol, phospholipids and most lipoproteins; and synthesis of fat from proteins and carbohydrates. Most (80%) of cholesterol synthesised in the liver is converted into bile salts, which are secreted into bile, with the remainder transported in lipoproteins and carried in blood to cells throughout the body. Phospholipids are similarly synthesised in the liver and transported mainly in lipoproteins. Cholesterol and phospholipids are used to make cell membranes, intracellular structures and chemical substances important for cell function. Following synthesis, fat is transported in lipoproteins to adipose tissue for storage.

Protein metabolism. The most important functions of the liver in protein metabolism are deamination of amino acids; formation of urea for removal of ammonia; formation of plasma proteins; and interconversion of amino acids and the synthesis of compounds (non-essential amino acids) from amino acids.

> **APPLIED PHYSIOLOGY:** Plasma protein depletion causes rapid mitosis of hepatic cells and growth of the liver, coupled with rapid output of plasma proteins until the plasma concentration returns to normal.

> **CLINICAL PHYSIOLOGY:** In chronic liver disease (cirrhosis) plasma proteins (albumin) can fall to very low levels, resulting in generalised oedema and ascites.

> **CLINICAL PHYSIOLOGY:** Death occurs within a few days without the liver's contribution to protein metabolism.

Other liver functions. The liver stores vitamins (A, D, B_{12}), iron (except for that in haemoglobin) in the form of ferritin, and substances important in coagulation (fibrinogen, prothrombin, accelerator globulin, factor VII), with vitamin K being required for the formation of prothrombin, factors VII, IX and X. In addition, the liver removes excess drugs (sulphonamides, penicillin, ampicillin, erythromycin), hormones (thyroxine, all steroids including oestrogen, cortisol and aldosterone) and other substances (calcium, which is secreted into bile and then lost in faeces).

> **CLINICAL PHYSIOLOGY:** Liver damage can lead to excess accumulation of hormones in body fluids causing over activity of the hormone systems.

URINARY SYSTEM

Embryologically the urinary and genital systems are anatomically intimately related, developing from a common mesodermal ridge (intermediate mesoderm) along the entire length of the posterior body wall, with the excretory ducts of both systems initially entering a common cavity (cloaca); however, they function as separate systems. The urinary system is concerned with the formation, concentration, storage and excretion of urine. It lies partly in the abdomen (kidneys, ureters) and partly in the pelvis (bladder), with the remainder passing through the perineum (urethra).

Kidney

DEVELOPMENT: The kidney develops from the nephrogenic cord of the intermediate cell mass and goes through three stages (pronephros, mesonephros and metanephros). The pronephros appears during the 4th week as a few cell clusters in the cervical region, which soon degenerate (Fig. 6.52A). Most of the pronephric ducts are incorporated into the developing mesonephros, which appears later in the 4th week caudal to the pronephros, as large ovoid structures on either side of the midline (Fig. 6.52A) containing 70–80 S-shaped tubules, each

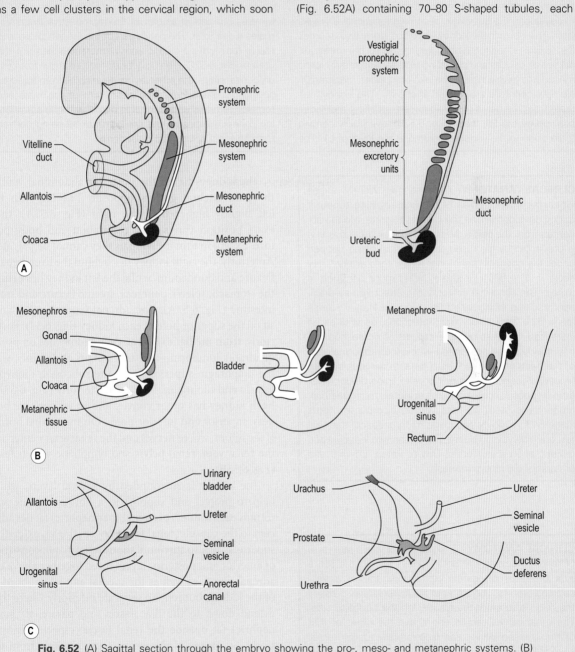

Fig. 6.52 (A) Sagittal section through the embryo showing the pro-, meso- and metanephric systems. (B) Ascent of the kidneys. (C) Development of the urogenital sinus into the urinary bladder.

Continued

being invaginated by a branch of the dorsal aorta to form an internal glomerulus at one end opening into the mesonephric (Wolffian) duct at the other. The mesonephros excretes urine during the embryonic and early foetal periods. By the end of the 9th week all that remains of the mesonephros are a few caudal tubules in both sexes and the mesonephric duct in males. The metanephros begins to develop in the 5th week, becoming functional 6 weeks later. The permanent kidney develops from two sources (Fig. 6.52B), the ureteric bud (giving rise to the ureter, renal pelvis, calyces and collecting tubules) and metanephric mesoderm (giving rise to the excretory units (nephrons)). No new nephrons are formed after birth. The kidneys migrate from the pelvis to the abdomen, attaining their adult position by the 9th week (Fig. 6.52B), eventually coming to lie close to the vertebral column at the level of L1. The kidneys become fully functional during the 2nd half of pregnancy, with urine passing into the amniotic cavity and forming the major part of the amniotic fluid. Because the placenta eliminates metabolic waste products from foetal blood the kidneys do not need to be functional before birth. The distal parts of the mesonephric ducts become incorporated into the bladder. The proximal parts degenerate in females but persist as part of the reproductive system in males (page 523). The pelvic part of the urogenital sinus in males forms the prostatic and membranous parts of the urethra (Fig. 6.52C). The bladder epithelium arises from the urogenital sinus, the other layers developing from adjacent splanchnic mesoderm. The epithelium of the male and female urethra is endodermal in origin, with the surrounding connective tissue and smooth muscle being derived from adjacent splanchnic mesoderm.

CLINICAL ANATOMY: A horseshoe kidney arises when the inferior poles of the kidneys fuse together during development as the kidneys migrate into the abdomen from the pelvis. Migration to their adult position is prevented by the fused part (isthmus) being trapped under the origin of the inferior mesenteric artery. They occur in 1 in 500 individuals, being more common in males. The abnormal anatomy can affect kidney drainage resulting in increased frequency of kidney stones (page 521) and urinary tract infections, as well as an increased risk of some renal cancers. A horseshoe kidney may also be associated with other abnormalities: of the heart (ventricular septal defect); nervous system (encephalocele, myelomeningocele, spina bifida); skeleton (kyphosis, scoliosis, hemivertebrae, micrognathia); urogenital system (septate vagina, bicornuate uterus (page 543), hypospadias (page 539), undescended testes, adult polycystic kidney, more than two kidneys) and genetic anomalies (Turner, Down, Patau, Edward and oro-cranial-digital syndromes).

CLINICAL ANATOMY: Crossed dystopia is a rare form of renal ectopia where both kidneys are on the same side, often fused together but retaining their own vessels and ureters. The ureter of the lower kidney crosses the midline to enter the bladder on the opposite side. The renal pelves can lie one above the other or that of the crossed kidney can face laterally (unilateral 'S' shaped kidney).

The kidneys lie on the posterior abdominal wall in the paravertebral gutters opposite T12–L3, with the left slightly higher than the right (Fig. 6.53A); their exact position varies with respiration and body posture. Except in thin individuals they cannot be palpated. Anteriorly, the right kidney lies behind the liver, hepatic flexure and duodenum, while the left kidney lies behind the stomach, spleen, pancreas, splenic flexure and small intestine (Fig. 6.53A). The adrenal (suprarenal) glands sit on the superior pole of each kidney (Fig. 6.34). Posteriorly, from medial to lateral, each kidney lies on psoas, quadratus lumborum and transversus abdominis, with the diaphragm superiorly and the subcostal, iliohypogastric and ilioinguinal nerves posteriorly (Fig. 6.53A). Each kidney has outer convex and inner concave borders, superior and inferior poles. On the medial border is the hilum, where nerves and the renal artery enter and the renal vein, renal pelvis and lymphatic vessels leave (Fig. 6.53B).

The kidney is surrounded by several layers, which help to protect and support it: a fibrous capsule surrounds each kidney; perirenal (perinephric) fat lies adjacent to the capsule; renal fascia covers the fat, extending superiorly to also surround the adrenal gland, consisting of anterior and posterior layers fused together above the adrenal gland, as well as the medial and lateral borders of the kidney, but remain separate inferiorly where they extend down to the iliac fascia and pararenal (paranephric) fat outside the renal fascia, especially posteriorly. By means of numerous septa crossing from the renal fascia to the capsule through the perirenal fat, the

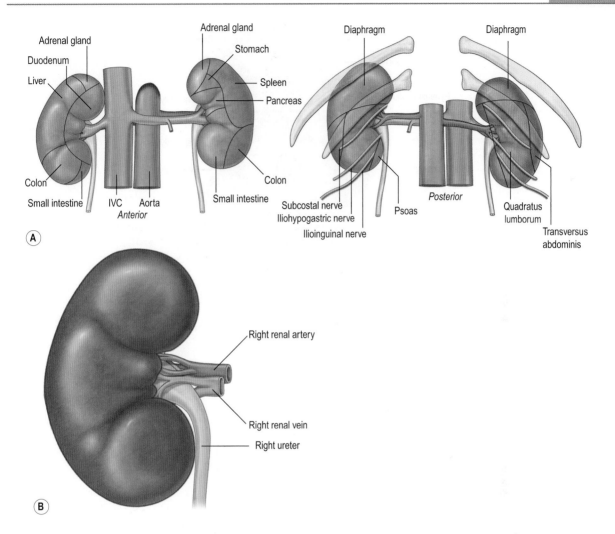

Fig. 6.53 (A) Anterior and posterior relations of the kidneys. (B) Anterior aspect of the right kidney showing the arrangement of structures at the hilum. *IVC,* Inferior vena cava.

kidney is held in place through its attachment to the diaphragmatic and psoas fascia. In addition, neighbouring viscera also contribute to supporting the kidney.

Within the thin fibrous capsule is a darker outer cortex containing many renal corpuscles and tubule cross-sections and an inner medulla consisting of 8–12 renal pyramids, comprising straight, aligned structures separated by renal columns (cortex) (Fig. 6.54). Each pyramid and its adjacent cortex constitutes a renal lobe. The renal papillae project into a minor calyx which collects urine formed in the tubules of the pyramid. In turn, the minor calyces drain into a major calyx, which drains into the upper expanded end (pelvis) of the ureter (Fig. 6.54).

Each kidney contains in excess of 1 million functional units (nephrons) that consist of simple, single-layered epithelium along their entire length. Each nephron comprises: a renal corpuscle consisting of a glomerulus (tuft of capillary loops), the site of blood filtration, surrounded by Bowman's capsule located in the cortex; a long convoluted proximal tubule in the cortex, with a shorter part that enters the medulla; a loop of Henle (nephron loop) in the medulla, with a thin descending and ascending limbs; a distal part consisting of a thick straight part ascending back into the cortex; and a convoluted part within the cortex (Fig. 6.55). Each collecting tubule receives connecting tubules from several

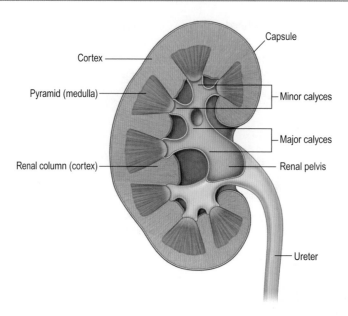

Fig. 6.54 Coronal section through the kidney showing its internal organisation.

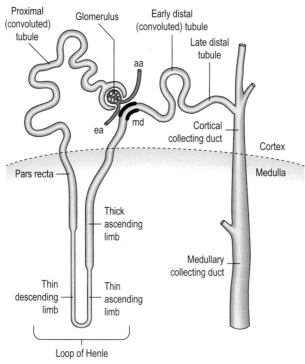

Fig. 6.55 Organisation of a nephron.

nephrons and merge to form collecting ducts (Fig. 6.55), which converge onto the renal papilla.

> **APPLIED ANATOMY:** Cortical nephrons are located almost completely in the cortex, while juxtamedullary nephrons (~15%) lie close to the medulla and have long loops of Henle.

> **CLINICAL ANATOMY:** Polycystic kidney disease is an inherited disorder in which the normal organisation of both kidneys is lost due to the formation of large fluid-filled cysts, which can arise from any epithelial cells of the nephron. It can lead to gross kidney enlargement and loss of function.

The large blood supply to the kidney is well organised and closely associated with all components of the nephron. The renal artery (direct branch of the aorta) divides into two or more segmental arteries at the hilum, which then further divide into interlobar arteries around the renal pelvis. Interlobar arteries extend between the pyramids towards the corticomedullary junction, where they divide into arcuate arteries. Smaller cortical lobar arteries radiate from the arcuate arteries extending deep into the cortex (Fig. 6.56). Microvascular afferent arteries arise from the cortical lobular arteries and divide forming a plexus of capillary loops (glomerulus), each located within a renal corpuscle. Blood leaves the glomerulus in efferent arterioles, which branch again forming another capillary network (peritubular capillaries) distributed throughout the cortex. Efferent arterioles from juxtamedullary nephrons branch repeatedly forming parallel bundles of capillaries (vasa recta) which penetrate deep into the medulla in association with the loops of Henle and collecting ducts. Blood leaves the kidney in similarly named veins and follows the same course as the arteries, eventually draining into the renal vein and then the inferior vena cava.

> **CLINICAL PHYSIOLOGY:** Bacterial infections of the urinary tract can lead to inflammation of the renal pelvis and calyces (pyelonephritis). In acute pyelonephritis bacteria often move from one or more minor calyx into the associated renal papilla, causing an accumulation of neutrophils in the collecting ducts.

Renal Physiology

The kidneys have several functions besides the formation of urine; however, their primary role is maintaining homeostasis. During the formation of urine the kidneys regulate various body activities concerned with homeostasis. The formation of urine involves: filtration, whereby water and solutes in the blood leave the vascular space and enter the lumen of the nephron; tubular secretion, by which substances move from epithelial cells of the tubules into the lumen, usually after uptake from the surrounding interstitium and capillaries; and tubular reabsorption, in which substances move from the tubular lumen across the epithelium into the interstitium and surrounding capillaries.

Homeostasis

Excretion. The kidneys are the primary means of eliminating the waste products of metabolism no longer needed by the body and must do so as rapidly as they are produced: urea, the end product of amino acid metabolism; uric acid, the end product of nucleic acid metabolism; creatinine, the end product of muscle metabolism; bilirubin, the end product of haemoglobin metabolism and metabolites from various hormones. Most toxins and other foreign substances produced by the body or ingested (pesticides, drugs, food additives) are also eliminated by the kidneys.

Regulation. *Body fluid osmolality and electrolyte concentrations.* The kidneys maintain water and electrolyte balance. Although water intake is largely governed by an individual's eating and drinking habits, the kidneys adjust their excretion rates to match intake. Within 2–3 days of an excess intake of sodium the kidney increases its sodium excretion, re-establishing the balance between intake and excretion. During this time there is a small increase in extracellular fluid volume and/or plasma sodium concentration (due to a small accumulation of sodium), triggering hormonal changes and other compensatory mechanisms that signal the kidneys to increase sodium excretion. The kidneys respond in a similar way for water and other electrolytes (chloride, potassium, calcium, hydrogen, magnesium and phosphate ions).

Acid-base balance. The body is under constant threat of developing acidosis due to the large amounts of acid produced during metabolism. Together with the lungs and body fluid buffers, the kidneys contribute to acid-base balance by excreting acids and regulating the body fluid buffer stores. The kidneys play a major role in

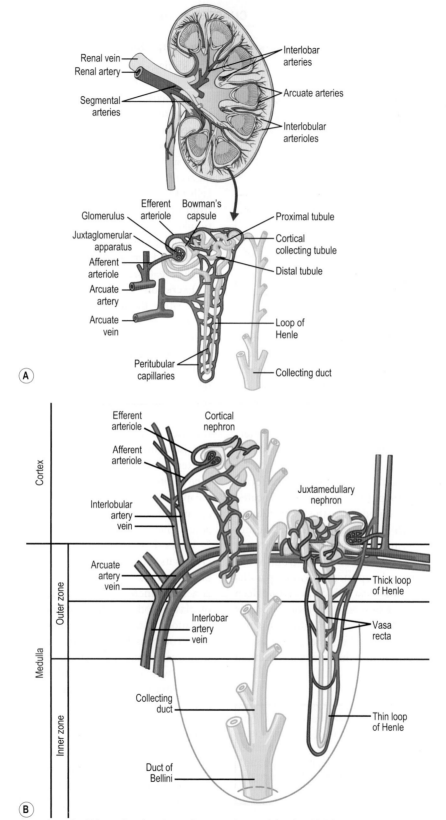

Fig. 6.56 (A) Coronal section of a kidney showing the major vessels supplying it with blood and the microcirculation of a cortical nephron. (B) Relationship between blood vessels and tubular structures in cortical and juxtamedullary nephrons.

preventing acidosis. Only the kidneys can eliminate the sulphuric and phosphoric acid generated by the metabolism of proteins.

Blood pressure. The kidneys play an important role in the long-term regulation of arterial blood pressure by regulating the volume of extracellular fluid (excreting variable amounts of sodium and water); and through the renin-angiotensin mechanism (page 516). They also contribute to short-term regulation by secreting hormones and vasoactive factors or substances (renin) leading to the formation of vasoactive products (angiotensin II).

Haematopoiesis. Erythropoietin secreted by the kidneys stimulates the production of red blood cells by haematopoietic stem cells in bone marrow, an important stimulus being hypoxia. Almost all erythropoietin secreted into the circulation is by the kidneys. The kidneys also secrete thrombopoietin which stimulates the production of thrombocytes.

> **CLINICAL PHYSIOLOGY:** Decreased erythropoietin production in individuals with severe kidney disease or who have had a kidney removed and are undergoing dialysis can lead to severe anaemia.

Endocrine function. The kidneys secrete many hormonal substances in addition to erythropoietin and thrombopoietin, including renin, calcitriol (1,25-dihydroxycholecalciferol) and prostaglandins. Calcitriol is essential for normal calcium deposition in bone and calcium reabsorption by the digestive tract, by hydroxylating vitamin D. Calcitriol also plays an important role in calcium and phosphate regulation.

Gluconeogenesis. The kidneys synthesise glucose from amino acids and other precursors during prolonged fasting. The capacity to add glucose to the blood in such times is similar to that of the liver.

Urine Formation

Renal corpuscle. Blood filtration occurs in the renal corpuscle at the beginning of the nephron. The renal corpuscle comprises the glomerulus surrounded by a double layered (Bowman's) capsule, the visceral layer envelops the glomerular fenestrated capillaries and the parietal layer forms the capsule surface. Between the layers is the capsular (urinary) space which receives the fluid filtered through the capillary wall (Fig. 6.57A). The visceral layer

consists of stellate epithelial cells (podocytes), which, with the capillary endothelial cells, allows for renal filtration. Each podocyte projects primary processes curving around the capillary, as well as giving rise to many parallel interdigitating secondary processes (pedicels) covering much of the capillary surface (Fig. 6.57B). Between pedicels are elongated spaces (filtration slit pores), while spanning adjacent pedicels bridging the slit pores, are slit diaphragms.

The most substantial part of the filtration barrier separating blood from the capsular space is the glomerular basement membrane between the fenestrated endothelial cells and covering podocytes. Filtration, therefore, occurs through a structure with three parts: the fenestrations, which block blood cells and platelets; the glomerular basement membrane, which restricts large proteins and some organic anions; and the filtration slit diaphragms, which restrict some small proteins and organic anions (Fig. 6.57C).

> **CLINICAL PHYSIOLOGY:** In diabetes mellitus and glomerulonephritis, the glomerular filter becomes more permeable to proteins, with the subsequent loss of proteins into the urine (proteinuria). Proteinuria is an indicator of a number of potential kidney disorders.

In addition to capillary endothelial cells and podocytes, the renal corpuscle also contains mesangial cells. They and their surrounding matrix (mesangium) fill the spaces between capillaries that lack podocytes (Fig. 6.58). Their functions include: physically supporting the capillaries; adjusting contractions in response to blood pressure changes, thereby helping to maintain optimal filtration; phagocytosis of protein aggregates adhering to the glomerular filter, including antibody-antigen complexes present in many pathological conditions; and secretion of several cytokines, prostaglandins and other factors important for immune defence and glomerular repair.

Juxtaglomerular apparatus. A specialised organ near the glomerulus comprising macula densa, extraglomerular mesangial (agranular) and juxtaglomerular (granular) cells (Fig. 6.59). The macula densa is the end part of the thick ascending segment before it opens into the distal convoluted tubule and is situated between the afferent and efferent arterioles of the same nephron. It consists of tightly packed cuboidal epithelial cells. The

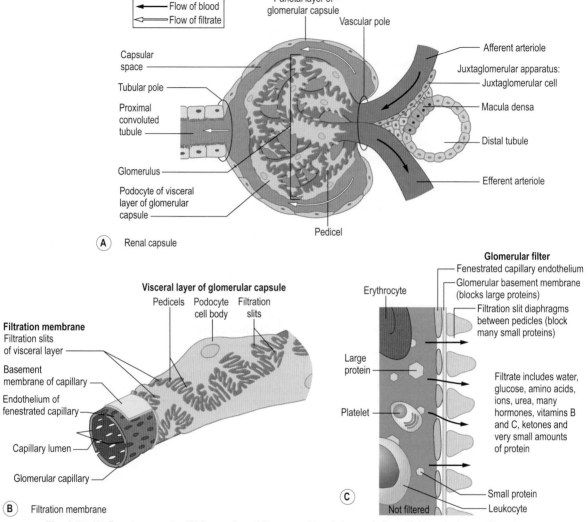

Fig. 6.57 (A) Renal corpuscle. (B) Formation of filtrate as blood plasma is forced through the capillary fenestrations. (C) The glomerular filter and its major functions.

extraglomerular mesangial cells are situated between the afferent and efferent arterioles and macula densa (Fig. 6.59); the juxtaglomerular cells are specialised smooth muscle cells situated in the wall of the afferent capillary before it enters Bowman's capsule (Fig. 6.59), being present in the tunica media and adventitia.

The primary function of the juxtaglomerular apparatus is the secretion of hormones (renin, prostaglandin), as well as regulating glomerular blood flow and filtration rate. The extraglomerular cells secrete cytokines (interleukin-2, tumour necrosis factor) and the macula densa thromboxane A_2. The stimuli for renin secretion

are a fall in blood pressure; reduction in the volume of extracellular fluid; increased sympathetic activity; and decreased concentration of sodium and chloride in the macula densa.

Renin-angiotensin system. When renin is released into blood it acts on a specific plasma protein (angiotensinogen) converting it into angiotensin I, which is then converted to angiotensin II. Most of the conversion of angiotensin I to angiotensin II occurs in the lungs by angiotensin-converting enzyme (ACE) secreted by the lungs. Angiotensin II is rapidly converted to angiotensin III by angiotensinases present in red blood cells and most tissue capillaries. Angiotensin III is then converted into angiotensin IV (Fig. 6.60).

Angiotensin I is physiologically inactive.

Angiotensin II is the most active form. On blood vessels it increases arterial blood pressure by acting directly on the blood vessels causing vasoconstriction and indirectly increases blood pressure by increasing the release of noradrenaline (epinephrine) from post-ganglionic sympathetic fibres. It stimulates the zona glomerulosa of the adrenal cortex (page 343) to secrete aldosterone, which acts on the renal tubules and increases sodium retention (which also raises blood pressure), regulating glomerular filtration rate by constricting efferent arterioles and causing contraction of the glomerular

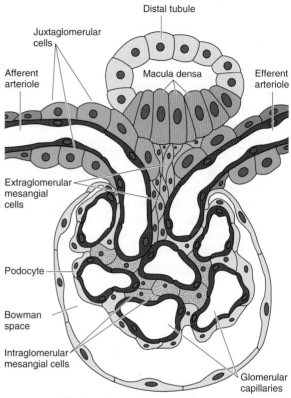

Fig. 6.59 Juxtaglomerular apparatus.

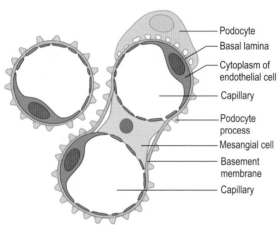

Fig. 6.58 Mesangial cells between capillaries in the renal corpuscle, cover the capillary surface not covered by podocytes.

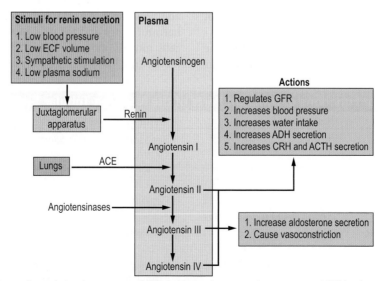

Fig. 6.60 The renin-angiotensin system. *ACE*, Angiotensin-converting enzyme; *ACTH*, adrenocorticotropic hormone; *ADH*, antidiuretic hormone; *CRH*, corticotropin-releasing hormone; *ECF*, extracellular fluid; *GFR*, glomerular filtration rate.

mesangial cells decreasing the surface area of the capillaries and therefore filtration. It also increases sodium reabsorption from the proximal tubules. On the brain it: inhibits the baroreceptor reflex indirectly increasing blood pressure; increases water intake by stimulating the thirst centre; increases the secretion of CRH from the hypothalamus (page 255), which in turn increases the secretion of adrenocorticotropic hormone (ACTH) from the pituitary (page 335); and increases secretion of antidiuretic hormone (ADH) from the hypothalamus. Angiotensin II also acts as a growth factor in the heart causing muscular hypertrophy and cardiac enlargement.

Angiotensin III increases blood pressure and stimulates aldosterone secretion from the adrenal cortex.

Angiotensin IV has adrenocortical stimulating and vasopressor actions.

Prostaglandins. These have a variety of physiological actions. They mainly act by the formation of 2nd messenger cyclic adenosine monophosphate (AMP).

On the kidney they stimulate the juxtaglomerular apparatus enhancing the secretion of renin, diuresis and natriuresis.

On blood they accelerate the capacity of red blood cells to pass through minute blood vessels. On blood vessels prostaglandin (PGE_2) causes vasodilation.

On the digestive tract they reduce gastric secretion; some prostaglandins are antilipolytic, inhibiting the release of free fatty acids from adipose tissue.

On the respiratory system PGE_2 causes bronchodilation.

In the brain they control or change the actions of neurotransmitters.

On reproduction they play a role in regulating the reproductive cycle causing degeneration of the corpus luteum (luteolysis) and increase the receptive capacity of cervical mucosa for sperm and cause reverse peristaltic movement of the uterus and fallopian tubes during intercourse increasing the rate of sperm movement in the female genital tract. They also play an important role in parturition and facilitate labour by increasing the force of uterine contractions by elevating the concentration of calcium ions in uterine smooth muscle fibres. Prostaglandins secreted from uterine tissues, foetal membranes and the placenta increasing their concentration in maternal blood and amniotic fluid.

Proximal convoluted tubule. The long tortuous proximal convoluted tubules fill most of the cortex. The cells are specialised for both reabsorption and secretion. More than half of the water and electrolytes and all of the organic nutrients (glucose, amino acids, vitamins) filtered from plasma in the renal corpuscle are normally reabsorbed in the proximal convoluted tubule (Table 6.7). They are transferred directly across the tubular wall for immediate uptake into the plasma of the peritubular capillaries.

In the first part of the proximal tubule sodium is reabsorbed, together with glucose, amino acids and other solutes; but in the second part little glucose and amino acids remain to be absorbed, while sodium is reabsorbed mainly with chloride ions. The proximal tubule is also an important site for the secretion of organic acids and bases (bile salts, oxalate, urate, catecholamines), the end products of metabolism, which must be rapidly removed from the body (Fig. 6.61). In addition, the proximal tubules secrete many potentially harmful drugs and toxins directly through the tubular cells into the tubules, rapidly clearing them from the blood. In addition to their major roles in reabsorption

TABLE 6.7	**Major Functions of Different Parts of the Nephron Tubular System**	
Region	Location	Major Function
Proximal convoluted tubule	Cortex	Reabsorption of all organic nutrients, all proteins, most water and electrolytes; secretion of organic anions and cations, H^+, NH_4
Loop of Henle		
Thin limb	Medulla	Passive reabsorption of Na^+, Cl^-
Thick ascending limb	Medulla and medullary rays	Active reabsorption of various electrolytes
Distal convoluted tubule	Cortex	Reabsorption of electrolytes
Collecting system		
Principal cells	Medullary rays and medulla	Regulated reabsorption of water and electrolytes; regulated secretion of K^+
Intercalated cells	Medullary rays	Reabsorption of K^+; helps maintain acid-base balance

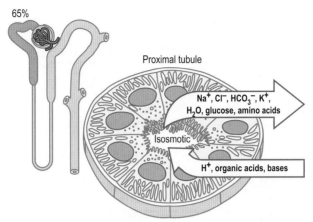

Fig. 6.61 Cellular structure and primary transport characteristics of the proximal tubule.

and secretion, the cells of the proximal tubule hydroxylate vitamin D and release it into the capillaries. Fibroblastic interstitial cells in cortical areas near the proximal tubules produce erythropoietin in response to a prolonged decrease in local oxygen concentration.

> **APPLIED PHYSIOLOGY:** The rapid clearance of some drugs (penicillin, salicylates) creates a problem in maintaining a therapeutically effective drug concentration.

Loop of Henle. This consists of three functionally distinct segments: thin descending and ascending limbs and thick ascending limb. The thin descending segment is highly permeable to water and moderately permeable to most solutes, including urea and sodium, with 20% of the filtered water being reabsorbed. The thin and thick ascending limb is almost impermeable to water, an important characteristic for concentrating the urine (Fig. 6.62). The thick ascending segment reabsorbs 25% of the filtered sodium, chloride and potassium, together with considerable amounts of other ions (calcium, bicarbonate, magnesium).

The counter-current flow of the filtrate in the parallel limbs establishes an osmolarity gradient in the interstitium of the medullary pyramids, which is multiplied at deeper levels in the medulla, with counter-current blood flow in the descending and ascending limbs of the vasa recta helping to maintain the interstitium hyperosmotic.

Distal convoluted tubule. Where the initial straight part of the distal tubule contacts the arterioles at the vascular pole its cells form the macula densa, part of the juxtaglomerular apparatus (page 515), which utilises feedback mechanisms to regulate glomerular blood flow, keeping the glomerular filtration rate relatively constant. The convoluted part of the distal tubule has many of the absorptive characteristics of the thick ascending loop of Henle, reabsorbing most ions (sodium, potassium, chloride), but is almost impermeable to water and urea (Fig. 6.63). 5% of the filtered sodium chloride is reabsorbed in the early distal tubule, with the sodium-chloride co-transporter moving sodium chloride from the lumen of the tubule into the cell, and the sodium-potassium ATPase pump transporting it out of the cell.

> **APPLIED PHYSIOLOGY:** Thiazide diuretics inhibit the sodium-chloride co-transporter; they are widely used in hypertension and heart failure.

The second part of the distal tubule and the subsequent connecting tubule have similar functional characteristics: the principal cells reabsorb sodium and water from the lumen and secrete potassium ions into the lumen; the intercalating cells reabsorb potassium and bicarbonate ions and secrete hydrogen ions into the lumen. The permeability of the late distal tubule and cortical collecting ducts is controlled by the concentration of ADH. With high levels they are permeable to water, but in the absence of ADH they are almost impermeable to water. This, therefore, provides an important mechanism for controlling the dilution/concentration of urine.

Medullary ducts. Although the medullary collecting ducts reabsorb less than 10% of the filtered water and sodium, they are the final site for processing urine. They play an important role in determining the final urine output of water and solutes (Fig. 6.64).

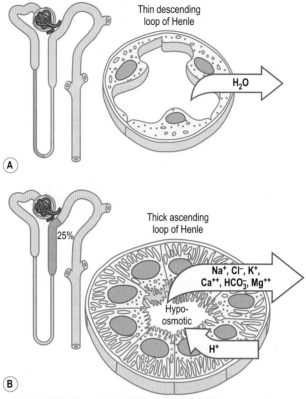

Fig. 6.62 Cellular structure and transport characteristics of the thin descending segment (A) and thick ascending segment (B) of the loop of Henle.

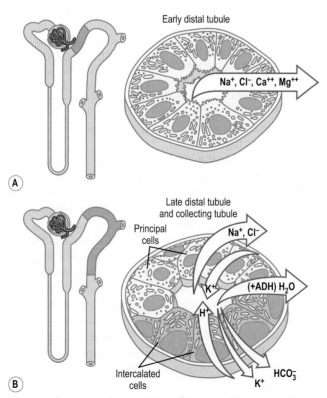

Fig. 6.63 Cellular structure and transport characteristics of the early (A) and late (B) distal convoluted tubule.

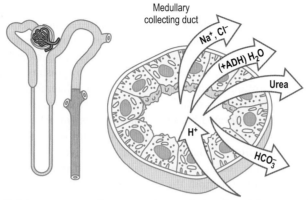

Fig. 6.64 Cellular structure and transport characteristics of medullary collecting ducts.

The permeability of the medullary collecting ducts to water is controlled by the level of ADH (as in the later part of the distal tubule and cortical connecting tubule), reducing urine volume and concentrating most of the solutes; however, the medullary collecting duct is permeable to urea. The ducts are also capable of secreting hydrogen ions against a large concentration gradient (as in the cortical connecting tubules), therefore playing a key role in regulating acid-base balance.

Dilute or concentrated urine. The kidneys can excrete a large volume of dilute urine or a small volume of concentrated urine without major changes in the rates of secretion of sodium and potassium. When there is excess water in the body and extracellular osmolarity is reduced, the secretion of ADH by the posterior pituitary decreases, reducing the permeability of the distal tubule and collecting ducts to water, resulting in large amounts of dilute urine being excreted.

When there is a water deficit in the body, the kidney forms concentrated urine by continuing to excrete solutes while at the same time increasing water reabsorption, decreasing the volume of urine formed.

The kidneys minimise fluid loss during water deficiency through the osmoreceptor-antidiuretic feedback system. Adequate fluid intake is necessary to counterbalance fluid loss through sweating, breathing and via the digestive tract. It does this by the thirst mechanism, as well as the feedback mechanism to maintain and control extracellular fluid osmolarity and sodium concentration. Stimuli for increasing fluid intake include increased plasma osmolarity and angiotensin II, decreased blood volume and blood pressure, and dryness of the mouth. Stimuli for decreasing fluid intake include decreased plasma osmolarity and angiotensin II, increased blood volume and blood pressure, and gastric distension.

CLINICAL PHYSIOLOGY: Urinary tract stones (renal calculi) develop when small variations in the pH of urine cause salts within the urine (calcium, phosphate, oxalate, urate and other soluble salts) to precipitate, forming polycrystalline aggregates within an organic matrix. They occur more frequently in males, being most common in individuals aged 20–60. Individuals report pain radiating from the infrascapular region to the groin, and sometimes into the scrotum or labia majora. It may be accompanied by blood in the urine (haematuria). Complications include infection; urinary obstruction and renal failure. Stones can also develop in the bladder producing marked irritation, pain and discomfort.

CLINICAL PHYSIOLOGY: Most tumours that arise in the kidney are renal cell carcinomas. They develop from the proximal tubular epithelium. These tumours grow outward from the kidney invading the fat and fascia, as well spreading into the renal vein. They may be spread into the inferior vena cava and, rarely, into the right atrium across the tricuspid valve into the pulmonary artery. However, 5% of tumours are transitional cell tumours arising from the transitional epithelium (urothelium) of the renal pelvis, presenting anywhere from the calyces to the urethra. Individuals with transitional carcinomas in the bladder may also have similar tumours in the upper part of the urinary tract.

Diuretics

These enhance urine formation and output by increasing the excretion of water, sodium and chloride and act by influencing the processes involved in urine formation. They are generally used in treating disorders involving an increase in extracellular fluid volume (hypertension, congestive heart failure, oedema). The adverse effects of diuretics include dehydration; electrolyte imbalance; potassium deficiency; headache; dizziness; renal damage; cardiac arrhythmia and heart palpitations. Diuretics are classified into six types:

Osmotic diuretics (urea, mannitol, sucrose, glucose) inhibit water and sodium reabsorption by increasing osmolarity of tubular fluid, which occurs mainly in the proximal convoluted tubules. Elevated blood sugar levels can also cause osmotic diuresis.

Diuretics inhibiting active reabsorption of electrolytes: some (furosemide, torsemide, bumetanide) inhibit sodium and chloride reabsorption from the thick ascending loop of Henle, some (chlorothiazide, metolazone, chlortalidone) inhibit sodium reabsorption in the proximal part of the distal tubule, while others (triamterene, amiloride) inhibit sodium and potassium excretion in the distal part of the distal convoluted tubule and collecting ducts.

Diuretics inhibiting aldosterone action (spironolactone, eplerenone) inhibit sodium reabsorption and potassium excretion in the distal convolutes tubule and collecting ducts.

Diuretics inhibiting carbonic anhydrase activity (acetazolamide) prevent reabsorption of bicarbonates from the renal tubules.

Diuretics increasing glomerular filtration rate (caffeine, theophylline) work by decreasing sodium reabsorption.

Diuretics inhibiting ADH secretion (water, ethanol).

Kidney Diseases

Kidney disease is an important cause of death and disability, with severe kidney disease being: acute renal failure, in which the kidneys abruptly stop working entirely or almost entirely, but may eventually recover nearly normal function; or chronic renal failure, in which there is progressive loss of function of more and more nephrons that gradually decreases kidney function. There are many specific kidney diseases that can affect the blood vessels, glomeruli, tubules, renal interstitium and parts of the urinary tract (ureters, bladder) outside the kidneys. Kidney failure is always accompanied by other complications: deficiency of calcitriol (activated vitamin D), resulting in reduced calcium absorption from the intestines and hypocalcaemia, which can cause secondary hyperparathyroidism in some individuals; deficiency of erythropoietin, resulting in anaemia; and disturbances in acid-base balance.

Acute renal failure. This can lead to sudden life-threatening reactions requiring emergency treatment. It can be caused by acute nephritis (kidney inflammation) usually developing as an immune reaction; damage to renal tissue by poisons (lead, mercury, carbon tetrachloride); renal ischaemia following circulatory shock; acute tubular necrosis caused by burns, haemorrhage, snake bites, toxins (insecticides, heavy metals, carbon tetrachloride) and drugs (diuretics, aminoglycosides, platinum derivatives); severe transfusion reactions; sudden falls in blood pressure during haemorrhage, diarrhoea, severe burns and cholera; and ureter blockage due to the presence of a kidney stone or tumour.

The features of acute renal failure include decreased urine output (oliguria); cessation of urine formation in severe cases (anuria); the presence of proteins in the urine (proteinuria), including albuminuria (excretion of albumin); blood in the urine (haematuria); increased extracellular fluid volume caused by sodium and water retention (oedema); increased extracellular fluid volume within a few days (hypertension); retention of metabolic end products (acidosis) and coma, due to severe acidosis resulting in death within 10–14 days.

Chronic renal failure. As nephrons cease functioning the remaining nephrons can compensate to some extent; however, as more and more cease functioning the compensatory mechanisms fail leading to chronic renal failure. The causes include chronic nephritis; polycystic kidney disease; kidney stones; urethral constriction; hypertension; atherosclerosis; tuberculosis and slow poisoning by drugs or metals.

The features of chronic renal failure include uraemia, an excess accumulation of the end products (urea, nitrogen, creatinine in blood) of protein metabolism and of some toxic substances (organic acids, phenols) that is accompanied by anorexia, lethargy, drowsiness, nausea and vomiting, skin pigmentation, muscle twitching, tetany, convulsions, confusion and mental disorders and coma; acidosis, leading to coma and death; oedema, due to failure of the kidneys to excrete sodium and electrolytes increasing extracellular fluid volume; blood loss, due to gastrointestinal bleeding accompanied by platelet dysfunction; anaemia, due to decreased red blood cell production leading to normocytic normochromic anaemia (page 169); and hyperparathyroidism (page 342), due to calcitriol deficiency increasing the removal of calcium from bones, leading to osteomalacia.

Ureter

DEVELOPMENT: The ureter arises as a hollow ureteric bud from the lower end of the mesonephric duct. It grows dorsally and cranially coming into contact with the metanephric cap of the mesoderm, which then ascend together to the lumbar region. The upper end expands and repeatedly divides forming the renal pelvis, major and minor calyces and collecting tubules of the kidney. The caudal part of the mesonephric duct is absorbed into the wall of the urogenital sinus, becoming incorporated and opening directly into the bladder. Two ureteric buds may develop from the mesonephric duct on one side giving rise to double ureters, with one leaving the kidney at the hilum and the other at the lower pole. Splitting of the upper end of the ureteric bud (cleft pelvis) gives rise to a bifid ureter at its upper end.

A muscular tube, the continuation of the renal pelvis terminating at the bladder: its upper part is in the abdomen and lower part in the pelvis. Each ureter passes downwards over psoas behind the peritoneum along the tips of the lumbar transverse processes and crosses the pelvic brim anterior to the bifurcation of the common iliac artery to enter the pelvis, where it passes medially to enter the bladder obliquely at the upper lateral angle of the trigone (Fig. 6.65). In the abdomen, the right ureter lies to the right of the inferior vena cava, with its upper part lying behind the third part of the duodenum: it is crossed anteriorly (from above down) by the gonadal (testicular/ovarian), right colic and ileocolic vessels, root of the mesentery, superior mesenteric vessels and terminal part of the ileum. In the abdomen, the upper part of the left ureter lies behind the stomach: it is crossed anteriorly (from above down) by the left gonadal (testicular/ovarian), superior and inferior colic vessels, with the lower part being crossed by the sigmoid colon and mesocolon. Close to the bladder each ureter is crossed by the vas deferens in males but lies below the broad ligament in females (see Fig. 6.79).

The blood supply to the ureter is from several sources: the upper one-third from the renal artery, middle one-third from the gonadal artery and lower one-third from the internal iliac and inferior vesicle arteries (Fig. 6.66). In females, there is also an additional supply from the uterine artery.

APPLIED ANATOMY: The upper end of the ureters lie on the transpyloric plane at the tip of the 9th costal cartilage on the left and 1.5 cm lower on the right. From this point the ureter extends down to the pubic tubercle.

CLINICAL ANATOMY: Along its length the ureter has three constrictions: where the renal pelvis joins the ureter at the lower end of the kidney; where it crosses the pelvic brim and as it passes through the bladder wall (the narrowest part). There may be an additional constriction where it is crossed by the vas deferens in males or inferior to the root of the broad ligament in females. These constrictions represent regions where kidney stones can become lodged, causing intense pain.

Bladder

DEVELOPMENT: The bladder develops from three parts: the vesicourethral canal, which forms the major part; the proximal part of the allantois forming the apex, with the distal part of the allantois (urachus) forming the median umbilical ligament and the proximal part of the mesonephric ducts, which are absorbed into the bladder wall (trigone). Absorption of the mesonephric ducts frees the ureter, allowing it to open directly into the bladder.

CLINICAL ANATOMY: Failure of formation of the anterior bladder wall, as well as the infra-umbilical part of the anterior abdominal wall, leads to the cavity of the bladder opening onto the body surface just above the symphysis pubis (ectopia vesicae). Failure of obliteration of a localised part, the distal part or all of the urachus after birth gives rise to a urachal cyst, sinus and fistula, respectively. A urachal fistula is accompanied by urine leakage from the umbilicus.

A hollow muscular organ varying in shape, size and position depending on the amount of urine contained. When empty it lies in the pelvis, but as it fills (up to 500–600 mL) it enlarges upwards into the abdominal cavity. It has outer longitudinal, middle circular and

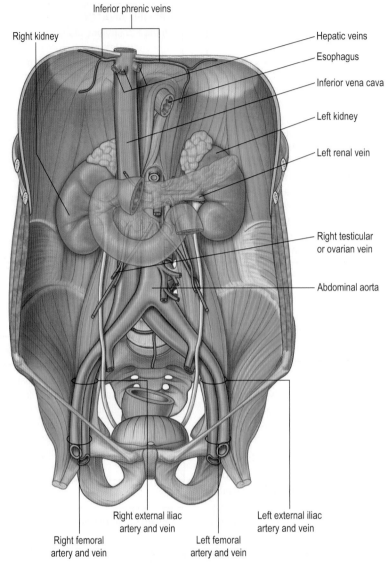

Inferior phrenic veins

Right kidney

Hepatic veins

Esophagus

Inferior vena cava

Left kidney

Left renal vein

Right testicular
or ovarian vein

Abdominal aorta

Right external iliac
artery and vein

Left external iliac
artery and vein

Right femoral
artery and vein

Left femoral
artery and vein

Fig. 6.65 The course and relationships of the ureters in the abdomen and pelvis.

inner longitudinal muscle layers (detrusor muscle), with the lining mucous membrane (transitional epithelium) thrown into folds due to its loose attachment to the underlying tissue, except at the trigone between the openings of the ureters and urethra, where it is firmly attached and appears smooth (Fig. 6.67B).

Empty, the bladder has four pyramidal sides: a posterior base, and superior and two inferolateral surfaces which meet at the apex (Fig. 6.67A), which lies behind the symphysis pubis. The superior surface has coils of small intestine resting on it in males, as well as the uterus in females; the inferolateral surfaces rest on the pelvic floor (levator ani) and against obturator internus posteriorly; and the base is related to the uterus and vagina in females and seminal vesicles and vas deferens in males, with the rectum further posteriorly (Fig. 6.67C). Where the urethra leaves the bladder neck, the bladder is relatively immobile, being fixed by ligaments in both sexes. It is also firmly adherent to the prostate in males.

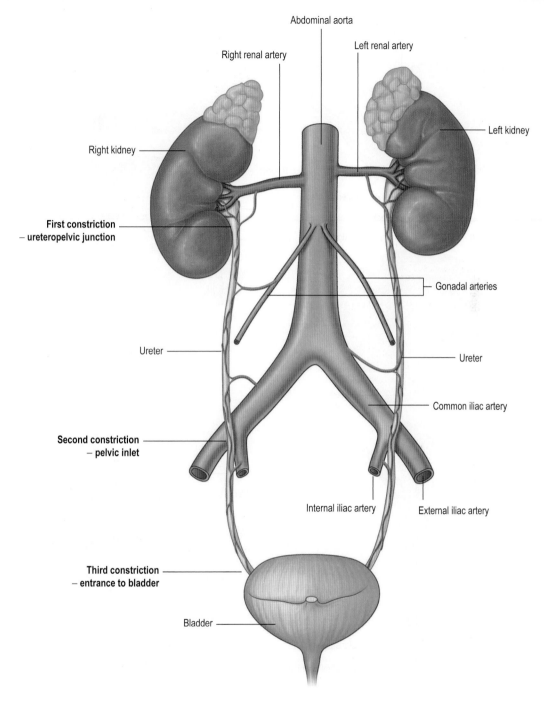

Fig. 6.66 The arterial supply to the ureters, also showing regions where the ureter is constricted.

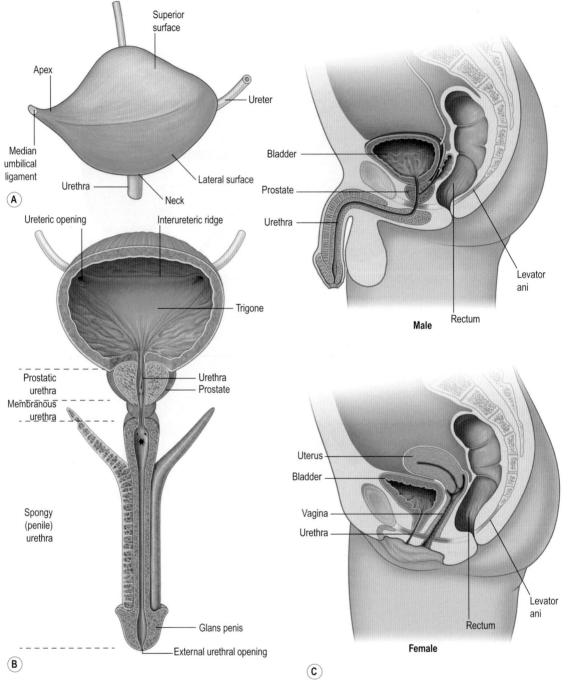

Fig. 6.67 (A) The bladder viewed obliquely. (B) Internal aspect of the bladder showing the trigone and urethra in males. (C) Coronal sections through the abdomen and pelvis showing the position and relations of the bladder in males and females.

Bladder Filling

Urine is continuously formed by nephrons, flowing into the bladder through the ureters. Urine collecting in the renal pelvis initiates a contraction, which is transmitted through the rest of the ureter as a peristaltic wave. A valve at the entrance of the ureters into the bladder opens when peristaltic waves push urine towards it allowing urine to flow through into the bladder. When the detrusor muscle contracts the valve closes preventing backflow of urine.

APPLIED ANATOMY: In infants, the bladder lies in the abdomen and can be palpated in the hypogastrium (page 461) when full. A completely full bladder in adults is potentially palpable above the pubis; however, rectus abdominis makes this difficult.

CLINICAL PHYSIOLOGY: Urinary tract infections involving coliform bacteria (Chlamydia) often produce urethritis, which in females often leads to cystitis because of the short urethra. Infections (urethritis) are usually accompanied by a persistent or more frequent urge to urinate. Urethritis may produce pain or difficulty during urination (dysuria).

CLINICAL PHYSIOLOGY: Inflammation of the bladder lining (cystitis) is common during urinary tract infections; however, it can also be caused by immunodeficiency, urinary catheterisation, radiation and chemotherapy. Chronic cystitis can lead to an unstable urothelium, with benign urothelial changes involving hyperplasia or metaplasia. Bladder cancer usually arises from unstable urothelium.

CLINICAL PHYSIOLOGY: Bladder cancer begins in the epithelial lining, with the most common (90%) type being transitional (urothelial) bladder cancer. Other types are squamous cell bladder cancer (5%), adenocarcinoma (2%), small cell bladder cancer and sarcoma, which involves the muscle or other supporting tissues. The main symptom in 80% of cases is blood in the urine (haematuria), which usually looks bright red or occasionally brown. Other symptoms include passing urine very often and/or very suddenly; pain or burning when passing urine; weight loss; pain in the back, lower abdomen or bones; and feeling tired and generally unwell. Bladder cancer can be secondary to prostatic, rectal, ovarian, cervical or uterine cancer.

Urethra

The urethra is much longer in males (20 cm) than in females (4 cm) (Fig. 6.67B, C). In females, it runs from the neck of the bladder through the pelvic floor and perineal membrane, opening into the vestibule (region between the labia minora) firmly attached to the anterior wall of the vagina.

In males, the urethra passes from the neck of the bladder through the prostate (prostatic urethra), an external sphincter, the pelvic floor and perineal membrane (membranous urethra) and penis enclosed within erectile tissue (penile/spongy urethra), ending at the external urethral opening at the tip of the glans penis (Fig. 6.67B). The prostatic urethra receives the ejaculatory and prostatic ducts (page 535).

The internal urethral sphincter (smooth muscle thickening of the detrusor muscle) is situated between the bladder neck and upper part of the urethra. The external urethral sphincter (circular skeletal muscle) is located in the urogenital diaphragm (page 550) and is under voluntary control.

CLINICAL ANATOMY: Injury to/rupture of the male urethra can occur at well-defined sites, with the commonest being at the proximal penile urethra below the perineal membrane. It is usually torn when perineal structures are caught between a hard object and the inferior pubic arch, with urine escaping through the rupture into the superficial perineal pouch (page 550), descending into the scrotum and up onto the anterior abdominal wall deep to the superficial fascia. (Fluid does not track into the anal triangle (page 555) or thigh because the membranous layer of fascia fuses with the deep tissues at the borders of these regions [Fig. 6.68].) When associated with pelvic fractures, the urethra can rupture at the prostatomembranous junction above the deep perineal pouch (page 550), with urine tracking into the true pelvis. In serious pelvic injuries there can be complete disruption of the puboprostatic ligaments, causing superior displacement of the prostate reinforced by haematoma formation within the true pelvis.

Continued

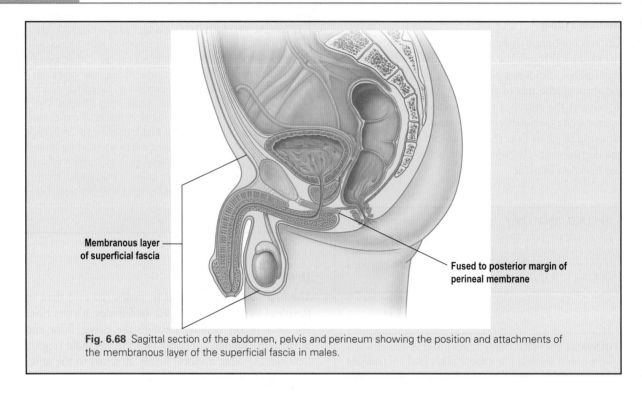

Fig. 6.68 Sagittal section of the abdomen, pelvis and perineum showing the position and attachments of the membranous layer of the superficial fascia in males.

Nerve Supply to the Bladder and Urethral Sphincters

The bladder and internal urethral sphincter are innervated by both sympathetic fibres from the L1 and L2 segments of the spinal cord, and parasympathetic fibres from the S1, S2 and S3 segments, whereas the external urethral sphincter is innervated by somatic fibres from the S2, S3 and S4 segments via the pudendal nerve. Sympathetic stimulation (hypogastric nerve) causes relaxation of detrusor, constriction of the internal urethral sphincter and filling of the bladder. In contrast, parasympathetic stimulation causes contraction of detrusor, relaxation of the internal urethral sphincter and emptying of the bladder, provided the external urethral sphincter is relaxed. If the external urethral sphincter remains in a state of tonic contraction micturition does not occur.

> **APPLIED ANATOMY:** Contraction of the internal urethral sphincter prevents retrograde movement of semen into the bladder during ejaculation.

Micturition

The process by which urine is voided from the bladder. It is a reflex process, which can be overridden and controlled voluntarily in adults and older children. When the bladder contains more than 300–400 mL of urine the desire to micturate increases as the pressure within the bladder starts to rise rapidly (Fig. 6.69). Although some individuals can retain 600 mL, there comes a point at which the bladder will empty involuntarily.

Once a micturition reflex begins it is self-regenerative, activating stretch receptors causing a greater increase in sensory impulses from the bladder and posterior urethra, in turn causing a further increase in reflex bladder contraction. The cycle is repeated again and again until the bladder has attained a strong degree of contraction. After a short time (few seconds to more than a minute), the self-regenerative reflex fatigues and the cycle ends, enabling the bladder to relax. Following a micturition reflex that has not succeeded in emptying the bladder, the associated nerves are inhibited for up to an hour before another reflex can be initiated. Once the need to

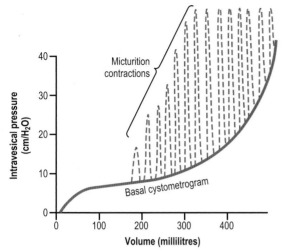

Fig. 6.69 Normal cystometrogram showing micturition contractions caused by micturition reflexes.

micturate becomes powerful enough it causes another reflex, the pudendal nerves to the external urethral sphincter inhibit micturition. However, if inhibition is more potent in the brain than the voluntary constrictor signals to the external sphincter, urination does not occur, in which case the bladder continues filling until the micturition reflex becomes more powerful.

Facilitation or Inhibition by the Brain

The micturition reflex is an autonomic spinal cord reflex, which can be facilitated or inhibited by centres in the brain (facilitative and inhibitory centres mainly in the pons and a centre within the cerebral cortex that are inhibitory but can become excitatory). The reflex is the basic cause of micturition. However, higher centres normally exert the final control by: keeping the micturition reflex partially inhibited, except when micturition is desired; preventing micturition by tonic contraction of the external urethral sphincter until it is convenient to do so; and facilitating the sacral micturition centres to help initiate a micturition reflex when it is appropriate, at the same time inhibiting the external urethral sphincter to enable urination to occur.

Voluntary Urination

This initially involves contraction of the abdominal muscles and diaphragm, raising intra-abdominal pressure, followed by contraction of detrusor and relaxation of the sphincter mechanisms in the proximal part of

the urethra in males and along most of the urethra in females. Towards the end of micturition, the abdominal muscles again contract then relax, detrusor relaxes and the sphincters contract. During micturition, the neck of the bladder becomes funnel-shaped due to relaxation of the pelvic floor.

Abnormalities of Micturition

Atonic bladder. Loss of tone in detrusor occurs when the sensory fibres from the bladder to the spinal cord are destroyed. The individual loses bladder control despite intact efferent fibres from the spinal cord and intact neurogenic connections within the brain. Rather than emptying periodically, the bladder fills to capacity and overflows a few drops at a time through the urethra (overflow incontinence). A common cause of atonic bladder is crush injury to the sacral part of the spinal cord. Some diseases (syphilis) can damage the dorsal root nerve fibres (page 220) entering the spinal cord.

> **CLINICAL ANATOMY:** In individuals unable to empty the bladder, a suprapubic catheter can be passed through the lower part of the anterior abdominal wall immediately above the symphysis pubis to gain access to the bladder to empty the contents.

Automatic bladder. This is characterised by a hyperactive micturition reflex with loss of voluntary control, with small amounts of urine collected in the bladder eliciting the micturition reflex and bladder emptying. It occurs if the spinal cord is damaged above the sacral region with the sacral segments still intact; however, micturition is no longer controlled by the brain. During the initial stage (a few days to several weeks) of spinal shock the bladder loses tone, becoming atonic with overflow incontinence. If the bladder is periodically emptied by catheterisation, to prevent bladder injury caused by overstretching, the micturition reflex gradually increases until typical micturition reflexes return. This is the second stage of spinal shock in which periodic, but often unannounced, bladder emptying occurs.

> **CLINICAL ANATOMY:** Some individuals can still control urination by stimulating the skin in the genital region, eliciting a micturition reflex.

Uninhibited neurogenic bladder. Characterised by frequent and relatively uncontrollable urination. It is the result of partial damage to the spinal cord or brainstem, interrupting most of the inhibitory signals. The facilitative impulses continually passing down the spinal cord keep the sacral centres extremely excitable, so that even a small quantity of urine elicits an uncontrollable micturition reflex, resulting in frequent urination.

Nocturnal micturition. Enuresis (bed wetting) is the involuntary voiding of urine during the night due to the absence of voluntary control. It is a common and normal process in children under 3 years of age.

> **CLINICAL ANATOMY:** Nocturnal micturition in later childhood may be due to neurological (lumbosacral defects) or psychological factors. Loss of voluntary control can also occur following impairment of the motor area of the cerebral cortex.

REPRODUCTIVE SYSTEM

> **DEVELOPMENT:** The early genital systems of both sexes are similar. Under the influence of the testis-determining factor (SRY gene) on the Y chromosome a series of events later occur determining the fate of the rudimentary sexual organs. The gonads appear as a pair of longitudinal (genital) ridges, from which primary sex cords develop and, after the 6th week, primordial germ cells. Up to week 7 the gonads of both sexes are identical (indifferent gonads). In males the primary sex cords form the testes which become connected to the epididymis. In females the primary sex cords degenerate; however, secondary sex cords extend from the surface epithelium of the developing ovary into the underlying mesenchyme incorporating the primary germ cells. As the ovary separates from the regressing mesonephros it becomes suspended by its own ligament (mesovarium). Initially, both males and females have two pairs of ducts (mesonephric, paramesonephric): in males, the mesonephric duct gives rise to the epididymis, ductus (vas) deferens, seminal vesicle, ejaculatory duct, ureteric bud and trigone of the bladder, and the paramesonephric duct degenerates; in females, the paramesonephric ducts form the main genital duct with three recognisable parts, with the first two parts forming the uterine (fallopian) tubes and the fused third parts becoming the body and cervix of the uterus (Fig. 6.70). The surrounding mesenchyme forms the myometrium of the uterus and its peritoneal covering (perimetrium). The fibromuscular wall of the vagina develops from mesenchyme with the epithelial lining derived from the urogenital sinus. Until late in foetal life the lumen of the vagina is separated from the cavity of the urogenital sinus by a membrane (hymen). It usually ruptures during the perinatal period.

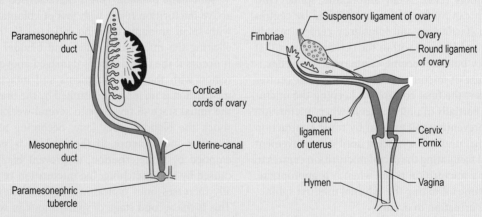

Fig. 6.70 Diagrammatic representation of the female genital ducts at 8 weeks and their contribution to the female genital system.

Sex Determination

This is accomplished by a complex system of genes, the proteins coded by them and their functions on various target organs, which cumulatively determine the development of an individual's sexual characteristics. The process begins with the development of male and female reproductive structures during embryonic development. It is switched on depending on the type of sex chromosomes present, initiating a cascade of events comprising protein synthesis and activation, muting of genes and synthesis of various proteins (factors) which act differently on various organs leading to their sex-specific development.

There are 46 chromosomes (arranged in 23 pairs) in human cells: 44 (22 pairs) are autosomes, which carry genes for characters not related to the formation of the reproductive organs, and 2 sex chromosomes, X and Y. Females have 22 pairs of autosomes and 2 X chromosomes and males have 22 pairs of autosomes and 1 X and 1 Y chromosome. The gametes produced in the ovaries of females contain X chromosomes, while sperm can contain either an X or a Y chromosome, with female offspring being produced when an X-containing chromosome fertilises the ovum and male offspring when a Y-containing chromosome fertilises the ovum. The sex of the child is determined by the type of sex chromosome contributed by the father. The X chromosome contains genes for characteristics such as colour vision, anti-haemophilic factor and the development of mental ability. In the early stage of development in females one X chromosome is permanently inactivated so that gene expression of only 1 X chromosome occurs, ensuring that the number of proteins produced by gene expression of the X chromosome is the same in males and females. The Y chromosome contains the SRY gene, which when activated cells create testosterone and anti-Müllerian hormone which typically ensures the development of a single male reproductive system, with many genes required to develop testes. In XX embryos, cells secrete oestrogen driving the body towards the female pathway.

Abnormalities in the number of X and Y chromosomes are responsible for a number of conditions:

Klinefelter syndrome (karyotype (44+XXY)) is a condition occurring in males with a frequency of 1–2 in 2000. Some individuals have no obvious symptoms, while others may have varying degrees of cognitive, social, behavioural and learning difficulties; adults may also have decreased testosterone production (primary hypogonadism), small and/or undescended testes (cryptorchidism), enlarged breast tissue (gynecomastia), tall stature, as well as an abnormality of the penis (hypospadias, page 539) and a small penis (micropenis). Individuals have a small risk of developing breast cancer and systemic lupus erythematosus.

Triple X (Trisomy X) syndrome (karyotype 44+XXX) affects 1 in 1000 females; however, signs and symptoms vary greatly among individuals, with many having no noticeable effects or only mild symptoms. The most typical physical feature is that individuals are taller than average. Most females undergo normal sexual development and can become pregnant; some have intelligence in the normal range, but slightly lower compared to their siblings, while others have intellectual disabilities and occasionally behavioural problems. Other signs and symptoms include: delayed development of speech, language (difficulty with reading, understanding, mathematics) and motor (sitting up, walking) skills; behavioural problems (attention-deficit hyperactivity disorder (ADHD), autism); psychological problems (anxiety, depression); problems with fine and gross motor skills, memory, judgement and information. Other potential signs and symptoms include vertical folds of skin covering the inner corners of the eyes (epicanthal folds); widely spaced eyes; abnormally curved little finger; flat feet; abnormally shaped sternum; weak muscle tone (hypotonia); seizures; kidney abnormalities and premature ovarian failure or ovarian abnormalities.

Turner's syndrome (karyotype 44+X0) is a chromosomal disorder affecting 1 in 2000 females. Most individuals are infertile. Signs and symptoms include: short stature; a wide webbed neck; low hairline at the back of the neck; swelling (lymphedema) of the hands and feet; skeletal abnormalities (scoliosis, broad chest with widely spaced nipples, arms turned out at the elbow); kidney problems; congenital heart defects or heart murmur; an underactive thyroid; increased risk of developing diabetes, especially when older or overweight; and osteoporosis, due to lack of oestrogen. Most individuals have normal intelligence, but some have developmental delays, learning disabilities and/or behavioural problems. In early childhood middle ear infections are common and can lead to hearing loss; most girls do not produce the necessary sex hormones for puberty, so they do not have a pubertal growth spurt, start their periods or develop breasts without hormone treatment.

XYY syndrome (karyotype 44+XYY) is a chromosomal disorder occurring in 1 in 1000 males. For some the symptoms are barely noticeable, but for others there may be learning and attention difficulties, delayed motor skill development (writing), delayed or difficult speech, low muscle tone (hypotonia), emotional or behavioural issues, hand trembling or involuntary muscle movements, being taller than expected and a diagnosis of autism.

Male Reproductive System

The male reproductive system includes the testes, epididymis, vas deferens, seminal vesicles, prostate, scrotum and penis.

Testis

DEVELOPMENT: The testis develops from three sources: the genital ridge forms the connective tissue and its covering (tunica albuginea); the coelomic epithelium gives rise to the Sertoli cells of the sex cords and the primordial germ cells give rise to spermatogonia (see also page 351). The primitive sex cords branch and anastomose to form the testis cords, which lose their connection with the surface epithelium and canalise to become the seminiferous tubules, the straight ends of which anastomose at the hilum of the testis forming the rete testis. The rete testis becomes connected to the epididymis via the vasa efferentia (mesonephric tubules). The testis develops opposite L1 being initially anchored to the diaphragm by the cranial suspensory ligament and to the inferior portion of the scrotum by the gubernaculum testis. During the 7th week the gubernaculum shortens pulling the testis down towards the deep inguinal ring (page 456), reaching it by the 7th month (Fig. 6.71A). The cranial suspensory ligament degenerates. Further shortening of the gubernaculum pulls the testis through the inguinal canal (page 456) during the 8th month, taking 2–3 days, passing outside the peritoneum and processus vaginalis so that at 9 months it lies at the superficial inguinal ring (page 456). At birth the testis lies within the scrotum (Fig. 6.71B).

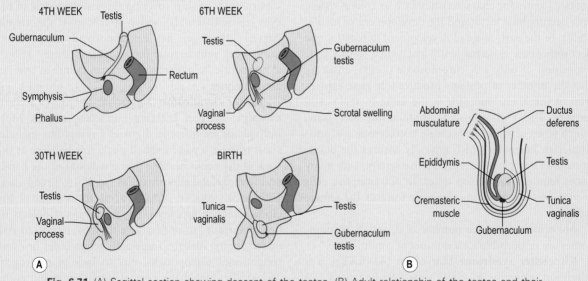

Fig. 6.71 (A) Sagittal section showing descent of the testes. (B) Adult relationship of the testes and their coverings.

> **CLINICAL ANATOMY:** An undescended testis can remain in the abdomen, inguinal canal (page 456) or superficial ring (cryptorchidism: individuals with cryptorchidism have a higher risk of testicular cancer and can become irreversibly sterile) or can descend to an abnormal position (perineum, root of the penis, femoral triangle).

> **CLINICAL ANATOMY:** Failure of the processus vaginalis to become obliterated after the testis has moved into the scrotum leaves a connection with the peritoneal cavity, which can give rise to a hydrocele (swelling of the scrotum due to an accumulation of peritoneal fluid, becoming more obvious when standing) or the presence of a congenital indirect inguinal hernia (page 458).

As the testis migrates into the scrotum it takes with it the testicular artery (branch of the abdominal aorta) and a serous sac (processus vaginalis) derived from the peritoneum. The peritoneal connection to the abdomen becomes obliterated, except around the testis (tunica vaginalis). The tunica vaginalis has an outer parietal layer lining the scrotum and an inner visceral layer covering the tunica albuginea on the anterior and lateral sides of the testis (Fig. 6.72).

Each testis is surrounded by a dense connective tissue capsule (tunica albuginea) from which fibrous septa divide it into some 250 pyramidal lobules (Fig. 6.72), each containing sparse connective tissue with endocrine interstitial (Leydig) cells, which secrete testosterone, and between one and four convoluted seminiferous tubules in which sperm production occurs. Details of spermatogenesis can be found on page 351.

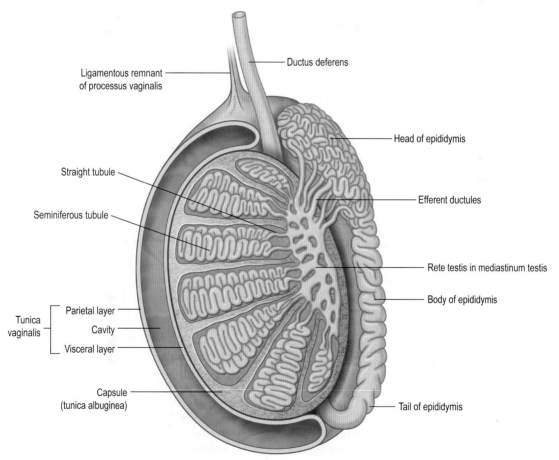

Fig. 6.72 The testis and seminiferous tubules.

Because spermatocytes, spermatids and developing sperm are isolated from plasma proteins and nutrients by the blood-testis barrier, they depend on Sertoli cells for the production and/or transport of metabolites and nutrients into the lumen of the seminiferous tubules. While protecting spermatogenic cells from circulating immune components Sertoli cells supply many plasma factors required for cell growth and differentiation.

APPLIED ANATOMY: Some molecular events involved in sperm production cannot occur at core body temperature (37°C), consequently a temperature of about 34°C is maintained in the scrotum by a number of mechanisms including: the pampiniform plexus of veins surrounding the testicular artery removes heat by a counter-current heat-exchange system; evaporation of sweat from the scrotum; and relaxation/contraction of dartos in the scrotum and cremaster of the spermatic cord (page 457) move the testes away from/towards the body.

CLINICAL ANATOMY: Testicular torsion occurs when a testicle twists within the scrotum, also twisting the spermatic cord, leading to a reduction in blood flow to the testis. It is most common between ages 12 and 18, but can occur at any age, including before birth. It usually requires emergency surgery. If treated quickly the testicle can be saved, but when the blood supply has been cut off for too long the testis can become damaged and has to be removed. Signs and symptoms include sudden, severe pain in the scrotum; swelling of the scrotum; abdominal pain; nausea and vomiting; one testicle much higher than the other or at an unusual angle; frequent urination and fever. Young boys who have testicular torsion typically wake up in the middle of the night or early morning due to scrotal pain.

CLINICAL ANATOMY: Acute or chronic inflammation of the testis (orchitis) usually involves ducts connecting the testis to the epididymis. Common forms of orchitis are produced by infective agents occurring secondarily to a urinary tract or sexually transmitted pathogen (*Chlamydia*, gonorrhoea) entering the testis from the epididymis or via the lymphatics.

Sertoli cells. They continuously release water into the seminiferous tubules carrying new sperm out of the testis. The production of nutrients and androgen-binding protein (ABP), which concentrates testosterone to levels necessary for spermiogenesis, is promoted by follicle-stimulating hormone (FSH). Sertoli cells secrete inhibin, which suppresses FSH synthesis and release by the anterior pituitary gland (page 335). They also secrete anti-Müllerian hormone causing regression of the embryonic paramesonephric (Müllerian) ducts, which if they persist become part of the female reproductive tract. In addition to their endocrine and exocrine function, Sertoli cells phagocytose and digest excess cytoplasm shed as residual bodies during spermiogenesis. No proteins from sperm normally pass back across the blood-testis barrier.

Excretory Genital Ducts

These are the epididymis, ductus (vas) deferens and urethra. They transport sperm from the testis to the penis during ejaculation.

Epididymis. The long, coiled duct of the epididymis lies in the scrotum along the superior and posterior sides of the testis (Fig. 6.72). It has a head, where the efferent ductules enter, body and tail opening into the ductus deferens. While passing through the epididymis, sperm become motile, with their surfaces and acrosomes undergoing final maturation. Fluid within the epididymis contains glycolipid decapacitation factors that bind sperm cell membranes and block acrosomal reactions until the factors are removed as part of the capacitation process in the female reproductive tract. The principal cells of the epididymis secrete glycolipids and glycoproteins, but also absorb water and remove residual bodies and other debris not removed earlier by Sertoli cells. Peristaltic contractions of the inner and outer longitudinal muscle layers, as well as the circular muscle layer in the tail, move the sperm along the duct and empty the body and tail during ejaculation.

CLINICAL ANATOMY: Acute epididymitis is a result of sexually transmitted infection (gonorrhoea, *Chlamydia*) causing intrascrotal pain and tenderness. Persistent inflammation of the epididymis involves massive invasion by leukocytes into the infected duct, stimulating fibrosis obstructing the duct. It is a common cause of male infertility.

Ductus (vas) deferens. Continuation of the epididymis, the ductus (vas) deferens is a long, straight tube with a thick muscular wall and small lumen, which continues towards the prostatic urethra where it empties (Fig. 6.73). Within the prostate the ampulla merges with the duct of the seminal vesicle forming the ejaculatory duct which opens into the prostatic urethra.

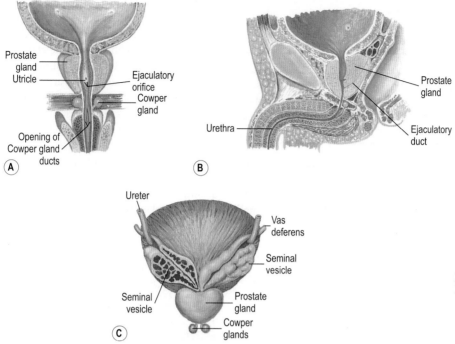

Fig. 6.73 Coronal (A), sagittal (B) sections and posterior aspect (C) showing the accessory glands of the male reproductive system; (B) sagittal section showing the ejaculatory duct passing through the prostate.

CLINICAL ANATOMY: Accessibility to the vas deferens enables vasectomy to be undertaken, in which the vas is exposed, cut, cauterised and tied. Following vasectomy sperm are still produced but degenerate and are removed by macrophages in the epididymis. Adverse effects of vasectomy are minimal, although inflammatory and other changes occur in the mucosa of the epididymis. The procedure may be reversed by reconnecting the cuts ends; however, it often fails to restore fertility due to incomplete sperm maturation in the epididymis changed by post-vasectomy inflammation.

Accessory Glands

The accessory glands produce secretions that are mixed with sperm during ejaculation to produce semen, being essential for reproduction. The glands are the paired seminal vesicles, prostate and paired bulbourethral glands (Fig. 6.73).

Seminal vesicles. The paired seminal vesicles are exocrine glands which secrete a viscid yellowish fluid which makes up 70% of the ejaculate. Secretion is dependent on the presence of testosterone. The fluid contains fructose, a major energy source for sperm, as well as inositol, citrate and other metabolites; prostaglandins, which stimulate activity in the female reproductive tract; and fibrinogen, which allows semen to coagulate after ejaculation.

The efferent duct from each seminal vesicle joins with the ductus deferens after the ampulla to form the ejaculatory duct, which passes through the prostate to empty its contents into the prostatic urethra (Fig. 6.73).

Prostate. A relatively small (about the size of a walnut), dense gland, surrounded by a fibroelastic capsule from which septa extend into the gland dividing it into distinct lobes. It surrounds the urethra below the bladder lying posterior to the symphysis pubis and anterior to the rectum (Fig. 6.73). The prostate comprises 30–50 individual tubuloacinar glands embedded in a dense fibromuscular stroma, in which the smooth muscle contracts during ejaculation. Ducts from individual glands run through the centre of the prostate and may converge, but all empty directly into the prostatic urethra. The tubuloacinar glands produce fluid containing various glycoproteins, enzymes and small molecules (prostaglandins), which are stored until ejaculation. Prostate-specific antigen (PSA) helps liquefy coagulated semen for the slow release of sperm following ejaculation.

APPLIED ANATOMY: The prostate reaches its mature size at puberty. After age 50, its size and secretions decrease.

CLINICAL PHYSIOLOGY: Small amounts of PSA normally leak into the prostatic vasculature. Elevated levels of PSA indicate abnormal glandular mucosa typically due to prostatic carcinoma or inflammation.

The prostate consists of four zones (Fig. 6.74A): the transition, central and peripheral zones surrounded by the fibromuscular zone (stroma). The transition zone occupies only 5% of prostatic volume and surrounds the proximal urethra and is the growth region throughout life, being responsible for benign prostatic hyperplasia (see below): 10%–20% of prostatic cancers originate in the periurethral mucosal glands in this zone. The central zone comprises 25% of the gland's tissue and surrounds the ejaculatory ducts; 2.5% of prostate cancers arise in this zone, and they tend to be more aggressive and are more likely to invade the seminal vesicles. The peripheral zone surrounds the distal urethra and lies immediately deep to the capsule, it comprises 70% of the organ's tissue and contains the main glands: 70%–80% of prostatic cancers originate from this zone. The prostate can also be considered as consisting of a number of lobes: anterior (isthmus), posterior, median (middle) and right and left lateral lobes (Fig. 6.74B).

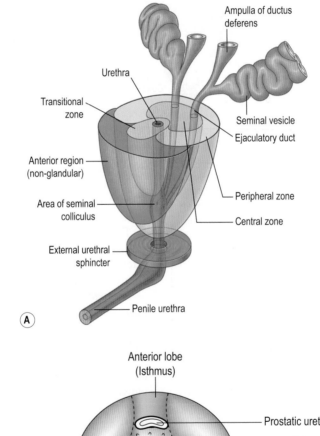

Fig. 6.74 Zones (A) and lobes (B) of the prostate. *M,* Median lobe.

Bulbourethral (Cowper's) glands. Paired round glands situated in the urogenital diaphragm (page 550) which empty into the proximal part of the penile urethra. During sexual arousal the glands, together with many other small and similar glands along the penile urethra, are responsible for releasing a clear mucus-like secretion pre-ejaculate fluid (Cowper's fluid) that neutralises the acidity of the urethra and lubricates it in preparation for the passage of sperm.

Semen

The white/grey fluid comprises 10% sperm and 90% fluid (seminal plasma) from the testes, seminal vesicles, prostate and bulbourethral glands. It is ejaculated through the penis at the climax of male sexual arousal. Immediately following ejaculation, the sperm are non-motile due to the viscosity of the coagulum, but as the coagulum dissolves the sperm become motile. The seminal vesicles contribute 60% (ascorbic acid, fibrinogen, flavin, fructose, inositol, pepsinogen, phosphorylcholine, PGE_2, citrate, citric acid) and the prostate 30% (acid phosphatase, cholesterol, clotting enzymes, fibrinolysin, glucose, lactate dehydrogenase, phospholipids, plasminogen activator, seminin, spermine, bicarbonate, calcium, citrate, sodium, zinc) to seminal plasma.

Sperm. Sperm consists of four parts (Fig. 6.75): an oval head comprising a condensed nucleus with a thin cytoplasm, of which the anterior two-thirds is the acrosome containing hyaluronidase and proteolytic enzymes essential to enable the sperm to fertilise the ovum; a short neck, which with the body is the midpiece; a cylindrical body with a central core (axial filament) surrounded by a closely wound spiral filament consisting of mitochondria; and tail consisting of two pieces, chief (main) piece and terminal (end) piece.

To maximise the chance of fertilisation the sperm count must be at least 20 million/mL, with the number of sperm in the ejaculate being at least 40 million. In addition, 75% of sperm must be alive, 50% must be motile, and 30% have a normal shape and structure. Fewer than 35% have head, 20% midpiece and 20% tail defects.

Anomalies of sperm and semen. A number of anomalies are associated with sperm and semen, which will have a profound effect on the ability to fertilise the egg (ovum): a lack of sperm in semen (azoospermia), a congenital disease caused by corticosteroids and androgens; a sperm count of less than 20 million/mL (oligozoospermia); sperm with abnormal morphology (teratozoospermia), which can occur in Crohn's, Hodgkin and coeliac disease; lack of semen (aspermia) due to retrograde ejaculation into the bladder, which can be caused by prostatic surgery or excess drug use; a low volume of sperm (oligospermia); and the appearance of blood in semen (haematospermia) due to infection of the urethra or prostate, also being common in congenital bleeding disorders.

Parts of sperm   Structure of different parts of sperm

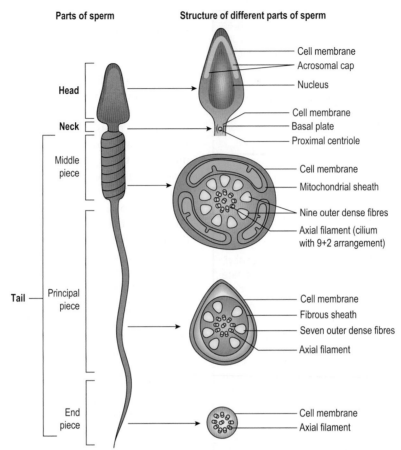

Fig. 6.75 Human sperm.

Penis

Because the penis houses the continuation of the prostatic urethra, where the secretions of the reproductive system enter the urethra prior to their ejaculation, it can be considered as part of both the urinary and reproductive systems.

The penis consists of three cylindrical masses of erectile tissue surrounded by skin (Figs 6.76 and 6.77A), with the corpora cavernosa dorsal and corpus spongiosum, containing the urethra, ventral which is expanded at its end (gland penis). Each corpus cavernosum is covered by a dense fibroelastic layer (tunica albuginea). The penis has two parts: the root comprising the two crura, which are the proximal parts of the corpora cavernosa attached to the pubic arch, and bulb of the penis, the proximal part of the corpus spongiosum attached to the perineal

membrane; and body (shaft) which is formed by tethering the three parts together (Fig. 6.77). All three erectile tissues consist of numerous venous cavernous spaces separated by trabeculae, with smooth muscle and connective tissue continuous with the surrounding tunic. Central arteries in the corpora cavernosa branch to form nutritive arterioles and small coiling helicine arteries, which lead to the vascular spaces of erectile tissue. There are arteriovenous shunts between the central arteries and dorsal veins. Erection involves blood filling the cavernous spaces in the three masses of erectile tissue.

Each corpus cavernosus, including its crus, is covered by the ischiocavernosus muscle, and the corpus spongiosum, including the bulb, by the bulbospongiosus muscle (Fig. 6.67B). Ischiocavernosus forces blood from the crus into the body of the erect penis, while

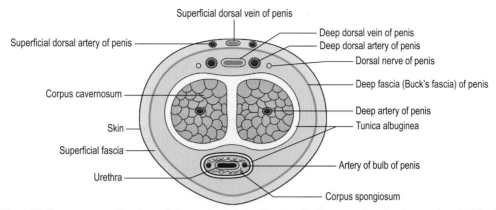

Fig. 6.76 Transverse section through the penis showing the erectile tissue, tunica albuginea and major blood vessels.

bulbospongiosus forces more blood into more distal regions, especially the glans penis.

> **APPLIED ANATOMY:** In males, bulbospongiosus also facilitates emptying of the bulbous part of the penile urethra following urination, while its reflex contractions during ejaculation are responsible for the pulsatile emission of semen from the penis.

> **APPLIED ANATOMY:** In uncircumcised males the glans penis is covered by the prepuce (foreskin), a retractable fold of thin skin with sebaceous glands on its inner surface.

> **CLINICAL ANATOMY:** Hypospadias is a birth defect in which the opening of the urethra is not located at the tip of the penis but is on the ventral surface between the end of the penis and scrotum, due to failure of the urethral folds to fuse together. There are different degrees of hypospadias, some of which can be minor (subcoronal, where the opening is near the glans penis) and some more severe (midshaft, where the opening is on the shaft; penoscrotal, where the opening is at the junction of the penis and scrotum). In addition to an abnormal opening, other symptoms include downward curve of the penis (chordee), a hooded appearance of the penis because only the top half is covered by foreskin; and abnormal spraying during urination. Individuals may experience erectile problems, especially when associated with a chordee. There is usually minimal interaction with the ability to ejaculate provided the opening remains distal; however, there can be pain on ejaculation and/or a weak/dribbling ejaculation. The condition can be surgically corrected.

> **CLINICAL ANATOMY:** Epispadias is a rare birth defect in which the external urethral opening is somewhere on the dorsal surface of the penis. In glandular epispadias the opening is on the top of the glans rather than at the tip; in penile epispadias the opening is anywhere before the glans but above where the shaft meets the body wall; and in penopubic epispadias the opening is close to the body wall near the pubis at the base of the penis. The condition can occur alone, but is more commonly associated with other conditions ranging from additional alterations to the way urine exits the body, bladder issues (bladder exstrophy), and incomplete abdominal wall formation. Ten percent of individuals have no additional problems; however, 90% have an epispadias-related condition (exstrophy-epispadias complex). Other conditions commonly appearing with epispadias include small genitalia; gaping of the pubic bones; pelvic floor alterations; atypical position of the anus; and inguinal hernia (page 458).

Erection and ejaculation. Triggered by external stimuli to the CNS, erection is controlled by autonomic nerves. Parasympathetic stimulation relaxes the trabecular muscle dilating the helicine arteries enabling blood to flow and fill the cavernous spaces in the erectile tissue, enlarging them, and causing compression of the dorsal veins against the dense tunica albuginea, blocking venous outflow and producing rigidity in the erectile tissue. At the start of ejaculation, sympathetic stimulation constricts the helicine arteries and trabecular muscle decreasing blood flow into the spaces allowing the veins to drain most blood from the erectile tissue.

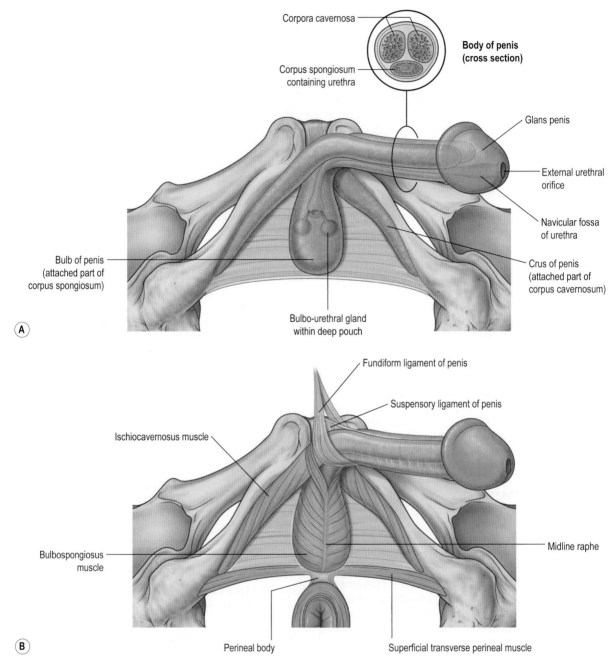

Fig. 6.77 (A) Erectile tissue of the penis. (B) Muscles in the superficial perineal pouch covering the erectile tissue.

CLINICAL ANATOMY: Erectile dysfunction is the inability to initiate or maintain an erection. It increases with age, being a risk factor for coronary heart disease. It is frequently associated with cardiovascular disease, anxiety, diabetes, spinal cord injuries, multiple sclerosis and nerve damage due to pelvic surgery or pelvic radiation.

Ejaculation of semen from the penis is generated by the reflex contraction of bulbospongiosus (innervated by the pudendal nerve), forcing semen from the base of the penis out of the external urethral orifice. Contraction of the internal urethral sphincter and periurethral smooth muscle prevents retrograde ejaculation into the bladder; they are innervated by sympathetic nerves.

CLINICAL ANATOMY: Delayed or absent ejaculation can be due to nerve damage associated with diabetes, Parkinson's disease, spinal cord injuries, multiple sclerosis, pelvic surgery complications and pelvic irradiation. Although ejaculation may be absent following radical prostatectomy for prostate cancer (which also removes the seminal vesicles), orgasm is still possible as the pudendal nerve is spared. Premature ejaculation is when the male ejaculates too quickly during sexual intercourse. It can be due to various physical (prostate problems, under or overactive thyroid, use of recreational drugs) and psychological (depression, stress, relationship problems, anxiety about sexual performance) factors.

Female Reproductive System

The greater part of the female reproductive system (ovaries, uterine (fallopian) tubes, uterus, upper part of the vagina) lies in the pelvis, with the lower part of the vagina lying in the perineum. The ovary is the female gonad (analogous to the testis in males); the uterine tube conveys the ovum (egg) to the uterus where, following fertilisation, the zygote becomes implanted; development into an embryo and foetus occurs in the uterus. The vagina connects the uterus to the exterior, enabling sperm to enter the uterus and uterine tubes, as well as acting as the birth canal. Details of the development of the female reproductive system can be found on page 530.

Ovary

Each ovary lies in the posterior layer of the broad ligament close to the opening (infundibulum) of the uterine tube (Fig. 6.78). The lower pole is connected to the uterus by the round ligament of the ovary, which is continuous with the round ligament of the uterus, which passes through the inguinal canal to the labia majora (page 552). At approximately monthly intervals a single ovum (Graafian follicle) is shed by one ovary and enters the peritoneal cavity, where it is immediately engulfed by the infundibulum and conveyed to the uterus; the journey takes 4 days. Further details of the ovary and ovulation can be found on pages 356 and 358, respectively.

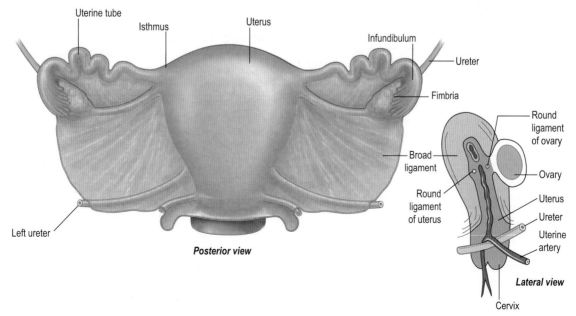

Fig. 6.78 Posterior and lateral aspects of the broad ligament showing the uterus and ovary.

APPLIED ANATOMY: Up until age 6 the ovary lies in the iliac fossa, after which it moves into the pelvis.

APPLIED ANATOMY: In children the surface of the ovary is smooth, becoming more irregular with successive ovulations, resulting in areas of fibrous tissue. Following the menopause, the ovary becomes smaller.

CLINICAL ANATOMY: During pregnancy the ovary is pulled upwards by the enlarging uterus, returning to the pelvis after childbirth; however, its position is more variable and no longer vertical.

CLINICAL ANATOMY: An ovarian cyst is a fluid-filled sac that develops on the ovary. Most occur naturally and disappear after a few months without requiring treatment. Cysts usually only cause symptoms if they rupture, are very large or obstruct the blood supply to the ovary. Symptoms include pelvic pain (ranging from a dull heavy sensation to a sudden, severe and sharp pain), pain during intercourse, difficulty emptying the bowels, frequent need to urinate, heavy/irregular/lighter periods than normal, bloating and a swollen abdomen, a feeling of being full after eating only small amounts and difficulty getting pregnant (fertility is usually unaffected).

CLINICAL ANATOMY: Ovarian tumours commonly originate in the germinal epithelium at the transition zone continuous with the peritoneum of the mesovarium. They can occur at any age but are more frequent in older women. The cancer can spread via the blood and lymphatics, frequently metastasising directly into the peritoneal cavity, allowing the spread of tumour cells along the paracolic gutters to the liver, from where the disease can easily disseminate. At the time of diagnosis many individuals already have metastatic and diffuse disease. The risk of ovarian cancer is increased in women who have ovulated more over their lifetime, either by starting at a younger age or reaching menopause later. Other risk factors include hormone therapy after menopause, fertility medication and obesity; however, few/no menstrual cycles, hormonal birth control, multiple pregnancies, an early pregnancy, tubal ligation

and breast feeding reduce the risk. Approximately 10% of cases are related to an inherited genetic risk. Individuals with mutations in the BRCA1 and BRCA2 genes have a 50% chance of developing the disease. Early signs and symptoms may be absent, subtle and painless, but include: bloating; abdominal and/or pelvic pain or discomfort; back pain; irregular menstruation or postmenopausal vaginal bleeding; pain during or after sexual intercourse; loss of appetite; fatigue; diarrhoea; indigestion; heartburn; constipation; nausea; feeling full and frequent or urgent urination. Late symptoms include: pain caused by the growing mass or metastases pressing on abdominopelvic organs; menometrorrhagia (irregular, but frequent, prolonged or excessive bleeding); abnormal vaginal bleeding after menopause; hirsutism; virilisation and an adnexal mass (a lump in tissue closely related, both structurally and functionally, to the uterus).

Uterine (Fallopian) Tubes

Each extends laterally from the junction of the fundus and body of the uterus (see Fig. 6.80), with the lumen communicating with that of the uterus (Fig. 6.79). The narrowest part (isthmus) is where it joins the uterus, widening (ampulla) as it passes laterally, ending as the funnel-shaped infundibulum fringed with fimbria, one of which attaches to the superior pole of the ovary. The layers of the uterine tube are continuous with their counterparts in the uterus (see below).

APPLIED ANATOMY: Fertilisation takes place in the uterine tube at the ampulla, with the fertilised ovum moved by contraction of its smooth muscular wall, as well as by the action of cilia, towards the uterus.

CLINICAL ANATOMY: A tubal pregnancy occurs when there is a delay in the passage of the fertilised (and dividing) ovum so that it becomes lodged in the uterine tube. Rupture of the tube, with severe haemorrhage, usually occurs within 4–6 weeks; it can be fatal.

CLINICAL ANATOMY: Tubal ligation is a simple and effective form of birth control preventing sperm from reaching the ovum.

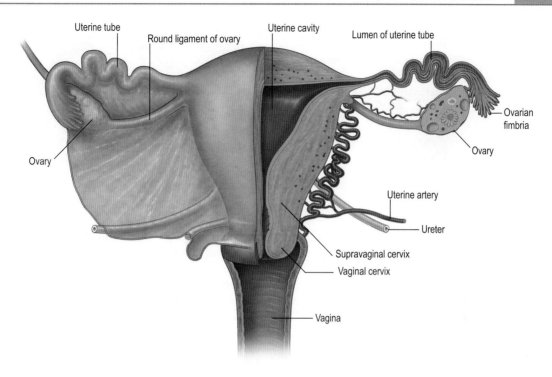

Fig. 6.79 Posterior aspect of the uterus with the broad ligament (left side) and a coronal section through the uterus, uterine tube and ovary (right side).

Uterus

A thick-walled muscular organ lying in the pelvic cavity. It can be divided into three parts, fundus above the opening of the uterine tubes, body narrowing inferiorly and neck (cervix) projecting into the vagina. The cavity is triangular mediolaterally and slit-like anteroposteriorly, being continuous with the cervical canal through the isthmus and opening into the vagina through the external os (Fig. 6.80A). Except for the vaginal part of the cervix, the uterus is relatively free and mobile. In most women the body lies over the superior surface of the bladder (anteverted); however, the uterus is also bent forwards along its own axis (anteflexed) (Fig. 6.80B). The uterus is separated from the bladder by the uterovesical pouch; posteriorly, it is separated from the middle third of the rectum by the rectouterine pouch (of Douglas) (Fig. 6.67C). Inferiorly the cervix is supported by the muscular pelvic floor and condensations of pelvic fascia forming three ligaments (transverse cervical, pubocervical, sacrocervical).

CLINICAL ANATOMY: A bifid (bicornuate) uterus is more or less completely divided into two, often with lateral horns, resulting from imperfect union of the paramesonephric ducts (Fig. 6.81). The cervix can be single (uterus bicornis unicollis) or double (uterus bicornis bicollis); in 25% of cases, it is associated with a longitudinal vaginal septum. The most common symptomatic presentation is early pregnancy loss and cervical incompetence. Infertility is usually not a problem because embryo implantation is not impaired.

CLINICAL ANATOMY: The fibromuscular perineal body (associated with levator ani) is important in maintaining the pelvic floor. If it becomes damaged during childbirth, prolapse of the uterus and other pelvic viscera may occur, including the bladder in severe cases.

The cervical region around the external os projects into the upper vagina. Under the influence of progesterone the consistency of cervical mucous changes

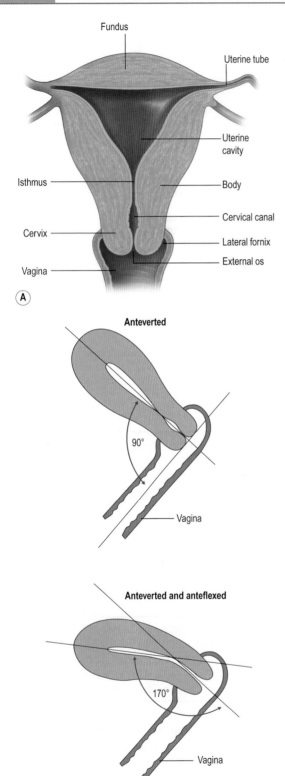

(A)

Anteverted

90°

Vagina

Anteverted and anteflexed

170°

Vagina

(B)

Fig. 6.80 (A) Coronal section through the uterus. (B) Sagittal sections showing the 'normal' position of the uterus.

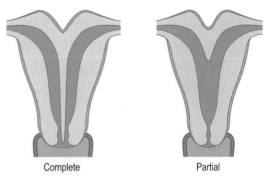

Complete   Partial

Fig. 6.81 Complete and partial bifid (bicornuate) uterus.

cyclically, playing a significant role in fertilisation and early pregnancy. At ovulation, the mucous secretion is watery, facilitating movement of sperm into the uterus; in the luteal phase the mucous is more viscous, hindering the passage of sperm; during pregnancy the cervical glands proliferate and secrete highly viscous mucous which forms a plug in the cervical canal. The cervix becomes relatively rigid during pregnancy, helping to retain the foetus in the uterus. Prior to parturition the cervix softens and the cervical canal dilates.

CLINICAL PHYSIOLOGY: Periodic exposure of the epithelial junction zone immediately outside the external os can lead to epithelial dysplasia and squamous cell neoplasia (most common type of cervical cancer). The human papillomavirus (HPV) is implicated in its pathogenesis.

The main blood supply to the uterus is from the uterine artery (Fig. 6.79), a branch of the anterior division of the internal iliac artery, with the fundus (and uterine tube) also receiving a supply from the ovarian (gonadal) artery (a direct branch from the abdominal aorta), and the cervix from the vaginal artery (a branch of the anterior division of the internal iliac).

The uterus has three major layers: an outer connective tissue layer (perimetrium) continuous with the supporting ligaments; a thick layer of highly vascularised smooth muscle (myometrium) and a mucosa (endometrium), which is influenced cyclically by the changing levels of ovarian hormones (Fig. 6.82).

Myometrium. The myometrium has bundles of smooth muscle fibres separated by connective tissue containing venous plexuses and lymphatics. The smooth muscle is arranged in layers (outer, inner)

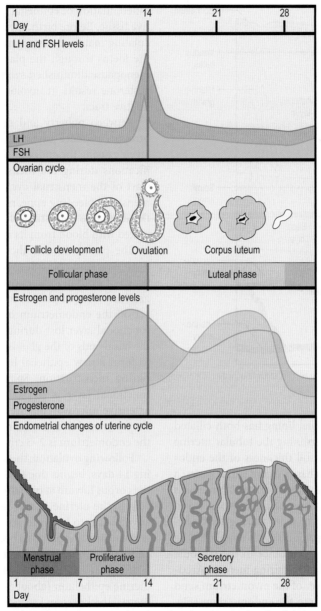

Fig. 6.82 Correlation of ovarian and menstrual cycles also showing the levels of their controlling hormones and changes in the endometrium.

parallel to the long axis of the uterus. During pregnancy the myometrium goes through a period of extensive growth involving hyperplasia, cell hypertrophy and increased collagen production by the muscle cells strengthening the uterine wall. This well-developed myometrium forcefully contracts during parturition to expel the infant from the uterus. Following pregnancy the smooth muscle cells shrink, with many undergoing apoptosis, with removal of unneeded collagen, with the uterus returning to its pre-pregnancy size.

CLINICAL ANATOMY: Benign tumours (fibroids) can develop in the myometrium. They can become sufficiently large to cause painful pressure and unexpected bleeding.

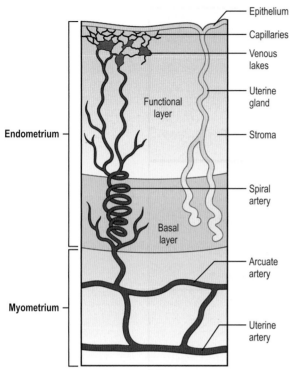

Epithelium
Capillaries
Venous lakes
Uterine gland
Stroma
Spiral artery
Arcuate artery
Uterine artery

Functional layer

Basal layer

Endometrium

Myometrium

Fig. 6.83 Arterial supply to the endometrium.

Endometrium. The epithelial lining has both ciliated and secretory cells, the latter lining the tubular uterine glands which penetrate the full thickness of the endometrium. The endometrium has two concentric zones: a basal layer adjacent to the myometrium, which remains relatively unchanged, and a superficial functional layer, which undergoes profound changes during the menstrual cycle (Fig. 6.82). The blood vessels supplying the endometrium have special significance in the periodic sloughing of the functional layer during menses. Arcuate arteries in the middle layer of the myometrium send two sets of smaller arteries into the endometrium (Fig. 6.83): straight arteries, which supply only the basal layer; and long, progesterone-sensitive spiral arteries, which extend further and supply blood throughout the functional layer. The spiral arteries branch providing a rich superficial capillary bed which includes many dilated, thin-walled vascular lacunae drained by venules. The cervix lacks spiral arteries and is therefore not shed during menstruation.

Menstrual cycle. Throughout the menstrual cycle oestrogens and progesterone control the growth and differentiation of epithelial cells and associated connective tissue. Before birth, these cells are influenced by circulating maternal oestrogen and progesterone reaching the foetus through the placenta (page 548). Following menopause diminished synthesis of oestrogen and progesterone results in involution of tissues in the reproductive tract.

Between puberty and menopause pituitary gonadotropins produce cyclic changes in ovarian hormone levels causing the endometrium to undergo cyclic modifications during the menstrual cycle (Fig. 6.82). The start of the menstrual cycle is taken as the day when menstrual bleeding appears, which lasts 3–4 days, with the discharge consisting of degenerating endometrium mixed with blood from its ruptured microvasculature.

The proliferative (follicular, oestrogen) phase lasts 8–10 days and coincides with rapid growth of a small group of ovarian follicles, which actively secrete oestrogen increasing its plasma concentration. The oestrogens act on the endometrium inducing regeneration of the functional layer lost during menstruation, with cells in the basal ends of the glands proliferating and migrating to form a new epithelial lining of the surface exposed during menstruation. Spiral arteries lengthen as the functional layer is re-established and grows, with an extensive microvasculature forming near the surface of the functional layer. At the end of the proliferative phase the endometrium is 2–3 cm thick.

Following ovulation, the secretory (luteal) phase, lasting 14 days, begins due to the progesterone secreted by the corpus luteum at ovulation stimulating the epithelial cells of the uterine glands (formed during the proliferative phase) to begin to secrete and accumulate glycogen, causing the glands to become coiled (Fig. 6.82). The endometrium now reaches its full thickness (5 mm). If fertilisation has occurred the embryo attaches to the uterine epithelium (about 5 days later) when the endometrial thickness and secretions are optimal for implantation and nutrition, with the major source of nutrients for the embryo before and during implantation being the uterine secretions. Progesterone also inhibits strong contractions of the myometrium that could interfere with implantation.

If fertilisation and implantation do not occur the menstrual phase begins. The corpus luteum regresses and circulating levels of progesterone and oestrogens start to decrease 8–10 days following ovulation, causing menstruation. The reduction in progesterone produces muscle spasms in the small spiral arteries of the functional layer, interrupting normal blood flow, and increased synthesis by arterial cells of prostaglandins, producing vasoconstriction and local hypoxia. Cells undergoing hypoxic injury release cytokines, which increase vascular permeability and immigration of leukocytes, which release collagenase and other matrix metalloproteinases that degrade the basement membranes and other extracellular matrix components. As the basal layer is not dependent on the progesterone-sensitive spiral arteries it remains relatively unaffected; however, the functional layer (including the surface epithelium, most of each uterine gland, the stroma and blood-filled lacunae) become detached from the endometrium and slough away as the menstrual flow (menses) begins. Arterial constriction usually limits blood loss during menstruation, but some blood is lost from the open ends of the venules. At the end of the menstrual phase the endometrium is reduced to a thin layer ready to begin a new cycle as its cells begin dividing to reconstitute the mucosa.

APPLIED PHYSIOLOGY: The amount of endometrium and blood lost in menstruation varies between individuals, as well as in the same individual at different times.

CLINICAL PHYSIOLOGY: Viable endometrial tissue can enter or pass through the uterine tubes, leading, in some individuals, to endometrial tissue growing on the ovaries, uterine tubes and elsewhere (endometriosis). The endometrial tissue undergoes the same cyclic changes induced by oestrogen and progesterone; however, the degenerated tissue cannot effectively be removed from the body. Endometriosis produces pelvic pain, inflammation, ovarian cysts (page 542), adhesions and scar tissue that can cause infertility.

APPLIED ANATOMY: During pregnancy the uterus (and foetus) enlarges upwards occupying more and more of the abdominal cavity (Fig. 6.84). By 12 weeks it has reached the symphysis pubis (page 569); by 24 weeks the umbilicus; by 36 weeks the xiphisternum (page 69).

In the final 4 weeks the foetal head may descend into the pelvis (engagement of the head). At the end of labour (page 365), the uterus returns almost to its former size within 6 weeks.

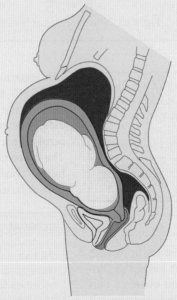

Fig. 6.84 Sagittal section showing the size and position of the uterus and foetus near full-term.

CLINICAL ANATOMY: Fibroids are benign (non-cancerous) growths consisting of muscle and fibrous tissue that can develop anywhere in the uterus, and can vary considerably in size under the influence of oestrogen and progesterone. They are usually slow growing and new fibroids can develop over time; after menopause they usually begin to shrink in line with hormonal changes. The main types of fibroids are intramural (most common), which develop in the myometrium; submucosal, which develop in the myometrium deep to the endometrium and grow into the uterine cavity; subserosal, which develop outside the uterus into the pelvis and can become very large; and pedunculated, which are submucosal or subserosal fibroids attached to the uterus by a narrow stalk (Fig. 6.85). Symptoms include: heavy periods that can last a long time, which can lead to anaemia with feelings of tiredness, dizziness and shortness of breath; painful periods (dysmenorrhoea); abdominal swelling; pain and/or pressure in the pelvis; bloating or constipation; increased frequency of urination and fertility problems (difficulty in becoming pregnant).

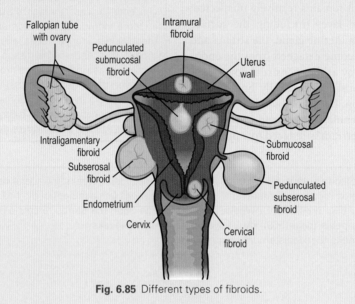

Fig. 6.85 Different types of fibroids.

CLINICAL ANATOMY: Surgical removal of the uterus (hysterectomy) may be performed in individuals with reproductive malignancy (cancer), endometriosis and/or excessive bleeding. The procedure usually removes the fundus, body and cervix, although the cervix may be left *in situ*. It may also include removal of the ovaries (oophorectomy) or both the ovaries and fallopian tubes (salpingo-oophorectomy).

Placenta. The placenta connects the developing foetus to the uterine wall and contains tissues from both foetus and mother, the embryonic part being the chorion (derived from the trophoblast) and maternal part from the decidua basalis (part of the endometrium). It is the site of exchange of nutrients, wastes, O_2 and CO_2 between mother and foetus. Exchange occurs between embryonic blood in chorionic villi outside the embryo and maternal blood in lacunae of the decidua basalis (Fig. 6.86). Suspended in pools of maternal blood in the decidua, the chorionic villi provide an enormous surface area for metabolic exchange, with diffusion occurring across the trophoblast layer and capillary endothelium. The placenta is also an endocrine organ, producing human chorionic gonadotropin (hCG), relaxin, various growth factors, oestrogen and progesterone.

CLINICAL ANATOMY: Implantation of the fertilised ovum usually occurs on the ventral or dorsal walls of the body of the uterus; however, sometimes it attaches close to the internal os, in which case the placenta becomes interposed between the foetus and vagina (placenta previa) obstructing the passage of the foetus during parturition. In this situation the foetus should be delivered by caesarean section to avoid the potential of foetal death.

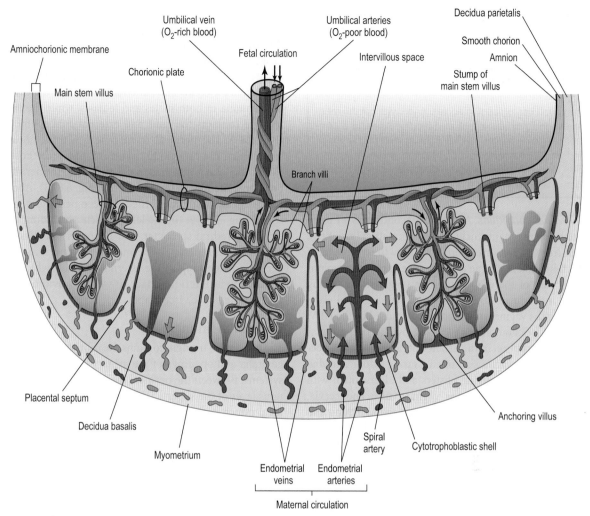

Fig. 6.86 Following implantation, the endometrium develops three regions (decidua basalis/capsularis/parietalis): chorionic stem villi contain a branch from the umbilical artery and vein, with the entire villus bathed in maternal blood circulated by endometrial arteries and veins.

Vagina

Terminal part of the female reproductive tract continuous with the uterine cavity through the external os and opening into the vestibule between the labia minora (page 552), lying parallel with the pelvic inlet (page 573), it is an elastic, muscular canal with a soft flexible lining that provides lubrication and sensation. The space between the cervix and vagina (fornix) is divided into anterior, posterior and lateral parts (Fig. 6.80). The anterior and posterior walls are usually opposed, becoming distended and elongated during childbirth. The posterior wall is longer than

the anterior so that the posterior fornix is deeper than the anterior.

The vagina is surrounded by levator ani. It is related to the base of the bladder, to which it is bound anteriorly, to the rectouterine pouch and ampulla of the rectum posteriorly, and inferiorly to the perineal body. The upper part of the vagina is related to the broad ligament containing the ureter and uterine artery (Fig. 6.79).

The mucous membrane lining is firmly attached to the underlying muscular layer, being thick and corrugated by transverse elevations (vaginal rugae). Longitudinal ridges form anterior and posterior rugal columns in the corresponding walls. The musculature is arranged longitudinally, with a thin layer of erectile tissue between the mucosal and muscular layers.

> **CLINICAL ANATOMY:** Gartner's duct can swell forming a Gartner's (vaginal wall) cyst, which is generally benign. It can present in adolescence with painful menstruation (dysmenorrhea) or difficulty inserting a tampon. Typically it does not have any symptoms, although individuals may complain of infection, bladder dysfunction, abdominal pain, vaginal discharge, urinary incontinence and discomfort during intercourse.

Vaginal conditions. A number of conditions are associated with the vagina including inflammation (vaginitis), often from a yeast or bacterial overgrowth, symptoms of which include discharge and a change of odour; involuntary spasm of the vaginal muscles (vaginismus) during sexual intercourse, due to emotional stress; genital warts affecting the vagina, vulva and cervix, caused by the HPV; infection (trichomoniasis), caused by the trichomonas parasite; disruption in the balance of healthy vaginal bacteria (bacterial vaginosis), often causing odour and discharge; painful, recurring blisters and ulcers, often with no symptoms, affecting the vagina, vulva and cervix, caused by the herpes simplex virus; vaginal itching and discharge due to bacterial infection (gonorrhoea), there may be no symptoms but it can cause pelvic inflammatory disease and infertility; vaginal discharge and/or vaginal or abdominal pain caused by chlamydia, it can also cause pelvic inflammatory disease and infertility; vaginal bleeding and/or discharge caused by cancer and vaginal prolapse due to weakened pelvic muscles, often following childbirth, in which the uterus, rectum or bladder push on the vagina (in severe cases the vagina protrudes out of the perineum).

PERINEUM

Together with the pelvis, the perineum contains and supports the terminal parts of the digestive tract (anal canal), urinary system (urethra) and reproductive system (penis and scrotum in males, vagina and vulva in females). Details of the penis can be found on page 538, of the urethra in males and in females on page 527, and of the vagina on page 549.

The perineum is a diamond-shaped region separated from the pelvis by the pelvic floor between the thighs. Its peripheral boundary is the pelvic outlet (page 573) and narrow lateral walls, the walls of the pelvic cavity below the attachment of levator ani. It is divided into anterior urogenital and posterior anal triangles. The anterior triangle is associated with the openings of the reproductive and urinary systems and functions to anchor the external genitalia in both males and females, while the anal triangle contains the anus and external anal sphincter (Fig. 6.87). The perineal membrane is a thick fibrous sheet filling the urogenital triangle. It has a free posterior border and is attached in the midline to the perineal body and laterally to the pubic arch (Fig. 6.87B). Above the perineal membrane is the thin deep perineal pouch containing a layer of skeletal muscle, including the external urethral sphincter, and neurovascular tissues. The strong fibromuscular perineal membrane and deep perineal pouch support the external genitalia, which are attached to its inferior surface, as well as providing support for the pelvic viscera above.

Urogenital Triangle

The urogenital triangle contains the roots of the external genitalia and openings of the urinary and reproductive systems. Between the perineal membrane and membranous layer of the superficial fascia is the superficial perineal pouch containing the erectile tissues of the penis or clitoris and their associated muscles (Figs 6.77 and 6.88). The clitoris comprises two corpora cavernosa and the glans clitoris; details of the penis can be found on page 538.

> **APPLIED ANATOMY:** The glans clitoris is exposed in the perineum. The body of the clitoris can be palpated through the skin.

The greater vestibular (Bartholin's) glands are small mucous glands on each side of the vagina in the superficial perineal pouch; however, the bulbourethral glands lie within the deep perineal pouch. The duct of the greater vestibular glands opens into the vestibule of the perineum along the posterolateral margin of the vaginal opening.

Paired superficial transverse perineal muscles lie parallel to the posterior margin of the inferior surface of the perineal membrane (Figs 6.77B and 6.88B). They help to stabilise the perineal body.

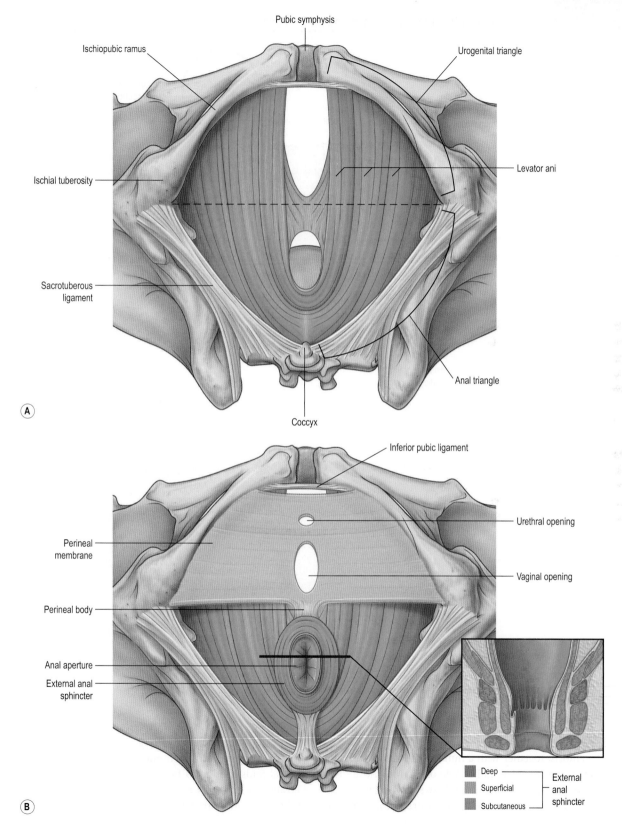

Fig. 6.87 The perineum in males (A) and females (B). (B) also shows the perineal membrane.

Pubic symphysis

Ischiopubic ramus

Urogenital triangle

Levator ani

Ischial tuberosity

Sacrotuberous ligament

Anal triangle

Coccyx

Ⓐ

Inferior pubic ligament

Urethral opening

Perineal membrane

Vaginal opening

Perineal body

Anal aperture

External anal sphincter

Deep

Superficial

Subcutaneous

External anal sphincter

Ⓑ

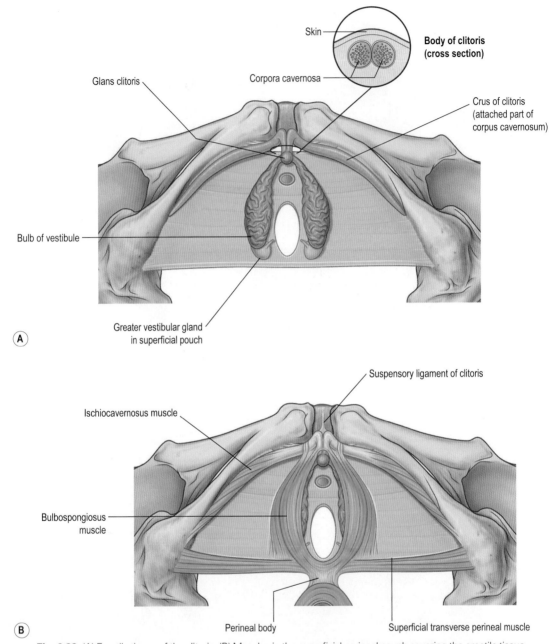

Skin

Body of clitoris (cross section)

Glans clitoris

Corpora cavernosa

Crus of clitoris (attached part of corpus cavernosum)

Bulb of vestibule

Greater vestibular gland in superficial pouch

(A)

Suspensory ligament of clitoris

Ischiocavernosus muscle

Bulbospongiosus muscle

Perineal body

Superficial transverse perineal muscle

(B)

Fig. 6.88 (A) Erectile tissue of the clitoris. (B) Muscles in the superficial perineal pouch covering the erectile tissue.

Female External Genitalia

The clitoris, together with a number of folds of skin and tissue form the vulva. Either side of the midline are two thin folds of skin (labia minora) between which is the vestibule containing the openings of the urethra anterior and vagina posterior (Fig. 6.89). Anteriorly, the labia minora bifurcate into medial and lateral folds, with the medial folds uniting to form the frenulum of the clitoris and the lateral folds uniting to form the prepuce of the clitoris. Posteriorly, the labia minora unite forming a transverse fold (frenulum of the labia minora/fourchette).

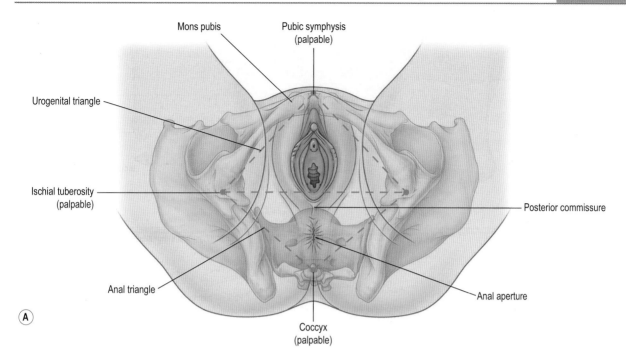

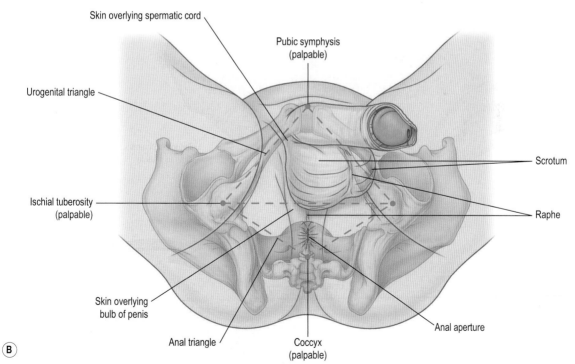

Fig. 6.89 Superficial features of the perineum in females (A) and males (B).

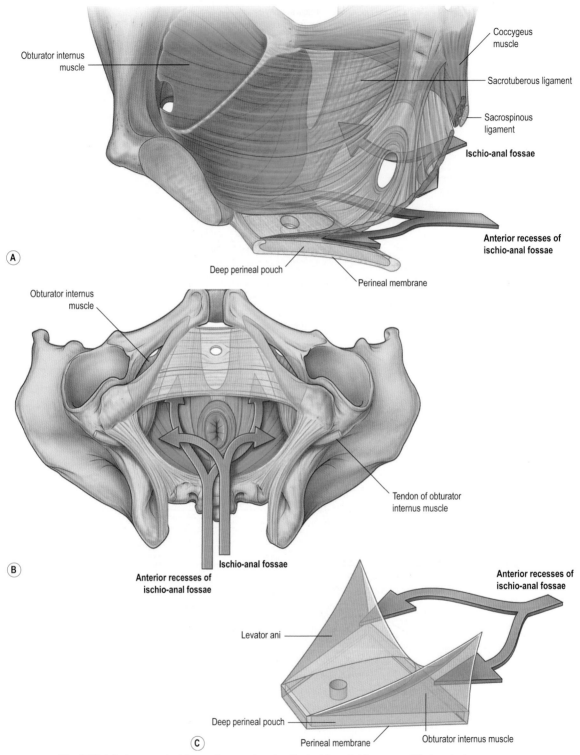

Obturator internus
muscle

Coccygeus
muscle

Sacrotuberous ligament

Sacrospinous
ligament

Ischio-anal fossae

**Anterior recesses of
ischio-anal fossae**

A

Deep perineal pouch

Perineal membrane

Obturator internus
muscle

Tendon of obturator
internus muscle

Ischio-anal fossae

**Anterior recesses of
ischio-anal fossae**

B

**Anterior recesses of
ischio-anal fossae**

Levator ani

Deep perineal pouch

Perineal membrane

Obturator internus muscle

C

Fig. 6.90 Inferior aspect of the perineum showing the ischiorectal fossae and their anterior recesses.

Lateral to the labia minora are two broad folds (labia majora), which unit anteriorly forming the mons pubis. Posteriorly the labia majora remain separated by a depression (posterior commissure) overlying the perineal body.

Male External Genitalia

The superficial components of the external genitalia comprise the scrotum and penis. The scrotum is the homologue of the labia majora in females.

> **DEVELOPMENT:** During development, in males the labioscrotal swellings fuse across the midline, giving rise to the scrotum housing the testes, their associated musculofascial coverings, blood vessels, nerves, lymphatics and drainage ducts, all of which have migrated from the abdomen. The line of fusion can be seen as a longitudinal midline raphe extending from the anus over the scrotum to the lower aspect of the body of the penis.

Superficial Fascia

The perineal fascia is continuous with the superficial fascia on the anterior abdominal wall, having a membranous layer (Colles' fascia) on its deep surface, attached to the perineal membrane posteriorly and ischiopubic rami laterally. The attachments of the membranous layer define the limits of the superficial perineal pouch. Anteriorly the membranous layer is continuous over the symphysis pubis and pubic bones with the membranous layer on the anterior abdominal wall. In the lower lateral part of the abdominal wall, the membranous layer attaches to the deep fascia of the thigh below the inguinal ligament (Fig. 6.68).

> **APPLIED ANATOMY:** As the membranous layer of fascia encloses the superficial perineal pouch and continues up the anterior abdominal wall, fluids or infectious material that accumulate in the pouch can track out of the perineum into the lower abdominal wall. It does not track into the anal triangle or thigh because the fascia fuses with the deep tissues at the borders of these regions.

Anal Triangle

The anal triangle faces posteroinferiorly, being defined laterally by the medial margins of the sacrotuberous ligaments (page 570), anteriorly by a line between the ischial tuberosities (page 567) and posteriorly by the coccyx (page 569). The anal opening is located centrally, related on either side to the fat-filled wedge-shaped ischiorectal (ischioanal) fossae, with anterior extensions passing between the deep perineal pouch and levator ani on each side (Fig. 6.90). The space is poorly vascularised.

> **CLINICAL ANATOMY:** An infection or tumour in the ischiorectal fossa (Fig. 6.91) can be extremely painful. It can occur spontaneously, but is often secondary to an anal fissure, thrombosed haemorrhoids or other diseases of the anus (Crohn's disease). An abscess on one side may spread to the opposite side behind the anal canal, as well as anteriorly to the deep perineal pouch. Symptoms include a severe throbbing pain near the anus, swelling and fever; it may cause an anal fistula. Pus can be drained via a surgical incision.

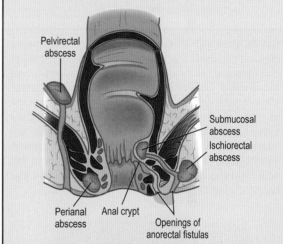

Fig. 6.91 Coronal section showing the location of ischiorectal and other abscesses in the perianal region.

External Anal Sphincter

The external anal sphincter comprises skeletal muscle surrounding the anal canal. It consists of three parts (deep, superficial, subcutaneous) arranged sequentially from superior to inferior (Fig. 6.92). The deep part blends with levator ani, the superficial part is attached to the perineal body anteriorly, coccyx and anococcygeal ligament posteriorly, and the subcutaneous part surrounds the anal opening. The sphincter is innervated by the inferior rectal branch of the internal pudendal nerve and by direct branches from S4.

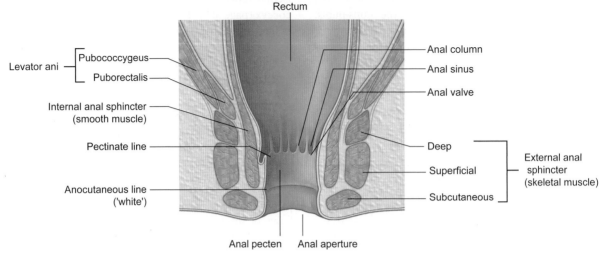

Fig. 6.92 Longitudinal section through the lower rectum and anal canal showing the components of the external anal sphincter.

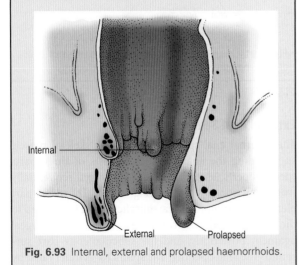

CLINICAL ANATOMY: Engorgement of the venous plexus at or inside the anal sphincter (haemorrhoids) is common and can be caused by straining during bowel movements, obesity and a sedentary lifestyle. Symptoms include irritation, pain and swelling. Haemorrhoids at the distal boundary of the anal canal are typically called external haemorrhoids, while those inside are internal haemorrhoids, which tend to bleed. Prolapsed internal haemorrhoids form lumps protruding from the anal canal (Fig. 6.93); they can undergo thrombosis and become painful.

Fig. 6.93 Internal, external and prolapsed haemorrhoids.

Neurovascular Supply of the Perineum
Nerves
Somatic nerves. The major nerve of the perineum is the pudendal nerve (S2–S4) from the sacral plexus. It enters the perineum through the lesser sciatic foramen having left the pelvis through the greater sciatic foramen and passed around the ischial spine (page 567). It runs in the pudendal canal in the fascia covering obturator internus. The pudendal nerve has three terminal branches: the inferior rectal and perineal nerves and the dorsal nerve of the penis/clitoris. Other somatic nerves are mainly sensory.

Autonomic nerves. These enter the perineum via two routes: post-ganglionic sympathetic fibres come with fibres supplying the skin; pelvic splanchnic (parasympathetic) nerves to the erectile tissues pass through the deep perineal pouch from the hypogastric plexus in the pelvis.

Arteries
The most significant artery is the internal pudendal artery (branch of the internal iliac artery), with others being the external pudendal artery (branch of the femoral artery), and the testicular (from the abdominal aorta) and cremasteric (from the external iliac artery) arteries (in males). The internal pudendal artery has a similar course to the pudendal nerve from the pelvis to perineum and gives similar branches.

Veins

The veins generally accompany the arteries joining to form the internal pudendal vein, which drains into the internal iliac vein. The exception is the dorsal vein of the penis/clitoris, which passes through the gap between the inferior pubic ligament and deep perineal pouch to join the venous plexus around the prostate (males) and bladder (females).

Lymphatics

Lymphatics from the deep parts of the perineum accompany the arteries draining mainly into the internal iliac nodes. Those from superficial tissues of the penis/clitoris drain mainly into the superficial inguinal nodes, together with vessels from the scrotum and labia majora (Fig. 6.94). The glans penis/clitoris, labia minora and terminal part of the vagina drain to deep inguinal nodes and then to the external iliac nodes. The lymphatic drainage of the testes is to lateral aortic, lumbar and pre-aortic nodes around the aorta.

> **APPLIED ANATOMY:** Diseases from the testes track superiorly to nodes high on the posterior abdominal wall and NOT to inguinal or iliac nodes.

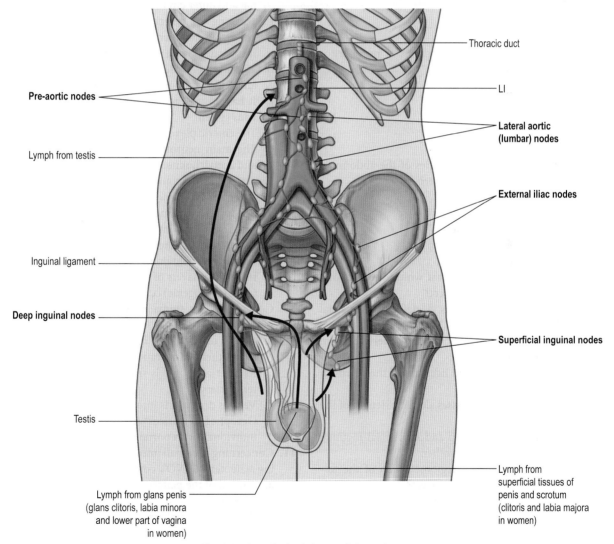

Fig. 6.94 Lymphatic drainage of the perineum.

SELF-TEST QUESTIONS

1. Which of the following muscles is NOT part of the anterior abdominal wall?
   a. External oblique
   b. Rectus abdominis
   c. Transversus abdominis
   d. Internal oblique
   e. Quadratus lumborum

2. Which of the following is NOT a boundary of the abdominal cavity?
   a. Pelvic floor
   b. Diaphragm
   c. Vertebral column
   d. Sternum
   e. Sacrum

3. Which of the following structures is retroperitoneal?
   a. Liver
   b. Pancreas
   c. Transverse colon
   d. Stomach
   e. Sigmoid colon

4. Which of the following muscles of the abdominal wall has a free posterior border?
   a. External oblique
   b. Rectus abdominis
   c. Transversus abdominis
   d. Internal oblique
   e. Pyramidalis

5. Concerning the inguinal canal, which of the following statements is NOT correct?
   a. The superficial ring is a defect in external oblique.
   b. The internal spermatic fascia is derived from internal oblique.
   c. It transmits the round ligament of the uterus in females.
   d. An indirect hernia passes along the length of the inguinal canal.
   e. In the young the deep and superficial inguinal rings lie opposite each other.

6. Concerning abdominal regions, which of the following statements is NOT correct?
   a. The caecum and appendix lie in the right iliac fossa.
   b. The stomach lies in the left hypochondrium.
   c. The gallbladder lies in the epigastrium.

   d. The ascending colon lies in the right lumbar region.
   e. The pancreas lies in the upper left quadrant.

7. Concerning the digestive tract, which of the following statements is correct?
   a. The muscularis layer consists of skeletal muscle.
   b. The mucosa contains blood vessels and lymphatics.
   c. The submucosa contains a plexus of somatic nerves.
   d. The serosa is a thick layer of loose connective tissue.
   e. The muscularis is organised as inner longitudinal and outer circular muscle cells.

8. Concerning the enteric nervous system, which of the following statements is NOT correct?
   a. It is located in the walls of the digestive tract.
   b. The myenteric plexus mainly controls peristalsis and gut secretions.
   c. It has no interactions with the autonomic nervous system.
   d. The enteric plexus is absent in Chagas disease.
   e. The main neurotransmitters are noradrenaline and acetylcholine.

9. Concerning the stomach, which of the following statements is NOT correct?
   a. The pyloric sphincter controls the passage of gastric contents into the duodenum.
   b. It is attached to the liver by the lesser omentum.
   c. Gastric pits contain five functional cell types.
   d. It has three layers of muscle fibres.
   e. Chief (zymogenic) cells secrete hydrochloric acid.

10. Concerning the stomach, which of the following statements is correct?
   a. Gastric ulcers are the result of bacterial infection.
   b. Sympathetic innervation is via the vagus nerves.
   c. Its arterial supply is from the superior mesenteric artery.
   d. Venous drainage is into the portal vein.
   e. Oesophageal varices are commonly found in individuals with portal hypertension.

11. Concerning the small intestine, which of the following statements is NOT correct?
   a. The tail of the pancreas lies within the C-shaped duodenum.
   b. Pancreatic secretions drain into the second part of the duodenum.
   c. The mucosa and submucosa have plica circulares.

d. Coeliac disease is an immune reaction against gluten.

e. Paneth cells release lysozyme which breaks down bacterial cell walls.

12. Which of the following is NOT secreted by entero-endocrine cells of the small intestine.

a. Serotonin

b. Hydrophobic peptides

c. Substance P

d. Gastric inhibitory peptide

e. Motilin

13. Concerning the colon, which of the following statements is NOT correct?

a. It is associated with peritoneal-covered accumulations of fat.

b. Ulcerative colitis affects the descending and sigmoid colon.

c. The base of the appendix lies at the junction of the lateral two-thirds and medial one-third of a line connecting the anterior superior iliac spine and umbilicus.

d. The transverse colon is suspended from the posterior abdominal wall.

e. The lamina propria is rich in lymphoid cells.

14. Which of the following are NOT potential sites of portosystemic anastomosis?

a. Lower one-third of the oesophagus

b. Rectum

c. Around the umbilicus

d. Sigmoid colon

e. Ascending colon

15. Concerning the liver, which of the following statements is NOT correct?

a. It lies mainly in the left hypochondrium.

b. It is held in place by the hepatic veins.

c. 75% of blood entering the liver is from the portal vein.

d. The free edge of the falciform ligament contains the ligamentum teres.

e. Functionally the caudate lobe is part of the left lobe.

16. Concerning the liver, which of the following statements is correct?

a. Each lobule is arranged around a central artery.

b. Hepatocytes line the walls of the sinusoids.

c. The basal surfaces of hepatocytes form bile canaliculi.

d. Hepatocytes intermittently secrete bile.

e. Stellate cells recognise and phagocytose old erythrocytes.

17. Concerning the biliary system, which of the following statements is NOT correct?

a. Bilirubin is a breakdown product of haem.

b. Fatty liver disease is an abnormal accumulation of large lipid deposits in hepatocytes.

c. The common bile duct empties into the second part of the duodenum.

d. The gallbladder stores and concentrates bile.

e. The fundus of the gallbladder lies at the tip of the left 9th costal cartilage.

18. Concerning the pancreas, which of the following statements is NOT correct?

a. It is a mixed endocrine and exocrine gland.

b. Pancreatic cancer is usually associated with the duct cells.

c. In acute pancreatitis proenzymes may be activated and digest pancreatic tissue.

d. The islets of Langerhans are mainly situated in the tail.

e. The activity of α and β cells is mainly regulated by blood glucose levels.

19. Concerning digestion, which of the following statements is NOT correct?

a. The hypothalamus receives sensory information about stomach filling.

b. Decreases in amino acid and lipid levels in blood increase the desire for food.

c. Most stored energy is in the form of fat.

d. Anorexigenic substances stimulate feeding.

e. When more energy is consumed than expended body weight increases.

20. Concerning digestion, which of the following statements is correct?

a. Polypeptides are released in the stomach in the absence of food.

b. Glucose is not present in the saliva of individuals with diabetes mellitus.

c. Only 5% of saliva is water.

d. Adrenaline decreases the secretion of saliva.

e. Reduced salivary secretion occurs during pregnancy.

21. Which of the following is NOT a function of the stomach?

a. Storage of large amounts of food.

b. Mixing of food with gastric secretions to form chyme.

c. Release of chyme into the small intestine for its digestion and absorption.

d. Acute gastritis can be caused by excess alcohol consumption.

e. The secretion of highly alkaline gastric juice enhances stomach emptying.

22. Concerning secretions into the digestive tract, which of the following statements is NOT correct?
   a. Pancreatic secretions contain lipolytic enzymes.
   b. Bile has a laxative action through the action of bile salts.
   c. Sympathetic stimulation increases secretions from the small intestine.
   d. No digestive enzymes are secreted into the large intestine.
   e. Gallstones are associated with the absorption of water from bile.

23. Concerning the movement of food through the digestive tract, which of the following statements is NOT correct?
   a. Chyme is propelled through the small intestine by peristaltic action.
   b. Contraction of the mucosa in the small intestine is largely initiated by the autonomic nervous system.
   c. An inflamed appendix can cause spasm of the ileocaecal sphincter.
   d. Irritation of the colon can initiate intense mass movements.
   e. Distension of the rectum initiates the defaecation reflex.

24. Which of the following is NOT considered to be associated with nutrition?
   a. Assimilation
   b. Excretion
   c. Digestion
   d. Anabolism
   e. Biosynthesis

25. Concerning carbohydrates, which of the following statements is NOT correct?
   a. The major product of carbohydrate digestion is glucose.
   b. They are absorbed from the small intestine as disaccharides.
   c. Glucose is transported into epithelial cells by sodium cotransport.
   d. Glucagon is secreted by α cells in the pancreas in response to low blood glucose levels.
   e. Following absorption most galactose is rapidly converted to glucose in the liver.

26. Concerning fats/lipids, which of the following statements is NOT correct?
   a. Trans fats increase the risk of coronary heart disease.
   b. Monounsaturated fats decrease the risk of coronary heart disease.
   c. Cholesterol is rapidly absorbed from the digestive tract into intestinal lymph.
   d. High-density lipoproteins prevent the deposition of cholesterol on arterial walls.
   e. Thyroid hormone causes rapid mobilisation of fat.

27. Concerning proteins, which of the following statements is NOT correct?
   a. The principal constituents are amino acids.
   b. Most proteins are digested in the duodenum and jejunum.
   c. There is a constant exchange of amino acids between tissue cells and blood.
   d. Albumin is a plasma protein.
   e. Insulin decreases the formation of tissue proteins.

28. Concerning proteins, which of the following statements is correct?
   a. Whole protein molecules are rarely absorbed into the blood.
   b. Amino acid molecules diffuse through cell membranes.
   c. Proteins constitute 25% of body solids.
   d. Saliva contains proteolytic enzymes.
   e. Cancer cells rarely use amino acids.

29. Which of the following is NOT an essential amino acid?
   a. Proline
   b. Serine
   c. Asparagine
   d. Arginine
   e. Glutamine

30. Concerning vitamins, which of the following statements is NOT correct?
   a. Vitamin K increases calcium absorption from the digestive tract.
   b. Thiamine (B$_1$) is required for the final metabolism of carbohydrates.
   c. Riboflavin (B$_2$) deficiency can result in digestive disturbances.
   d. Vitamin B$_{12}$ is important in promoting red blood cell formation and maturation.
   e. Vitamin A is needed to form visual pigments.

31. Which of the following minerals is essential for brain and nervous system development?
    a. Iodine
    b. Zinc
    c. Copper
    d. Manganese
    e. Calcium

32. Concerning liver function, which of the following statements is NOT correct?
    a. It converts galactose and fructose to glucose.
    b. Amino acids and glycerol are converted to glucose.
    c. It synthesises fat from proteins and carbohydrates.
    d. It removes excess hormones.
    e. It stores vitamin K.

33. Concerning the kidney, which of the following statements is NOT correct?
    a. The presence of a horseshoe kidney is more common in males.
    b. It has outer concave and inner convex borders.
    c. The right is slightly lower than the left.
    d. The outer cortex contains renal corpuscles.
    e. The functional unit is the nephron.

34. Which of the following statements is NOT a function of the kidney?
    a. Helps maintain acid-base balance
    b. Excretion
    c. Haematopoiesis
    d. Accumulates toxins
    e. Gluconeogenesis

35. Concerning the nephron, which of the following statements is NOT correct?
    a. The glomerulus is surrounded by a single layered capsule.
    b. The main function of the juxtaglomerular apparatus is the secretion of hormones.
    c. In diabetes mellitus the glomerular filter becomes more permeable to proteins.
    d. The medullary ducts play a key role in regulating acid-base balance.
    e. The thin descending segment of the loop of Henle is highly permeable to water.

36. Concerning the renin-angiotensin system, which of the following statements is NOT correct?
    a. Angiotensin II increases arterial blood pressure.
    b. Angiotensin I is physiologically inactive.
    c. Acting on the brain angiotensin II stimulates the thirst centre.
    d. Renin converts angiotensinogen into angiotensin I.
    e. Angiotensin IV has vasoconstriction actions.

37. Concerning prostaglandins, which of the following statements is correct?
    a. They inhibit renin secretion by the kidneys.
    b. They increase gastric secretions in the digestive tract.
    c. They can change the actions of neurotransmitters.
    d. They cause bronchoconstriction in the respiratory system.
    e. They reduce the capacity of red blood cells to pass through very small blood vessels.

38. Concerning the nephron, which of the following statements is correct?
    a. The distal convoluted tubule is located in the medulla.
    b. The principal cells of the collecting system regulate the reabsorption of electrolytes.
    c. The proximal convoluted tubule is located in the medulla.
    d. Active reabsorption of sodium and chlorine occurs in the thin limb of the loop of Henle.
    e. The permeability of the distal tubule is not influenced by the concentration of antidiuretic hormone.

39. Concerning diuretics, which of the following statements is NOT correct?
    a. Osmotic diuretics decrease the osmolarity of tubular fluid.
    b. They enhance urine formation.
    c. Furosemide inhibits sodium reabsorption.
    d. Dehydration is an adverse effect.
    e. They are used in treating congestive heart failure.

40. Concerning kidney diseases, which of the following statements is NOT correct?
    a. It is an important cause of death.
    b. In chronic renal failure there is progressive loss of nephrons.
    c. Acute renal failure can occur following a severe transfusion reaction.
    d. They do not affect blood vessels.
    e. Chronic renal failure can occur in hypertension.

41. Concerning the urinary system, which of the following statements is NOT correct?
    a. The ureter is constricted in three places.
    b. It has blood supply from the gonadal artery.
    c. The upper end of the ureter lies on the transcristal plane.
    d. The bladder has three muscle layers.
    e. Bladder cancer begins in the epithelium.

42. Concerning the urinary system, which of the following statements is correct?
    a. In males the urethra is 40 cm long.
    b. Cystitis is common during urinary tract infections.
    c. The formation of urine is intermittent.
    d. Enuresis is the voluntary voiding of urine during the night.
    e. Sympathetic stimulation causes relaxation of the internal urethral sphincter.

43. Concerning the male reproductive system, which of the following statements is NOT correct?
    a. The testis migrates through the inguinal canal immediately prior to birth.
    b. Testicular torsion most commonly occurs between ages 12 and 18.
    c. Sertoli cells release water into the seminiferous tubules.
    d. The tunica albuginea covers the anterior and lateral sides of the testis.
    e. The ejaculatory duct is formed by the duct of the seminal vesicle and epididymis.

44. Concerning the male reproductive system, which of the following statements is correct?
    a. The prostate consists of four zones.
    b. Elevated levels of prostate-specific antigen are normal.
    c. After age 50 prostatic secretions increase.
    d. Prostate cancer is one of the most common cancers in young men.
    e. Semen consists of 90% sperm.

45. Concerning the female reproductive system, which of the following statements is NOT correct?
    a. Each ovary lies in the posterior layer of the broad ligament.
    b. Fertilisation takes place in the ampulla of the uterine tube.
    c. The cavity of the uterus is triangular mediolaterally.
    d. The uterus is separated from the bladder by the rectouterine pouch.
    e. The uterus comprises three layers.

46. Concerning the female reproductive system, which of the following statements is correct?
    a. During pregnancy the ovary is pulled downwards by the enlarging uterus.
    b. The risk of ovarian cancer is increased in women who have had fewer ovulations.
    c. Approximately 10% of ovarian cancers are related to an inherited risk.
    d. Damage to the pelvic floor during childbirth is not a precursor to prolapse of the uterus.
    e. Fibroids can develop in the endometrium.

47. Concerning the menstrual cycle, which of the following statements is NOT correct?
    a. Oestrogens and progesterone control the growth and differentiation of epithelial cells.
    b. Oestrogen induces regeneration of the functional layer of the endometrium.
    c. Viable endometrial tissue can occur outside the uterus.
    d. Pituitary gonadotropins produce cyclic changes in ovarian hormone levels.
    e. Following ovulation, the proliferative phase begins with rapid growth of a few ovarian follicles.

48. Concerning the perineum, which of the following statements is NOT correct?
    a. It lies below the pelvic floor.
    b. The urogenital triangle contains the opening of the urinary and reproductive tracts.
    c. The deep perineal pouch lies between the perineal membrane and membranous layer of superficial fascia.
    d. Infection of the ischiorectal fossa is often secondary to an anal fissure.
    e. The external anal sphincter consists of skeletal muscle.

49. Which of the following decreases blood cholesterol?
    a. Cream
    b. Fatty meat
    c. Coconut oil
    d. Peanuts
    e. Butter

50. Concerning the liver, which of the following statements is NOT correct?
    a. The bare area is in direct contact with the diaphragm.
    b. It is the interface between the digestive system and blood.
    c. A portal triad comprises a bile ductule, arteriole and lymphatics.
    d. It synthesises and secretes the major plasma proteins.
    e. Hepatitis can lead to liver failure and death.

Lower Limb

CONTENTS

Key Concepts, 564
Learning Outcomes, 564
Overview, 565
Introduction, 565
Pelvic Girdle, 567
  Innominate, 567
   Ilium, 567
   Ischium, 567
   Pubis, 567
  Symphysis Pubis, 569
   Movements, 569
  Sacrum and Coccyx, 569
  Sacroiliac Joint, 570
   Movements, 573
  Lumbosacral Joint, 573
   Movements, 573
  Sacrococcygeal Joint, 573
  Function of the Pelvic Girdle, 574
  Relations, 574
   Internal Iliac Artery and Vein, 578
   External Iliac Artery and Vein, 579
   Lumbosacral Plexus, 580
  Gluteal Region/Buttocks, 580
   Blood Vessels, 581
Thigh, 582
  Femur, 582
  Hip Joint, 584
   Movements, 586
   Relations, 588
  Femoral Triangle, 588
   Lymph Nodes, 589
  Compartments of the Thigh, 589
   Anterior Compartment, 590
   Medial Compartment, 593
   Posterior Compartment, 593
   Muscles, 594

Calf/Leg, 594
  Tibia, 596
  Fibula, 598
  Patella, 598
  Knee Joint, 598
   Collateral Ligaments, 601
   Cruciate Ligaments, 602
   Menisci, 604
   Movements, 605
  Popliteal Fossa, 608
  Tibiofibular Joints, 611
   Superior Tibiofibular Joint, 611
   Inferior Tibiofibular Joint, 612
  Compartments of the Calf/Leg, 612
   Anterior Compartment, 612
   Lateral Compartment, 614
   Posterior Compartment, 614
   Muscles, 615
Ankle, 615
  Ankle Joint, 616
   Movements, 618
Foot, 624
  Tarsus, 625
  Metatarsals and Phalanges, 626
  Joints of the Foot, 626
  Subtalar joint, 626
  Transverse (Mid) Tarsal Joint, 626
   Movements at the Subtalar and Transverse (Mid)
    Tarsal Joints, 626
  Tarsometatarsal Joints, 627
   Movements, 627
  Metatarsophalangeal Joints, 627
   Movements, 628
  Interphalangeal Joints, 629
   Movements, 629
  Dorsum of the Foot, 629

Plantar Aspect (Sole) of the Foot, 634
Function of the Foot, 636
Walking, 636
    Walking (Gait) Cycle, 636
Summary of Nerves and Muscles, 638
Major Nerves of the Lower Limb and the Muscles
    They Innervate, 638
    Femoral Nerve, 638
    Obturator Nerve, 638
    Superior Gluteal Nerve, 638
    Inferior Gluteal Nerve, 638

Sciatic Nerve, 638
Tibial Nerve, 640
Common Fibular/Peroneal Nerve, 640
Muscles of the Lower Limb Supplied by Each Nerve
    Root, 641
Movements in Each Region of the Lower Limb, the
    Muscles Responsible and Their Innervation, 642
    Hip Joint, 642
    Knee Joint, 642
    Ankle Joint, 643
    Joints of the Foot, 643

KEY CONCEPTS

- The lower limb is adapted for weight bearing and locomotion.
- The foot acts as a locomotor prop and lever during walking.
- Bones of the lower limb are more robust than those of the upper limb.
- Joint stability is through articular surface shape, ligaments and muscle activity.
- Muscles function to stabilise joints; producing movement is secondary.
- Muscles crossing several joints promote coordinated movement and function.
- A wide range of movements is achieved by combinations of muscle actions.

- Muscles of the anterior thigh are innervated by the femoral nerve; the anterior calf/leg and dorsum of the foot by the deep peroneal/fibular nerve; the posterior thigh by the sciatic nerve; the posterior calf/leg and plantar surface of the foot by the tibial nerve; and the lateral calf/leg by the superficial peroneal/fibular nerve.
- Skin of the anterior thigh is innervated by L1/L2/L3; the anterior calf/leg and dorsum of the foot by L4/L5; the posterior thigh by S2; the posterior calf/leg by S2/S1; and plantar surface of the foot by S1 (lateral part), L4/L5 (medial part).
- The foot is the interface between the body and the supporting surface during walking and other locomotor activities.

LEARNING OUTCOMES

By the end of this chapter, you should be able to:
- Identify, palpate and examine the pelvis, femur, tibia, fibula, tarsus, metatarsals and phalanges.
- Examine and assess movements of the pelvic girdle, the hip, knee, tibiofibular and ankle joints, and joints of the foot.
- Appreciate the influence of pathology and/or trauma on the function of the pelvic girdle, the hip, knee, tibiofibular and ankle joints, and joints of the foot.
- Locate, palpate and examine muscles associated with the pelvic girdle, thigh, calf/leg and foot.

- Appreciate the influence of pathology and/or trauma on the muscles of the lower limb.
- Describe the location of the femoral triangle and popliteal fossa and the significance of their contents.
- Appreciate the influence of pathology and/or trauma to the femoral triangle and popliteal fossa and their contents.
- Describe the formation, course and distribution of the lumbar, lumbosacral and sacral plexuses and their branches.

- Appreciate the influence of pathology and/or trauma to the lumbar, lumbosacral and sacral plexuses and their branches.
- Describe the origin, course and distribution of the major blood vessels of the lower limb.

- Assess the femoral, popliteal, posterior tibial and dorsalis pedis pulse.
- Describe the lymphatic drainage of the lower limb.
- Describe and understand events within the gait cycle.

OVERVIEW

This chapter considers the lower limb and is organised into five sections (pelvic girdle, thigh, calf/leg, ankle, foot), and within each section, the anatomy, function, and relevant applied and clinical anatomy are considered. At the end of the chapter is a summary of the major nerves of the lower limb and the muscles supplied by each; the muscles supplied by each nerve root of the nerve plexuses; and the movements possible in each region (pelvic girdle, hip, knee, ankle, foot) and the muscles producing them, together with their innervation.

INTRODUCTION

The lower limb is adapted for weight bearing, locomotion and maintaining the upright bipedal posture: for all these functions a greater degree of strength and stability are required than in the upper limb. The bones of the lower limb are larger and more robust than those in the upper limb, varying in their characteristics in relation to muscle development and body build; some bones (innominate, sacrum) show sexual differences, with the female pelvis being adapted for childbearing. The form and structure of individual bones have adapted to supporting and resisting mechanical stresses, with their internal architecture arranged to resist stresses and forces in all directions. As the stresses change during growth and throughout life, continuous modifications are made to maintain the functions of support and resistance. The foot can be considered a locomotor prop and lever during walking, even though some non-locomotor function is still possible; the joints are much less mobile than those in the hand.

The lower limb is attached to the trunk by the pelvic girdle (innominate, sacrum), with the point of articulation being the sacroiliac joint. The uppermost limit of the lower limb is a line joining the iliac crest, inguinal ligament, symphysis pubis, ischiopubic ramus,

sacrotuberous ligament and dorsum of the sacrum and coccyx. The thigh lies between the hip and knee joints, the calf/leg between the knee and ankle joints and the foot beyond the ankle; the foot has plantar and dorsal surfaces (Fig. 7.1).

DEVELOPMENT: The lower limb develops as a swelling of the body wall projecting at right angles to the surface opposite the lower lumbar and sacral segments. It has ventral and dorsal surfaces and cephalic (preaxial, marked by the big toe) and caudal (postaxial, marked by the little toe) borders (see Figs 5.2 and 5.3 (i)). As the limb grows in length (see Fig. 5.3 (ii)), it becomes segmented (thigh, calf/leg, foot) and folded ventrally so that the ventral surface becomes medial (see Fig. 5.3 (iii)), with the convexity of the knee directed laterally (see Fig. 5.3 (iv)). At a later stage, the lower limb undergoes a process of adduction and rotation so that the preaxial border becomes medial and the postaxial border lateral, with the convexity of the knee lying on the anterior aspect of the limb (see Fig. 5.3 (v)). As a result, the flexor surface of the lower limb comes to lie posterior and the extensor surface anterior.

Functionally, there are two types of fascia in the lower limb (superficial, deep). The superficial fascia merges with and acts as a base for the skin, permitting it to move freely over the underlying tissue, being continuous with that of the abdominal wall, perineum and back. The two layers in the lower part of the abdominal wall and perineum continue into the upper part of the anterior thigh. The deeper membranous layer crosses superficial to the inguinal ligament entering the thigh and fusing with the deep fascia along a line just below and parallel to the inguinal ligament; this attachment prevents the spread of fluid into the thigh from the perineum or deep to the superficial abdominal fascia. Over the ischial tuberosity, the fascia contains many

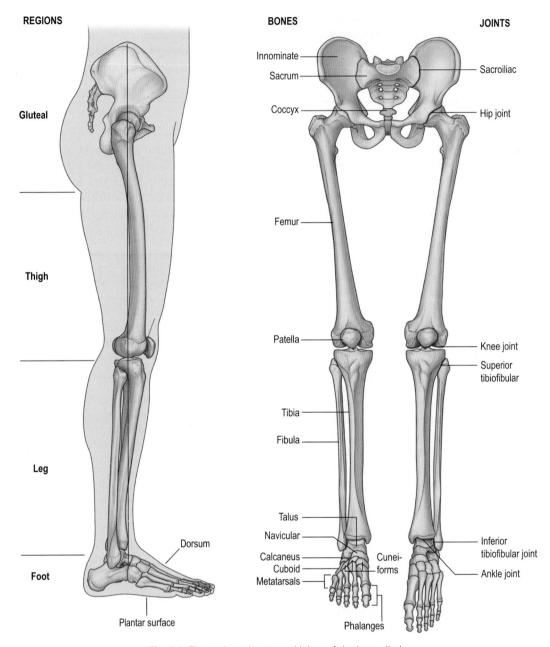

Fig. 7.1 The regions, bones and joints of the lower limb.

dense strands enclosing fat, helping to prevent tissue damage when seated. In the sole of the foot, the superficial fascia is characterised by its thickness and the presence of fat pads under the heel and the balls and pads of the toes.

The deep (investing layer) fascia comprises dense, tough, fibrous tissue which passes over and attaches to bony projections. Its fibres tend to lie in the same direction as the applied stresses. From its deep surface sheets of similar tissue (intermuscular septa) pass between groups of muscles; these help maintain the shape of the limb, as well as exerting a compressive force on the contents of the osseofascial compartments, aiding venous return.

PELVIC GIRDLE

The pelvic girdle is a ring of bone (two innominates, sacrum) providing articulation of the lower limbs with the trunk at the hip joint: the innominates articulate posteriorly with the sacrum at the sacroiliac joint and anteriorly with each other at the symphysis pubis. It is essentially a basin, with that part above the pelvic brim being the greater (false) pelvis containing abdominal viscera and that part below being the lesser (true) pelvis. The pelvis is arranged to provide strength for transferring weight from the trunk to the lower limbs when standing or via the ischial tuberosities when seated. This is achieved by loss of mobility at the sacroiliac joint and symphysis pubis.

Innominate

> **DEVELOPMENT:** Each innominate ossifies from three primary centres, which appear during the third (ilium), fourth (ischium) and fifth (pubis) months *in utero*. At birth the individual bones are separate, but by age 13 or 14 they are separated by a Y-shaped triradiate cartilage at the acetabulum; three secondary centres appear in the triradiate cartilage between ages 8 and 9, fusing with the ilium, ischium and pubis between 16 and 18 years. Secondary centres appear in the iliac crest, anterior inferior iliac spine, ischial tuberosity and pubic symphysis at puberty, fusing with the innominate between 20 and 22 years.

An irregularly shaped bone consisting of two triangular blades twisted 90 degrees to each other in the region of the acetabulum, it comprises three bones (ilium, ischium, pubis) fused at the acetabulum so that in adults it appears as a single bone (Fig. 7.2).

Ilium

Upper part of the innominate: the anterior two-third forms the smooth concave iliac fossa, part of the lateral and posterior abdominal wall; the thicker posterior one-third has the auricular surface for articulation with the sacrum (sacroiliac joint), behind which is the iliac tuberosity. The curved upper border (iliac crest) is convex superiorly and anteroposteriorly: the crest ends at the anterior and posterior superior iliac spines (Fig. 7.2). The arcuate line, part of the pelvic brim, separates the iliac fossa from the sacropelvic surface of the ilium; the iliopubic eminence is the junction between the ilium and pubis.

Ischium

Angulated posteroinferior part of the innominate with a blunt rounded apex (ischial tuberosity); the tuberosity passes upwards being continuous with the inferior pubic ramus forming the ischiopubic ramus. The posterior border of the body is continuous above with the ilium forming the greater sciatic notch; inferiorly it ends as a blunt medially projecting ischial spine, below which is the lesser sciatic notch (Fig. 7.2). The greater and lesser sciatic notches are transformed into the greater and lesser sciatic foramen by the sacrotuberous and sacrospinous ligaments (Fig. 7.5D). The pelvic surface of the body is continuous with the pelvic surface of the ilium, forming part of the lateral wall of the pelvis.

Pubis

The anterior lower part of the innominate, the bodies articulate in the midline (symphysis pubis); above the body is the pubic crest with the pubic tubercle laterally. The superior ramus joins the ilium and ischium at the acetabulum, while the inferior ramus extends below the obturator foramen to join the ischium (Fig. 7.2).

Acetabulum. A hemispherical hollow on the lateral surface of the innominate: the anterior fifth is formed by the pubis, the posterosuperior two-fifths by the

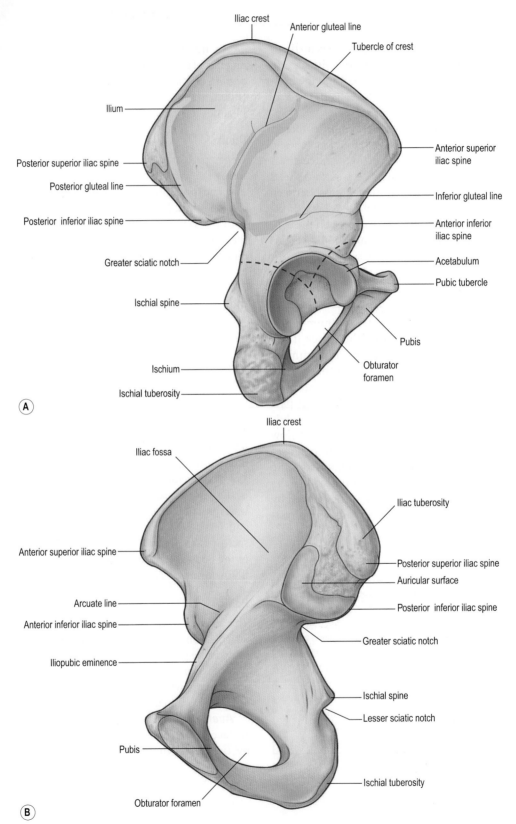

Fig. 7.2 (A) Lateral aspect of the left innominate; (B) medial aspect of the right innominate.

body of the ilium, the posteroinferior two-fifths by the body of the ischium (Fig. 7.2A). The prominent rim is deficient inferiorly (acetabular notch) and gives attachment to the acetabular labrum and synovial membrane of the hip joint. The floor of the acetabulum is partly articular (smooth auricular surface open inferiorly) with a deep central thinner portion (acetabular fossa).

Obturator foramen. A large opening surrounded by the sharp margins of the pubis and ischium (Fig. 7.2); it is covered by the obturator membrane, except superiorly at the obturator groove which is converted into a canal by a specialisation of obturator fascia.

APPLIED ANATOMY: In females, the anterior superior iliac spines are further apart, the pubic arch is less everted, and the greater sciatic notch is shallower and wider than in males; the subpubic angle is also greater (120 degrees) than in males (90 degrees).

APPLIED ANATOMY: The whole of the iliac crest can be felt from the anterior to the posterior superior iliac spines, with the iliac tubercle 5 cm from the anterior superior iliac spine. The bodies of the right and left pubic bones can be felt anteriorly where they separate the anterior abdominal wall from the genitalia.

APPLIED ANATOMY: The highest point of the iliac crest lies opposite the spine of L4; the tubercle of the iliac crest lies opposite the spine of L5; the posterior superior iliac spine lies opposite the spine of S2 at the level of the sacroiliac joint.

Symphysis Pubis

Secondary cartilaginous joint between the medial surfaces of each pubic bone between which is an interpubic fibrocartilaginous disc (Fig. 7.3A and B), thicker in females than males; a small fluid-filled cavity appears in the upper part of the disc, which in females may eventually extend throughout its whole length. The joint has superior and arcuate pubic ligaments, with decussations of tendinous fibres of rectus abdominis, external oblique and adductor longus (Fig. 7.3C) providing additional support.

Movements

Normally, there is no movement at the joint; however, during childbirth (parturition) the joint can widen by as much as 2 mm, increasing the circumference of the pelvic inlet. Occasionally, the bone adjacent to the joint can be absorbed, facilitating separation of the symphysis.

CLINICAL ANATOMY: Slipping of one pubic body with respect to the other can occur (osteitis pubis) in females following childbirth, with the associated pain being referred to the hip joint; it can also affect professional footballers (possibly due to abnormal stresses across the symphysis pubis). The unevenness of the pubic arch is clearly visible on radiographs.

Sacrum and Coccyx

DEVELOPMENT: Primary centres appear between the third and eighth month *in utero*, one for each body, one for each half of the vertebral arch and one for each costal element. By age 5 the costal elements have fused with the arches, with the arches fusing with the body slightly later; the two parts of the arch fuse between ages 7 and 10. The lateral mass segments fuse together during puberty, with secondary centres appearing in the bodies at the same time; the epiphyses fuse with the bodies between 18 and 25 years. Secondary centres appear in the ends of the costal and transverse processes forming two epiphyses; these fuse with the remainder of the sacrum between 18 and 25 years.

A triangular bone with the apex inferior: it consists of five fused vertebrae broadened by the incorporation of large costal elements and transverse processes (lateral masses), which lie lateral to the transverse tubercles on the dorsum, extending between the anterior sacral foramina onto the front of the bone; the auricular surface lies

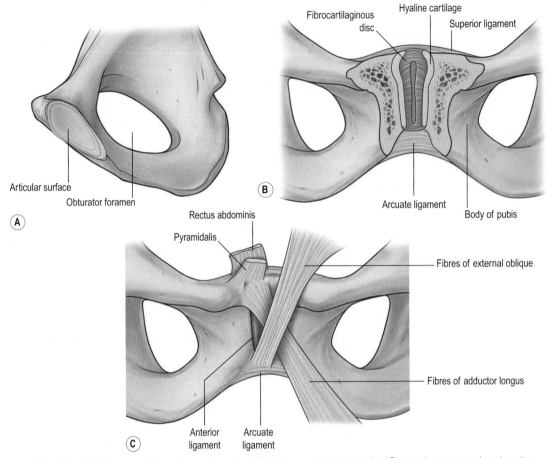

Fig. 7.3 Medial aspect (A) and coronal section (B) of the symphysis pubis; (C) anterior aspect showing the principle relations.

entirely on the lateral masses (Fig. 7.4). The pelvic (anterior) surface is smooth and concave, while the dorsal (posterior) surface is convex and highly irregular; posteriorly in the midline is the median sacral crest (spinous processes), medial to the posterior sacral foramina is the intermediate sacral crest (fused articular processes) and lateral to the foramina is the lateral sacral crest (transverse processes) (Fig. 7.4B). The superior articular facets on S1 (Fig. 7.4B) articulate with the inferior facets on L5; the body of S1 articulates with the body of L5 (lumbosacral joint). The inferior articular facets on S5 form the sacral cornua, which articulate with the cornua of the coccyx.

The coccyx consists of four fused vertebrae forming two bones. The pelvic surface is concave and smooth, while the dorsal surface has a row of tubercles (rudimentary articular processes).

APPLIED ANATOMY: When viewed laterally the sacrum is J-shaped in males, while in females it has a gentle smooth concavity.

Sacroiliac Joint

Between the L-shaped irregular auricular surfaces of the ilium and sacrum (Fig. 7.5A), with the region behind the joint being united by powerful interosseous ligaments; the anterior part of the joint is synovial while posteriorly it is more fibrous, giving the joint increased stability. Extremely strong posterior and weaker anterior sacroiliac ligaments surround the joint (Fig. 7.5B and C); accessory ligaments (sacrotuberous, sacrospinous) provide additional stability (Fig. 7.5D).

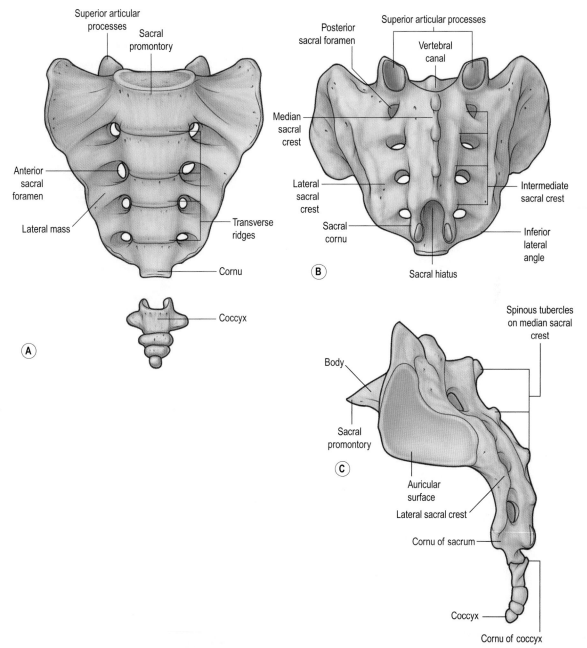

Fig. 7.4 Anterior (A); posterior (B) and lateral (C) aspects of the sacrum and coccyx.

APPLIED ANATOMY: With increasing age, especially in males, the joint cavity becomes partially (or completely) obliterated by fibrous bands or fibrocartilaginous adhesions between the articular surfaces; in old age, there may be a bony fusion between the articular surfaces.

APPLIED ANATOMY: The joint line can be represented by a curved line, with the posterior superior iliac spine at its apex, running at an angle of 25 degrees from superolateral to inferomedial for 2 cm in each direction.

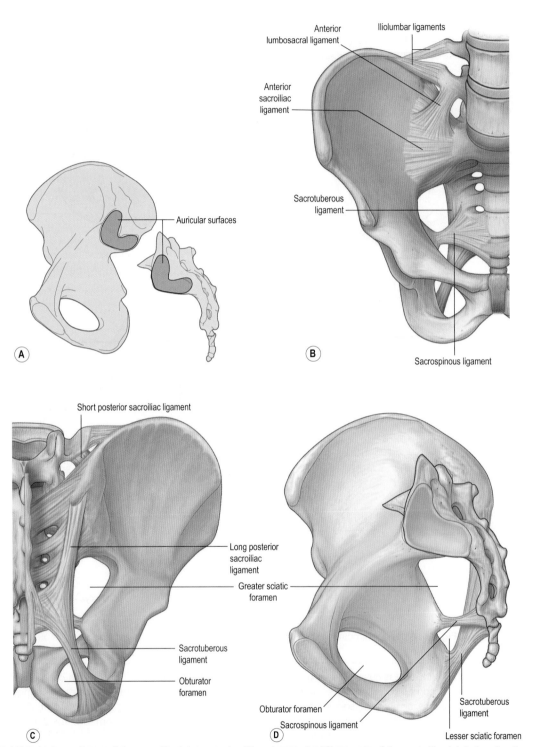

Fig. 7.5 (A) Articular surfaces of the sacroiliac joint; anterior (B) and posterior (C) aspects of the sacroiliac joint showing the anterior and posterior sacroiliac ligaments; (D) accessory sacrotuberous and sacrospinous ligaments.

The joint is extremely stable due to the superincumbent weight of the trunk, head and upper limbs; however, this has a tendency to push the sacral promontory forwards and downwards into the pelvis with an associated upward tilt of the lower part of the sacrum and coccyx, resisted by the sacrotuberous and sacrospinous ligaments.

Movements

Normally, there is little movement at the joint; however, during childbirth (parturition) the sacrum undergoes a complex movement (nutation) which initially increases the diameter of the pelvic inlet by 3 to 13 mm and then of the pelvic outlet by 15 to 18 mm (Fig. 7.6): movement is possible due to softening of the associated ligaments.

> **APPLIED ANATOMY:** Sudden forward bending can tear the posterior ligaments and can lead to joint dislocation; both are extremely painful in trunk flexion and may be disabling.

Lumbosacral Joint

Secondary cartilaginous joint between the bodies of S1 and L5 and synovial joints between their articular processes (Fig. 7.7A); the superior surface of the sacrum is inclined 30 degrees to the horizontal, with the lumbosacral angle between the axes of S1 and L5 being 140 degrees. The stability of the joint depends on the overlapping of the articular facets and the spinous and iliolumbar ligaments. Details of vertebral articulations can be found on pages 195 and 199.

Movements

Flexion and extension (18 degrees), and lateral flexion (0 to 7 degrees) are possible, with the range varying with age and between individuals.

> **CLINICAL ANATOMY:** Fracture or destruction of the pars interarticularis (part of the vertebral arch between the superior and inferior articular processes) is spondylolysis; the buttressing of L5 on S1 no longer occurs so that the body of L5 slips anteroinferiorly (spondylolisthesis) (Fig. 7.7B). The condition can arise as a slowly developing fracture, being more common in adolescents who participate in contact sports and gymnastics. Incomplete fracture at diagnosis may heal by avoiding repetitive bending stresses, but once disrupted the joint becomes unstable; spinal fusion may be the only option to regain stability at the joint.

Sacrococcygeal Joint

Secondary cartilaginous joint between S5 and the first coccygeal segment; it is surrounded and reinforced by

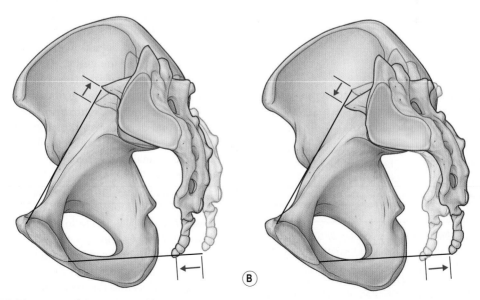

Fig. 7.6 Movement of the sacrum with respect to the innominate at the sacroiliac joint increasing the diameter of the pelvic inlet (A) and outlet (B).

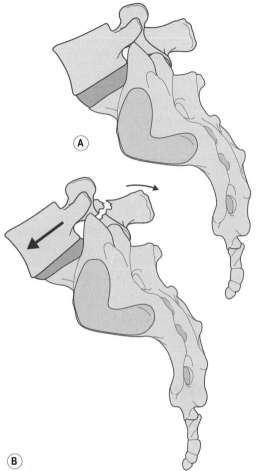

Fig. 7.7 (A) Normal anatomy of the lumbosacral joint; (B) fracture of the vertebral arch leading to spondylolisthesis.

longitudinal fibrous bands (sacrococcygeal ligaments). Flexion and extension at the joint are passive, occurring during defaecation and childbirth.

> **APPLIED ANATOMY:** The line of the joint can be felt as a groove between the apex of the sacrum and the coccyx deep in the natal cleft.

> **CLINICAL ANATOMY:** Dislocation of the sacrococcygeal joint can occur following a backward fall onto the buttocks (the coccyx can move anteriorly or posteriorly with respect to the sacrum) causing inflammation and/or pain, especially when seated; the dislocation can be reduced by digital rectal manipulation.

Function of the Pelvic Girdle

The pelvic girdle has a number of functions, including: (1) support and protection of the pelvic viscera; (2) support of body weight when standing and sitting; (3) attachment of muscles of the trunk and lower limb and (4) bony support for the birth canal in females.

> **CLINICAL ANATOMY:** Pelvic fractures can occur in isolation; however, they are more commonly associated with trauma. The pelvis essentially consists of a series of bony and fibro-osseous rings of tissue, with fractures on one side often being accompanied by a fracture(s) on the opposite side. As the pelvis has a large bony surface area it can give rise to significant bleeding producing a large haematoma, which compresses internal structures (bladder, ureters); rapid blood loss can lead to hypovolaemia and shock. Pelvic fractures can also lacerate blood vessels, causing internal bleeding and further blood loss, rupture of internal organs (bowel) and nerve damage.

Relations

At the level of the lumbosacral joint, the common iliac artery divides into its terminal branches (external and internal iliac). The external iliac artery leaves the pelvis deep to the inguinal ligament (page 455) (when it becomes the femoral artery) accompanied by the external iliac vein; the internal iliac artery passes over the pelvic brim into the true pelvis where it divides to supply pelvic viscera, as well as structures in the gluteal region (Fig. 7.8). Iliacus also passes into the thigh deep to the inguinal ligament lateral to psoas major. The external iliac vessels lie in the gutter between iliacus and psoas major. The lumbar plexus (Fig. 7.9) is formed within the substance of psoas major, giving rise to motor (femoral, obturator (page 578)) and sensory branches (Fig. 7.10); the femoral nerve leaves the pelvis by passing deep to the inguinal ligament and the obturator nerve by the obturator canal in the upper part of the obturator foramen (Fig. 7.11).

Emerging from the anterior sacral foramina are the S1 to S5 nerve roots: S1, S2 and S3 join with the lumbosacral trunk (L4, L5) to form the sciatic nerve, which leaves the pelvis through the greater sciatic foramen (Fig. 7.8) to enter the gluteal region (Fig. 7.12A and B). Structures passing through the greater sciatic foramen from the pelvis into the lower limb are: superior gluteal vessels; superior gluteal nerve; piriformis; sciatic nerve; inferior gluteal vessels; inferior gluteal nerve; pudendal

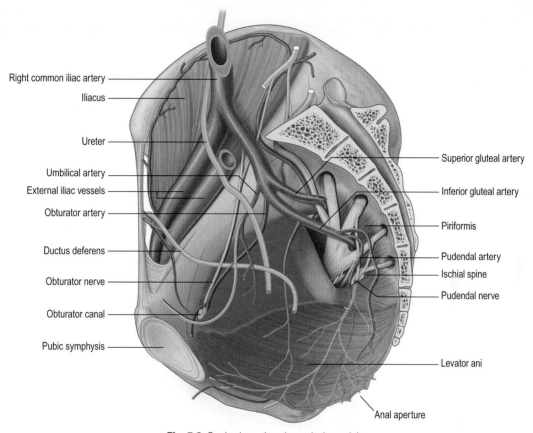

Fig. 7.8 Sagittal section through the pelvis.

Right common iliac artery

Iliacus

Ureter

Umbilical artery

External iliac vessels

Obturator artery

Ductus deferens

Obturator nerve

Obturator canal

Pubic symphysis

Superior gluteal artery

Inferior gluteal artery

Piriformis

Pudendal artery

Ischial spine

Pudendal nerve

Levator ani

Anal aperture

TABLE 7.1	The Attachments, Action and Innervation of Muscles Acting at the Hip Joint		
Muscle	**Attachments**	**Action**	**Innervation (Root Value)**
Psoas major[a]	From the adjacent margins of the bodies of T12 to L5 and medial part of the transverse processes to the lesser trochanter of the femur	Flexes the thigh at the hip joint: it can also flex and laterally flex the lumbar spine if the femur is fixed	(L1, L2, L3, (L4))
Iliacus[a]	From the upper posterior two-thirds of the iliac fossa, ala of the sacrum and anterior sacroiliac ligament to the lesser trochanter of the femur	Flexes the thigh at the hip joint; tilts the pelvis forwards if the femur is fixed	Femoral nerve (L2, L3)
Pectineus[a]	From the superior ramus of the pubis, iliopubic eminence and pubic tubercle to a line running from the lesser trochanter to the linea aspera of the femur	Flexes and adducts the thigh at the hip joint	Femoral nerve (L2, L3); occasionally also the obturator or accessory obturator nerve (L3)

Continued

TABLE 7.1   The Attachments, Action and Innervation of Muscles Acting at the Hip Joint (cont'd)

Muscle	Attachments	Action	Innervation (Root Value)
Rectus femoris[a] (see Table 7.2)			
Sartorius[a] (see Table 7.2)			
Gluteus maximus[a]	From the gluteal surface of the ilium medial to the posterior gluteal line, posterior border of the ilium, adjacent iliac crest, and upper part of the sacrotuberous ligament to the gluteal tuberosity of the femur (one-fourth) and iliotibial tract (three-fourth)	Powerful extensor of the thigh at the hip joint (as in stepping, climbing, running) at the same time laterally rotating the thigh; the upper fibres can adduct and lower fibres abduct the thigh at the hip joint; via the iliotibial tract it extends the calf/leg at the knee joint and supports the lateral aspect of the knee	Inferior gluteal nerve (L5, S1, S2)
Gluteus medius[a]	From the gluteal surface of the ilium between the posterior and anterior gluteal lines to the greater trochanter of the femur	With the pelvis fixed it abducts the thigh at the hip joint; the anterior fibres medially rotate the thigh at the hip joint; with the femur fixed the opposite side of the pelvis is rotated forwards	Superior gluteal nerve (L4, L5, S1)
Gluteus minimus[a]	From the gluteal surface of the ilium between the inferior and anterior gluteal lines to the greater trochanter of the femur	With the pelvis fixed it abducts the thigh at the hip joint; the anterior fibres medially rotate the thigh at the hip joint; with the femur fixed the opposite side of the pelvis is rotated forwards	Superior gluteal nerve (L4, L5, S1)
Semitendinosus[b]	From the ischial tuberosity to the medial surface of the medial condyle of the tibia	Extends the thigh at the hip joint, as well as aiding flexion of the calf/leg at the knee joint; with the knee semiflexed it produces medial rotation of the calf/leg at the knee joint; with the foot fixed it laterally rotates the thigh and pelvis on the tibia	Sciatic nerve via its tibial part (L5, S1, S2)
Semimembranosus[b]	From the ischial tuberosity to the posteromedial surface of the medial tibial condyle	Extends the thigh at the hip joint, as well as aiding flexion of the calf/leg at the knee joint; with the knee semiflexed it produces medial rotation of the calf/leg at the knee joint; with the foot fixed it laterally rotates the thigh and pelvis on the tibia	Sciatic nerve via its tibial part (L5, S1, S2)

TABLE 7.1 The Attachments, Action and Innervation of Muscles Acting at the Hip Joint (cont'd)

Muscle	Attachments	Action	Innervation (Root Value)
Biceps femoris[b]	From the ischial tuberosity and sacrotuberous ligament (*long head*) and the lower half of the linea aspera and upper half of the lateral supracondylar ridge of the femur (*short head*) to the head of the fibular	Extends the thigh at the hip joint, especially when the trunk is to be raised to the erect position; with the knee semiflexed it produces lateral rotation of the calf/leg at the knee joint; with the foot fixed it medially rotates the thigh and pelvis on the tibia	Sciatic nerve (L5, S1, S2): the *long head* by the tibial part; and *short head* by the common fibular/peroneal part
Tensor fascia lata[a] (see Table 7.2)			
Adductor magnus[a]	From the ischiopubic ramus and ischial tuberosity to the linea aspera, medial supracondylar ridge and adductor tubercle of the femur	Adducts the thigh at the hip joint, with the posterior part aiding extension of the thigh at the hip joint	Obturator nerve (L2, L3) and sciatic nerve via its tibial part (L4)
Adductor longus[a]	From the obturator crest and body of the pubis to the middle part of the linea aspera	Adducts the thigh at the hip joint; it also flexes the extended thigh and extends the flexed thigh	Obturator nerve (L2, L3, L4)
Adductor brevis[a]	From the body and inferior ramus of the pubis to the upper half of the linea aspera	Adducts the thigh at the hip joint	Obturator nerve (L2, L3, L4)
Gracilis[a] (see Table 7.2)			
Piriformis[a]	From the front of S2–S4 to the greater trochanter of the femur	Laterally rotates the thigh at the hip joint; when seated it is important when moving sideways	(L5, S1, S2)
Obturator internus[a]	From the internal surface of the obturator membrane and surrounding margins to the greater trochanter	Laterally rotates the thigh at the hip joint	Nerve to obturator internus (L5, S1, S2)
Gemellus superior[a]	From the gluteal surface of the ischial spine to the greater trochanter	Laterally rotates the thigh at the hip joint	Nerve to obturator internus (L5, S1, S2)
Gemellus inferior[a]	From the ischial tuberosity to the greater trochanter	Laterally rotates the thigh at the hip joint	Nerve to quadratus femoris (L4, L5, S1)
Quadratus femoris[a]	From the ischial tuberosity to the quadrate tubercle on the intertrochanteric crest of the femur	Laterally rotates the thigh at the hip joint; with the hip flexed it can abduct the thigh at the hip joint	Nerve to quadratus femoris (L4, L5, S1)
Obturator externus[a]	From the outer surface of the obturator membrane and surrounding margins to the trochanteric fossa of the femur	Laterally rotates the thigh at the hip joint; with the hip flexed it can abduct the thigh at the hip joint	Obturator nerve (L3, L4)

[a]Shown in Fig. 7.23.
[b]Hamstrings.

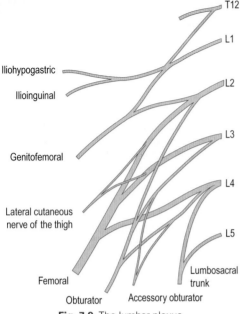

Fig. 7.9 The lumbar plexus.

vessels; pudendal nerve; nerve to obturator internus; and posterior cutaneous nerve of the thigh. The tendon of obturator internus passes through the lesser sciatic foramen from the pelvis into the lower limb, while the pudendal vessels, pudendal nerve and nerve to obturator internus re-enter the pelvis from the gluteal region. Once inside the pelvis, the pudendal vessels and nerve enter the pudendal canal (page 556) to be distributed to structures in the perineum (page 550).

Internal Iliac Artery and Vein

Terminal branch of the common iliac artery arising at the level of L5/S1 anteromedial to the sacroiliac joint. It passes over the pelvic brim and divides into anterior and posterior branches at the upper border of the greater sciatic foramen: posterior branches (iliolumbar, lateral sacral and superior gluteal arteries) supply the lower posterior abdominal wall, posterior pelvic wall and gluteal region; anterior branches (umbilical, superior vesical, inferior vesical (in males) or vaginal (in females),

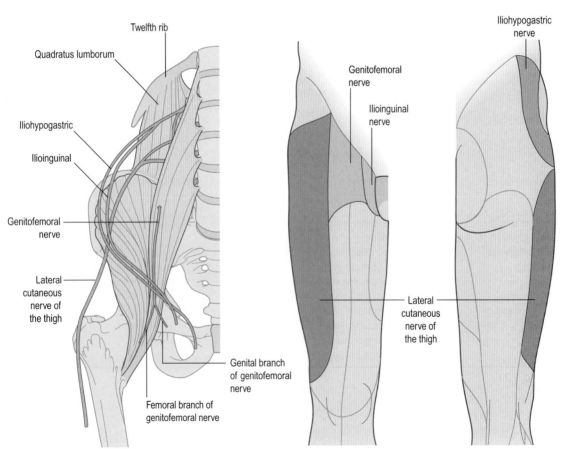

Fig. 7.10 Cutaneous nerves arising from the lumbar plexus together with their distribution.

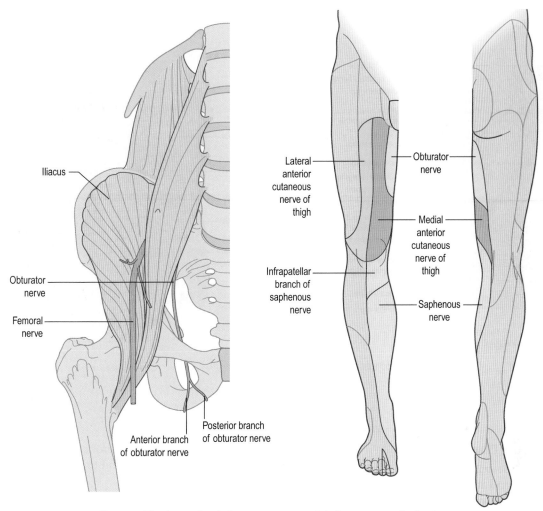

Fig. 7.11 The femoral and obturator nerves and their cutaneous distribution.

middle rectal, obturator, internal pudendal, inferior gluteal and uterine (in females) arteries) supply pelvic viscera, the perineum, gluteal region and adductor region of the thigh.

CLINICAL ANATOMY: In the foetus, the large umbilical artery carries de-oxygenated blood from the foetus to the placenta; two umbilical veins carry oxygenated blood from the placenta to the foetus. After birth, the umbilical artery closes distal to the origin of the superior vesical artery becoming a solid fibrous cord (medial umbilical ligament), which raises a fold of peritoneum (medial umbilical fold) on the anterior abdominal wall.

The internal iliac vein receives the corresponding veins and leaves the pelvic cavity to join the external iliac vein to form the common iliac vein superolateral to the pelvic inlet.

External Iliac Artery and Vein

Terminal branch of the common iliac artery at the level of L5/S1 anteromedial to the sacroiliac joint. It passes through the pelvis giving no branches to enter the thigh deep to the inguinal ligament together with the external iliac vein enclosed within an extension of the iliac and transversalis fascia (femoral sheath).

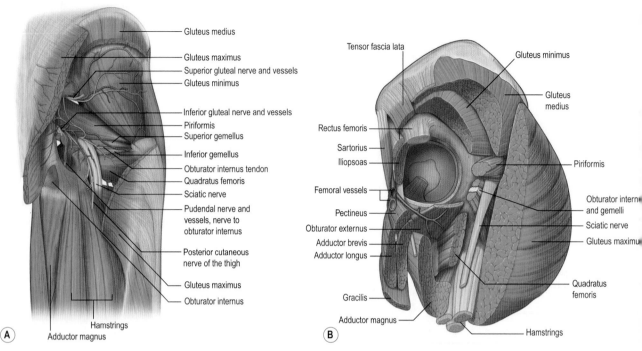

Fig. 7.12 Posterior (A) and lateral (B) aspects of the pelvis and gluteal region.

Lumbosacral Plexus

Lying on the posterior wall of the pelvis between piriformis and its fascia the lumbosacral plexus is formed by the ventral rami of L4 to S4 (Fig. 7.13); each ramus divides into anterior and posterior divisions as they approach the greater sciatic foramen. The anterior divisions give rise to: nerve to quadratus femoris (L4, L5, S1); nerve to obturator internus (L5, S1, S2); pelvic splanchnic nerves (S2, S3, S4); posterior femoral cutaneous nerve (S2, S3) and pudendal nerve (S2, S3, S4). The posterior divisions give rise to: branches to piriformis ((L5), S1, (S2)), coccygeus (S3, S4) and levator ani (S3, S4); superior gluteal nerve (L4, L5, S1); inferior gluteal nerve (L5, S1, S2); perforating cutaneous nerve (S2, S3); and a perineal branch (S4). The sciatic nerve consists of the medial tibial (anterior divisions L4 to S3) and

lateral common fibular/peroneal (posterior divisions L4 to S2) nerves bound together in a common sheath.

> **CLINICAL ANATOMY:** The sciatic nerve can bifurcate into the tibial and common fibular/peroneal nerves in the pelvis: the common fibular/peroneal nerve can pass either below piriformis with the tibial nerve, through or above piriformis. If it passes through piriformis, it can be subject to compression by piriformis leading to 'foot drop' (page 613) and an inability to evert the foot (page 626).

Gluteal Region/Buttocks

The superficial fascia in the gluteal region is thick and fatty, contributing to the shape of the buttocks: in females, there is usually fat deposition over the lateral

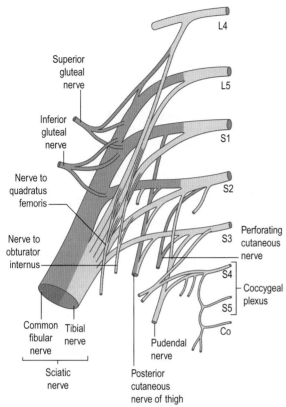

Fig. 7.13 The lumbosacral plexus. *Light blue,* anterior divisions; *dark blue,* posterior divisions.

thigh (secondary sexual characteristic). The outer (gluteal) surface of the ilium follows the curve of the iliac crest. It has three curved lines (posterior, anterior, inferior) demarcating the attachment of the gluteal muscles (Fig. 7.2A), with gluteus maximus attaching behind the posterior gluteal line, gluteus medius between the posterior and anterior gluteal lines, and gluteus minimus between the anterior and inferior gluteal lines.

The majority of the buttocks consists of muscles, which cross the hip joint, with deeper vascular and neural structures passing out of the pelvis into the lower limb, mainly through the greater sciatic foramen (Fig. 7.12A); some structures (pudendal vessels, pudendal nerve, nerve to obturator internus) re-enter the pelvis via the lesser sciatic foramen, while the tendon of obturator internus leaves to enter the lower limb. Details of the muscles in the gluteal region are given in Table 7.1.

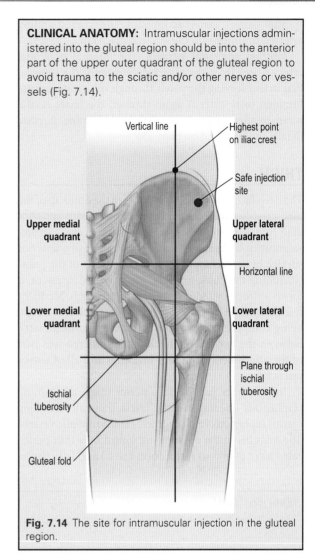

CLINICAL ANATOMY: Intramuscular injections administered into the gluteal region should be into the anterior part of the upper outer quadrant of the gluteal region to avoid trauma to the sciatic and/or other nerves or vessels (Fig. 7.14).

Fig. 7.14 The site for intramuscular injection in the gluteal region.

Blood Vessels

Superior and inferior gluteal vessels. The superior gluteal artery arises from the posterior division and the inferior from the anterior division of the internal iliac artery; both arteries leave the pelvis to enter the lower limb (gluteal region) via the greater sciatic foramen. Together they supply muscles in the gluteal region, with the inferior gluteal artery descending into the posterior thigh supplying adjacent structures, as well as giving a branch to the sciatic nerve.

The gluteal veins accompany the corresponding arteries, draining into the internal iliac vein.

Internal pudendal vessels. The internal pudendal artery arises from the anterior division of the internal iliac artery leaving the pelvis through the greater sciatic foramen to re-enter it again through the lesser sciatic foramen after passing around the ischial spine. Further details can be found on page 556.

THIGH

The deep fascia of the thigh attaches to the outer lip of the iliac crest between the anterior and posterior superior iliac spines, posterior aspect of the ilium and sacrum, sacrotuberous ligament and ischial tuberosity, anterior surface of the ischiopubic ramus and body of the pubis (including the pubic tubercle) and inguinal ligament; it forms a strong cylinder surrounding the thigh. Medially, it is thin, while laterally it is extremely thick and tough, being composed of two distinct layers (iliotibial tract); between the two layers, the iliotibial tract receives part of the attachment of gluteus maximus and all of tensor fascia lata.

In the upper part of the anterior thigh, an opening (saphenous opening) in the fascia transmits the long (great) saphenous vein (page 592) and lymphatic vessels. The margins of the opening are joined by a thin perforated layer of fibrous (cribriform fascia) and fatty tissue.

> **APPLIED ANATOMY:** The saphenous opening lies three finger breadth below and lateral to the pubic tubercle.

In the fascia in the lower part of the thigh intermuscular septa pass from its deep surface to the femur dividing the thigh into three compartments (anterior, medial, posterior). The septa are prolonged downwards onto the medial and lateral supracondylar ridges as far as the medial and lateral femoral condyles. In the upper part of the anteromedial thigh, a thickening of the fascial septum deep to sartorius forms the roof of the adductor canal (page 588).

Femur

> **DEVELOPMENT:** A primary ossification centre appears in the shaft at 7 weeks *in utero*. Secondary centres appear in the lower end shortly before birth, in the head at 1 year, in the greater and lesser trochanters at 4 and 12 years, respectively. The upper epiphysis fuses with the shaft at 18 years, with the last being the head, and the lower epiphysis at 20 years; the femoral neck ossifies from the shaft and not the upper epiphysis.

The longest and strongest bone in the body, the femur transmits body weight from the ilium to the upper end of the tibia; it has a shaft and two extremities (Fig. 7.15). The proximal end has a spherical head, with a hollow (fovea capitis to which the ligamentum teres (ligament of the head of the femur) is attached) just below its centre (see Fig. 7.17), connected to the shaft by a long (5 cm) neck (flattened anteroposteriorly) forming an angle of 125 degrees (angle of inclination) with the shaft (Fig. 7.16A). The head and neck are twisted anteriorly with respect to the shaft (angle of retroversion) by 10 degrees (Fig. 7.16C).

> **CLINICAL ANATOMY:** In some pathological conditions (congenital dysplasia of the hip (CDH)), the angle of inclination can be as much as 140 degrees (producing a coxa valga) and the angle of anteversion can be a large as 40 degrees; both increase the risk of hip dislocation. In contrast, the angle of inclination can be reduced (acquired dislocation of the hip) or there may be a reduced or reversed angle of anteversion. If the angles of inclination and anteversion exceed 130 degrees and 15 degrees, respectively, there is reduced contact between the joint surfaces decreasing stability at the hip.

The almost cylindrical shaft is gently convex anteriorly being narrowest in the central region: it has a rough posterior border (linea aspera) with medial and lateral lips for muscle attachments. Inferiorly, the medial and lateral lips diverge (supracondylar lines), between which is the

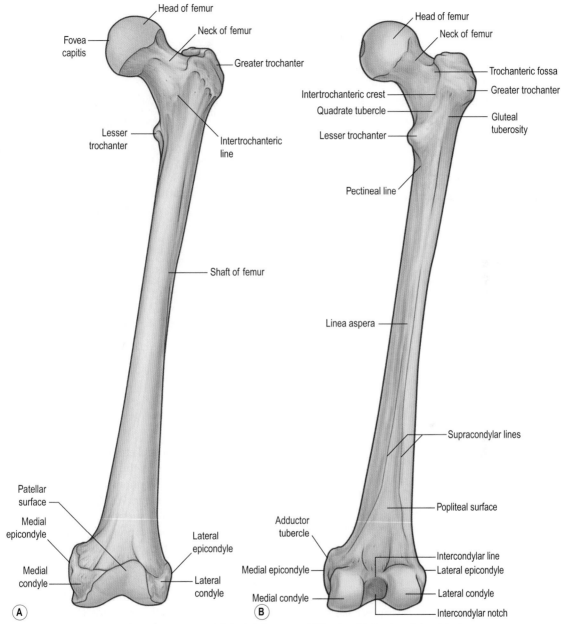

Fovea capitis

Head of femur

Neck of femur

Greater trochanter

Lesser trochanter

Intertrochanteric line

Shaft of femur

Patellar surface

Medial epicondyle

Medial condyle

Lateral epicondyle

Lateral condyle

(A)

Head of femur

Neck of femur

Trochanteric fossa

Intertrochanteric crest

Greater trochanter

Quadrate tubercle

Gluteal tuberosity

Lesser trochanter

Pectineal line

Linea aspera

Supracondylar lines

Popliteal surface

Adductor tubercle

Intercondylar line

Medial epicondyle

Lateral epicondyle

Medial condyle

Lateral condyle

Intercondylar notch

(B)

Fig. 7.15 (A) Anterior aspect of the left femur and (B) posterior aspect of the right femur.

popliteal surface; the medial supracondylar line ends at the adductor tubercle (Fig. 7.15B). A large quadrilateral greater trochanter sits on the upper lateral aspect of the shaft, with a smaller conical lesser trochanter situated medially below the neck. The lower end consists of two large smooth condyles continuous anteriorly with the triangular patellar surface; each condyle projects posteriorly beyond the shaft, with the medial being smaller than the lateral. The outer surface of each condyle is marked by a roughened area (epicondyle) (Fig. 7.15).

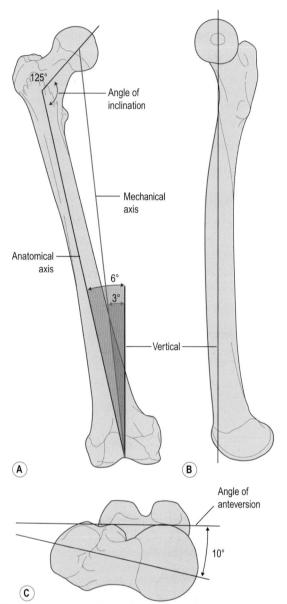

Fig. 7.16 Anterior (A), medial (B) and superior (C) aspects of the right femur showing the relationship between the anatomical and mechanical axes of the femur with the vertical, as well as the angles of inclination and anteversion.

CLINICAL ANATOMY: In fractures of the upper one-third of the femoral shaft, the proximal segment is flexed, abducted and laterally rotated, with the distal fragment being displaced superomedially.

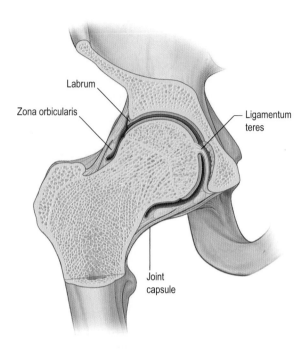

Fig. 7.17 Coronal section showing the femoral head within the acetabulum.

Hip Joint

A synovial ball-and-socket joint between the hemispherical acetabulum of the pelvis (page 567), deepened by the fibrocartilaginous acetabular labrum, and the head of the femur (Fig. 7.17); because of the reciprocally curved articular surfaces, the joint is extremely stable. A strong fibrous capsule, thicker anteriorly, surrounds the joint attaching proximally to the margin of the acetabulum and transverse ligament at the acetabular notch, and distally to the intertrochanteric line and junction of the neck with the trochanters anteriorly and to the femoral neck posteriorly (Fig. 7.18A–C). The majority of the capsular fibres pass from the innominate to the femur longitudinally or obliquely, but some (arcuate fibres) only attach to the innominate, while others (zona orbicularis) have no bony attachment (Fig. 7.18D). The anterior capsule forms part of the articular surface of the hip joint and is lined by fibrocartilage. The capsule is strengthened anteriorly by the iliofemoral and pubofemoral ligaments and posteriorly by the ischiofemoral ligament (Fig. 7.19).

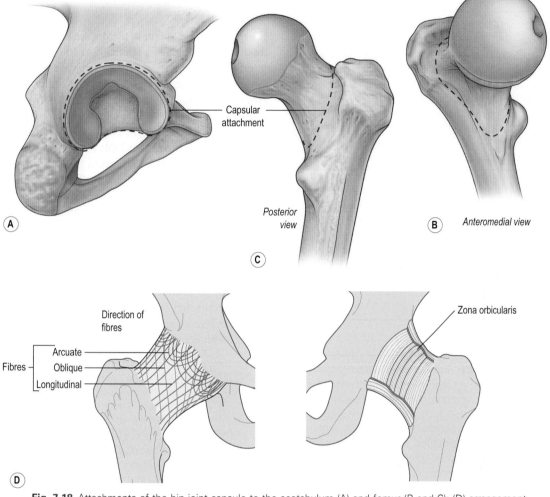

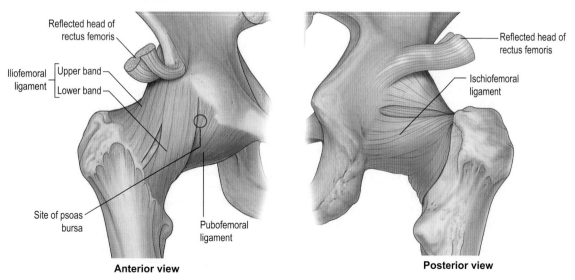

Fig. 7.18 Attachments of the hip joint capsule to the acetabulum (A) and femur (B and C); (D) arrangement of the capsular fibres.

Fig. 7.19 Capsular ligaments associated with the hip joint.

APPLIED ANATOMY: The capsular ligaments help limit movement, except flexion, of the thigh at the hip joint; when standing all three ligaments are under moderate tension. In extension all ligaments become taut, with the lower part of the iliofemoral ligament being under the greatest tension; abduction is limited by the pubofemoral and ischiofemoral ligaments; adduction by the upper part of the iliofemoral ligament; lateral rotation by the iliofemoral and pubofemoral ligaments and medial rotation by the ischiofemoral ligament.

APPLIED ANATOMY: The hip joint centre lies on a horizontal plane through the top of the greater trochanters, with the centre lying 1 cm below the middle one-third of the inguinal ligament. The greater trochanter lies 7 to 10 cm below the middle of the iliac crest and can be felt moving during flexion and extension of the thigh at the hip joint.

CLINICAL ANATOMY: Traumatic dislocation of the hip joint is not common, except in car accidents; posterior dislocation is more common, being due to the direction of the dislocating force in such accidents. The joint capsule is ruptured and the femoral head lies in the posterior iliac fossa; the limb is shortened, adducted and medially rotated, with the knee on the affected side overlying the non-affected knee. In contrast, in femoral neck fractures, the limb is shortened but laterally rotated.

CLINICAL ANATOMY: The vascular supply to the head of the femur can be disrupted following femoral fracture and lead to avascular necrosis; the head and neck are frequently replaced with a prosthesis (hemiarthroplasty). (In osteoarthritis, total hip replacement (arthroplasty) replaces both articular components.)

CLINICAL ANATOMY: Perthes' disease may also result from a disrupted blood supply to the head of the femur in early childhood. The initial necrosis is followed by revascularisation and distorted growth of the head, which is typically flattened (coxa plana) or enlarged (coxa magna).

Movements

The movements possible at the hip are flexion/extension about a transverse axis, abduction/adduction about an anteroposterior axis, and medial/lateral rotation about the mechanical axis (Fig. 7.16) of the femur, with the axes intersecting at the centre of the head of the femur; all movements involve conjoint rotation of the head within the acetabulum. For details of the muscles producing each movement see Table 7.1.

Flexion and extension. Flexion of the joint is free, being limited by contact between the thigh and anterior abdominal wall with the knee flexed, and with the knee extended tension in the hamstrings and posterior capsular structures. The total range of flexion and extension is 135 to 140 degrees, with flexion being freer (120 degrees) than extension (15–20 degrees); passive movement can increase both ranges (Fig. 7.20).

Flexion is produced by psoas major, iliacus, pectineus, rectus femoris and sartorius; extension is by gluteus maximus and the hamstrings (semitendinosus, semimembranosus, biceps femoris).

APPLIED ANATOMY: The hamstrings play an important role in balancing the pelvis on the lower limb when standing, particularly when the trunk is moved from the vertical. Together with the abdominal muscles anteriorly and gluteus maximus posteriorly, the anteroposterior tilt of the pelvis can be adjusted influencing lumbar lordosis (page 189). The hamstrings are also involved in decelerating the forward motion of the tibia when the swinging calf/leg is extended during walking, preventing the knee from snapping into extension.

Abduction and adduction. These movements each have a range of 45 degrees, except for adduction in the anatomical position (Fig. 7.21). Adduction is easier with the hip joint flexed, being limited by the opposite limb, tension in the abductors and joint capsule; abduction is greatest with the hip joint partly flexed, being limited by tension in the adductors and joint capsule.

Abduction is produced by gluteus maximus, medius and minimus, and tensor fascia lata; adduction is produced by adductors magnus, longus and brevis, gracilis and pectineus.

Medial and lateral rotation. Rotation occurs about the mechanical axes of the femur (Fig. 7.16). In medial rotation, the shaft moves anteromedially so that the toes point medially and in lateral rotation, it moves

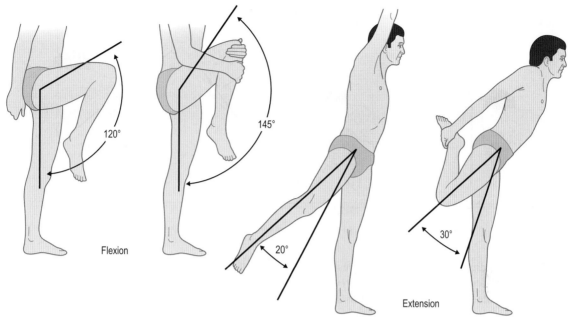

Fig. 7.20 The ranges of active and passive flexion and extension of the thigh at the hip joint.

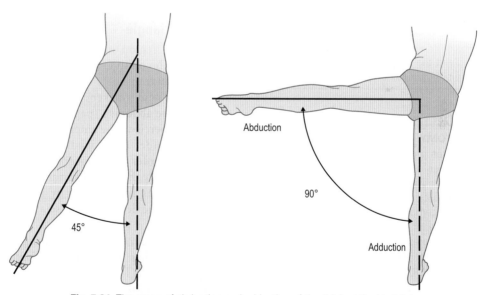

Fig. 7.21 The range of abduction and adduction of the thigh at the hip joint.

posterolaterally so that the toes point laterally. The total range of medial and lateral rotation is 90 degrees, 45 degrees each way (Fig. 7.22), being freer when combined with flexion. Lateral rotation is limited by tension in the medial rotators and anterior joint capsule and associated ligaments, and medial rotation by tension in the abductors and posterior joint capsule and associated ligaments.

Muscles producing medial rotation have their line of action passing in front of the mechanical axis of the femur, while those producing lateral rotation pass behind it. Medial rotation is produced by the anterior

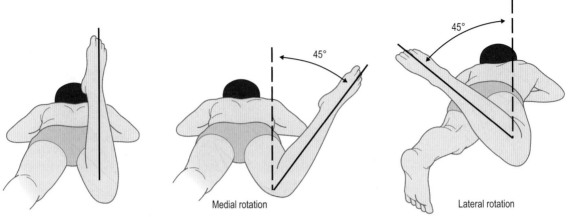

Fig. 7.22 The range of medial and lateral rotation of the thigh at the hip joint.

parts of gluteus medius and minimus, tensor fascia lata, psoas major and iliacus; lateral rotation by gluteus maximus, piriformis, obturator internus, gemellus superior and inferior, quadratus femoris and obturator externus.

> **APPLIED ANATOMY:** Gluteus maximus can be developed to produce a functional extension of the knee when quadriceps femoris is paralysed, enabling the knee to extend and the lower limb to become weight bearing during walking or standing.

> **CLINICAL ANATOMY:** Paralysis of gluteus medius and minimus causes dropping of the pelvis to the unsupported side when standing on one leg and during walking (positive Trendelenburg sign); when walking individuals compensate by moving the trunk to the affected side in an attempt to maintain the pelvis level. Damage to the superior gluteal nerve may be associated with pelvic fractures, space-occupying lesions extending into the greater sciatic foramen or hip surgery following disruption of the attachments of gluteus medius and minimus to the greater trochanter.

> **CLINICAL ANATOMY:** There may be loss of medial rotation at the hip in the osteitis pubis and loss of lateral rotation in upper femoral epiphysiolysis (slipping of the upper femoral epiphysis).

Relations

The hip joint is completely surrounded by muscles (Figs 7.12 and 7.23), with important blood vessels and nerves lying anteriorly (femoral vessels and nerve) and posteriorly (sciatic nerve, superior and inferior gluteal vessels and nerves) (Figs 7.12 and 7.23).

Femoral Triangle

A triangular region in the upper one-third of the anterior thigh continuous within the adductor (sub-sartorial) canal distally: the base is formed by the inguinal ligament (thickened lower border of external oblique of the abdomen (page 455)), extending from the pubic tubercle to the anterior superior iliac spine; the lateral border is the medial border of sartorius; the medial border is the medial border of adductor longus; medially the floor is formed by pectineus and adductor longus and laterally by iliopsoas; the roof is formed by the deep fascia (fascia lata) of the thigh (Fig. 7.23).

Just below the medial end of the inguinal ligament, the fascia lata has an opening (saphenous opening) through which the long (great) saphenous vein passes, draining superficial structures of the lower limb into the femoral vein; also passing through the opening are superficial vessels to the lateral iliac and genital regions, as well as superficial lymphatic vessels.

The femoral artery, vein and nerve and lymphatics pass between the abdomen and lower limb deep to the inguinal ligament (Fig. 7.24). The artery, vein and lymphatics are enclosed within the femoral sheath,

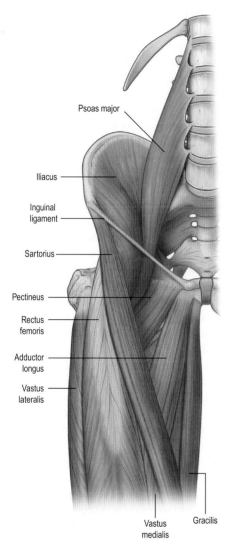

Fig. 7.23 Anterior relations of the hip joint.

Psoas major

Iliacus

Inguinal ligament

Sartorius

Pectineus

Rectus femoris

Adductor longus

Vastus lateralis

Vastus medialis

Gracilis

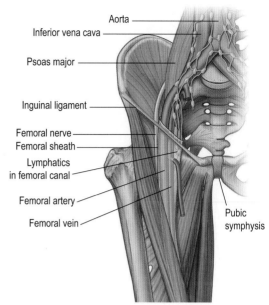

Aorta

Inferior vena cava

Psoas major

Inguinal ligament

Femoral nerve

Femoral sheath

Lymphatics in femoral canal

Femoral artery

Femoral vein

Pubic symphysis

Fig. 7.24 Boundaries and contents of the femoral triangle.

each within a separate compartment. The femoral sheath is a fascial extension continuous superiorly with the transversalis fascia and iliac fascia of the abdomen; 3 to 4 cm inferior to the inguinal ligament the sheath blends with the adventitia of the femoral vessels.

APPLIED ANATOMY: The femoral pulse can be felt as the artery passes over the femoral head.

Lymph Nodes

In the superficial fascia over the femoral triangle are two groups of lymph nodes (vertical, horizontal (Fig. 7.25)): the vertical group are associated with the long (great) saphenous vein near the saphenous opening and drain the superficial aspects of the medial side of the lower limb; the horizontal group lie parallel and below the inguinal ligament, with the lateral nodes receiving lymph from skin below the level of the umbilicus, and medial nodes lymph from the lower part of the anal canal and external genitalia (excluding the testes in males). The efferent vessels from both groups of superficial nodes drain through the cribriform fascia of the saphenous opening into the deep inguinal and external iliac nodes.

From the deep and superficial inguinal nodes, lymphatics leave the lower limb by passing under the inguinal ligament through the femoral canal (medial compartment of the femoral sheath) to the external iliac nodes; one deep inguinal node (of Cloquet) may be situated in the femoral canal.

Compartments of the Thigh

The thigh has three compartments: anterior, medial and posterior.

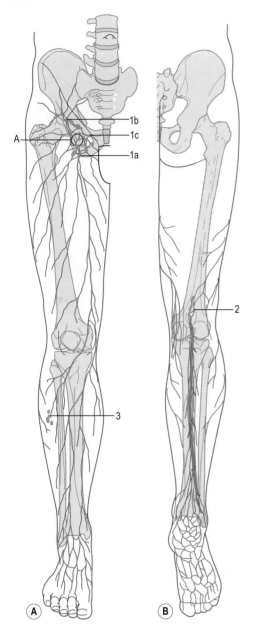

Fig. 7.25 Anterior (A) and posterior (B) aspects of the right lower limb showing the major lymphatics and groups of lymph nodes. 1, superficial inguinal lymph nodes (1a, vertical group; 1b, lateral group; 1c, medial group); 2, popliteal nodes; 3, anterior tibial nodes; *A*, saphenous opening.

Anterior Compartment

The anterior compartment contains the flexor muscles of the hip (psoas major, iliacus, pectineus) and extensor

muscles of the knee (quadratus femoris: rectus femoris, vastus lateralis, vastus intermedius, vastus medialis; sartorius), the femoral and profunda femoris arteries, the femoral and long (great) saphenous veins, and the femoral and saphenous nerves.

Femoral artery. The main arterial supply to the lower limb, being a continuation of the external iliac artery after passing deep to the inguinal ligament (Fig. 7.26A); within the femoral triangle it passes medially crossing the femoral vein to enter the adductor (subsartorial) canal. It leaves the anterior compartment of the thigh through a fibrous arch (adductor hiatus) in adductor magnus to enter the popliteal fossa (page 608) as the popliteal artery. It gives branches to the lateral iliac and gluteal regions (superficial circumflex iliac artery), the epigastric region (superficial epigastric artery), the genital region (superficial and deep external pudendal arteries), the descending genicular artery which participates in the anastomosis around the knee, and the profunda femoris supplying deep structures in the thigh and (Fig. 7.26).

Profunda femoris. Largest branch of the femoral artery arising from its lateral side 5 cm below the inguinal ligament. It passes behind the femoral artery to leave the femoral triangle between pectineus and adductor longus to lie on adductors brevis and magnus; it ends as the fourth perforating artery passing through adductor magnus (Fig. 7.26). It gives the medial and lateral circumflex femoral arteries which participate in the cruciate and trochanteric anastomoses supplying the gluteal region and hip joint. The descending branch of the lateral circumflex artery contributes to the anastomosis around the knee joint.

> **APPLIED ANATOMY:** The lateral and medial circumflex femoral arteries (from the profunda femoris) anastomose with the superior and inferior gluteal arteries around the neck of the femur (cruciate anastomosis), while the lateral and medial circumflex femoral arteries, inferior gluteal and first perforating branch of the profunda femoris anastomose below the level of the lesser trochanter (trochanteric anastomosis); both anastomoses contribute to the arterial supply to the hip joint.

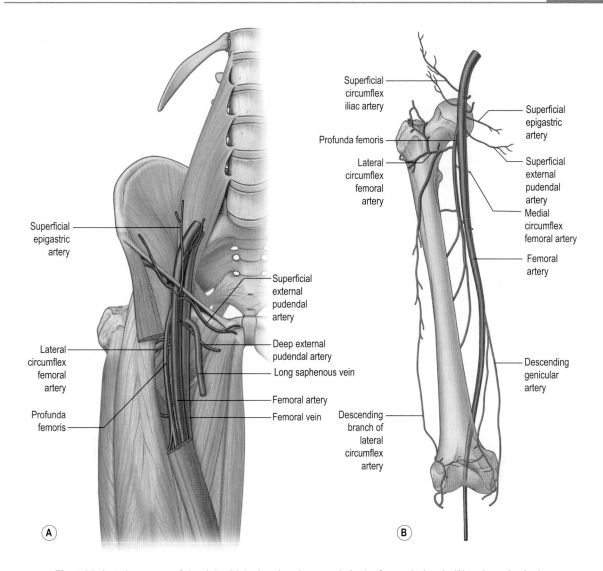

Fig. 7.26 Anterior aspect of the right thigh showing the vessels in the femoral triangle (A) and arteries in the thigh (B).

Femoral vein. Continuation of the popliteal vein after passing through the adductor hiatus. It ascends in the adductor canal to enter the femoral triangle ending by becoming the external iliac vein as it passes deep to the inguinal ligament. It receives the profunda femoris and long (great) saphenous veins (Fig. 7.26A); the long (great) saphenous vein passes through the saphenous opening in the deep fascia entering the femoral vein 3 cm below the inguinal ligament before it enters the femoral sheath.

CLINICAL ANATOMY: As the femoral vessels are relatively superficial below the inguinal ligament catheters can be placed in the artery or vein to obtain access to vessels in the ipsilateral or contralateral limb, abdomen, thorax and cerebral vessels. Using the femoral artery catheters can be placed in vessels around the aortic arch and into the coronary arteries to perform coronary angiography and angioplasty, while using the femoral vein catheters can be manoeuvred into the renal and gonadal veins, the right atrium and right side of the heart (including the pulmonary artery), superior vena cava and veins of the neck.

CLINICAL ANATOMY: A number of conditions can give rise to 'lumps in the groin': enlarged lymph nodes; direct or indirect inguinal hernia (page 458); femoral hernia (page 458); aneurysm; abscess; skin cyst; lipoma. Some lumps are mobile and their relationship to the inguinal ligament can help differentiate different 'lumps'.

Long (great) saphenous vein. Arising from the medial side of the venous network on the dorsum of the foot, initially as the medial marginal vein, the long saphenous vein ascends obliquely up the posteromedial aspect of the calf/leg towards the knee (Fig. 7.27), lying posteromedial to the femoral and tibial condyles it continues superiorly and anterolaterally in the thigh (Fig. 7.27A). It passes through the cribriform fascia of the saphenous opening to join the femoral vein. During its course, it has 8 to 20 bicuspid valves preventing backflow of blood. Before passing through the saphenous opening, it receives the superficial circumflex iliac, superficial external pudendal and superficial epigastric veins. In the calf/leg, it freely communicates with the short (small) saphenous vein and through the deep fascia with deep intermuscular veins, especially near the ankle and knee joints.

CLINICAL ANATOMY: The superficial and deep venous systems are connected by 'perforating veins', with the direction of blood flow (superficial to deep) controlled by unidirectional valves. Incompetent valves allow blood to flow from deep to superficial resulting in enlarged, swollen and painful superficial veins (varicose veins). Muscle contraction compresses the deep veins forcing blood towards the heart; however, it also tends to push blood into the superficial veins when valves in the perforating vessels are incompetent.

Femoral nerve. Arising from the posterior divisions of L2 to L4 it emerges from the lateral border of psoas major (Fig. 7.11) and runs in the grove between psoas and iliacus deep to the iliac fascia; in the abdomen it supplies iliacus. It enters the thigh deep to the inguinal ligament lateral to the femoral sheath where it immediately divides into a number of branches loosely grouped into anterior and posterior divisions which pass anterior or posterior to the lateral circumflex femoral artery. The anterior division supplies sartorius and gives the

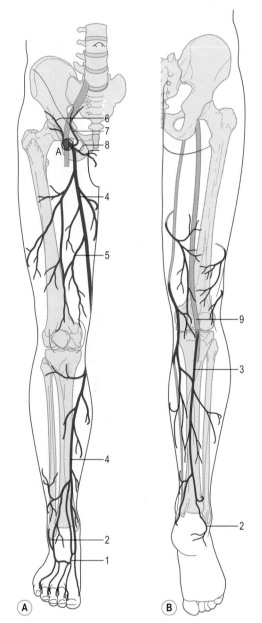

Fig. 7.27 Superficial veins on the anterior (A) and posterior (B) aspects of the lower limb.
1, dorsal venous arch; 2, lateral marginal vein; 3, short saphenous vein; 4, long saphenous vein; 5, lateral accessory vein; 6, superficial circumflex iliac vein; 7, superficial epigastric vein; 8, superficial external pudendal vein; 9, popliteal vein; A, saphenous opening.

medial and lateral branches of the anterior cutaneous nerve of the thigh (Fig. 7.11); the posterior division supplies quadriceps femoris (rectus femoris, vastus lateralis, vastus intermedius, vastus medialis) and pectineus, as well as giving the saphenous nerve (Fig. 7.11).

Saphenous nerve. Arises 3 cm below the inguinal ligament and passes through the femoral triangle to enter the adductor canal lateral to the femoral vessels: it pierces the roof of the canal becoming cutaneous between sartorius and gracilis posteromedial to the knee joint, which it supplies. It descends behind the femoral and tibial condyles and down the medial side of the calf/leg with the long (great) saphenous vein crossing anterior to the medial malleolus; it then passes along the medial side of the foot as far as the head of the first metatarsal. It supplies skin and fascia on the front and side of the knee, the calf/leg and foot as far as the base of the first (great) toe (Fig. 7.11).

Medial Compartment

The medial compartment contains the muscles (gracilis, adductors brevis, longus and magnus) involved in adducting the thigh at the hip joint and the obturator and accessory obturator (when present) nerves.

Obturator nerve. Arising from the anterior divisions of L2 to L4 it emerges from the medial border of psoas major onto the lateral surface of the sacrum. It crosses the sacroiliac joint and obturator internus to enter the obturator canal below the superior pubic ramus above the obturator membrane (Fig. 7.11). On leaving the canal it divides into anterior and posterior branches: the anterior branch supplies adductor longus, gracilis, adductor brevis (usually) and pectineus (occasionally) and is sensory to the medial side of the thigh (Fig. 7.11); the posterior branch supplies obturator externus and adductor magnus and ends by piercing the oblique popliteal ligament of the knee supplying the posterior part of the joint capsule including the cruciate ligaments (page 602).

Accessory obturator nerve. When present, it arises from the anterior divisions of L3 and L4 between the obturator and femoral nerves. It emerges from the medial border of psoas major and descends between the pelvic brim and external iliac vessels to enter the thigh between the pubis and femoral vessels. It supplies pectineus, the hip joint and communicates with the anterior branch of the obturator nerve.

Posterior Compartment

The posterior compartment contains the flexor muscles crossing the knee joint and the sciatic (tibial, common fibular/peroneal nerves) nerve and perforating cutaneous nerve of the thigh; at its lower end is the diamond-shaped popliteal fossa.

Sciatic nerve. Arises from the anterior rami of L4 to S3 it leaves the pelvis through the greater sciatic foramen to enter the gluteal region below piriformis (Figs 7.12 and 7.28); it passes down the back of the thigh deep to biceps femoris. In the lower one-third of the thigh,

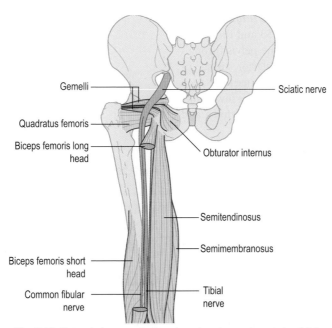

Gemelli

Quadratus femoris

Biceps femoris long head

Sciatic nerve

Obturator internus

Semitendinosus

Semimembranosus

Biceps femoris short head

Common fibular nerve

Tibial nerve

Fig. 7.28 The sciatic nerve in the gluteal region and posterior thigh.

it usually divides into its terminal branches (tibial and common fibular/peroneal nerves). It supplies the hamstrings (semitendinosus, semimembranosus, biceps femoris and hamstring part of adductor magnus).

> **APPLIED ANATOMY:** The sciatic nerve may divide at a higher level in the thigh or the components of the sciatic nerve may leave the pelvis separately. In the latter case, the tibial nerve always exits below piriformis, while the common fibular/peroneal nerve may leave below, above or pass through piriformis.

> **APPLIED ANATOMY:** The course of the sciatic nerve follows a line from midway between the ischial tuberosity and greater trochanter of the femur to where the hamstrings diverge in the lower one-third of the thigh.

> **CLINICAL ANATOMY:** When the common fibular/peroneal nerve pierces piriformis it may be subject to compression by contraction of the muscle giving rise to piriformis syndrome manifesting as pain and numbness in the buttocks and down the back of the calf/leg. There may be a degree of lateral rotation of the thigh at the hip joint if piriformis goes into spasm.

Perforating cutaneous nerve of the thigh. Arising from the anterior divisions of S2 and S3 and the posterior divisions of S1 and S2 it leaves the pelvis through the greater sciatic foramen on the posterior surface of the sciatic nerve as far as the back of the knee joint deep to the fascia lata. It supplies the skin over the lower buttock, posterior aspect of the thigh, popliteal fossa and upper part of the calf/leg (Fig. 7.29).

Muscles

The main action of the muscles in the thigh is to produce extension (quadriceps femoris) or flexion (hamstrings) of the calf/leg at the knee joint: however, with the knee flexed some muscles (semitendinosus, semimembranosus, gracilis, sartorius) produce medial rotation and others (biceps femoris) lateral rotation. Some anterior muscles (psoas major, iliacus, rectus femoris, sartorius, gracilis) produce flexion of the thigh at the hip joint, while others (hamstrings) are involved in extending the thigh at the hip joint; the principal role of the medial

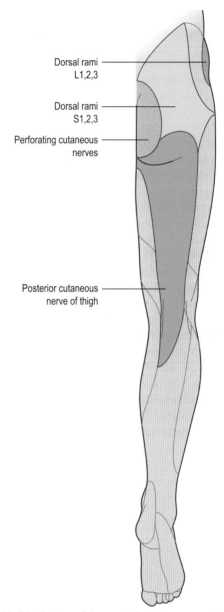

Fig. 7.29 Distribution of the posterior cutaneous nerve of the thigh and cutaneous branches of the lumbosacral plexus.

group (adductors, gracilis) is to adduct the thigh at the hip joint. Details of the attachments, action and innervation of the muscles of the thigh are given in Table 7.2.

CALF/LEG

The calf/leg is that part of the lower limb between the knee and ankle joints. Around the knee, the deep fascia

TABLE 7.2   The Attachments, Action and Innervation of Muscles in the Thigh and at the Knee Joint

Muscle	Attachments	Action	Innervation (Root Value)
Semitendinosus[b] (see Table 7.1)			
Semimembranosus[b] (see Table 7.1)			
Biceps femoris[b] (see Table 7.1)			
Gastrocnemius[b] (see Table 7.3)			
Plantaris[b] (see Table 7.3)			
Popliteus[c]	From the lateral femoral epicondyle inside the joint capsule to the posterior surface of the tibia above the soleal line	Laterally rotates the femur on the tibia with the foot fixed, flexes the calf/leg at the knee joint	Tibial nerve (L5)
Gracilis[b]	From the body of the pubis and its ramus to the medial surface of the shaft of the tibia	With the knee semiflexed it flexes the calf/leg at the knee joint; it aids medial rotation of the calf/leg at the knee joint; also contributes to adduction of the thigh at the hip joint	Obturator nerve (L2, L3)
Sartorius[b]	From the anterior superior iliac spine to the medial side of the shaft of the tibia	Flexes the calf/leg at the knee joint, medially rotates the tibia on the femur; flexes, laterally rotates and abducts the thigh at the hip joint	Femoral nerve (L2, L3)
Rectus femoris[a,b]	From the anterior inferior iliac spine (*straight head*) and area above the acetabulum (*reflected head*) to the upper border of the patella and ligamentum patellae	Extends the calf/leg at the knee joint; flexes the thigh at the hip joint	Femoral nerve (L2, L3, L4)
Vastus lateralis[a,b]	From the intertrochanteric line, greater trochanter, gluteal tuberosity, upper half of the lateral lip of the linea aspera and lateral intermuscular septum to the base and lateral border of the patella and ligamentum patellae	Extends the calf/leg at the knee joint	Femoral nerve (L2, L3, L4)
Vastus intermedius[a,b]	From the anterior and lateral surfaces of the upper two-third of the femur to the base of the patella: the articularis genu fibres arise from the lower one-third of the anterior surface of the femur to the suprapatellar bursa	Extends the calf/leg at the knee joint: articularis genu prevents the synovial membrane of the suprapatellar bursa becoming trapped between the articulating bones during movement	Femoral nerve (L2, L3, L4)
Vastus medialis[a,b]	From the intertrochanteric line, medial aspect of the upper end of the femoral shaft, medial lip of the linea aspera, medial supracondylar line and medial intermuscular septum to the medial patella border, medial tibial condyle and ligamentum patellae	Extends the calf/leg at the knee joint: the oblique medial fibres help prevent lateral displacement of the patella	Femoral nerve (L2, L3, L4)

Continued

TABLE 7.2   The Attachments, Action and Innervation of Muscles in the Thigh and at the Knee Joint (cont'd)

Muscle	Attachments	Action	Innervation (Root Value)
Tensor fascia lata	From the iliac crest between the iliac tubercle and anterior superior iliac spine to the lateral tibial condyle via the iliotibial tract	Extends the calf/leg at the knee joint; helps flex, abduct and medially rotate the hip	Superior gluteal nerve (L4, L5)

[a]Part of quadriceps femoris.
[b]Can be seen in Fig. 7.50.
[c]Can be seen in Fig. 7.33.

is continuous with that of the thigh above and calf/leg below, attaching to the medial and lateral condyles of the tibia, head of the fibula and patella anteriorly; the patella is attached to the tibial tuberosity by the ligamentum patellae and to the tibial condyles by thickened bands of deep fascia (medial and lateral patellar retinacula). Behind the knee, over the popliteal fossa, the fascia is reinforced by transverse fibres. Below the knee, the deep fascia encloses the calf/leg attaching to the anterior and medial borders of the tibia and the medial and lateral malleoli; where the tibia and fibula are subcutaneous, the deep fascia blends with the periosteum of the bone. Septa pass from the deep fascia to attach to the tibia and fibula dividing the calf/leg into three compartments (lateral, anterior, posterior). A further septum separates the superficial and deep muscles of the posterior compartment.

Tibia

DEVELOPMENT: The primary ossification centre appears in the shaft during the seventh week *in utero*. Secondary centres for the proximal end (including the tibial tuberosity, although it can develop from its own centre) appear at birth spreading into the tuberosity after age 10; for the distal end, the secondary centre appears during the second year. The distal epiphysis fuses with the shaft between ages 17 and 19, and proximal between ages 19 and 21.

Large medial bone of the calf/leg consisting of a shaft with proximal and distal ends (Fig. 7.30). The proximal end is expanded in all directions, but especially posteriorly where it projects beyond the shaft; it has two condyles (medial, lateral), which articulate with the femoral condyles forming the knee joint. Between the condyles is a non-articular area for attachment of the cruciate ligaments (anterior, posterior) and anterior and posterior horns of the medial and lateral menisci.

The triangular shaft tapers from the condyles for two-thirds its length, then widens again. It has three borders (anterior, medial, interosseous) and three surfaces (medial, lateral, posterior): the medial surface (shin) is subcutaneous throughout its length. The slightly expanded distal end has the prominent medial malleolus projecting inferiorly, the lateral surface of which is continuous with the smooth concave inferior surface for articulation with the talus (page 625), forming the ankle joint.

APPLIED ANATOMY: The tibial tuberosity can be felt at the upper end of the shin, with the ligamentum patellae attaching to its upper part, while the subcutaneous medial and lateral condyles can be felt 2 cm higher: the upper edge of the condyles indicates the knee joint line. The whole length of the medial surface (shin) can be felt as can the medial malleolus.

CLINICAL ANATOMY: Soreness, pain and swelling at the tibial tuberosity are characteristic of Osgood-Schlatter disease. It usually presents between ages of 9 and 16 in physically active individuals, as well as during 'growth spurts'. The pain is due to the pull of the quadriceps tendon (ligamentum patellae) on the tibial tuberosity, creating high stresses across the metaphysis (junction of the proximal epiphysis and shaft).

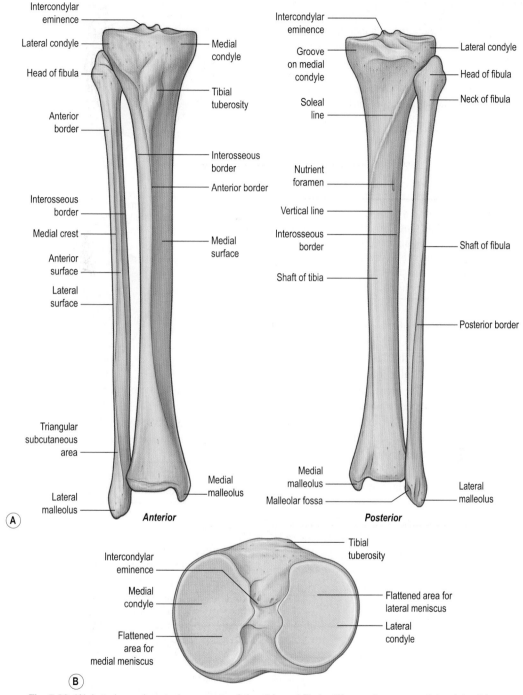

Intercondylar eminence

Lateral condyle

Head of fibula

Anterior border

Interosseous border

Medial crest

Anterior surface

Lateral surface

Triangular subcutaneous area

Lateral malleolus

Medial condyle

Tibial tuberosity

Interosseous border

Anterior border

Medial surface

Medial malleolus

Anterior

Intercondylar eminence

Groove on medial condyle

Soleal line

Nutrient foramen

Vertical line

Interosseous border

Shaft of tibia

Medial malleolus

Malleolar fossa

Lateral condyle

Head of fibula

Neck of fibula

Shaft of fibula

Posterior border

Lateral malleolus

Posterior

(A)

Tibial tuberosity

Intercondylar eminence

Medial condyle

Flattened area for medial meniscus

Flattened area for lateral meniscus

Lateral condyle

(B)

Fig. 7.30 (A) Anterior and posterior aspects of the tibia and fibula; (B) superior aspect of the right tibia.

CLINICAL ANATOMY: Because the medial surface of the tibia is subcutaneous, there is increased risk of damage and fracture of the bone, with the likelihood of infection and delayed or non-union being high and a common complication. The most common area of damage is at the thinnest part of the shaft (junction between the upper two-thirds and lower one-third), which also has a poor blood supply.

Fibula

DEVELOPMENT: The primary centre appears in the shaft during the seventh week *in utero*. Secondary centres for the proximal end appear during the third or fourth year, fusing with the shaft between ages 19 and 21, and for the distal end during the second year, fusing with the shaft between ages 17 and 19.

Long slender lateral bone of the calf/leg with proximal and distal ends (Fig. 7.30). The expanded proximal end (head) articulates with the lateral tibial condyle forming the superior tibiofibular joint; the apex of the head projects superiorly. The shaft has three borders (anterior, interosseous, posterior) and three surfaces (lateral, anterior, posterior). The expanded flattened distal end projects inferiorly as the lateral malleolus, projecting further distally than the medial malleolus; its medial surface articulates with the talus as part of the ankle joint. The fibula is not weight bearing but contributes to ankle joint stability.

APPLIED ANATOMY: The head of the fibula can be felt posterolaterally below the knee joint, while the lateral malleolus can be felt on the lateral side of the ankle, projecting 2.5 cm below the level of the joint.

Patella

DEVELOPMENT: At birth the patella is cartilaginous ossifying from a single centre between age 3 and puberty; occasionally, it is absent.

Triangular sesamoid bone formed in the tendon of quadriceps femoris, with superior (base), medial and lateral borders; it is flattened front to back, having anterior

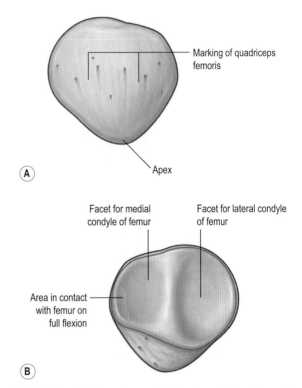

Fig. 7.31 Anterior (A) and posterior (B) surfaces of the right patella.

and posterior surfaces, with the posterior surface having larger lateral and smaller medial facets (Fig. 7.31).

APPLIED ANATOMY: The margins and anterior surface of the patella can be felt at the front of the knee.

Knee Joint

A modified synovial hinge joint between the medial and lateral condyles of the femur and those of the tibia, and between the femur and patella anteriorly. The femoral condyles are convex anteroposteriorly and transversely (Fig. 7.32), while the oval tibial condyles are relatively flat (Fig. 7.30B).

The knee joint has no complete, independent fibrous capsule but is surrounded by a thick ligamentous sheath composed mainly of muscle tendons and their expansions and ligaments (oblique popliteal, arcuate popliteal, medial (tibial) collateral, ligamentum patellae) reinforcing the true capsular fibres (Fig. 7.33). The capsule is deficient anteriorly where it is replaced by the patella. The joint cavity has an irregular shape lined by synovial membrane (Fig. 7.34), which is reflected onto

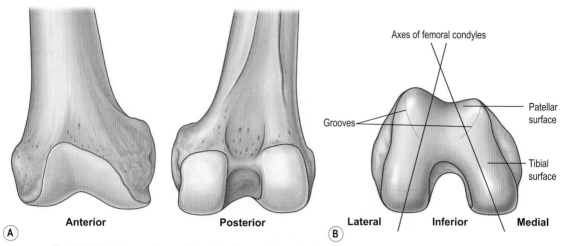

Fig. 7.32 Articular surfaces of the right femur viewed anteriorly and posteriorly (A) and inferiorly (B).

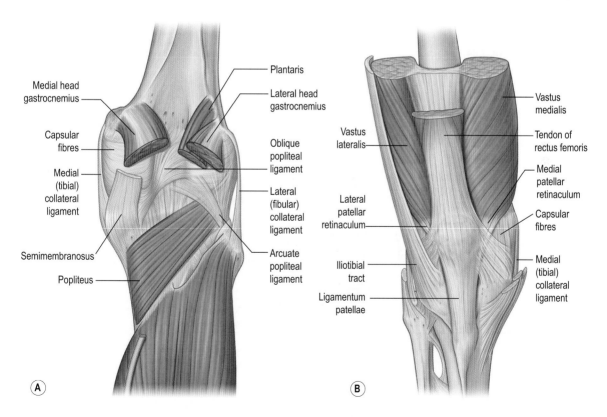

Fig. 7.33 Posterior (A) and anterior (B) aspects of the right knee showing the joint capsule and the contributions to the ligamentous sheath from muscles and ligaments crossing the joint.

the bone at the articular margins; an extension of the joint space (suprapatellar bursa) extends from the central part of the joint cavity deep to the quadriceps tendon, supported by articularis genu (Fig. 7.35).

APPLIED ANATOMY: The knee joint line can be felt on either side of the joint between the femoral and tibial condyles and followed anteriorly.

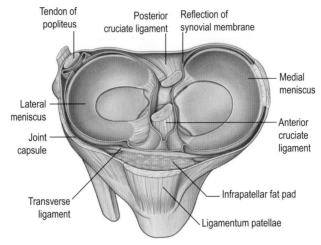

Fig. 7.34 Reflections of the synovial membrane on the superior aspect of the right tibia.

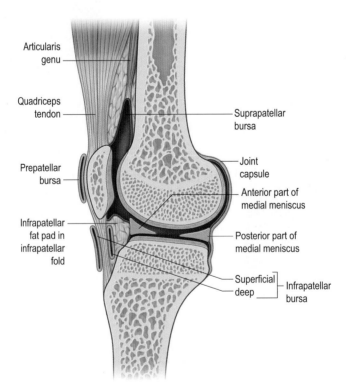

Fig. 7.35 Paramedian section through the knee showing reflections of the synovial membrane and bursa associated with the patella and ligamentum patellae.

CLINICAL ANATOMY: Malalignment of the femur and tibia at the knee joint can be a causative factor in the development of osteoarthritis, as the medial and lateral compartments are subject to unequal and high stresses. In a varus (bowlegs) deformity (Fig. 7.36), the medial side of the joint is subject to greater stresses, while in a valgus (knock knees) deformity (Fig. 7.36) it is the lateral side.

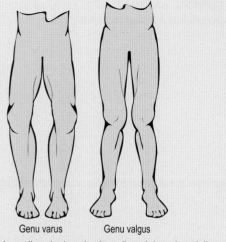

Genu varus   Genu valgus

Fig. 7.36 Varus (bowleg) and valgus (knock knee) malalignment of the femur and tibia at the knee.

Collateral Ligaments

The medial (tibial) collateral ligament is a strong flat band extending from the medial epicondyle of the femur to the medial tibial condyle and medial side of the shaft (Fig. 7.37), with the shorter deeper fibres attaching to the medial meniscus (page 604); it blends with the medial patellar retinaculum. The rounded cord-like lateral (fibular) collateral ligament extends from the lateral epicondyle of the femur to the head of the fibula (Fig. 7.37); the popliteus tendon passes deep to the ligament.

APPLIED ANATOMY: The collateral ligaments provide mediolateral stability at the knee, becoming tense during extension, thereby contributing to the 'locking' mechanism of the knee.

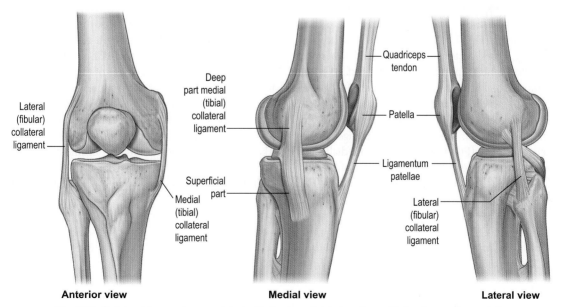

Anterior view   Medial view   Lateral view

Fig. 7.37 Collateral ligaments associated with the knee joint, together with the ligamentum patellae.

CLINICAL ANATOMY: With the knee extended (or hyperextended) lateral and medial displacement of the tibia is associated with disruption of the medial and lateral collateral ligament, respectively (Fig. 7.38).

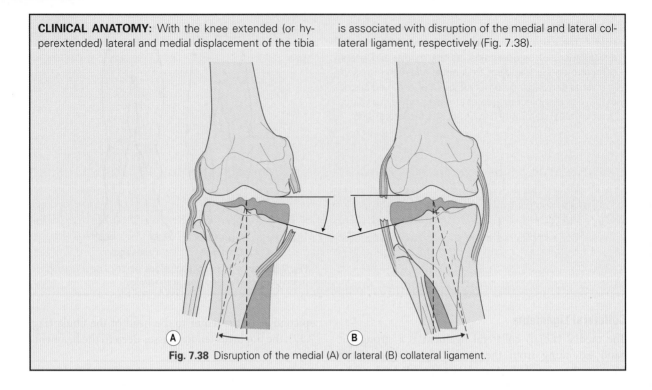

Fig. 7.38 Disruption of the medial (A) or lateral (B) collateral ligament.

Cruciate Ligaments

The cruciate ligaments lie within the knee joint capsule but are extrasynovial; they are named according to their tibial attachments (Fig. 7.34). The anterior cruciate ligament (ACL) passes posteriorly, laterally and superiorly from the anterior tibial spine to the medial surface of the lateral femoral condyle (Fig. 7.39), spiralling 110 degrees medially during its course: anatomically it is in two parts, an anteromedial band tense in flexion and a posterolateral band tense in extension. The shorter and stronger posterior cruciate ligament (PCL) runs anteriorly, medially and superiorly from the posterior intercondylar area of the tibia to the lateral surface of the medial femoral condyle (Fig. 7.39). Anatomically it is in two parts, an anterolateral band tense in extension and a posteromedial band tense in flexion. Functionally, each ligament should be considered as a continuum with part of it being tense throughout the whole range of movement, thus having a restraining influence at all positions of the joint. The ACL provides 86% of the restraint to anterior displacement of the tibia with respect to the femur and 30% of the resistance to its medial displacement, whereas the PCL provides 94% of the restraint to posterior displacement of the tibia with respect to the femur and 36% of the resistance to its lateral displacement. The blood supply to the cruciate ligaments is from the middle genicular artery, which forms a periligamentous sheath around them from which small penetrating vessels arise.

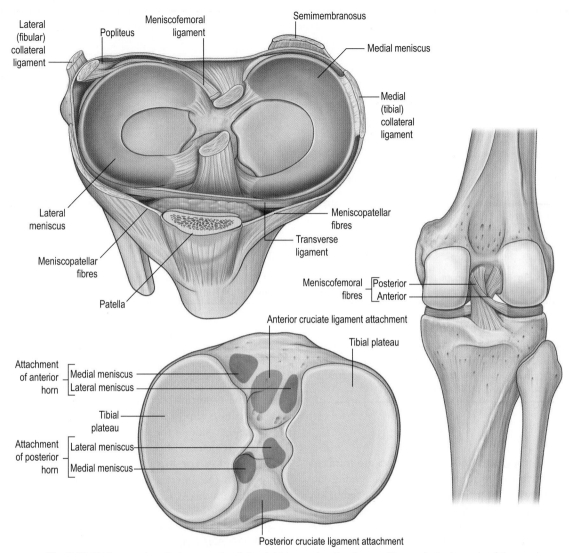

Fig. 7.39 Oblique and posterior aspects of the right knee showing the position and attachments of the cruciate ligaments and menisci and their relationship.

APPLIED ANATOMY: ACL rupture results in a small increase in anterior drawer (anterior tibial displacement at 90 degrees), whereas rupture of the PCL results in a drawer of up to 25 mm (Fig. 7.40).

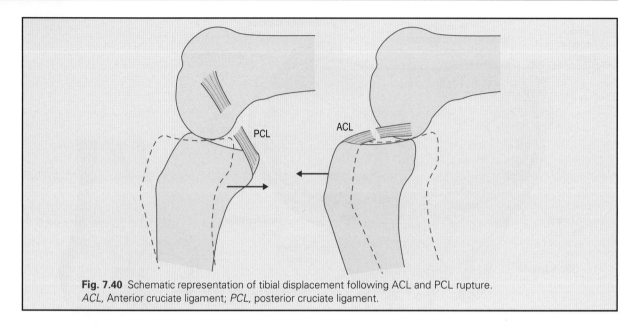

Fig. 7.40 Schematic representation of tibial displacement following ACL and PCL rupture. *ACL,* Anterior cruciate ligament; *PCL,* posterior cruciate ligament.

CLINICAL ANATOMY: Rupture of a cruciate ligament results in haematoma in the extrasynovial joint space, with the knee adopting a semiflexed position.

Menisci

The fibrocartilaginous crescentic menisci are intracapsular, intrasynovial structures (Fig. 7.34) increasing congruence between the articular surfaces of the femur and tibia, participating in weight bearing, acting as shock absorbers and aiding lubrication; their thick convex outer borders are attached to the deep surface of the joint capsule. The menisci are attached to the intercondylar area of the tibia by anterior and posterior horns (Fig. 7.39). The larger semicircular medial meniscus is broader posteriorly, while the lateral meniscus forms four-fifths of a circle of uniform breadth. Except at their periphery, the menisci are avascular and aneural.

In addition to their capsular attachments the menisci are attached anteriorly by the transverse ligament, and occasionally (20%) by a posterior transverse ligament. The posterior part of the lateral meniscus gives a ligamentous slip to the PCL (Fig. 7.39), which splits to run either side of the ligament (anterior and posterior meniscofemoral ligaments); posteriorly the lateral meniscus gives rise to some fibres of popliteus. A few fibres from the anterior horn of the medial meniscus may run with the ACL.

APPLIED ANATOMY: During movements of the knee joint, the menisci follow the movements of the femur with respect to the tibia, with the lateral meniscus being the more mobile. The menisci move forwards in extension and backwards in flexion; in rotation, one moves forwards and the other backwards depending on the direction of rotation.

CLINICAL ANATOMY: Severe strain on a meniscus, usually involving rotation, may cause longitudinal, or occasionally transverse, splitting of the fibrocartilage (Fig. 7.41). Because of its attachment to the medial collateral ligament, the medial meniscus is more frequently injured, with the thinner inner part separating from the thicker outer part (bucket-handle rupture). The detached part can move into the centre of the joint preventing full extension of the knee.

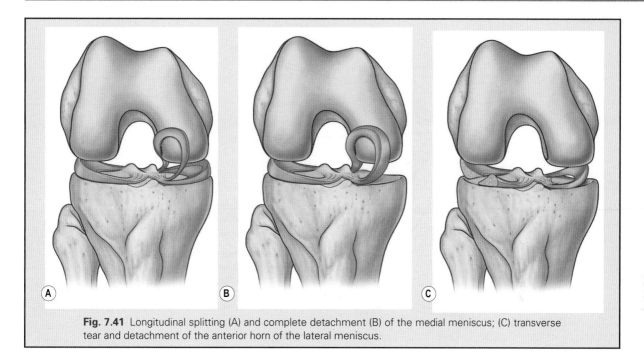

Fig. 7.41 Longitudinal splitting (A) and complete detachment (B) of the medial meniscus; (C) transverse tear and detachment of the anterior horn of the lateral meniscus.

Movements

Two separate articulations must be considered with movements of the knee; that between the femur and tibia is the most important in determining the length of the lower limb, and that between the femur and patella, with the patella acting as a pulley for the quadriceps tendon changing its line of action. The main movement at the knee joint is flexion and extension (Fig. 7.42); with the knee semiflexed medial and lateral rotation of the tibia with respect to the femur is possible, but with the feet on the ground, the rotation is taken up by the femur, which rotates about its

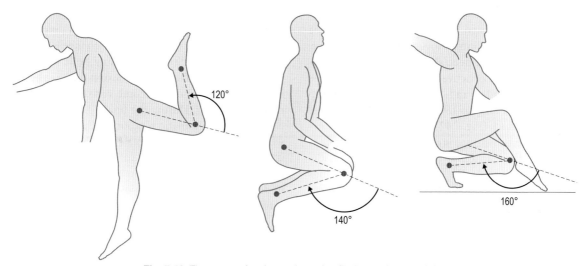

Fig. 7.42 The range of active and passive flexion at the knee joint.

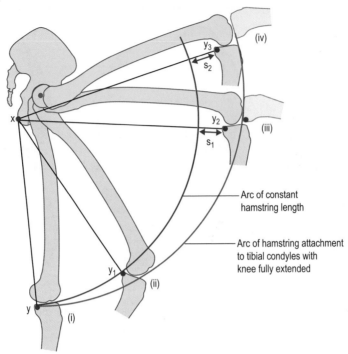

Fig. 7.43 The influence of hip position on the effectiveness of the hamstrings in flexing the knee. *S*, extent of lengthening, *x* and *y*, hamstring attachments to the ischial tuberosity and tibia.

mechanical axis (Fig. 7.16A) running through the intercondylar eminence: the intercondylar eminence of the tibia lodging in the intercondylar notch of the femur acts as the pivot.

Flexion and extension. Flexion is movement of the calf/leg bringing its posterior aspect towards the posterior aspect of the thigh. Extension brings the calf/leg back to the neutral position; movement, usually passive, of the tibia beyond the neutral position, is hyperextension. The total range of active movement is 120 degrees with the hip extended and 140 degrees with the hip flexed; the passive range is 160 degrees enabling the heel to touch the buttock (Fig. 7.42).

Because the hamstrings are hip extensors as well as knee flexors, their action at the knee depends on the position of the hip. As the hip flexes the hamstrings become wrapped around the ischial tuberosity effectively shortening them (Fig. 7.43). With hip flexion greater than 90 degrees it becomes difficult to keep the knee fully extended (Fig. 7.43(iii)); however, with stretching their efficiency as knee flexors increases. Similarly, knee extension increases the efficiency of the hamstrings as hip extensors.

Movement of the femoral condyles over the tibial plateaux is a combination of rolling and gliding: initially rolling then gliding (Fig. 7.44). This change is important for knee joint function in providing both stability and mobility; beyond 20 degrees of flexion the knee becomes looser as the ligaments become relaxed enabling axial rotation to occur. During the final 20 degrees of active extension, an automatic rotation of the knee occurs in which the femur medially rotates on the tibia if the foot is fixed, or the tibia laterally rotates on the femur if the foot is free. To enable flexion to occur the knee must undergo rotation in the opposite direction to that in extension.

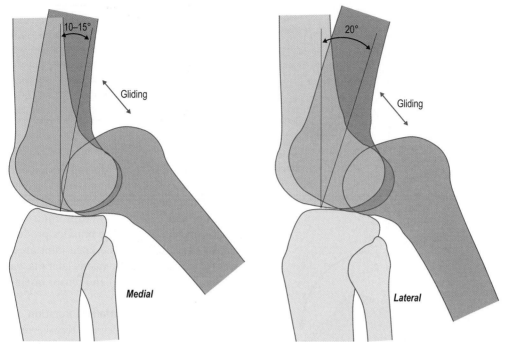

Fig. 7.44 The extent of rolling and gliding of the femoral condyles over the tibial plateaux.

APPLIED ANATOMY: The Helfet test can be used to determine whether lateral rotation of the tibia occurs during knee extension with the foot free. The medial and lateral borders of the patella are marked on the skin and lines drawn on the middle of the patella and tibial tuberosity and their alignment checked: with knee extension the tibial tuberosity should move laterally, becoming aligned with the lateral border of the patella (Fig. 7.45).

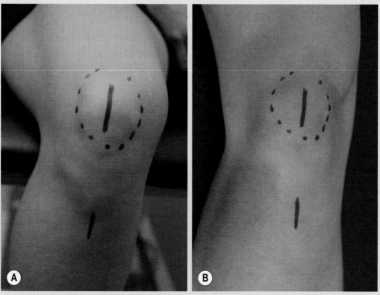

Fig. 7.45 The Helfet test: (A) knee flexed; (B) knee extended.

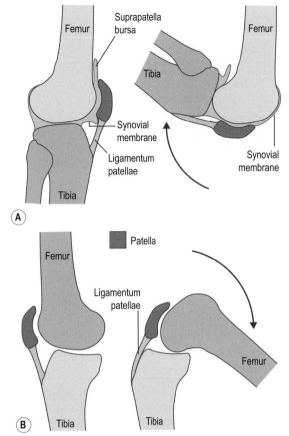

Fig. 7.46 Movement of the patella with the femur (A) and tibia (B) fixed.

The patella changes its relationship with the femur; its movement depending on whether the femur or tibia is fixed (Fig. 7.46).

APPLIED ANATOMY: Normally, there is no transverse movement of the patella during flexion/extension, being held against the femur by the quadriceps tendon (ligamentum patellae); lateral displacement is prevented by the lateral lip of the patellar surface of the femur and the horizontal fibres of vastus medialis. An underdeveloped lateral lip or weakness of vastus medialis may allow lateral patella displacement in extension. A severely underdeveloped lateral lip may lead to displacement during flexion, this is the underlying mechanism of recurrent patella dislocation.

APPLIED ANATOMY: When the knee is fully extended the collateral and cruciate ligaments are fully taut making the joint extremely stable.

CLINICAL ANATOMY: If the capsular recesses (suprapatellar bursa, parapatellar recesses) associated with the patella are obliterated by inflammatory adhesions, the patella is held firmly against the femur so that it cannot move down towards the intercondylar notch; this is one cause of post-traumatic or post-infective 'stiff knee'.

The main muscles producing flexion of the calf/leg at the knee joint are the hamstrings (semitendinosus, semimembranosus, biceps femoris), gastrocnemius and popliteus (Table 7.2), with contributions from gracilis and sartorius. The muscles producing extension of the calf/leg at the knee joint are quadriceps femoris (rectus femoris, vastus lateralis, vastus intermedius, vastus medialis) and tensor fascia lata (Table 7.2).

Medial and lateral rotation. Rotation occurs about the long axis of the calf/leg in a transverse plane, being influenced by the degree of joint flexion; medial and lateral rotation bring the toes to face medially or laterally, respectively (Fig. 7.47). The range of rotation is influenced by the degree of knee extension: active medial and lateral rotation are 30 degrees and 40 degrees, which can be increased passively to 35 degrees and 50 degrees, respectively. During axial rotation the patella moves in a frontal plane with respect to the tibia (Fig. 7.48).

The main muscles responsible for producing medial rotation of the calf/leg at the knee joint are semitendinosus, semimembranosus, gracilis, sartorius, with a contribution from popliteus (Table 7.2). The only muscle producing lateral rotation of the calf/leg at the knee joint is biceps femoris (Table 7.2). Muscles crossing the knee joint are shown in Fig. 7.49.

Popliteal Fossa

Diamond-shaped space at the lower end of the posterior thigh behind the knee. The upper boundaries are the tendons of semitendinosus and semimembranosus medially and biceps femoris laterally, the medial and lateral heads of gastrocnemius form the lower boundaries (Fig. 7.50); the floor (from above down) is the popliteal surface of the femur (Fig. 7.15B), the posterior knee joint capsule and popliteus (Fig. 7.33A); the roof is formed by the popliteal fascia continuous with the fascia of the thigh and calf/leg.

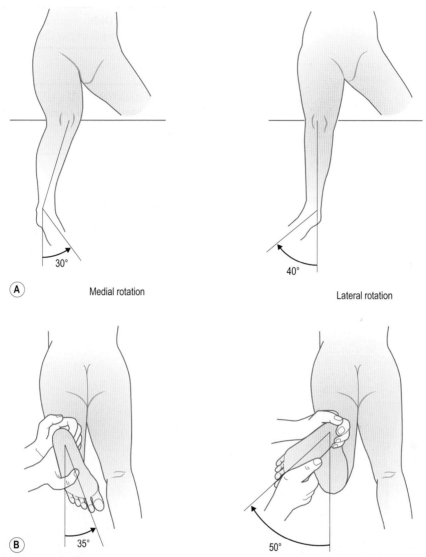

Fig. 7.47 Active (A) and passive (B) ranges of medial and lateral rotation at the knee.

APPLIED ANATOMY: With the knee flexed the boundaries of the popliteal fossa can be felt; superomedially the tendons of semitendinosus and gracilis, superolaterally the tendon of biceps femoris, inferomedially and inferolaterally the medial and lateral heads of gastrocnemius, respectively.

Immediately deep to the fascia are the tibial and common fibular/peroneal nerves and posterior cutaneous nerve of the thigh. Above the popliteal fossa, the femoral vessels lie opposite the posterior border of the femur and lower end of the adductor canal against the tendon of adductor magnus. When they pass through the adductor hiatus (in adductor magnus) they become the popliteal vessels, with the popliteal artery lying directly on the popliteal surface of the femur. Within the fossa the popliteal artery gives five genicular branches (Fig. 7.51) supplying the knee joint and participating in the genicular anastomosis. The popliteal artery terminates at the level of the tibial tuberosity by dividing into anterior and posterior tibial arteries.

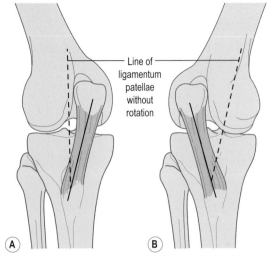

Fig. 7.48 Movement of the patella during (A) medial and (B) lateral rotation of the tibia with respect to the femur.

APPLIED ANATOMY: Applying deep pressure with the knee flexed the popliteal pulse can be felt.

CLINICAL ANATOMY: The popliteal artery is protected from external trauma but is vulnerable to supracondylar fractures of the femur, or occasionally during knee joint surgery.

The popliteal vein, formed by the anterior and posterior tibial veins at the lower border of popliteus ascends through the fossa crossing from medial to lateral posterior to the artery, bound to it by a dense fascial sheath; it also receives the short (small) saphenous vein, which pierces the fascial roof of the fossa. The popliteal vessels

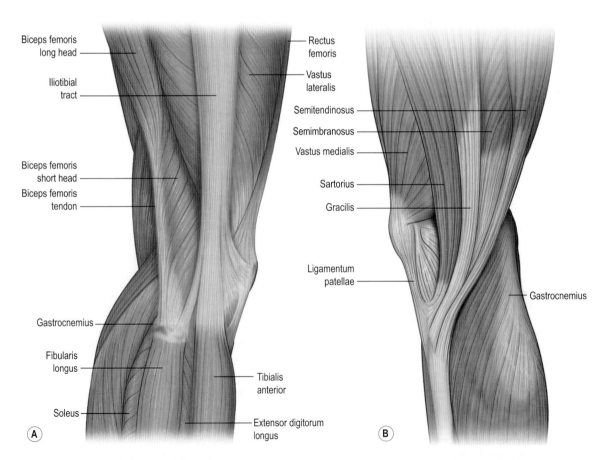

Fig. 7.49 Lateral (A) and medial (B) aspects of the right knee showing muscles crossing the joint.

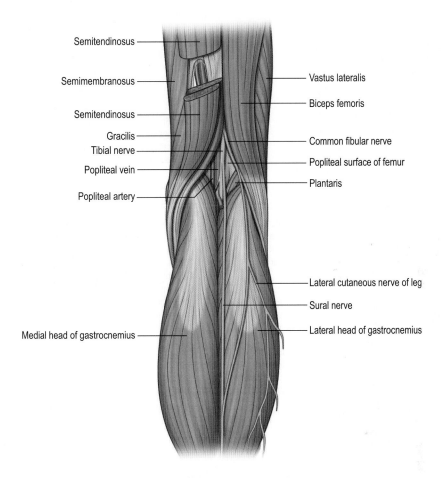

Fig. 7.50 Posterior aspect of the right knee showing the boundaries and contents of the popliteal fossa.

Labels (left side, top to bottom): Semitendinosus, Semimembranosus, Semitendinosus, Gracilis, Tibial nerve, Popliteal vein, Popliteal artery, Medial head of gastrocnemius

Labels (right side, top to bottom): Vastus lateralis, Biceps femoris, Common fibular nerve, Popliteal surface of femur, Plantaris, Lateral cutaneous nerve of leg, Sural nerve, Lateral head of gastrocnemius

are embedded in fat and areolar connective tissue, which also contains the popliteal lymph nodes (Fig. 7.25).

Tibiofibular Joints

Below the knee, the deep fascia encloses the calf/leg attaching to the anterior and medial borders of the tibia and the medial and lateral malleoli; where the tibia and fibula are subcutaneous the deep fascia blends with the periosteum. Intermuscular septa pass to the fibula separating the fibularis/peroneal muscles from the extensors anteriorly and flexors posteriorly; a further septum separates the superficial and deep flexors. Around the ankle, the fascia thickens forming retaining bands (retinaculae) preventing the tendons of muscles crossing the joint from bowstringing.

The tibia and fibula are connected along their shafts by an interosseous membrane, whose fibres run predominantly inferolaterally from tibia to fibula (Fig. 7.52). The upper margin does not reach the superior tibiofibular joint, allowing the anterior tibial vessels to gain access to the anterior compartment of the calf/leg. It is continuous with the interosseous ligament of the inferior tibiofibular joint. The interosseous membrane separates the muscles of the anterior (extensor) and posterior (flexor) compartments, as well as giving attachment to some muscles.

Superior Tibiofibular Joint

Plane synovial joint, surrounded by a fibrous capsule strengthened by ligaments, between the head of the

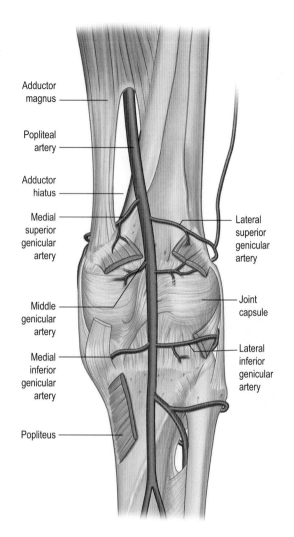

Fig. 7.51 Posterior aspect of the right knee showing its arterial supply.

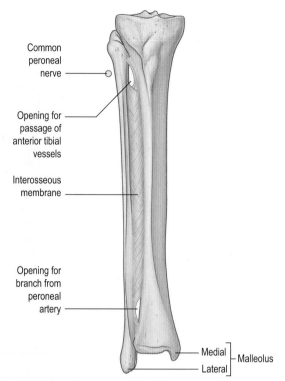

Fig. 7.52 Anterior aspect of the right tibia and fibula showing the interosseous membrane.

fibula and underside of the lateral tibial condyle (Fig. 7.53A). There is no active movement at the joint; however, slight movement accompanies movement at the ankle joint.

Inferior Tibiofibular Joint

Fibrous joint (syndesmosis) between the medial surface of the fibula and lateral side of the tibia (Fig. 7.53B); the bones are united by a strong interosseous ligament. It provides a firm union between the tibia and fibula contributing significantly to the stability of the ankle joint.

Compartments of the Calf/Leg

The calf/leg has three compartments (anterior, posterior, lateral) separated by an interosseous membrane attached to the interosseous borders of the tibia and fibula, and intermuscular septa (Fig. 7.54).

Anterior Compartment

The anterior (extensor) compartment contains the extensor muscles of the ankle (tibialis anterior, fibularis/peroneus tertius) and toes (extensor hallucis longus, extensor digitorum longus), the anterior tibial artery and its vena comitantes and the deep fibular/peroneal nerve, with the terminal branches of the superficial fibular/peroneal and saphenous nerves and long (great) saphenous vein in the superficial fascia (Fig. 7.4).

Anterior tibial artery. Terminal branch of the popliteal artery passing into the anterior compartment through an opening above the interosseous membrane

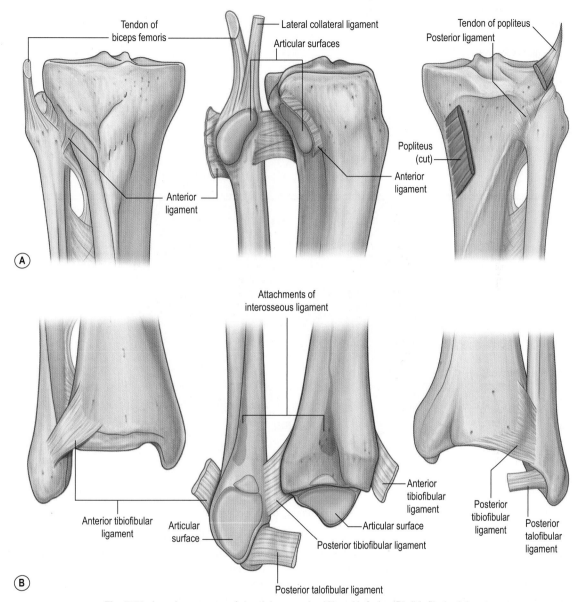

Fig. 7.53 Anterior aspects of the right superior (A) and inferior (B) tibiofibular joints.

to run on its anterior surface becoming the dorsalis pedis artery at the ankle joint (Figs 7.55 and 7.58).

Deep fibular/peroneal nerve. Terminal branch of the common fibular/peroneal nerve as it passes around the neck of the fibula (Fig. 7.52). It passes inferomedially into the anterior compartment joining the anterior tibial vessels on the anterior surface of the interosseous membrane entering the foot deep to the superior and inferior extensor retinaculae (Fig. 7.55).

CLINICAL ANATOMY: The common fibular/peroneal nerve is vulnerable to injury at the neck of the fibula, where it can be crushed by direct trauma (kick, car bumper) or pressure (tight immobilising cast or bandage). The superficial and deep branches are both affected resulting in 'foot drop', having a profound effect on walking, which may require splinting to enable the foot to clear the ground during the swing phase (page 636); there is also extensive, but less significant, sensory loss.

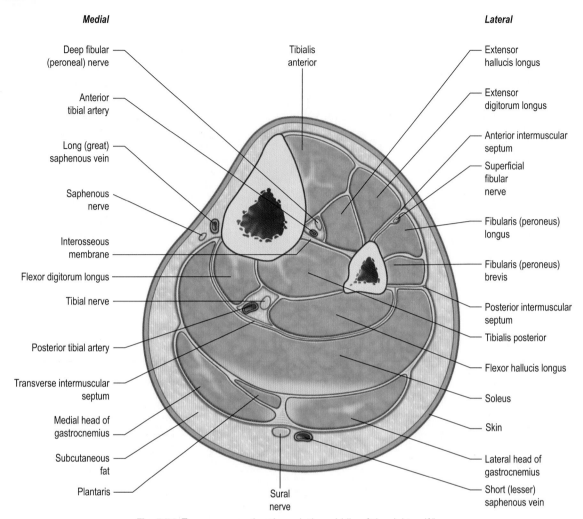

Medial

Deep fibular (peroneal) nerve

Anterior tibial artery

Long (great) saphenous vein

Saphenous nerve

Interosseous membrane

Flexor digitorum longus

Tibial nerve

Posterior tibial artery

Transverse intermuscular septum

Medial head of gastrocnemius

Subcutaneous fat

Plantaris

Tibialis anterior

Sural nerve

Lateral

Extensor hallucis longus

Extensor digitorum longus

Anterior intermuscular septum

Superficial fibular nerve

Fibularis (peroneus) longus

Fibularis (peroneus) brevis

Posterior intermuscular septum

Tibialis posterior

Flexor hallucis longus

Soleus

Skin

Lateral head of gastrocnemius

Short (lesser) saphenous vein

Fig. 7.54 Transverse section through the middle of the right calf/leg.

Saphenous nerve. Cutaneous branch of the femoral nerve supplying skin over the medial side of the calf/leg and ankle (Fig. 7.11).

Long (great) saphenous vein. Arises from the dorsal venous arch anterior to the medial malleolus ascending obliquely up the posteromedial aspect of the calf, behind the tibial and femoral condyles to continue superiorly and anterolaterally in the thigh towards the saphenous opening (Figs. 7.27 and 7.54).

Lateral Compartment

The lateral compartment contains muscles which evert the foot (fibularis/peroneus longus and brevis), the superficial fibular/peroneal nerve and fibular/peroneal artery (Fig. 7.54).

Superficial fibular/peroneal nerve. Terminal branch of the common fibular/peroneal nerve, it descends almost vertically anterior to the fibula, becoming superficial after piercing the deep fascia dividing into its terminal branches (see Fig. 7.56), which supply the dorsum of the foot.

Fibular/peroneal artery. A branch of the posterior tibial artery (see Fig. 7.58), which anastomoses with the anterior tibial and dorsalis pedis arteries.

Posterior Compartment

The posterior compartment contains the flexor (plantarflexor) muscles of the ankle (gastrocnemius, soleus, plantaris, tibialis posterior) and toes (flexor hallucis longus, flexor digitorum longus), the tibial nerve and

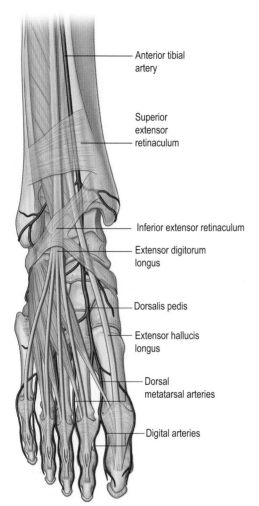

Anterior tibial artery

Superior extensor retinaculum

Inferior extensor retinaculum

Extensor digitorum longus

Dorsalis pedis

Extensor hallucis longus

Dorsal metatarsal arteries

Digital arteries

Fig. 7.55 Anterior tibial artery and arteries on the dorsum of the foot.

posterior tibial artery within the deep compartment, and the sural nerve and short (small) saphenous vein in the subcutaneous tissue (Fig. 7.54).

Tibial nerve. Terminal branch of the sciatic nerve arising in the lower one-third of the thigh; it passes through the popliteal fossa initially lateral to the popliteal vessels, but crossing them superficially to lie medial where it enters the calf/leg under the tendinous arch of soleus. It descends obliquely to pass behind the medial malleolus deep to the flexor retinaculum to enter the plantar aspect of the foot, dividing into its terminal branches (medial and lateral plantar nerves) as it does so (Fig. 7.57).

Posterior tibial artery. Larger terminal branch of the popliteal artery; it passes down the back of the calf/leg deep to soleus and gastrocnemius (Fig. 7.58). It crosses the ankle joint behind the medial malleolus deep to the flexor retinaculum, where it is covered only by skin and deep fascia, dividing immediately into its terminal branches (medial and lateral plantar arteries).

Short (small) saphenous vein. Arising from the lateral side of the dorsal venous arch passing behind the lateral malleolus it ascends on the posterior aspect of the calf/leg, pierces the roof of the popliteal fossa to drain into the popliteal vein (Figs. 7.27 and 7.54); it contains between 6 and 12 valves. During its course, it is accompanied by the sural nerve.

Sural nerve. Cutaneous branch of the tibial nerve supplying skin over the back of the calf/leg (Fig. 7.57).

Muscles

The main action of muscles of the calf/leg is to produce extension/dorsiflexion (tibialis anterior, fibularis/peroneus tertius) and flexion/plantarflexion (gastrocnemius, soleus, plantaris, tibialis posterior, fibularis/peroneus longus, fibularis/peroneus brevis) of the foot at the ankle joint, and extension (extensors hallucis longus and digitorum longus) and flexion (flexors hallucis longus and digitorum longus) of the toes; tibialis anterior and posterior also invert and fibularis/peroneus longus and brevis evert the foot at the subtalar and midtarsal joints (page 626).

ANKLE

The deep fascia around the ankle is thickened by transverse bands (retinaculae), which hold the tendons crossing the ankle joint in position preventing them from bowstringing (Fig. 7.59). As the tendons pass deep to the retinaculae they are enclosed within synovial sheaths, which facilitate sliding of the tendon under the retinacula; they are normally not evident.

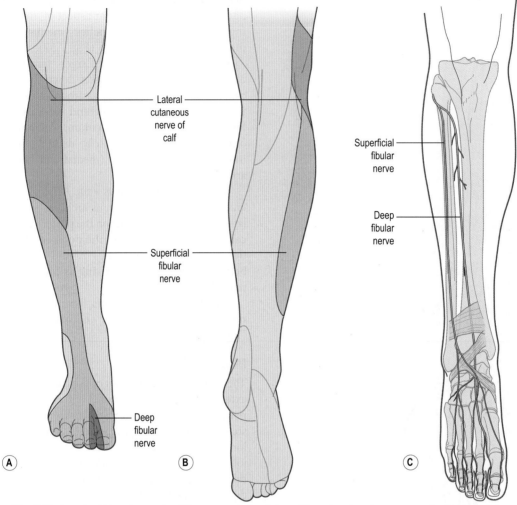

Fig. 7.56 Anterior (A) and posterior (B) aspects of the right calf/leg showing the sensory distribution of the superficial and deep fibular/peroneal nerve, as well as their course within the calf/leg (C).

APPLIED ANATOMY: When damaged (trauma, infection, overactivity), the tendon sheaths become swollen presenting as a 'sausage-like' swelling along the length of the sheath surrounding the tendon (tenosynovitis); it may be painful and incapacitating. The condition is often labelled 'repetitive strain injury'. It can occur anywhere in the body where tendons pass through sheaths in confined spaces.

Ankle Joint

Synovial hinge joint between the distal end of the tibia, lateral surface of the medial malleolus and medial surface of the lateral malleolus and the body of the talus (Fig. 7.60); the body of the talus is slightly wider in front than behind. The trochlear surface on the tibia is concave anteroposteriorly and slightly convex transversely, with that on the talus being reciprocally curved.

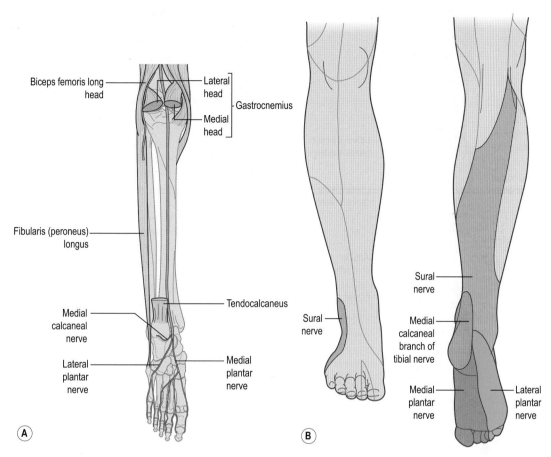

Fig. 7.57 The course (A) and cutaneous distribution (B) of the tibial nerve.

A fibrous capsule, lined by synovial membrane, completely surrounds the joint. It is thin and weak anteriorly and posteriorly permitting dorsiflexion and plantarflexion, but strengthened medially and laterally by collateral ligaments. Medially is the deltoid ligament, whereas laterally there are three separate bands (Fig. 7.61). Each set of ligaments radiates inferiorly from the respective malleolus, with both having a middle part/band attaching to the calcaneus and anterior and posterior parts/bands attaching to the talus.

Anteroposterior stability at the ankle joint depends on the effect of gravity, as well as the collateral ligaments and muscles crossing the joint, keeping the joint surfaces in contact. Mediolateral stability depends on the interlocking of its articular surfaces (Fig. 7.62A).

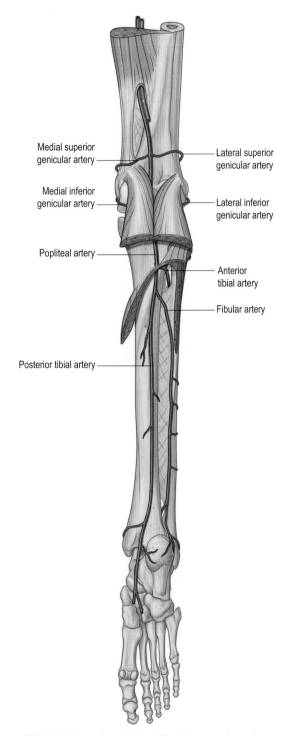

Medial superior genicular artery

Medial inferior genicular artery

Popliteal artery

Posterior tibial artery

Lateral superior genicular artery

Lateral inferior genicular artery

Anterior tibial artery

Fibular artery

Fig. 7.58 Posterior tibial and fibular/peroneal arteries.

CLINICAL ANATOMY: When the foot is forcibly moved laterally the lateral surface of the talus pushes against the lateral malleolus; the resulting outcome depends on the severity of the movement, the state of the bones and integrity of the ligaments. If the inferior tibiofibular ligament is ruptured, the grip of the malleoli on the talus is disrupted leading to widening of the joint (diastasis of the ankle (Fig. 7.62B and C)); if the deltoid ligament is also involved (Fig. 7.62D), the talus can rotate about its vertical axis against the posterior margin of the tibia, possibly fracturing it; if abduction continues, both malleoli may become fractured (Fig. 7.62E), one form of Pott's fracture, occasionally the lateral malleolus does not fracture with the fibular fracture occurring at the neck; if the inferior tibiofibular ligament does not fracture, there can still be fracture of both malleoli with the lateral malleolus fracturing through the inferior tibiofibular joint (Fig. 7.62G), another form of Pott's fracture; if there is violent adduction of the foot, both malleoli fracture (Fig. 7.62H), with the inferior tibiofibular and both collateral ligaments remaining intact. In all fractures, a chip of bone is often broken off the posterior margin of the tibia, which presents as a separate bone fragment or forms a single unit with the malleolar fragment.

All muscles, vessels and nerves entering the foot cross the ankle joint (Figs 7.59 and 7.63).

Movements

Movement is limited to plantarflexion (flexion) and dorsiflexion (extension) about a transverse axis. In normal standing, the foot is at right angles to the calf/leg; this is the neutral position of the joint (Fig. 7.64). In dorsiflexion, the foot is drawn up towards the calf/leg and in plantarflexion, it moves in the opposite direction (Fig. 7.64A). The range of dorsiflexion and plantarflexion is determined by the profiles of the articular surfaces (Fig. 7.64B).

During dorsiflexion the broader anterior part of the body of the talus is forced between the narrower part of the tibiofibular mortise causing movement of the fibula away from the tibia, accompanied by rotation about its long axis and upward movement (Fig. 7.65A). In plantarflexion, the opposite movements of the fibula occur (Fig. 7.65B). There is no resistance to movement at the synovial superior tibiofibular joint.

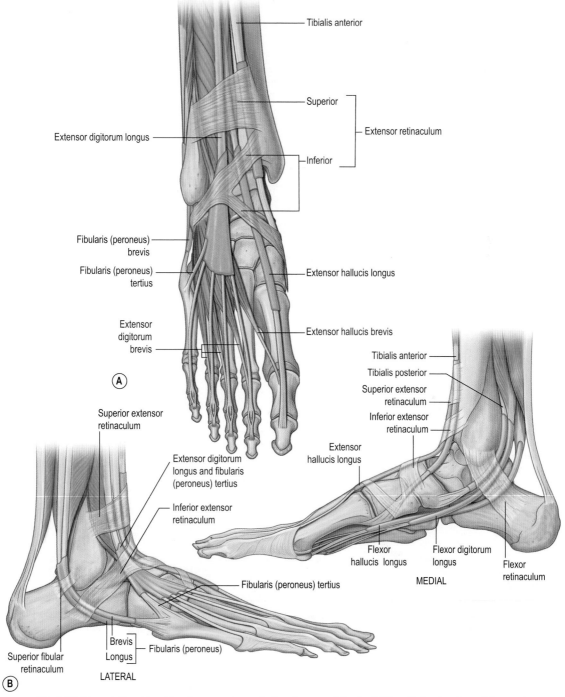

Fig. 7.59 The relationship of tendons passing onto the dorsum of the foot (A) and lateral and medial aspects (B), together with their associated synovial sheaths.

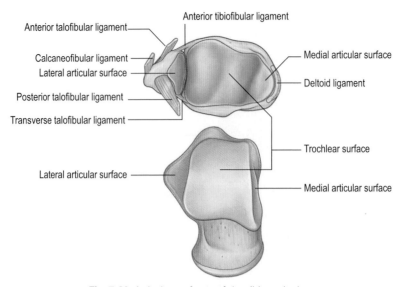

Fig. 7.60 Articular surfaces of the tibia and talus.

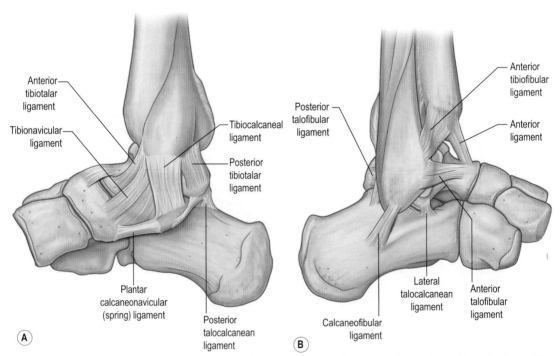

Fig. 7.61 Medial (A) and lateral (B) aspects of the right ankle showing the attachments of the medial and lateral collateral ligaments.

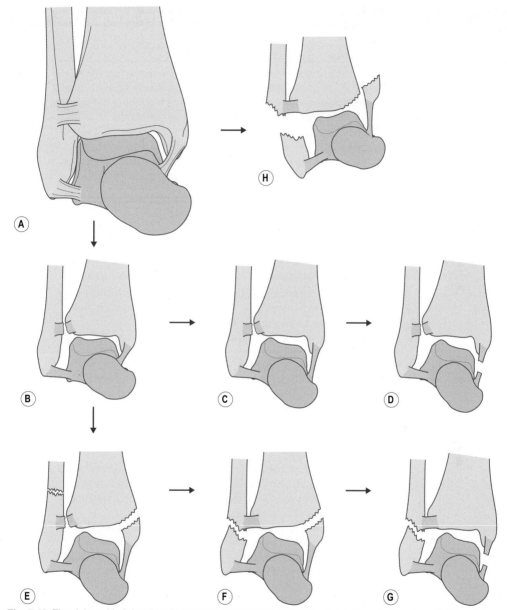

Fig. 7.62 The right ankle joint showing normal stability (A); instability due to ligament rupture (B–D) and combined ligament rupture and malleolar fracture (E–H).

The main muscle involved in dorsiflexing the foot at the ankle joint is tibialis anterior, aided by extensor hallucis longus, extensor digitorum longus and fibularis/peroneus tertius. The main muscles involved in plantarflexing the foot at the ankle joint are gastrocnemius, soleus and plantaris, aided by fibularis/peroneus longus and brevis, tibialis posterior, flexor digitorum longus and flexor hallucis longus. Details of the attachments, action and innervation of the muscles crossing the ankle joint are given in Table 7.3.

TABLE 7.3   The Attachments, Action and Innervation of Muscles Acting at the Ankle Joint

Muscle	Attachments	Action	Innervation (Root Value)
Tibialis anterior	From the upper two-third of the lateral surface of the tibia and adjacent interosseous membrane to the medial side of the medial cuneiform and base of the first metatarsal	Dorsiflexion of the foot at the ankle joint: with tibialis posterior it inverts the foot at the subtalar and midtarsal joints	Deep fibular/ peroneal nerve (L4, L5)
Fibularis/peroneus tertius	From the front of the lower one-fourth of the fibula to the medial and dorsal aspects of the base of the fifth metatarsal	Weak evertor and dorsiflexor of the foot at the ankle joint	Deep fibular/ peroneal nerve (L5, S1)
Extensor hallucis longus (see Table 7.4)			
Extensor digitorum longus (see Table 7.4)			
Gastrocnemius	From the medial supracondylar ridge, adductor tubercle, popliteal surface of the femur (medial head) and outer surface of the lateral femoral condyle (lateral head) to the posterior surface of the calcaneus via the tendocalcaneus (Achilles tendon)	Plantarflexion of the foot at the ankle joint: powerful flexor of the calf/leg at the knee joint	Tibial nerve (S1, S2)
Soleus	From the posterior surfaces of the tibia and upper one-third of the fibula to the posterior surface of the calcaneus via the tendocalcaneus (Achilles tendon)	Plantarflexion of the foot at the ankle joint	Tibial nerve (S1, S2)
Plantaris	From the lateral supracondylar ridge, popliteal surface of the tibia and knee joint capsule to the posterior surface of the calcaneus	Weak plantarflexor of the foot at the ankle joint: weak flexor of the calf/leg at the knee joint	Tibial nerve (S1, S2)
Tibialis posterior	From the upper half of the posterior surface of the tibia below the soleal line, interosseous membrane and posterior surface of the fibula to the medial side of the navicular and plantar surfaces of all tarsal bones	Main evertor of the foot at the subtalar and midtarsal joints; aids plantarflexion of the foot at the ankle joint	Tibial nerve (L4, L5)
Flexor hallucis longus (see Table 7.4)			
Flexor digitorum longus (see Table 7.4)			
Fibularis/peroneus longus (see Table 7.4)			
Fibularis/peroneus brevis (see Table 7.4)			

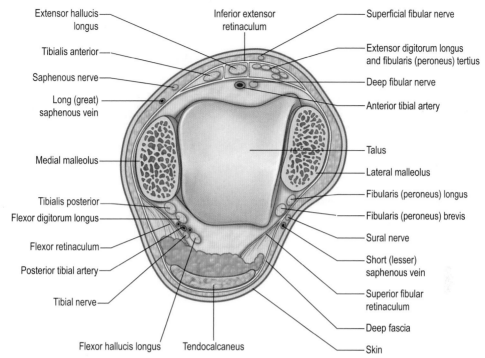

Extensor hallucis longus
Inferior extensor retinaculum
Superficial fibular nerve
Tibialis anterior
Extensor digitorum longus and fibularis (peroneus) tertius
Saphenous nerve
Deep fibular nerve
Long (great) saphenous vein
Anterior tibial artery
Talus
Medial malleolus
Lateral malleolus
Tibialis posterior
Fibularis (peroneus) longus
Flexor digitorum longus
Fibularis (peroneus) brevis
Flexor retinaculum
Sural nerve
Posterior tibial artery
Short (lesser) saphenous vein
Tibial nerve
Superior fibular retinaculum
Deep fascia
Flexor hallucis longus
Tendocalcaneus
Skin

Fig. 7.63 Transverse section through the right ankle showing the relationship of structures crossing the joint.

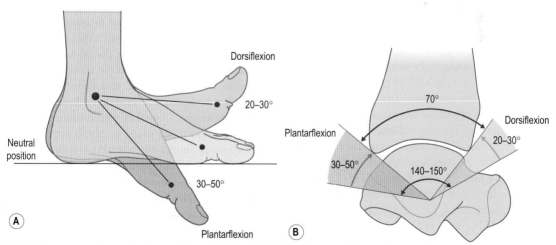

Fig. 7.64 (A) The ranges of dorsiflexion and plantarflexion; (B) tibial and talar articular surface profiles.

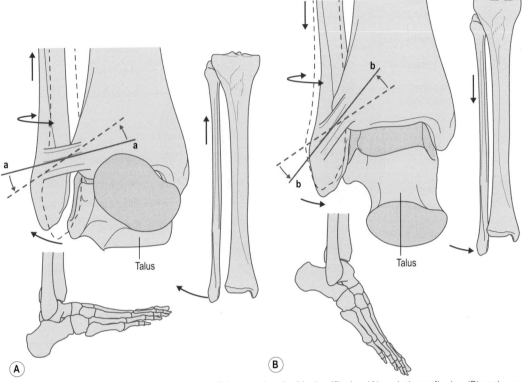

Fig. 7.65 Movements of the fibula with respect to the tibia associated with dorsiflexion (A) and plantarflexion (B) at the ankle joint.

FOOT

The foot is strong enough to support body weight but is also flexible and sufficiently resilient to absorb the shocks transmitted to it, as well as provide spring and lift during locomotor activities. These properties are achieved by a series of arches, convex above, formed by the bones of the foot (tarsus, metatarsals, phalanges); the medial longitudinal arch has a greater curvature and is more elastic than the lateral, which is flatter and more rigid providing a firm base for support (Fig. 7.66). The medial longitudinal arch comprises (from posterior to anterior) calcaneus, talus, navicular, the medial, intermediate and lateral cuneiforms, and the first, second and third metatarsals, their phalanges and intervening joints (Fig. 7.66D); the lateral longitudinal arch comprises (from posterior to anterior) calcaneus, cuboid, fourth and fifth metatarsals, their phalanges and intervening joints (Fig. 7.66C). The transverse arch is the result of the shape of the distal row of tarsal bones (medial, intermediate and lateral cuneiforms) and the metatarsal bases, which are broader dorsally, articulating in a domed arch. Maintenance of the arches depends on the integrity of the intertarsal and tarsometatarsal joints, supported by ligaments (especially those on the plantar aspect of the foot), together with muscle action, storing energy as they yield when weight is applied, recoiling and releasing energy when weight is removed.

The deep fascia of the foot is continuous with that of the calf/leg, being thin on the dorsum wrapping around either side of the foot becoming continuous with the plantar aponeurosis: anteriorly it splits covering the dorsum of the toes.

APPLIED ANATOMY: With the toes dorsiflexed, the slips of the aponeurosis wind around the metatarsal heads raising the longitudinal arches.

Tarsus

The arrangement of the tarsus is shown in Fig. 7.66, from which it can be seen that the calcaneus is the largest with the talus situated on top of it. The articulations between the tarsus (intertarsal joints), between the distal tarsus and metatarsals (tarsometatarsal joints) and between the metatarsals and phalanges (metatarsophalangeal (MTP) joints) are shown in Fig. 7.66C and D.

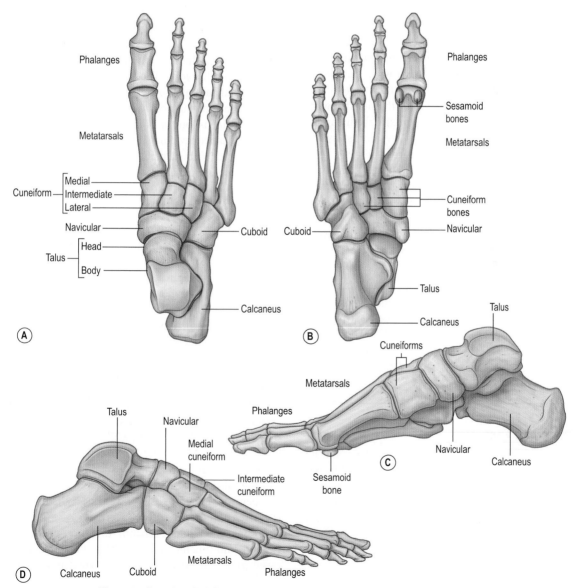

Fig. 7.66 Superior (A); inferior (B); medial (C) and lateral (D) aspects of the right foot.

Metatarsals and Phalanges

> **DEVELOPMENT:** A primary centre appears in the shaft of each metatarsal at 9 weeks *in utero*, with secondary centres appearing in the base of the first and heads of the remaining metatarsals during the second and third years; fusion of the epiphyses and shaft occurs between ages 15 and 18. Primary centres for the proximal and distal phalanges appear in the shafts during the fourth month *in utero*, and for the middle phalanx between 6 months *in utero* and birth. Secondary centres appear in the bases of all phalanges during the second and third years, fusing with the shaft between ages 15 and 20.

There are five metatarsals in each foot, with each having a proximal base, shaft and distal head: the bases articulate with the tarsal bones (first with the medial cuneiform, second with the intermediate cuneiform, third with the lateral cuneiform, fourth and fifth with the cuboid) and heads with the proximal phalanges of the toes (Fig. 7.66). The shafts are almost cylindrical narrowing as they pass towards the head. The first metatarsal is the stoutest and shortest, the second the longest, while the fifth has a large tubercle projecting posterolaterally from its base (Fig. 7.66B and C).

There are two phalanges in the great toe and three in each of the others; each has a shaft and proximal (base) and distal ends.

> **APPLIED ANATOMY:** Midway along the lateral border of the foot, the base of the fifth metatarsal and its prominent tubercle can be felt; the shafts and heads of the metatarsals can be felt on the dorsum of the foot, with the bases proximal and heads distal. With the toes extended the metatarsal heads, especially the first, can be felt under the forefoot.

Joints of the Foot

Within the foot the most important joints between the tarsus are the subtalar (calcaneus, talus) and midtarsal (talus, calcaneus and navicular medially; calcaneus and cuboid laterally) joints, with those between the distal tarsus and metatarsals (tarsometatarsal joints) and metatarsals and phalanges (MTP joints) also contributing to the mobility of the foot. Each joint is supported by dorsal and strong plantar ligaments (Fig. 7.67).

Subtalar Joint

Synovial joint between the concave inferior surface of the body of the talus and the convex superior surface of the calcaneus (Fig. 7.68); a thin loose fibrous capsule surrounds the joint being thickened posteriorly, medially and laterally by ligaments. Joint stability is maintained by the strong interosseous talocalcanean ligament lying directly below the long axis of the calf/leg. It acts as a fulcrum around which movements of the calf/leg and foot occur; it is continually subjected to twisting and stretching.

Transverse (Mid) Tarsal Joint

The combined medial talocalcaneonavicular and lateral calcaneocuboid joints (Fig. 7.69); although the joints do not communicate, they provide a distinctive movement pattern, which is an important contribution to the action of the foot. The talocalcaneonavicular joint is a synovial ball-and-socket joint between the head and lower surface of the neck of the talus, anterior surface of the calcaneus, posterior surface of the navicular and plantar calcaneonavicular ligament (Fig. 7.68). The calcaneocuboid joint is a plane synovial joint, even though its articular surfaces are reciprocally concavoconvex.

Movements at the Subtalar and Transverse (Mid) Tarsal Joints

In dorsiflexion and plantarflexion at the ankle joint, the talus moves within the tibiofibular mortise with the foot moving as a single unit; however, in other movements of the foot the calcaneus and navicular move on the talus, carrying with them the distal tarsal bones and metatarsals. Adduction and abduction of the foot occur about the long axis of the calf/leg at the subtalar joint, with supination and pronation occurring about the long axis of the foot mainly at the transverse tarsal joint (Fig. 7.70).

Inversion and eversion. The combined movements at the subtalar and midtarsal joints produce inversion and eversion of the foot, enabling it to be placed firmly on slanting or irregular surfaces, while still providing a firm base of support. Most inversion/eversion movements are carried out with the foot firmly anchored to the ground and the calf/leg and body inverting and everting above it; when walking across sloping surfaces the upper foot is everted and the lower foot inverted.

In inversion and eversion, the foot undergoes a twisting movement, mainly at the subtalar and midtarsal joints: inversion is the combined movement of

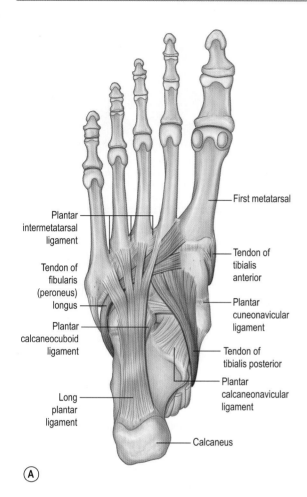

Plantar intermetatarsal ligament

First metatarsal

Tendon of fibularis (peroneus) longus

Tendon of tibialis anterior

Plantar cuneonavicular ligament

Plantar calcaneocuboid ligament

Tendon of tibialis posterior

Plantar calcaneonavicular ligament

Long plantar ligament

Calcaneus

(A)

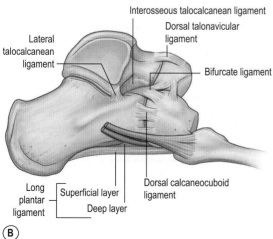

Interosseous talocalcanean ligament

Dorsal talonavicular ligament

Lateral talocalcanean ligament

Bifurcate ligament

Long plantar ligament
— Superficial layer
— Deep layer

Dorsal calcaneocuboid ligament

(B)

Fig. 7.67 Ligaments associated with the plantar (A) and lateral (B) aspects of the right foot.

adduction at the subtalar joint and supination at the midtarsal joint; eversion is the combined movement of abduction at the subtalar joint and pronation at the midtarsal joint. The combined movements in inversion and eversion cannot occur independently as the talus is part of both joints; inversion is often accompanied by plantarflexion at the ankle joint, and eversion by dorsiflexion. In inversion, the medial border of the foot is raised and the lateral border depressed turning the sole to face medially (Fig. 7.71B), while in eversion the lateral border of the foot is raised and the medial border depressed turning the sole to face laterally (Fig. 7.71A).

Inversion is produced by tibialis anterior and posterior, occasionally assisted by flexor and extensor hallucis longus, while eversion is produced by fibularis/peroneus longus, brevis and tertius. Details of the muscle producing inversion and eversion can be found in Table 7.4.

Tarsometatarsal Joints

Plane synovial joints between the distal tarsus (medial/intermediate/lateral cuneiforms, cuboid) and the metatarsal bases. The base of the second metatarsal is held in a mortise formed by the cuneiforms (Fig. 7.72). The surrounding joint capsules are reinforced by interosseous, plantar and dorsal ligaments (Fig. 7.72).

Movements

The joint line runs obliquely from medial, superior and anterior to lateral, inferior and posterior (Fig. 7.73A). Slight plantarflexion (flexion) and dorsiflexion (extension) are possible, with plantarflexion being accompanied by adduction of the metatarsals so that they move towards the long axis of the foot increasing the curvature of the transverse arch (Fig. 7.73B); the arch flattens in dorsiflexion as the metatarsals move away from the long axis of the foot.

> **APPLIED ANATOMY:** Immobility of the second metatarsal contributes to its 'spontaneous' fracture (March fracture), e.g., walking for long periods over hard surfaces.

Metatarsophalangeal Joints

Synovial condyloid joints between the rounded metatarsal heads and bases of the proximal phalanges. The loose joint capsule is reinforced by strong collateral ligaments, the plantar ligament on its plantar surface (Fig. 7.74A) and dorsally by fibres from the extensor tendons.

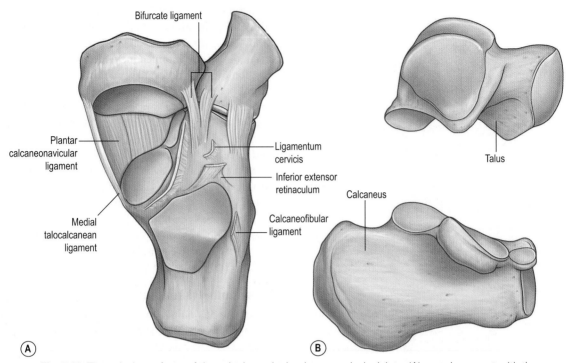

Fig. 7.68 The articular surfaces of the subtalar and talocalcaneonavicular joints: (A) superior aspect with the talus removed; (B) the bones separated.

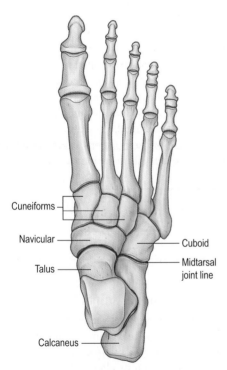

Fig. 7.69 The midtarsal joint.

The deep transverse metatarsal ligament connects the heads and joint capsules of all metatarsals (Fig. 7.74B).

> **APPLIED ANATOMY:** With the metatarsal joints plantarflexed the metatarsal heads can be felt on the dorsum of the foot.

Movements

The joints permit dorsiflexion, plantarflexion, abduction, adduction and circumduction. In dorsiflexion, the proximal phalanx is carried beyond the line of the metatarsal (Fig. 7.75), with the toes tending to spread apart and become slightly inclined laterally; dorsiflexion is carried out by the extensors. Plantarflexion is by the flexors passing into the toes (Fig. 7.75), with the toes tending to be pulled together. The total range of movement for the great toe (hallux) is 110 degrees, the majority of which is dorsiflexion: the remaining toes have a total range of between 80 degrees medially and 40 degrees laterally.

Because of the immobility of the second metatarsal and the arrangement of the interosseous muscles abduction and adduction occur with respect to the second

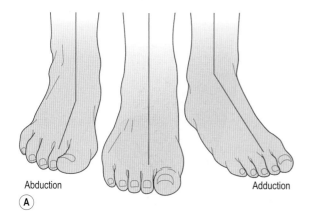

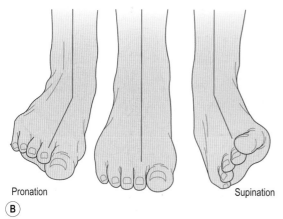

Fig. 7.70 (A) Adduction and abduction of the foot about the long axis of the calf/leg; (B) supination and pronation of the foot about the long axis of the foot.

toe. Abduction is produced by the dorsal interossei and abductors hallucis and digiti minimi, and adduction by the plantar interossei and adductor hallucis. Details of the intrinsic muscles of the foot producing movements of the toes can be found in Table 7.5.

Interphalangeal Joints

Synovial hinge joints between the head of the proximal phalanx and base of the succeeding phalanx. A loose fibrous capsule surrounds each joint strengthened laterally by collateral ligaments and partly replaced dorsally by the extensor tendon and on the plantar aspect by the plantar ligament.

> **APPLIED ANATOMY:** The distal interphalangeal (DIP) joint of the fifth (little) toe is often obliterated.

Movements

Due to the shape of the articular surfaces, only dorsiflexion and plantarflexion are possible: the range of movement for the hallux is 70 degrees dorsiflexion and 45 degrees plantarflexion; for the lesser toes the proximal interphalangeal (PIP) joints permit 50 degrees of dorsiflexion and 35 degrees of plantarflexion. Dorsiflexion away from the sole of the foot is produced by the extensor muscles, as well as the lumbricals and interossei; plantarflexion towards the sole of the foot by flexors digitorum longus and brevis (Table 7.4) at the distal and PIP joints, respectively.

Dorsum of the Foot

The tendons of muscles in the anterior compartment of the calf/leg enter the dorsum of the foot deep to the inferior extensor retinaculum (Fig. 7.59A), together with the deep fibular/peroneal nerve and dorsalis pedis artery. In the superficial fascia in front of the medial malleolus are the long (great) saphenous vein, arising from the medial end of the dorsal venous arch, and the saphenous nerve (Fig. 7.63).

Deep fibular/peroneal nerve. It enters the foot deep to the inferior extensor retinaculum and divides into medial and lateral branches. The medial branch supplies skin in the cleft between the first and second toes (Fig. 7.56) and the lateral branch supplies extensors digitorum and hallucis brevis.

Superficial fibular/peroneal nerve. After running in the superficial fascia over the anterior compartment of the calf/leg it enters the dorsum of the foot superficial to the extensor retinaculae supplying skin on the dorsum (Fig. 7.56).

Dorsalis pedis artery. The dorsalis pedis artery begins as the anterior tibial artery crosses the ankle joint, lying initially between the tendons of tibialis anterior and extensor hallucis longus, then passes deep to the tendon of extensor hallucis to lie on its lateral side (Fig. 7.55).

> **APPLIED ANATOMY:** The dorsalis pedis pulse can be felt on the dorsum of the foot distal to the ankle joint on the lateral side of the tendon of extensor hallucis longus.

Dorsal venous network. The superficial veins form a network on the dorsum of the foot, receiving venous

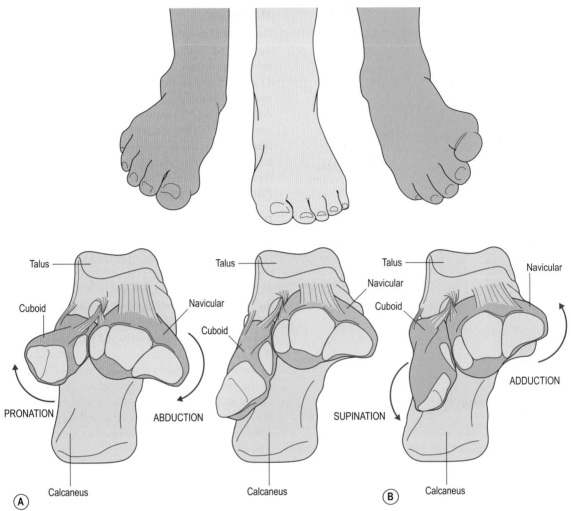

Fig. 7.71 Schematic representation of the right foot showing the changing relationship between the talus, calcaneus, cuboid and navicular during eversion (A) and inversion (B).

TABLE 7.4   Muscles of the Calf/Leg Whose Action Is on the Foot: Attachments, Action and Innervation

Muscle	Attachments	Action	Innervation (Root Value)
Extensor hallucis longus	From the middle half of the anterior surface of the fibula and adjacent interosseous membrane to the base of the distal phalanx of the first (great) toe	Extends all joints of the first (great) toe; it is also a powerful dorsi-flexor of the foot at the ankle joint	Deep fibular/ peroneal nerve (L5, S1)
Extensor digitorum longus	From the lateral condyle of the tibia, anterior surface of the fibula and upper part of the interosseous membrane, dividing into four tendons at the level of the ankle joint, to the base of the middle phalanx of each toe	Extends the metatarsophalangeal joints of the lateral four toes and assists extension at the interpha-langeal joints: it also aids dorsiflex-ion of the foot at the ankle joint	Deep fibular/ peroneal nerve (L5, S1)

TABLE 7.4 Muscles of the Calf/Leg Whose Action is on the Foot: Attachments, Action and Innervation (cont'd)

Muscle	Attachments	Action	Innervation (Root Value)
Flexor hallucis longus	From the lower two-third of the posterior surface of the fibula to the base of the distal phalanx of the first (great) toe	Flexes all joints of the great toe; it also aids plantarflexion of the foot at the ankle joint	Tibial nerve (S1, S2)
Flexor digitorum longus	From the posterior surface of the tibia, dividing into four tendons in the sole of the foot, to the base of the distal phalanx of the lateral four toes	Flexes all joints of the lateral four toes; it also aids plantarflexion of the foot at the ankle joint: with the ankle plantarflexed its action on the toes is diminished	Tibial nerve (L5, S1, S2)
Fibularis/peroneus longus	From the lateral tibial condyle and upper two-third of the lateral surface of the fibula to the plantar and lateral surfaces of the medial cuneiform and base of the first metatarsal	Everts the foot at the subtalar and midtarsal joints; it also aids plantarflexion of the foot at the ankle joint	Superficial fibular/peroneal nerve (L5, S1)
Fibularis/peroneus brevis	From the lower two-third of the lateral surface of the fibula to the tubercle and lateral side of the fifth metatarsal	Everts the foot at the subtalar and midtarsal joints; it also contributes to plantarflexion of the foot at the ankle joint	Superficial fibular/peroneal nerve (L5, S1)

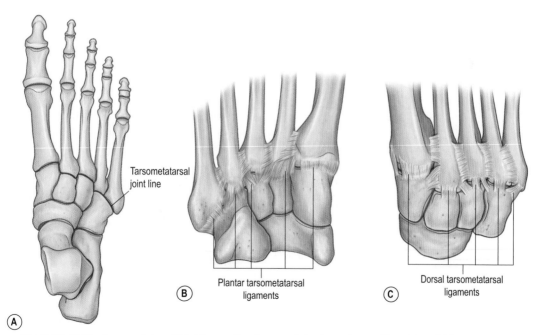

Fig. 7.72 (A) The tarsometatarsal joint line on the dorsum of the foot; plantar (B) and dorsal (C) tarsometatarsal ligaments.

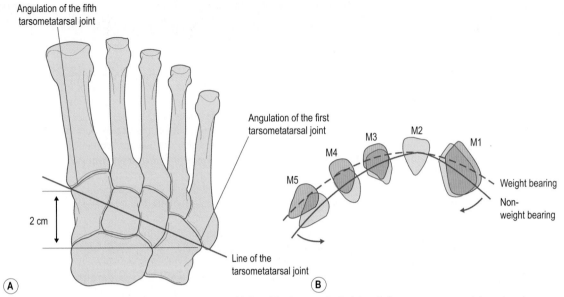

Fig. 7.73 (A) The line of the tarsometatarsal joint; (B) changes in height of the transverse metatarsal arch with weight bearing.

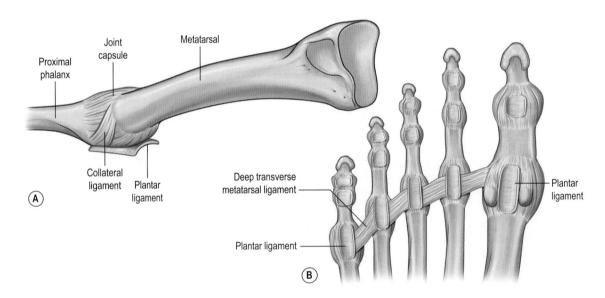

Fig. 7.74 (A) The collateral and plantar ligaments of the metatarsophalangeal joints; (B) the deep transverse metatarsal ligament.

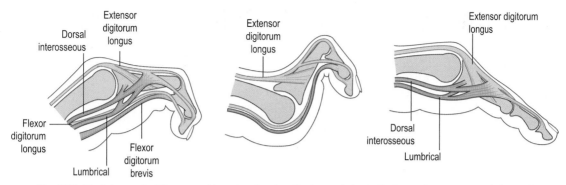

Fig. 7.75 Medial aspect of the second toe showing dorsiflexion and plantarflexion at the metatarsophalangeal and interphalangeal joints.

TABLE 7.5 Intrinsic Muscles of the Foot: Attachments, Action and Innervation

Muscle	Attachments	Action	Innervation (Root Value)
Extensor digitorum brevis	From the upper surface of the calcaneus to the extensor expansion of the second, third and fourth toes	Aids extensor digitorum longus dorsiflex the second, third and fourth toes at the metatarsophalangeal joints: it also helps the lumbricals dorsiflex the interphalangeal joints	Deep fibular/peroneal nerve (L5, S1)
Extensor hallucis brevis	From the upper surface of the calcaneus to the base of the proximal phalanx of the toe	Aids extensor hallucis longus dorsiflex the toe at the metatarsophalangeal joint	Deep fibular/peroneal nerve (L5, S1)
Lumbricals	From the medial sides of the tendons of flexor digitorum longus to the medial side of the extensor hood and base of the proximal phalanx of the same toe	Plantarflexion the toes at the metatarsophalangeal joints and dorsiflexion of the interphalangeal joints	First (medial) medial plantar nerve (S1, S2); second, third, fourth (lateral 3) lateral plantar nerve (S2, S3)
Flexor accessorius (quadratus plantae)	From the calcaneus and long plantar ligament to the tendon of flexor digitorum longus proximal to the attachment of the lumbricals	Aids the long flexor tendons plantarflex all joints of the lateral four toes: it is important during walking when flexor digitorum longus is already shortened	Lateral plantar nerve (S2, S3)
Flexor digitorum brevis	From the calcaneus and plantar aponeurosis the muscles splits into separate tendons to the lateral four toes	Plantarflexion of the proximal interphalangeal joints followed by plantarflexion of the metatarsophalangeal joints	Medial plantar nerve (S1, S2)
Flexor hallucis brevis	From the cuboid, lateral cuneiform and tendon of tibialis posterior to the base of the proximal phalanx of the first toe	Plantarflexion of the metatarsophalangeal joint of the first toe	Medial plantar nerve (S1, S2)
Flexor digiti minimi brevis	From the plantar surface of the base of the fifth metatarsal to the plantar surface of the proximal phalanx of the fifth toe	Plantarflexion of the metatarsophalangeal joint of the fifth toe: also helps support the lateral longitudinal arch of the foot	Lateral plantar nerve (S2, S3)

Continued

TABLE 7.5 Intrinsic Muscles of the Foot: Attachments, Action and Innervation (cont'd)

Muscle	Attachments	Action	Innervation (Root Value)
Abductor hallucis	From the plantar aspect of the calcaneus to the medial side of the base of the proximal phalanx	Abduction and helps plantarflexion of the first toe at the metatarsophalangeal joint	Medial plantar nerve (S1, S2)
Abductor digiti minimi	From the calcaneus to the base of the proximal phalanx of the fifth toe	Abduction and helps plantarflexion of the fifth toe at the metatarsophalangeal joint	Lateral plantar nerve (S2, S3)
Adductor hallucis	From the bases of the second, third and fourth metatarsals (*oblique head*) and plantar surfaces of the lateral three metatarsophalangeal joints (*transverse head*) to the lateral side of the base of the proximal phalanx of the first toe	Adduction of the first toe towards the second toe and plantarflexion of the first metatarsophalangeal joint	Lateral plantar nerve (S2, S3)
Dorsal interossei	From the sides of adjacent metatarsal to the side of the proximal phalanx of and capsule of the metatarsophalangeal joint	Abduction of the toes at the metatarsophalangeal joint: with the plantar interossei they plantarflex the metatarsophalangeal joint	Lateral plantar nerve (S2, S3)
Plantar interossei	From the medial side of the base of the metatarsal to the medial side of the base of the proximal phalanx	Adduction of the third, fourth and fifth towards the second: with the dorsal interossei they plantarflex the metatarsophalangeal joint of the lateral three toes	Lateral plantar nerve (S2, S3)

blood from the toes, either side of the foot and deep plantar areas via perforating veins. It is drained by medial and lateral marginal veins, which become the long (great) and short (small) saphenous veins, respectively (Fig. 7.27).

Plantar Aspect (Sole) of the Foot

The tendons of muscles in the posterior and lateral compartments of the calf/leg pass behind the medial and lateral malleoli to enter the sole of the foot (Fig. 7.59B), respectively. Also passing behind the medial malleolus are the tibial nerve and posterior tibial artery, both of which divide into medial and lateral branches as they do so. Once in the foot, the medial and lateral branches lie deep to the plantar aponeurosis, as do the intrinsic muscles of the foot. Behind the lateral malleolus are the tendons of fibularis/peroneus longus and brevis, while in the superficial fascia are the short (small) saphenous vein and sural nerve (Fig. 7.63).

Plantar aponeurosis. The triangular plantar aponeurosis is continuous with the dorsal fascia at the sides of the foot and the fascia over the heel, from where it spreads out anteriorly into five slips, which pass forwards to become continuous with the fibrous flexor sheaths of the toes.

> **APPLIED ANATOMY:** The plantar aponeurosis is important in maintaining the longitudinal arches of the foot.

Fibro-osseous tunnels. Continuous with the slips of the plantar aponeurosis, each tunnel runs under the toe and contains the flexor tendons, with arching fibres passing over the tendons: at the interphalangeal joints the fibres criss-cross from the head of one phalanx to the base of the adjacent phalanx. Each tunnel is lined with a double layer of synovial membrane facilitating movement of the tendons in the tunnel.

Medial and lateral plantar nerves. Terminal branches of the tibial nerve as it passes behind the medial malleolus in the tarsal tunnel (Fig. 7.58) between the medial malleolus and flexor retinaculum. The medial plantar nerve supplies abductor hallucis, flexor digitorum brevis, flexor hallucis brevis and the first lumbrical; the lateral plantar nerve supplies flexor accessorius (quadratus plantae), flexor digiti minimi brevis, abductor digiti minimi, adductor hallucis, the lateral three lumbricals and the dorsal and plantar interossei.

Medial and lateral plantar arteries. Terminal branches of the posterior tibial artery as it passes behind the medial malleolus in the tarsal tunnel. The larger lateral artery passes medially across the foot on the metatarsals as the plantar arch (Fig. 7.76).

> **APPLIED ANATOMY:** The posterior tibial pulse can be felt as the artery passes behind the medial malleolus. Occasionally two pulses may be detected, these being those of the medial and lateral plantar arteries.

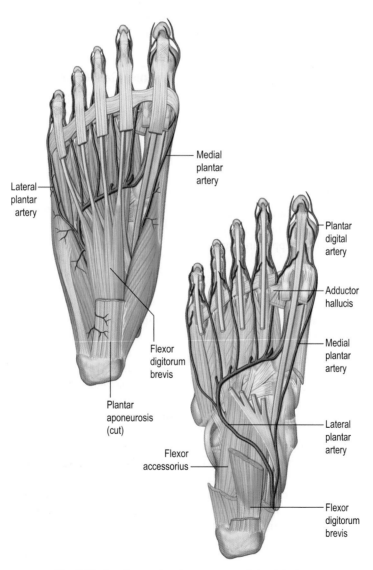

Fig. 7.76 Arteries on the plantar aspect of the right foot.

CLINICAL ANATOMY: In tarsal tunnel syndrome, individuals complain of numbness in the foot radiating to the medial three toes, pain, burning, electrical sensations, and tingling over the base of the foot and heel; depending on the area of entrapment, other areas can be affected. If the entrapment is proximal, the entire foot can be affected as branches of the tibial nerve become involved; ankle pain may also be present. Inflammation or swelling can occur within the tunnel as the flexor retinaculum has limited ability to stretch. Increased pressure can cause compression on the nerve within the tunnel, with an associated reduction in blood flow; the nerves respond with altered sensations (tingling, numbness). Fluid collects in the foot when standing and walking, making the condition worse. As the intrinsic muscles of the foot lose their nerve supply, they give rise to a cramping feeling.

Function of the Foot

The ankle and foot provide propulsion and restraint at each step so that equilibrium is maintained while the body is in motion. The ankle, subtalar and transverse (mid) tarsal joints, assisted by axial rotation at the knee, allowing the foot to take up any position in space and adapt to any irregularities in the supporting surface during walking.

APPLIED ANATOMY: The ankle, subtalar and transverse (mid) tarsal joints provide a high degree of stability without sacrificing mobility.

Walking

This involves the whole body, with changes in the pattern of movement of the upper body affecting the walking pattern. Each lower limb performs a cycle of similar events performed half a cycle out of phase with each other; the left limb will be weight bearing while the right is off the ground. As the toes of one limb push off, the heel of the other limb is making contact with the ground, and as one limb is moving forwards the other is drawn backwards. There are several determinates which influence the pattern of walking, these aim to improve the efficiency of walking by reducing energy expenditure. This is best visualised as reducing the motion of the body's centre of gravity (Fig. 7.77).

The main determinates which minimise motion of the centre of gravity are pelvic rotation in a transverse plane reducing the drop in its height; knee flexion in the supporting limb reducing the rise in its height; hip adduction moves the knees towards the midline reducing its lateral motion; and hip abduction (pelvic tilting) in the swinging limb reduces the rise in its height (Fig. 7.77).

Walking (Gait) Cycle

Numerous techniques (temporospatial, kinematic, kinetic, plantar pressure measurement, electromyography) are available for recording and analysing gait; however, these are outside the scope of this text. Parameters taken into account in gait analysis include step length, stride length, walking base, toe out angle (foot angle), speed, cadence (number of steps/strides per minute) and line of progression (Fig. 7.78).

When assessing temporal parameters the stance, swing and double support phases of the gait cycle (Fig. 7.79) can help to determine whether a gait pattern is considered 'normal' or pathological.

Normal gait can be permanent or transient, being modified or modulated by many factors: extrinsic (terrain, footwear, clothing, load carried); intrinsic (sex, weight, height, age); physical (physique); psychological (personality type, emotion); physiological (anthropometric characteristics) and pathology (trauma, neurological disease, musculoskeletal anomalies, psychiatric disorders).

CLINICAL ANATOMY: Pathological gait may reflect compensations for underlying pathologies or be the cause of the symptoms. It can enable diagnosis (cerebral palsy, stroke) and intervention strategies (physiotherapy, surgery) to be made and assessed.

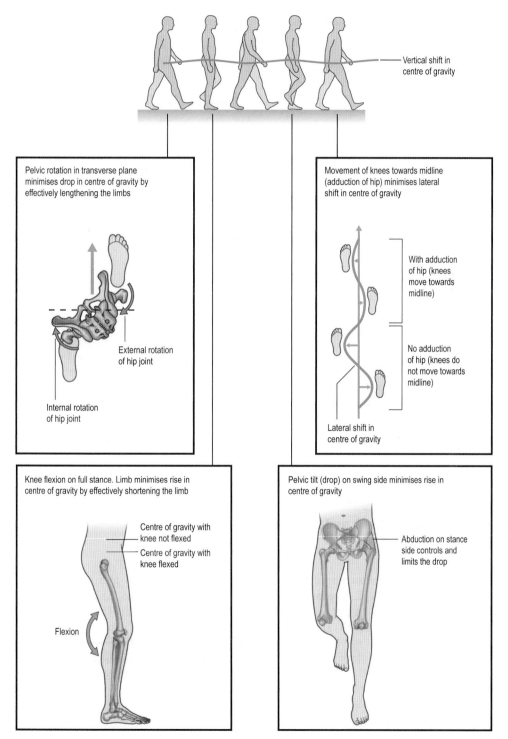

Vertical shift in centre of gravity

Pelvic rotation in transverse plane minimises drop in centre of gravity by effectively lengthening the limbs

External rotation of hip joint

Internal rotation of hip joint

Movement of knees towards midline (adduction of hip) minimises lateral shift in centre of gravity

With adduction of hip (knees move towards midline)

No adduction of hip (knees do not move towards midline)

Lateral shift in centre of gravity

Knee flexion on full stance. Limb minimises rise in centre of gravity by effectively shortening the limb

Centre of gravity with knee not flexed

Centre of gravity with knee flexed

Flexion

Pelvic tilt (drop) on swing side minimises rise in centre of gravity

Abduction on stance side controls and limits the drop

Fig. 7.77 Determinates of gait (walking).

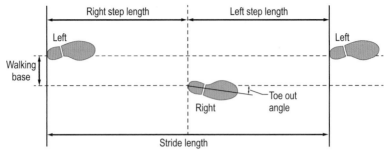

Fig. 7.78 Spatial parameters in gait analysis.

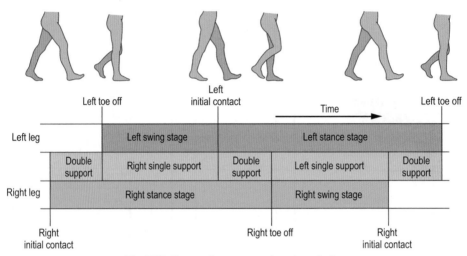

Fig. 7.79 Temporal parameters in gait analysis.

SUMMARY OF NERVES AND MUSCLES

Major Nerves of the Lower Limb and the Muscles They Innervate

Femoral Nerve

From the lumbar plexus (L2, L3, L4): it supplies iliacus (L2, L3), sartorius (L2, L3), pectineus (L2, L3), rectus femoris (L2, L3, L4), vastus medialis (L2, L3, L4), vastus intermedius (L2, L3, L4), vastus lateralis (L2, L3, L4) and gives the anterior medial and lateral cutaneous nerves of the thigh and the saphenous nerve (Figs. 7.11 and 7.80).

Obturator Nerve

From the lumbar plexus (L2, L3, L4): it supplies adductor longus (L2, L3, L4), adductor brevis (L2, L3, L4), adductor magnus (L2, L3), gracilis (L2, L3), obturator

externus (L3, L4), occasionally pectineus (L2, L3) and is sensory to skin on the medial side of the thigh (Figs. 7.11 and 7.80).

Superior Gluteal Nerve

From the lumbosacral plexus (L4, L5, S1): it supplies gluteus medius (L4, L5, S1), gluteus minimus (L4, L5, S1) and tensor fascia lata (L4, L5).

Inferior Gluteal Nerve

From the lumbosacral plexus (L5, S1, S2): it supplies gluteus maximus (L5, S1, S2).

Sciatic Nerve

From the lumbosacral plexus (L4, L5, S1, S2, S3): it supplies semitendinosus (L5, S1, S2), semimembranosus

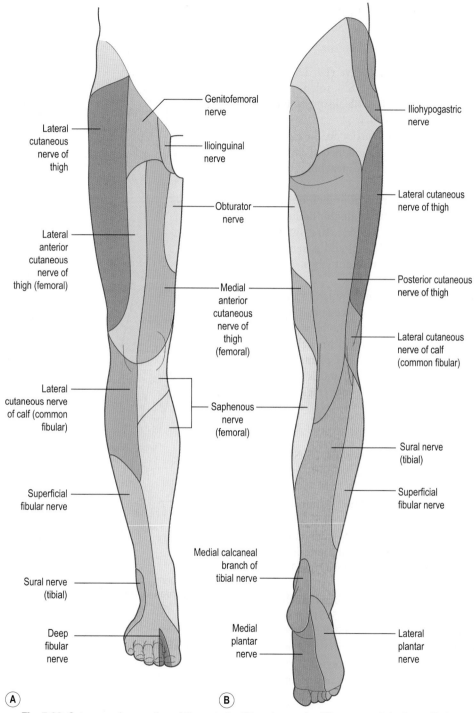

Lateral
cutaneous
nerve of
thigh

Lateral
anterior
cutaneous
nerve of
thigh (femoral)

Lateral
cutaneous nerve
of calf (common
fibular)

Superficial
fibular nerve

Sural nerve
(tibial)

Deep
fibular
nerve

Genitofemoral
nerve

Ilioinguinal
nerve

Obturator
nerve

Medial
anterior
cutaneous
nerve of
thigh
(femoral)

Saphenous
nerve
(femoral)

Medial calcaneal
branch of
tibial nerve

Medial
plantar
nerve

Iliohypogastric
nerve

Lateral cutaneous
nerve of thigh

Posterior cutaneous
nerve of thigh

Lateral cutaneous
nerve of calf
(common fibular)

Sural nerve
(tibial)

Superficial
fibular nerve

Lateral
plantar
nerve

(A)   (B)

Fig. 7.80 Cutaneous innervation of the anterior (A) and posterior (B) aspects of the lower limb.

(L5, S1, S2), biceps femoris (L5, S1, S2) and the hamstring part of adductor magnus (L4).

Tibial Nerve

Terminal branch of the sciatic nerve (L4, L5, S1, S2, S3): it supplies gastrocnemius (S1, S2), soleus (S1, S2), plantaris (S1, S2), popliteus (L5), tibialis posterior (L4, L5), flexor digitorum longus (L5, S1, S2), flexor hallucis longus (S1, S2) and is sensory to the posterior aspect of the thigh (sural nerve) and medial and posterior aspects of the heel (medial calcaneal branch) (Figs. 7.57 and 7.80).

Medial plantar nerve. Terminal branch of the tibial nerve (S1, S2, S3): it supplies abductor hallucis (S1, S2), flexor digitorum brevis (S2, S3), first lumbrical (S1), flexor hallucis brevis (S1, S2) and is sensory to the medial side of the sole of the foot (Figs. 7.57 and 7.80).

Lateral plantar nerve. Terminal branch of the tibial nerve (S1, S2, S3): it supplies flexor accessorius (quadratus plantae) (S2, S3), flexor digiti minimi brevis (S2, S3), abductor digiti minimi (S2, S3), adductor hallucis (S1, S2), lateral three lumbricals (S1, S2, S3), plantar interossei (S2, S3), dorsal interossei (S2, S3) and is sensory to the lateral aspect of the sole of the foot (Figs. 7.57 and Fig. 7.80).

Common Fibular/Peroneal Nerve

Terminal branch of the sciatic nerve (L4, L5, S1, S2): it gives the lateral cutaneous nerve of the calf/leg (see Fig. 7.80, see also Fig. 7.56).

Superficial fibular/peroneal nerve. Terminal branch of the common fibular/peroneal nerve (L5, S1): it supplies fibularis/peroneus longus (L5, S1), fibularis/peroneus brevis (L5, S1) and is sensory to the anterior aspect of the calf/leg and dorsum of the foot (Figs. 7.56 and 7.80).

Deep fibular/peroneal nerve. Terminal branch of the common fibular/peroneal nerve (L4, L5, S1): it supplies extensor digitorum longus (L5, S1), tibialis anterior (L4, L5), extensor hallucis longus (L5, S1), fibularis/peroneus tertius (L5, S1), extensor digitorum brevis (L5, S1) and is sensory to the cleft between the first and second toes (Figs. 7.56 and 7.80).

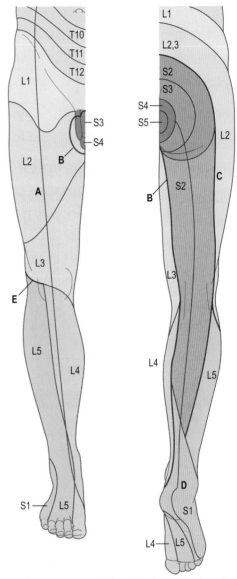

Fig. 7.81 Dermatomes of the right lower limb and foot: A, preaxial border; B, ventral (anterior) axial line; C, dorsal (posterior) axial line; D, postaxial border; E, extension from dorsal axial line.

While the sensory supply to the skin of the lower limb by named nerves is shown in Fig. 7.80, the innervation of the anterior and posterior aspects of the lower limb by individual nerve roots (dermatomes) is shown in Fig. 7.81.

Muscles of the Lower Limb Supplied by Each Nerve Root

Root value							
L1	L2	L3	L4	L5	S1	S2	S3
	Psoas	major					
	Iliacus						
	Sartorius						
	Pectineus						
	Rectus	femoris					
	Vastus	medialis					
	Vastus	intermedius					
	Vastus	lateralis					
	Adductor	longus					
	Adductor	brevis					
	Adductor	magnus					
		Obturator	externus				
			Tensor	fascia lata			
			Tibialis	anterior			
			Tibialis	posterior			
			Quadratus	femoris			
			Inferior	gemellus			
			Gluteus	minimus			
			Gluteus	medius			
				Popliteus			
				Fibularis/	peroneus longus		
				Fibularis/	peroneus brevis		
				Extensor	digitorum longus		
				Extensor	hallucis longus		
				Extensor	digitorum brevis		
				Fibularis/	peroneus longus		
				Fibularis/	peroneus tertius		
				Gluteus	maximus		
				Semi	membranosus		
				Semi	tendinosus		
				Biceps	femoris		
				Flexor	digitorum longus		
				Obturator	internus		
					Piriformis		
				Superior	gemellus		
					Gastrocnemius		
					Soleus		
					Plantaris		

Root value							
L1	L2	L3	L4	L5	S1	S2	S3
					Flexor hallucis longus		
					Flexor hallucis brevis		
					Abductor hallucis		
					Adductor hallucis		
					Lumbricals		
						Flexor digitorum brevis	
						Flexor accessorius	
						Flexor digiti minimi brevis	
						Abductor digiti minimi	
						Plantar interossei	
						Dorsal interossei	

Movements in Each Region of the Lower Limb, the Muscles Responsible and Their Innervation

Hip Joint

Movement	Muscles (Root Value of Innervation)
Flexion	Psoas major (L1, L2, L3)
	Iliacus (L2, L3)
	Pectineus (L2, L3)
	Rectus femoris (L2, L3, L4)
	Sartorius (L2, L3)
Extension	Gluteus maximus (L5, S1, S2)
	Hamstrings:
	Semitendinosus (L5, S1, S2)
	Semimembranosus (L5, S1, S2)
	Biceps femoris (L5, S1, S2)
Abduction	Gluteus maximus (L5, S1, S2)
	Gluteus medius (L4, L5, S1)
	Gluteus minimus (L4, L5, S1)
	Tensor fascia lata (L4, L5)
Adduction	Adductor magnus (L2, L3, L4)
	Adductor longus (L2, L3, L4)
	Adductor brevis (L2, L3, L4)
	Gracilis (L2, L3)
	Pectineus (L2, L3)
Medial rotation	Gluteus medius (L4, L5, S1)

Movement	Muscles (Root Value of Innervation)
	Gluteus minimus (L4, L5, S1)
	Tensor fascia lata (L4, L5)
Lateral rotation	Gluteus maximus (L5, S1, S2)
	Piriformis (L5, S1, S2)
	Obturator internus (L5, S1, S2)
	Obturator externus (L5, S1, S2)
	Superior gemellus (L5, S1, S2)
	Inferior gemellus (L4, L5, S1)
	Quadratus femoris (L4, L5, S1)

Knee Joint

Movement	Muscles (Root Value of Innervation)
Flexion	Hamstrings:
	Semitendinosus (L5, S1, S2)
	Semimembranosus (L5, S1, S2)
	Biceps femoris (L5, S1, S2)
	Gastrocnemius (S1, S2)
	Gracilis (L2, L3)
	Sartorius (L2, L3)
	Popliteus (L5)

Movement	Muscles (Root Value of Innervation)
Extension	Quadriceps femoris:
	Rectus femoris (L2, L3, L4)
	Vastus medialis (L2, L3, L4)
	Vastus intermedius (L2, L3, L4)
	Vastus lateralis (L2, L3, L4)
	Tensor fascia lata (L4, L5)
Medial rotation	Semitendinosus (L5, S1, S2)
	Semimembranosus (L5, S1, S2)
	Gracilis (L2, L3)
	Sartorius (L2, L3)
	Popliteus (L5)
Lateral rotation	Biceps femoris (L2, L3, L4)

Ankle Joint

Movement	Muscles (Root Value of Innervation)
Dorsiflexion/ extension	Tibialis anterior (L4, L5)
	Fibularis/peroneus tertius (L5, S1)
	Extensor digitorum longus (L5, S1)
	Extensor hallucis longus (L5, S1)
Plantarflexion/ flexion	Gastrocnemius (S1, S2)
	Soleus (S1, S2)
	Plantaris (S1, S2)
	Fibularis/peroneus longus (L5, S1)
	Fibularis/peroneus brevis (L5, S10)

Movement	Muscles (Root Value of Innervation)
	Tibialis posterior (L4, L5)
	Flexor digitorum longus (L5, S1, S2)
	Flexor hallucis longus (S1, S2)

Joints of the Foot

The first toe comprises two joints, MTP and interphalangeal (IP), while the lateral four toes comprise three joints, MTP, PIP and DIP joints.

Movement	Muscles (Root Value of Innervation)
Dorsiflexion/ extension	Extensor hallucis longus at IP and MTP (L5, S1)
	Extensor digitorum longus at DIP, PIP and MTP (L5, S1)
	Extensor digitorum brevis at DIP, PIP and MTP (L5, S1)
	Lumbricals at DIP and PIP (S1, S2, S3)
Plantarflexion/ flexion	Flexor hallucis longus at IP and MTP (S1, S2)
	Flexor hallucis brevis at MTP (S1, S2)
	Flexor digitorum longus at DIP, PIP and MTP (L5, S1, S2)
	Flexor accessorius at DIP, PIP and MTP (S2, S3)
	Flexor digitorum brevis at PIP and MTP (S2, S3)
	Flexor digiti minimi brevis at MTP (S2, S3)
	Interossei at MTP (S2, S3)
	Lumbricals at MTP (S1, S2, S3)
Abduction	Abductor hallucis at MTP (S1, S2)
	Abductor digiti minimi at MTP (S2, S3)
	Dorsal interossei at MTP (S2, S3)
Adduction	Adductor hallucis at MTP (S2, S3)
	Plantar interossei at MTP (S2, S3)

SELF-TEST QUESTIONS

1. Concerning the pelvic girdle, which of the following statements is NOT correct?
   a. Each innominate comprises the ilium, ischium and pubis.
   b. The bodies of the pubes articulate anteriorly by a synchondrosis.
   c. The sacrum is posterior.
   d. The articulation with the femur is at the acetabulum.
   e. It provides bony support for the birth canal.

2. Concerning the pelvic girdle, which of the following statements is NOT correct?
   a. The sacroiliac joint allows little movement.
   b. The obturator foramen is mostly filled by the obturator membrane.
   c. The anterior superior iliac spines are further apart in females.
   d. The lumbosacral joint is a symphysis.
   e. Spondylolisthesis can arise as a slowly developing fracture.

3. Concerning vessels and nerves associated with the pelvis, which of the following statements is NOT correct?
   a. The common iliac artery bifurcates at the level of L4/L5.
   b. The lumbar plexus is formed within the substance of psoas major.
   c. The obturator nerve innervates gracilis.
   d. The internal iliac artery gives the superior gluteal artery.
   e. The median umbilical ligament is the obliterated distal part of the superior vesical artery.

4. Which of the following nerves is NOT derived from the lumbar plexus?
   a. Femoral nerve
   b. Ilioinguinal nerve
   c. Genitofemoral nerve
   d. Obturator nerve
   e. Medial cutaneous nerve of the thigh

5. Concerning structures entering the thigh from the abdomen and pelvis, which of the following statements is correct?
   a. The femoral nerve is contained within the femoral sheath.
   b. The sciatic nerve passes through the lesser sciatic foramen.
   c. The pudendal nerve passes through the greater sciatic foramen.
   d. The internal iliac artery passes deep to the inguinal ligament.
   e. The inferior gluteal nerve passes through the greater sciatic foramen above the piriformis.

6. Concerning the gluteal region, which of the following statements is NOT correct?
   a. The superficial fascia is thick and fatty.
   b. The whole of the iliac crest can be palpated.
   c. Gluteus maximus has an attachment to the fascia lata.
   d. Intramuscular injections should be into the upper medial quadrant.
   e. Piriformis is a lateral rotator of the thigh at the hip joint.

7. Concerning the thigh, which of the following muscles laterally rotates the tibia on the femur?
   a. Semimembranosus
   b. Biceps femoris
   c. Popliteus
   d. Semitendinosus
   e. Gracilis

8. Which of the following muscles flex the thigh at the hip joint and extend the calf/leg at the knee joint?
   a. Gracilis
   b. Vastus intermedius
   c. Rectus femoris
   d. Vastus lateralis
   e. Vastus medialis

9. Which of the following muscles does NOT attach to the femur?
   a. Semitendinosus
   b. Biceps femoris
   c. Adductor magnus
   d. Popliteus
   e. Vastus intermedius

10. Which movement at the hip joint is the freest?
    a. Extension
    b. Medial rotation
    c. Abduction
    d. Adduction
    e. Flexion

11. Concerning the hip joint, which of the following statements is correct?
    a. The acetabulum is a complete bony ring.
    b. All capsular fibres associated with the joint capsule have an attachment to the femur.
    c. Anterior dislocation is more common than posterior dislocation.
    d. The hip joint centre lies on a horizontal line passing through the lesser trochanters.
    e. In adults the arterial supply to the femoral head is from the artery to the head of the femur.

12. Concerning movements at the hip joint, which of the following statements is NOT correct?
    a. Flexion is produced by sartorius.
    b. The hamstrings are involved in accelerating forward movement of the tibia during walking.
    c. Abduction is produced by tensor fascia lata.
    d. Rotation occurs about the mechanical axis of the femur.
    e. Extension is produced by biceps femoris.

13. What is the root value of the nerve supplying gluteus maximus?
    a. L1, L2, L3
    b. L2, L3, L4
    c. L3, L4, L5
    d. L4, L5, S1
    e. L5, S1, S2

14. Concerning the femoral triangle, which of the following statements is NOT correct?
    a. The lateral border is the medial border of sartorius.
    b. The roof is the fascia lata of the thigh.
    c. The short saphenous vein joins the femoral vein by passing through an opening in the roof.
    d. The femoral canal is the most medial compartment within the femoral sheath.
    e. The inguinal ligament is the lower free border of external oblique.

15. Concerning the thigh, which of the following statements is correct?
    a. It has anterior, posterior and medial compartments.
    b. The femoral vein is a continuation of the anterior tibial vein after passing through the adductor hiatus.
    c. The femoral artery is too deep to be able to be used for catheter insertion.
    d. The saphenous nerve arises directly from the lumbar plexus.
    e. The posterior compartment contains the obturator nerve.

16. Concerning the calf/leg, which of the following statements is NOT correct?
    a. It extends between the knee and ankle joints.
    b. The medial surface of the tibia is subcutaneous.
    c. It has anterior, lateral and posterior compartments.
    d. The fibula is weight bearing.
    e. Osgood-Schlatter disease usually presents between ages 9 and 16.

17. Concerning the popliteal fossa, which of the following statements is correct?
    a. The deepest structure is the sciatic nerve.
    b. The upper medial border is formed by biceps femoris.
    c. The popliteal artery gives four genicular branches.
    d. The floor is formed partly by the femur.
    e. The popliteal vein is formed at the lower border of adductor magnus.

18. Concerning the knee joint, which of the following statements is NOT correct?
    a. It is between the femur and tibia.
    b. It is surrounded by an independent fibrous capsule.

c. The cruciate ligaments are intracapsular but extrasynovial.
    d. The medial collateral ligament blends with the joint capsule.
    e. The femoral condyles are convex transversely.

19. Concerning ligaments associated with the knee joint, which of the following statements is NOT correct?
    a. The anterior cruciate ligament passes upwards, forwards and medially.
    b. The lateral collateral ligament is separated from the joint capsule by the tendon of the popliteus.
    c. The posterior cruciate ligament is stronger than the anterior.
    d. The deep part of the medial collateral ligament attaches to the medial meniscus.
    e. The posterior cruciate ligament prevents forward movement of the femur on the tibia.

20. Concerning the knee joint, which of the following statements is correct?
    a. The knee joint line cannot be palpated.
    b. In varus deformity the knee joints are closer together than normal.
    c. The joint capsule is deficient anteriorly.
    d. The anterior cruciate ligament helps resist lateral displacement of the femur on the tibia.
    e. The medial meniscus is almost circular.

21. Which of the following muscles does NOT cross the knee joint?
    a. Popliteus
    b. Gastrocnemius
    c. Semimembranosus
    d. Soleus
    e. Plantaris

22. Which of the following is NOT a function of the menisci?
    a. Shock absorption
    b. Lubrication
    c. Improve congruence between the articular surfaces
    d. Weight bearing
    e. Control movement

23. Concerning the knee joint, which of the following statements is NOT correct?
    a. The patella is a sesamoid bone within the quadriceps tendon.
    b. The anterior cruciate ligament is shorter than the posterior.

c. Malalignment of the femur and tibia can lead to osteoarthritis.
d. The medial meniscus is the more frequently damaged.
e. Knee extension is limited by hip flexion.

24. Concerning the tibiofibular joints, which of the following statements is NOT correct?
  a. The inferior joint is a syndesmosis.
  b. The superior joint is between the head of the fibula and lateral tibial condyle.
  c. During dorsiflexion of the ankle joint, the malleoli become approximated.
  d. The tibia and fibula are united by an interosseous membrane.
  e. Movement occurs at both joints simultaneously.

25. Concerning the calf/leg, which of the following statements is correct?
  a. The anterior tibial artery passes through an opening in the interosseous membrane.
  b. Muscles of the lateral compartment invert the foot.
  c. The anterior compartment muscles are innervated by the tibial nerve.
  d. Muscles of the posterior compartment evert the foot.
  e. Muscles of the lateral compartment are innervated by the deep fibular/peroneal nerve.

26. Concerning the tibial nerve, which of the following statements is NOT correct?
  a. It is a terminal branch of the sciatic nerve.
  b. It enters the foot behind the medial malleolus.
  c. It divides into medial and lateral terminal branches.
  d. It supplies skin on the lateral aspect of the calf/leg.
  e. It innervates fibularis/peroneus tertius.

27. Concerning the ankle joint, which of the following statements is NOT correct?
  a. It permits dorsiflexion and plantarflexion only.
  b. The flexor retinaculum attaches to the medial malleolus.
  c. It is supported on the lateral aspect by the anterior talofibular ligament.
  d. The deltoid ligament has deep and superficial parts.
  e. The collateral ligaments contribute to anteroposterior stability.

28. Which of the following structures does NOT pass immediately behind the medial malleolus?
  a. Tendon of extensor hallucis longus
  b. Posterior tibial artery
  c. Tibialis anterior
  d. Tibial nerve
  e. Tendon of extensor digitorum longus

29. Which of the following structures is NOT associated with the plantar surface of the foot?
  a. Plantar aponeurosis
  b. Dorsalis pedis
  c. Quadratus plantae
  d. Flexor digiti minimi
  e. Medial plantar artery

30. Concerning the foot, which of the following statements is correct?
  a. The cuboid lies medially.
  b. The deep fascia is not continuous with that of the calf/leg.
  c. The navicular contributes to the medial longitudinal arch.
  d. There are eight tarsal bones.
  e. All digits have three phalanges.

31. Concerning bones of the foot, which of the following statements is NOT correct?
  a. The calcaneus is the largest of the tarsus.
  b. The cuboid articulates with fourth metatarsal.
  c. The second metatarsal is the least mobile.
  d. The first metatarsal is the longest.
  e. The navicular articulates with the talus.

32. Concerning the foot, which of the following statements is correct?
  a. The subtalar joint is between the talus and cuboid.
  b. Inversion and eversion occur at the midtarsal and tarsometatarsal joints.
  c. The interphalangeal joints permit abduction and adduction.
  d. The big toe has the smallest range of movement.
  e. Abduction and adduction of the digits occur with respect to the second metatarsal.

33. Concerning the foot, which of the following statements is NOT correct?
  a. Eversion is a combination of adduction at the subtalar joint and supination at the midtarsal joint.
  b. Plantarflexion and dorsiflexion are possible at the tarsometatarsal joints.

c. The range of inversion can be increased with ankle plantarflexion.

d. Skin between the first and second toes is innervated by the deep fibular/peroneal nerve.

e. Inversion is produced by tibialis anterior and posterior.

34. Concerning the ankle and foot, which of the following statements is NOT correct?

a. The lateral malleolus projects further distally than the medial.

b. In the sole the tendon of fibularis/peroneus longus crosses from medial to lateral.

c. The total range of movement at the ankle joint is determined by the length of the articular surfaces.

d. The dorsal interossei abduct the toes.

e. The ankle and foot provide propulsion and restraint during walking.

35. Concerning the walking cycle, which of the following statements is NOT correct?

a. Stride length is the distance covered between successive heel contacts of the same foot.

b. During walking there is always a period of double support.

c. Pathology has little influence on walking parameters.

d. The walking base is a measure of steadiness during walking.

e. Cadence is the number of strides per minute.

Answers to Self-Test Questions

CHAPTER 1: CELLS, TISSUES AND ORGANS

1. Nucleolus
2. All cells have a nucleus.
3. Friable
4. Cardiac muscle cells are joined together by intercalated discs.
5. Epithelium
6. Hemidesmosome
7. In pseudostratified epithelium all cells are attached to the basal lamina.
8. Osmosis
9. The number in different cells varies.
10. Proteasomes are protein complexes found in the nucleus.
11. Anaphase
12. Propagation of impulses
13. Open
14. Osteoblasts are bone-forming cells.
15. Three or more breaks in the same bone with fragments at the fracture site.
16. Syndesmosis
17. Skeletal muscle with a fusiform arrangement of fibres is stronger than one with a pennate arrangement of fibres.
18. The enteric nervous system is part of the central nervous system.
19. Myelinated fibres conduct impulses faster than non-myelinated fibres.
20. Regenerated nerves always make the same connections as before they were damaged.
21. It is thinnest over posterior and extensor surfaces than over anterior and flexor surfaces.
22. Proliferating basal cells under the scab migrate at 0.05 mm/day.
23. Apocrine sweat glands only become functional after puberty.
24. The epidermal-dermal junction is smooth.
25. Fascicles within a peripheral nerve are bound together by the epineurium.

CHAPTER 2: THORAX (CHEST)

1. Clavicle
2. During inspiration the sternum moves forwards and upwards.
3. Vein, artery, nerve
4. The right side of the head and neck
5. The remnants of the thymus lie in the posterior mediastinum.
6. The bronchi are lined with pseudostratified ciliated cuboidal epithelium.
7. At the hilum the bronchus is the most posterior structure.
8. 12 to 16 breaths/min.
9. Expiratory reserve volume is the same as vital capacity.
10. In the alveoli oxygen diffuses from blood in the capillaries into the inspired air.
11. In carbon monoxide poisoning the oxygen-haemoglobin dissociation curve is irreversibly shifted to the right.
12. The dorsal respiratory group of cells in the respiratory centre are mainly responsible for expiration.
13. Polypnoea is slow shallow breathing in which the rate of breathing changes but not the force.
14. Atelectasis

15. Bronchiectasis is a temporary dilation of the bronchi and bronchioles.
16. The apex is in the right 5th intercostal space 9 cm from the midline.
17. In the foetus, blood returning to the heart from the superior vena cava passes directly to the left atrium.
18. The blood supply to the conducting system of the heart is mainly from the left coronary artery.
19. At all heart rates there is complete filing of the heart chambers.
20. The QRS complex is a repolarising complex spreading through the atrioventricular node, atrioventricular bundle and Purkinje fibres.
21. Sinus bradycardia is associated with a reduced R-R interval.
22. High concentrations of potassium ions in the blood are fatal.
23. It is the amount of blood ejected from each ventricle with each heartbeat.
24. The right atrial (Bainbridge) reflex increases heart rate when venous return decreases.
25. The superior vena cava is formed behind the left sternoclavicular joint.
26. The tunica adventitia mainly comprises collagenous tissue.
27. In varicose veins blood flows from the superficial to deep veins.
28. The regulation of arterial pressure is entirely dependent on local blood flow.
29. 120 mm Hg
30. Pressure gradient
31. It is higher in the morning than at midday.
32. β adrenoreceptor blockers inhibit vasodilation.
33. Histamine
34. The anacrotic limb is due to the fall in pressure during systole.
35. It decreases when tilting the body.
36. Intercellular clefts between cells allow substances to pass through the cell walls.
37. Capillary pressure increases.
38. In the first stage regulatory mechanisms are unable to successfully restore normal blood pressure and blood flow.
39. In right-sided congestive cardiac failure blood in the venae cavae continues to flow normally.
40. A route for protein absorption.
41. Lymph nodes contain lymphocytes and macrophages.
42. It conveys urea to the liver.
43. The lifespan of red blood cells is between 1 and 10 days.
44. Erythrocyte
45. In anaemia there are no changes in red blood cell morphology.
46. 0.5–1 day
47. Neutrophils contain histamine.
48. Platelet count increases following surgical interventions.
49. Antibodies comprise 50% of total plasma proteins.
50. Cushing disease

CHAPTER 3: VERTEBRAL COLUMN (BACK)

1. 24
2. Dissipates forces from other parts of the body
3. Idiopathic
4. 16
5. Short transverse processes
6. Rotation
7. 25%
8. The cartilage end plates act as impermeable membranes.
9. Posterior longitudinal
10. The single posterior spinal artery is formed by branches from the vertebral artery.
11. T1–L2
12. Quadratus lumborum
13. VII
14. L3–L4
15. Anterior median sulcus
16. Pia mater
17. Local anaesthetics injected close to spinal nerves outside the intervertebral foramen do not spread to adjacent nerves.
18. Central nucleus
19. Rubrospinal tract
20. Corticospinal
21. Intrafusal muscle fibres are innervated by α and β motor neurons.
22. Hemisection
23. They leave the vertebral canal via the intervertebral foramen.
24. The T1 nerve passes deep to the first rib.
25. Vasoactive intestinal peptide (VIP)
26. Preganglionic sympathetic fibres synapse in ganglia close to the target organ/structure.

27. The posterior spinocerebellar tract carries impulses from the opposite side of the body.
28. All corticonuclear fibres terminate around the nuclei of both sides of the body.
29. Lumbar cord transection is not associated with incontinence.
30. The lateral white column is the narrowest.

CHAPTER 4: HEAD AND NECK

1. The bregma is the region between the parietal and occipital bones.
2. Its blood supply is by numerous branches.
3. Middle meningeal artery
4. Facial nerve
5. Lesser occipital
6. Pterygopalatine canal
7. The optic canal communicates with the anterior cranial fossa.
8. Superior petrosal sinus
9. A tract is a collection of axons with different functions.
10. The medial lemniscus carries proprioceptive fibres and tactile impulses.
11. Lesions of the lateral segment of the lower pons lead to spastic hemiplegia.
12. The red nucleus sends efferent fibres to the frontal cortex.
13. Each cerebellar hemisphere controls the same side of the body.
14. Two pairs of peduncles connect the cerebellum to the brainstem.
15. The right and left thalamus are separated by the 4th ventricle.
16. The medial geniculate body is concerned with auditory sensation.
17. The parietal lobe is separated from the temporal lobe by the calcarine sulcus.
18. Ventral spinocerebellar
19. The putamen is an efferent nucleus.
20. They are part of the pyramidal system.
21. The choroid plexuses produce cerebrospinal fluid.
22. It occupies the subdural space.
23. Extrapyramidal tracts are not modulated by the central nervous system.
24. Visual processing
25. Sphenoid sinus
26. Arachnoid villi are projections of pia mater.

27. The anterior cerebral artery supplies the visual cortex.
28. The abducens nerve innervates superior oblique.
29. The superior alveolar nerves are branches of the maxillary nerve.
30. Side-to-side movements of the mandible are produced by masseter and temporalis.
31. Nasal cavity
32. The main function of the facial muscles is to facilitate facial expressions.
33. The roof of the orbit is formed by the greater wing of the sphenoid.
34. The outer layer is vascular.
35. Lacrimal fluid contains antimicrobial agents.
36. Parasympathetic secretomotor innervation is by the maxillary division of the trigeminal nerve.
37. The arterial supply to the lips does not anastomose across the midline.
38. The secretions of the parotid gland are mainly serous.
39. Tensor tympani dampens down movements of the stapes in response to loud noises.
40. Bony support is provided by eight cervical vertebrae.
41. The investing layer of fascia extends into the axilla as the axillary sheath.
42. The pharynx extends from the base of the skull to the level of the 6th cervical vertebra.
43. Thyroid secretion is controlled by the neurohypophysis.
44. The subclavian vein cross the 1st rib posterior to scalenus anterior.
45. Protein hormones are secreted by the adrenal medulla.
46. They coordinate and regulate body functions.
47. In males follicle stimulating hormone is known as interstitial cell stimulating hormone.
48. Diabetes insipidus
49. Cretinism occurs due to congenital absence of the parathyroid glands.
50. The adrenal cortex and medulla do not function independently.
51. Each islet is associated with several small blood capillaries.
52. Type II diabetes is associated with increased plasma insulin concentrations.
53. Decreased thyroxin secretion inhibits fertility.
54. Sexual function is controlled by the release of hormones by the pituitary.

55. Oligomenorrhea
56. Fertilisation occurs in the uterus.
57. Foetal membranes release large amounts of cortisol.
58. Dopamine
59. The superior petrosal sinus and transverse sinus form the internal jugular vein.
60. Posterior nuclei receive afferent fibres from other thalamic nuclei.

CHAPTER 5: UPPER LIMB

1. Brachioradialis extends the forearm at the elbow joint.
2. Brachialis
3. Adduction
4. The shoulder joint is part of the pectoral girdle.
5. In retraction the scapula moves forwards around the chest wall.
6. The medial and lateral epicondyles of the humerus can be palpated.
7. It commonly dislocates posteriorly.
8. Combined flexion and extension has a range of 180 degrees.
9. C5, C6, C7
10. Latissimus dorsi
11. The axillary vein is a continuation of the cephalic vein.
12. Flexor carpi ulnaris
13. Thoracodorsal
14. Pectoral
15. The median nerve lies on biceps brachii.
16. The ulnar articulates with the lunate.
17. Supracondylar fractures are common in children.
18. It contains, from medial to lateral, the tendon of biceps brachii, brachial artery and median nerve.
19. The basilic vein is a continuation of the lateral end of the dorsal venous network.
20. C5, C6
21. The midcarpal joint is between the radius, scaphoid and lunate.
22. Flexion and extension occur about a transverse axis through the lunate.
23. Trapezoid
24. Trigger finger is a localised swelling of a flexor digitorum superficialis tendon.
25. Rotation at the metacarpophalangeal joints of the fingers is passive.
26. The tendons of flexor digitorum profundus lie superficial to those of flexor digitorum superficialis.
27. Flexor digitorum profundus
28. Span
29. The individual's pulse should always be taken with the thumb.
30. Rhomboid major
31. C7
32. Serratus anterior
33. Supraspinatus
34. Flexor carpi radialis and extensor carpi radialis brevis
35. Biceps brachii is a powerful pronator.

CHAPTER 6: ABDOMEN, PELVIS AND PERINEUM

1. Quadratus lumborum
2. Sternum
3. Pancreas
4. External oblique
5. The internal spermatic fascia is derived from internal oblique.
6. The gallbladder lies in the epigastrium.
7. The mucosa contains blood vessels and lymphatics.
8. It has no interactions with the autonomic nervous system.
9. Chief (zymogenic) cells secrete hydrochloric acid.
10. Venous drainage is into the portal vein.
11. The tail of the pancreas lies within the C-shaped duodenum.
12. Hydrophobic peptides
13. The base of the appendix lies at the junction of the lateral two-thirds and medial one-third of a line connecting the anterior superior iliac spine and umbilicus.
14. Sigmoid colon
15. It lies mainly in the left hypochondrium.
16. Hepatocytes line the walls of the sinusoids.
17. The fundus of the gallbladder lies at the tip of the left 9th costal cartilage.
18. In acute pancreatitis proenzymes may be activated and digest pancreatic tissue.
19. Anorexigenic substances stimulate feeding.
20. Polypeptides are released in the stomach in the absence of food.
21. The secretion of highly alkaline gastric juice enhances stomach emptying.

22. Sympathetic stimulation increases secretions from the small intestine.
23. Contraction of the mucosa in the small intestine is largely initiated by the autonomic nervous system.
24. Anabolism
25. They are absorbed from the small intestine as disaccharides.
26. Cholesterol is rapidly absorbed from the digestive tract into intestinal lymph.
27. Insulin decreases the formation of tissue proteins.
28. Whole protein molecules are rarely absorbed into the blood.
29. Arginine
30. Vitamin K increases calcium absorption from the digestive tract.
31. Copper
32. It stores vitamin K.
33. It has outer concave and inner convex borders.
34. Accumulates toxins
35. The glomerulus is surrounded by a single-layered capsule.
36. Angiotensin IV has vasoconstriction actions.
37. They can change the actions of neurotransmitters.
38. The principal cells of the collecting system regulate the reabsorption of electrolytes.
39. Osmotic diuretics decrease the osmolarity of tubular fluid.
40. They do not affect blood vessels.
41. The upper end of the ureter lies on the transcristal plane.
42. Cystitis is common during urinary tract infections.
43. The ejaculatory duct is formed by the duct of the seminal vesicle and epididymis.
44. The prostate consists of four zones.
45. The uterus is separated from the bladder by the rectouterine pouch.
46. Approximately 10% of ovarian cancers are related to an inherited risk.
47. Following ovulation, the proliferative phase begins with rapid growth of a few ovarian follicles.
48. The deep perineal pouch lies between the perineal membrane and membranous layer of superficial fascia.
49. Peanuts
50. A portal triad comprises a bile ductile, arteriole and lymphatics.

CHAPTER 7: LOWER LIMB

1. The bodies of the pubes articulate anteriorly by a synchondrosis.
2. The lumbosacral joint is a symphysis.
3. The common iliac artery bifurcates at the level of L4/L5.
4. Medial cutaneous nerve of the thigh
5. The pudendal nerve passes through the greater sciatic foramen.
6. Intramuscular injections should be into the upper medial quadrant.
7. Biceps femoris
8. Rectus femoris
9. Semitendinosus
10. Flexion
11. The hip joint centre lies on a horizontal line passing through the lesser trochanters.
12. The hamstrings are involved in accelerating forward movement of the tibia during walking.
13. L5, S1, S2
14. The short saphenous vein joins the femoral vein by passing through an opening in the roof.
15. It has anterior, posterior and medial compartments.
16. The fibula is weight bearing.
17. The floor is formed partly by the femur.
18. It is surrounded by an independent fibrous capsule.
19. The anterior cruciate ligament passes upwards, forwards and medially.
20. The capsule is deficient anteriorly.
21. Soleus
22. Control movement
23. The anterior cruciate ligament is shorter than the posterior.
24. During dorsiflexion of the ankle joint, the malleoli become approximated.
25. The anterior tibial artery passes through an opening in the interosseous membrane.
26. It supplies skin on the lateral aspect of the calf/leg.
27. The collateral ligaments contribute to anteroposterior stability.
28. Tendon of extensor hallucis longus
29. Dorsalis pedis
30. The navicular contributes to the medial longitudinal arch.
31. The first metatarsal is the longest.
32. Abduction and adduction of the digits occur with respect to the second metatarsal.

33. Eversion is a combination of adduction at the subtalar joint and supination at the midtarsal joint.
34. In the sole the tendon of fibularis/peroneus longus crosses from medial to lateral.
35. Pathology has little influence on walking parameters.

Note: Page numbers followed by *b* indicate box, *f* indicate figures and *t* indicate tables.

A

'a' wave, 154
Abdomen, 381f, 450–508, 451b, 452f–454f, 453b
  arterial supply to, 88
  quadrants of, 461f
  regions of, 459–460, 460b, 461f
Abdominal aorta, 467f, 524f–525f
Abdominal cavity, 451f
Abdominal wall
  anterior and lateral, 453–458, 454b–456b, 455f–456f
  dermatomes of, 459f
  innervation of, 457t, 458, 459f
  layers of, 452f–453f
Abdominopelvic cavity, orientation and boundaries of, 451f
Abducens nerve, 272f, 275f, 276, 276b, 296f
Abduction
  axis of, 422f
  of metacarpophalangeal joints, 428–430
  of shoulder joint, 395, 395f–396f
  of wrist, 422–424, 424b
Abductor digiti minimi muscle, 421f, 433t, 633t–634t
Abductor hallucis muscle, 633t–634t
Abductor pollicis brevis muscle, 433t
Abductor pollicis longus muscle, 417f, 419f, 421f, 429t–430t
ABO system, 168, 168t–169t, 168b
ABP. *See* Androgen-binding protein
Accessory glands, of male reproductive system, 535–537
Accessory hemiazygos vein, 77f–78f, 89f
Accessory ligaments, 199–200, 199b–200b, 201f
Accessory nerves, 248, 248b, 280, 280b, 281f, 322f
Accessory obturator nerve, 578f, 593
Accessory phrenic nerve, 92
Accommodation reflex pathway, 273, 273b

ACE. *See* Angiotensin-converting enzyme
Acetabulum, 567–569, 568f, 585f
Acetylcholine, 151, 369
Achlorhydria, 467b
Acid-base balance, kidney and, 513–515
Acinar cells, 483f
Acromegalic gigantism, 339
Acromegaly, 339
Acromial angle, 385f
Acromial facet, 382f
Acromicria, 340
Acromioclavicular joint, 380f, 384, 384b, 386f–387f, 391f
Acromion, 318f, 385f–386f, 392f
Acrosome, 354f
Action potential, in nervous tissue, 50, 50f
Active immunisation, 179
Activin, 360f
Acute bronchitis, 114
Acute haemorrhage, 157
Acute heart failure, 160
Acute renal failure, 522
Adduction
  axis of, 422f
  of metacarpophalangeal joints, 428–430
  of shoulder joint, 395, 395f–396f
  of wrist, 422–424, 424b
Adductor brevis muscle, 575t–577t, 580f
Adductor hallucis muscle, 633t–634t, 635f
Adductor hiatus, 612f
Adductor longus muscle, 570f, 575t–577t, 580f, 589f
Adductor magnus muscle, 575t–577t, 580f, 612f
Adductor pollicis muscle, 433t
Adductor tubercle, of femur, 583f
Adenosine triphosphate (ATP), 497
Adhesiveness, 174

Adipocytes, in connective tissues, 25, 26f
Adipose tissue, 27–28, 28b, 367f, 502–503, 503b
Adrenal cortex, 343–344, 343b–344b, 344f
Adrenal (suprarenal) glands, 337f, 343–347, 483f, 510, 511f
  adrenal cortex, 343–344, 343b–344b, 344f
  cells in, function, 9t
  glucocorticoids, 345–347, 345b
  mineralocorticoids, 344–345
Adrenal medulla, 347
Adrenaline, 150
α adrenoceptor blockers, for hypertension, 148
β adrenoceptor blockers, for hypertension, 148
Adrenocorticoid secretion, abnormalities of, 346–347
Adrenocorticotropic hormone (ACTH), 339t
Adventitia, 139f
Afferent arteriole, 516f–517f
Afferent lymphatics, 162f
Afferent tracts, of spinal cord, 212–217, 212f
Age
  arterial blood pressure and, 148, 148t
  effect of, in respiratory physiology, 111
  heart rate and, 135
Agglutination, 174
Aggregation, 174
Agranulocytes, 173
Airway obstruction, 113–116
Airway resistance, breathing and, 103
Ala, 197f
Albumin, 146, 165, 504
Aldosterone, 151
  diuretics inhibiting, 522
  regulation of, 344–345, 345b
Allantois, 478f
Allergies, 180

Alpha granules, 174t
Alveolar air, 105, 105t
Alveolar bone, 310f
Alveolar ducts, 107, 107f, 115f
Alveolar pore, 108f
Alveolar respiratory membrane,
    ultrastructure of, 108f
Alveolar sacs, 107, 107f
Alveolar ventilation, 104, 104b
Alveoli, 107, 107f–108f, 115f, 367f
Amino acids, 503b–504b, 504f
    essential, 504
    non-essential, 504, 504b
Amniochorionic membrane, 549f
Amnion, 362f–363f, 549f
Amniotic cavity, 362f
Amniotic ectoderm, 362f
Ampulla, 367f
Amygdala, 263
Anacrotic pulse, 152b
Anaemia, 169–172, 170b
    aetiological classification of, 171t
    morphological classification of, 169t
    signs and symptoms of, 171
Anaemic hypoxia, 113
Anal aperture, 460f, 551f, 553f, 575f
Anal canal, 476–477
    arterial supply to, 477f, 477b
Anal column, 556f
Anal sinus, 556f
Anal triangle, 551f, 553f, 555–556,
    555b
Anal valve, 556f
Anaphase, 17
Anaphylactic reactions, 180
Anaphylactic shock, 159
Anastomoses, 138
Anatomical neck, 390f
Anatomical snuffbox, region
    of, 421f
Anaxonic neuron, 46, 46f
Anchoring villus, 549f
Anconeus muscle, 410t, 417f
Androgen-binding protein (ABP), 534
Androgenic effects, 356f
Androgens, 344f, 351
Aneurysm, 141–142, 142f, 142b
Angiogenesis, 137–138
Angiopoietins, 137–138
Angiotensin(s), 151
Angiotensin I, 517
Angiotensin II, 517–518, 517f

Angiotensin II receptor blockers, for
    hypertension, 148
Angiotensin III, 517f, 518
Angiotensin IV, 517f, 518
Angiotensin-converting enzyme
    (ACE), 516–517
    for hypertension, 148
Angular artery, 291f
Angular vein, 291f, 296f
Ankle, 615–621, 616b, 619f
Ankle joint, 566f, 616–621, 618b,
    619f–621f, 623f
    movements in, 618–621, 622t,
    623f–624f, 643
Annular ligament, 408f, 413f,
    415f–416f
Annulus fibrosis, 196–197, 198f, 202f
Anococcygeal body, 460f
Anocutaneous line, 556f
Anorectal junction, 476
Anorexia, 487
Anosmia, 272b
Ansa cervicalis, 325b
Anteflexed uterus, 543, 544f
Anterior arch, 193f
Anterior cardiac veins, 125–126
Anterior cerebral artery, 266f–268f,
    267–268, 268b, 272f
Anterior chamber, 298f
Anterior circumflex humeral artery,
    386f
Anterior column, of brain, 255f
Anterior communicating artery, 267f
Anterior cranial fossa, 242, 243f, 243t
Anterior cruciate ligament, 600f,
    603f–604f
Anterior ethmoidal artery, 296f, 307f
Anterior ethmoidal nerve, 296f, 309f
Anterior external plexus, 203f
Anterior fontanelle, 235b, 236f
Anterior funiculus, of spinal cord, 210f
Anterior glandular branch, of superior
    thyroid artery, 332f
Anterior gluteal line, 568f
Anterior head cap, 354f
Anterior horn, 261f, 603f
Anterior inferior cerebellar artery, 267f
Anterior inferior iliac spine, 568f
Anterior intercostal arteries, 76–77, 76f
Anterior intercostal vein, 77f
Anterior intermuscular septum, 614f
Anterior internal plexus, 203f

Anterior interosseous nerve, 417f, 440f
Anterior interosseous vessels, 417f
Anterior interventricular artery, 125f
Anterior jugular vein, 322f
Anterior ligament
    of ankle joint, 620f
    of symphysis pubis, 570f
    of tibiofibular joints, 613f
Anterior longitudinal ligament, 199,
    199f, 201f
Anterior lumbosacral ligament, 572f
Anterior median fissure, of spinal cord,
    208f, 210f, 249f
Anterior mediastinum, 83
Anterior nuclei, 253
Anterior pituitary, 338f, 356f, 360f
Anterior pulmonary plexus, 70f
Anterior radiate ligaments, 71f
Anterior sacral foramen, 197f
Anterior sacroiliac ligament, 572f
Anterior scalene, 318f, 321f, 333f
Anterior spinal artery, 209f, 267f
    occlusion, 219
Anterior sternoclavicular ligament,
    382f
Anterior superior iliac spine, 568f
Anterior superior pancreaticoduodenal
    artery, 467f
Anterior talofibular ligament, 620f
Anterior tibial artery, 612–613,
    614f–615f, 618f, 623f
Anterior tibial nodes, 590f
Anterior tibial vessels, passage of, 612f
Anterior tibiofibular ligament, 613f,
    620f
Anterior tubercle, 193f
Anterior vagal trunk, 88f
Anterior vein of forearm, 437f
Anterior ventral nucleus, 253
Anteverted uterus, 543, 544f
Antibodies, 178
Antibody-mediated reactions, 180
Anticoagulants, 176, 176b
Antidiuretic hormone, secretion of,
    immediate compensatory effects
    on, 158
Antidiuretic hormone (ADH)
    secretion of, diuretics inhibiting, 522
Anti-diuretic hormone (ADH), 339t
Antidromic vasodilator fibres, 150
Antigens, 177
Antihelix, 315f

Antihypertensive drugs, for hypertension, 148
Anti-Müllerian hormone, 534
Antral follicle, 357f
Antrum, 357f
Anus, 460f
Aorta, 76f, 93f, 136–137, 511f
    arch of, 83, 84f, 86f, 87b
    coarctation of, 136b
    femoral triangle and, 589f
Aortic arches, 138f
Aortic impression, 99f
Aortic plexus, 91f
Aortic regurgitation, peripheral pulses in, 153f
Aortic valve, 119f–121f, 121–122
Aorticorenal ganglion, 91f
Apical axillary lymph nodes, 402f
Apical lymph nodes, 403f
Aplastic anaemia, 171, 171t
Apneustic centre, 110, 110f, 110b
Apnoea, 112
Apocrine secretion, 23, 25f
Apocrine sweat glands, 61, 61b
Aponeurotic layer, of scalp, 237, 237f
Apoptosis, 19, 19b
Appendicitis, acute, 475b
Appendix, 471f, 472–475, 473f, 473b
Aqueous chamber, 297f
Arachnoid granulation, 265f
Arachnoid mater, 208f, 220f, 264, 264b, 265f, 315f
Arch of aorta, 83, 84f, 86f, 87b
Archicerebellum, 252, 253b
Arcuate artery, 546, 546f
Arcuate ligament, of symphysis pubis, 570f
Arcuate line, 568f
Arcuate popliteal ligament, 599f
Arm, 380f, 387–404
    axilla, 398–400, 398b, 399f
    compartments of, 402–404
        anterior, 402–404
            muscles, 404
        posterior, 404
    humerus, 387–391, 387b, 390f, 391b
    shoulder joint, 391–398, 392f–393f, 393b
Arrector pili muscle, 56f
Arrhythmias, 130–133
Arteria recta, 476f
Arterial anastomosis, 267b

Arterial arcades, 471f
Arterial blood pressure, 134, 147–151
    fall in, 150
    pathological variations in, 148–149
    physiological variations in, 148
    regulation of, 144, 149–151
Arterial pulse, 151–152, 152f
Arterial supply
    to brain, 264–269, 266f
    to chest wall, 75–77, 76f
    to face, 287–288, 288b
    of hand, 435, 437f
    of lateral and medial walls of nasal cavity, 307f
    to oesophagus, 87–88
    to orbit, 295, 296f
    of palate, 313
    of thyroid gland, 331, 331b
    of tongue, 311
Arteries
    development of, 136b
    function of, 143
    of lymph nodes, 162f
    of posterior triangle, 319
    structure of, 139f
Arteriolar constriction, angiotensin II and, 150
Arterioles, 143, 155f
Arteriosclerosis, 139–141
Arteriovenous shunts, 138, 141f
Articular cartilage, 419f
    of bone, 30f
    in synovial joints, 37f
Articular disc, 413f, 416f, 419f
Articular process, of vertebra, 191f
Articular surfaces, 382f, 392f, 431f
    of head, typical rib, 72f
    of sacroiliac joint, 572f
    of symphysis pubis, 570f
    of talus, 620f
    of tibia, 620f
    of tibiofibular joints, 613f
    of uncovertebral joints, 194f
Articularis genu, 600f
Arytenoid cartilages, 329
    muscular process of, 330f
    vocal process of, 330f
Ascending aorta, 83–84, 86f, 87b, 120f, 125f, 152f
Ascending cervical artery, 333f
Ascending colon, 471f, 473f
Ascending lumbar vein, 78f

Ascending (sensory) tracts, of spinal cord, 213–214, 213f
Ascorbic acid (vitamin C), 506
Aspermia, 537
Asphyxia, 113–114
Asthma, 115
Asymmetrical forces, of intervertebral disc, 202f
Atelectasis, 114
Atheroma, 138–139
Atheromatous plaques, 139, 141f
Atherosclerosis, 139, 500b, 501f
Atherosclerotic arteries, 142f
Atherosclerotic plaque, development of, 501f
Atmospheric pressure, changes in, 105t
Atonic bladder, 529, 529b
Atopic (extrinsic) asthma, 115
ATP. See Adenosine triphosphate
Atrial fibrillation, 132
Atrial flutter, 132
Atrial natriuretic peptide, 151, 368–369
Atrioventricular block, 131, 132b
Atrioventricular node, 120f, 126f
Atypical blood vessels, 138
Atypical ribs, 71, 71b
Auditory area, 269
Auditory pathway, 277, 277b
Auditory tube, 315f, 327–328, 328b
Auerbach plexus. See Myenteric plexus
Auricular surface
    of ilium, 568f, 572f
    of sacrum, 197f
Auriculotemporal nerve, 239f, 276f
Autocrine messenger, 336f
Autoimmune diseases, 180
Automatic bladder, 529, 529b
Autonomic nerves, of perineum, 556
Autonomic nervous system, 223–227, 224f
Autophagy, in lysosome, 12–13
Avascular cornea, 297
Avulsion fracture, of bone, 34, 34f
Axial rotation (opposition), of metacarpophalangeal joints, 430, 433t
Axilla, of arm, 398–400, 398b, 399f
    axillary artery, 398, 398b
    axillary vein, 398
    brachial plexus, 398–400, 400b, 401t
Axillary artery, 398, 398b, 399f, 437f
Axillary lymph nodes, 403f

Axillary nerve, 397f, 400f–401f, 401t, 438f
  of upper limb, 435, 438f
Axillary vein, 398, 399f, 402f, 437f
Axis, of movement, 387f
Axolemma, 47b, 48f
Axon, 245f
  in muscle contraction, 43f
  in neuron, 46f, 47–48, 47b
    myelination, 47–48, 47f–48f
Axonotmesis, 53
Azoospermia, 537
Azygos system, 78f
Azygos vein, 77f–78f, 81f, 88, 88b, 89f

B
B cells, 177
B lymphocytes, 178
Back muscle, 79f
Bacterial vaginosis, 550
Bainbridge reflex, heart rate and, 135b
Balance and equilibrium, 317
Ball-and-socket joint, of bone, 38
Barin, 154b
Baroreceptor reflex, heart rate and, 135, 135b
Baroreceptors, role of, 149–150
Bartholin's gland. *See* Greater vestibular gland
Basal ganglia, 245f, 260
Basal lamina, 367f, 483f
Basement membrane, 139f
Basilar artery, 266, 266f–268f
Basilar groove, 249
Basilar membrane, 316f
Basilic vein, 417f, 419f, 437f
  of arm, 402, 402f–403f, 412f
  of forearm, 414, 414b
Basivertebral vein, 203f
Basophils, 172f, 172t, 173
Behavioural effects, 356f, 360f
Bell's palsy, 294b
Benedikt syndrome, 251b
Benign hypertension, 148
Benign prostatic hyperplasia, 537b
Beriberi. *See* Thiamine deficiency
'Berry' aneurysms, 142b
Bezold-Jarisch reflex, 135b
Biceps, 412f
  long head of, 391f–393f
  short head of, 391f
  tendon, 412f

Biceps brachii muscle, 394t, 399f, 403f, 410t, 415t
Biceps brachii tendon, 417f
Biceps femoris muscle, 575t–577t, 595t–596t, 611f
  long head, 593f, 610f, 617f
  short head, 593f, 610f
Biceps femoris tendon, 610f
Bicipital aponeurosis, 412f
Biconvex lens, 299
Bifid gallbladder, 482b
Bifid spinous process, 193f
Bifid (bicornuate) uterus, 543b, 544f
Bifurcate ligament, in foot, 627f–628f
Bilaminar disc, 362f
Bile, 492, 492f, 493b
Bile canaliculi, 479f–480f, 480
Bile duct, 469f, 479f–480f
Biliary system, 469f, 477–482
  development of, 477b
Bilirubin, 480b
  water-insoluble yellow, conjugation of, 482b
Biot breathing, 112, 112f
Bipennate muscles, 44, 45f
Bipolar neuron, 46, 46f
Birth
  changes at, heart in, 124
  cranial cavity at, 235
Bisferiens pulse, 152b
Bladder, 473f, 523–527, 523b, 525f–526f
  cancer, 527b
  development of, 523b
  filling, 527, 527b
  nerve supply to, 528
Bleeding disorders, 176b
Blind spot, 299
Blink (corneal) reflex, 301b
Blocking reactions, 180
Blood, 38, 164–180, 165b
  constituents in, normal values of, 164t
  tumours of, 143
  viscosity of, 146
Blood capillary, 40f
Blood clots, 175, 175t
Blood flow, 144–147
  in capillaries, 155, 155b
  local, autoregulation of, 146–147, 147f
  rate of, to each tissue, 143–144
  velocity of, 146
  volume of, 147
Blood glucose regulation, 349–351

Blood groups, 168–169, 168t, 168b
Blood pressure, 144, 144f, 145t
  arterial, 134, 147–151
    fall in, 150
    pathological variations in, 148–149
    physiological variations in, 148
    regulation of, 149–151
  hormones and, 150–151, 151t
  venous, 153
    pathological variation in, 153
    physiological variation in, 153
    regulation of, 153
Blood supply, 308, 308b
  to conducting system, 127b
  to face, 287–292
  of hand, 435, 435b
  to heart, 124–127, 124b
  to pericardium, 86–87, 87b
  to pleurae, 97, 97b
  to retina, 299–300, 300b
  to scalp, 237–238, 237f
  to thalamus, 254b
  to thoracic cage, 75–79
  to trachea and bronchi, 95
Blood vessel, 352f
  in connective tissues, 26f
  in skeletal muscle, 40f
  in skin, 56f
Blood vessels
  characteristic features of, 140t–141t
  flow in, 146f
  of gluteal region, 581–582
  isolated, 147
  pathology of, 138–143
  structure of, 137–138
Blood volume, 134, 144, 144f, 145t
BMI. *See* Body mass index
Body mass index (BMI), 487
Body temperature, heart rate and, 135
Bone, 29–34, 29f, 29b
  cells, 30–31, 30b
  deposition, 31b
  development of, 31–32, 32b
  fractures of, 33
    repair, 34, 35f
    types of, 34, 34f
  growth and remodelling of, 32, 32b, 33f
  joints, 34–38
  long, structure of, 30f
  ossification of, 32–33, 33f, 33b

Bone *(Continued)*
  of scalp, 237f
  types of, 31, 31b
Bone lining cells, 30, 31f
Bones, of thoracic cage, 68–72
Bouveret-Hoffmann syndrome, 132
Bowman's capsule, 511–513, 517f
Brachial artery, 386f, 397f, 402–403, 403f, 403b, 412f–413f, 437f
Brachial plexus, 223, 223f, 321f, 334f–335f, 398–400, 400f, 400b, 401t, 440f
  lateral cord of, 439f
  medial cord of, 439f
  muscles supplied by each root, 441
Brachial veins, 402f
Brachialis impression, 405f
Brachialis muscle, 403f, 410t, 412f, 440f
Brachiocephalic artery, 83
Brachiocephalic node, 96f
Brachiocephalic trunk, 81f–82f
Brachiocephalic veins, 83b, 335f, 383f
Brachioradialis muscle, 410t, 412f, 415t, 417f
Bradycardia, electrocardiogram in, 131f
Bradykinin, 151
Bradypnoea, 111
Brain, 243–270
  adult morphology of, 247–263, 248f
  arterial supply to, 266f, 269
  base of, 262–263, 262f
  coronal sections of, 246f
  development of, 245b
  inferior aspect of, 267f
  outer part of, 244
  right lateral aspect of, 246f
  sagittal section of, 255f
  superior aspect of, 257f
  transverse section of, 245f
  venous drainage of, 269–270
Brain natriuretic peptide, 151, 369
Brainstem, 247–252, 269
  anterior, lateral, and posterior aspect of, 249f
  inferior aspect of, 267f
  left lateral aspect of, 254f
  sagittal section of, 255f
Breast (mammary gland), 366, 367f
  contralateral (left), 403f
  glands in, 61

Breast milk, composition of, 367, 367b, 368t
Breathing
  in expiration, 102
  factors influencing, 102–103
Bronchi, 81f–82f, 93b, 94–95, 95b, 99f
  anterolateral aspect of, 96f
  blood and nerve supply to, 95
  principal and segmental, distribution of, 100f
Bronchial asthma, 115–116
Bronchiectasis, 116
Bronchitis, 114
Bronchopulmonary segments, 98–99, 98b–99b, 100f
  pulmonary circulation within, 106, 106b
Brown adipose tissue, 502, 502b
Buccal artery, 291f
Buccal nerve, 276f
Buccinator muscle, 292, 293f, 294
Buccopharyngeal fascia, 326f
'Bucket-handle' movement, 101
Buck's fascia, 539f
Bulbar fascia, 295
Bulbospongiosus muscle, 539b, 540f, 552f
Bulbourethral gland, 540f. *See also* Cowper's gland
Bundle branch block, 131, 132b
Bursitis, 44b
Buttocks, 580–582

C
'c' wave, 154
C1, 335f
C2, 335f
C3, 335f
C4, 335f
C5, 335f
C6, vertebral body, 333f
Cachexia, 487
Caecum, 472–475, 473f, 478f
Calcaneofibular ligament, 620f, 628f
Calcaneus, 566f, 625f, 627f–628f, 630f
Calcarine sulcus, 257f
Calcitonin, 341f, 342, 342b
Calcitriol, 368, 515
Calcium, 507
Calcium channel blockers, for hypertension, 148
Calcium ions, on heart, 133

Calf, 594–615
  compartments of, 612–615, 614f
    anterior, 612–614
    lateral, 614, 614f
    muscles, 615
    posterior, 614–615
  fibula, 566f, 597f, 598, 598b
  knee joint, 566f, 598–608, 599f–601f, 600b–601b
    movements in, 605–608, 605f, 642–643
  patella, 566f, 598, 598f, 598b
    in knee joint, 601b, 603f
    movement of, with femur and tibia, 608f, 610f
  popliteal fossa, 608–611, 609b–610b, 611f–612f
  tibia, 566f, 596–598, 596b, 597f, 598b
    patella with, movement of, 608f, 610f
    reflections of synovial membrane on, 600f
  tibiofibular joints, 611–612, 612f
    inferior, 612, 613f
    superior, 611–612, 613f
Callosal commissure, 260
Calyces, 512f
Camper's fascia, 451, 452f–453f
Canaliculus, 32f
Canals of Hering, 480, 480f
Cancellous bone, 30f, 32f–33f
Capillaries, 107f–108f, 341f, 367f
  blood flow in, 155, 155b
  cross section of, 155f
  function of, 143, 156–157
  mean pressure in, 144
  structure of, 154–155, 154b
Capillary bed, 141f, 155f
Capillary loop, in dermal ridge, 55f
Capillary lumen, 155f
Capillary oncotic pressure, 156
Capillary pressure, 156
  regulation of, 156
Capillary refill time (CRT), 155b
Capillary system, 154–157
Capitate bone, 418f–419f
Capsular fibres
  arrangement of, hip joint capsule to, 585f
  of knee joint, 599f
Capsular ligaments, associated with hip joint, 585f

Capsular space, 516f
Capsule
    anterior part of, 392
    of kidney, 512f
Carbohydrates, 497–498
    absorption of, 497
    digestion of, 497, 497t
    metabolism of, 497–498, 498f
        insulin effect on, 347–348
        in liver, 508, 508b
Carbon dioxide, 109
Carbon monoxide poisoning, 113
Carbonic anhydrase, 507
    diuretics inhibiting, 522
Cardia, 465f
Cardiac arrest, 133
Cardiac cycle, 127–133, 127b, 129f
    electrocardiogram and, 129–130,
        129f
Cardiac function curves, 135–136, 137f
Cardiac muscle, 39, 39f, 39b
Cardiac nerves, from sympathetic
    trunk, 84f
Cardiac notch, 99f
Cardiac output, 133–136, 133b, 134f,
    144
Cardiac output curves, 135–136, 135f
Cardiac tamponade, 136b
Cardiac veins, 125–126
Cardiogenic shock, 159
Cardiovascular hypertension, 149
Cardiovascular system, 116–164, 117f,
    117b
    cardiac cycle, 127–133, 127b, 129f
    cardiac output, 133–136, 133b,
        134f
    circulation, 143–164
    great vessels, 136–143
    heart, 118–127, 119b
Carotid canal, 244t
Carotid sheath, 319f, 325
Carotid sinus branch, of
    glossopharyngeal nerve, 279f
Carotid triangle, 318f, 321–324
Carpometacarpal joints, 380f, 419f,
    426–427
    1st, 419f, 428f
Carpus, 420, 420f, 420b
Cartilage, 28–29, 28b, 31f
Cartilage end plate, 198, 198f
Cartilaginous joints, of bone, 35–36,
    36f, 36b

Catecholamines, secretion of,
    immediate compensatory effects
    on, 158
Cathelicidins, 179, 179t
Cauda equina, 222f
Caveolae, 154
Cavernous sinus, 270, 271f–272f, 292f,
    296f
CCK. See Cholecystokinin
Cecum, 471f, 473f
Cell(s), 9–19, 9f–10f
    of blood, 165–176, 166f
    cell membrane in, 9–12, 9f–10f
        transport across, 11–12, 11f, 12b
    cycle of, 17, 18f
    cytoplasm in, 9f–10f, 12–15
        cytoskeleton, 15, 15f
        endoplasmic reticulum, 12, 13f,
            15f–16f
        Golgi apparatus, 10f, 12, 13f
        lysosome, 10f, 12–13, 13f, 13b
        mitochondria, 10f, 14f, 14b
        peroxisome, 10f, 13–14, 14b
        proteasomes, 14, 14b
    nucleus in, 9f–10f, 15–17, 16f
        chromatin, 10f, 17
        nuclear membrane, 9f, 16–17
        nucleolus, 9f–10f, 16f, 17, 17b
    stem, 17–19, 18f
    in meiosis, 19
    types and their function, 9t
Cell membrane, 9–12, 9f–10f
    transport across, 11–12, 11f, 12b
Cell-mediated reactions, 180
Cell-to-cell adhesion, of epithelium,
    20–23, 22f
    adherent junctions, 22–23, 23b
    gap junctions, 23, 23b
    tight junctions, 22, 22b
Cellular immunity, development of,
    177
Cellular vesicles, formation of, 13f
Cementum, 310f
Central axillary lymph nodes, 402f
Central canal, of spinal cord, 210f
Central chemoreceptors, 111
Central grey matter, 210f
Central lymph nodes, 399f, 403f
Central nervous system, 356f, 360f
Central retinal artery, 296f
Central sulcus, 256–257, 257f
Central tendon, 75f

Centrilobular emphysema, 114, 115f,
    115b
Centroacinar cells, 483f
Centrosome, 10f
Cephalic phase, of gastric secretion,
    490f
Cephalic vein, 399f, 417f, 419f, 437f
    of arm, 402, 402f–403f, 412f
    of forearm, 414
Cerebellar peduncles, 249f
Cerebellum, 248f, 252–253, 253b, 255f,
    262f, 269
Cerebral aqueduct, 255f, 261f
Cerebral arteries, 267–269
Cerebral cortex, 265f, 269
Cerebral hemisphere, 257f
Cerebral medulla, 259–260, 259f, 259b
Cerebral peduncle, anterior part of, 250
Cerebral projections, 269
Cerebral veins, 269–270, 270b
Cerebrospinal fluid, 261–262, 262b
Cerebrum, 248f, 256–262, 259f
Cervical canal, 544f
Cervical cardiac nerves, 70f
Cervical curvature, 189, 189f
Cervical enlargement, 208f
Cervical fibroid, 548f
Cervical ganglia, 90f
Cervical pleura, 95
Cervical plexus, 223, 223f
Cervical region, 189f
    intervertebral disc of, 198f
    zygapophyseal joints of, 200f
Cervical sympathetic fibres, 248b
Cervical vertebrae, 193–194,
    193f–194f, 193b
    1st, 193–194, 193f
    2nd, 193f, 194
    7th, 193f, 194, 194b
    in neck, 317
Cervix, 544f, 548f
Chagas disease, 464b
Chemical messengers, different types
    of, 336f
Chemokines, 178, 179t
Chemoreceptors, 150
Chest wall
    arterial supply to, 76f
    venous drainage of, 77f
Cheyne-Stokes breathing, 112, 112f
Chief cells, 466f
Chloride, 507

Cholangiocytes, 480f
Cholecystokinin (CCK), 482, 486–487, 486f, 492f
Cholesterol, 500
Chondroblasts, 9t, 28b
Chondrocytes, 28b
Chorda tympani, 312f, 314b
Chorda tympani syndrome, 489
Chordae tendineae, 120f, 121
Chorion, 363f, 549f
Chorionic epithelium, 363f
Chorionic plate, 549f
Choroid, 297–298, 297f
Choroid plexus, 260–261, 261b, 269
Chromatin, 10f, 17
Chronic (intrinsic) asthma, 115
Chronic bronchitis, 114
Chronic disease anaemia, 171, 171t
Chronic gastritis, 491b
Chronic haemorrhage, 157
Chronic heart failure, 160
Chronic obstructive pulmonary disease, 114
Chronic renal failure, 522
Chylomicrons, 499
Cigarette smoke, respiratory epithelium and, 95b
Ciliary body, 298
Ciliary ganglion, 225, 226f, 295–297, 296f
Ciliary muscle, 226f, 298f
Ciliary process, 298f
Cingulum, 259
Circular muscle, 298f
Circulation, 143–164
    blood in, distribution of, 144f
    pressures in, 144, 145f
Circulatory shock, 158–159
Circumflex branch, of left coronary artery, 125f
Circumflex scapular artery, 386f
Circumflex subscapular artery, 397f
Circumvallate papilla, 311f
Cirrhosis, 481b, 508b
Cisterna chyli, 89–90, 89f, 96f
Citrates, 176
Clavicle, 318f, 321f, 323f, 379–381, 379b, 380f, 381b, 382f–383f, 386f, 399f
    movements of, 382–383, 384f
Clavicular notch, 68f
Clavipectoral fascia, 399f

Cleavage, 361–363, 361f
Cleavage lines, of skin, 57, 57f, 57b
Clitoris, 552, 552f
Cloacal membrane, 478f
Closed foramen ovale, 123f
Closed fracture, of bone, 33
Coagulation, 175–176, 175t
Cobalt, 507
Coccygeal plexus, of lumbosacral plexus, 581f
Coccygeus muscle, 460f, 460t, 554f
Coccyx, 195, 195b, 197f, 551f, 553f, 566f, 569–570, 569b–570b, 571f
Cochlea, 316f
Cochlear duct, 316f
Cochlear nerve, 316f
Coeliac disease, 20b, 471b
Coeliac ganglion, 91f
Coeliac trunk, 91f
Colic artery, 476f
Collagen fibres
    in connective tissues, 26–27, 26f
    in interstitium, 157f
    in muscle contraction, 43f
Collapsing (water hammer) pulse, 152b
Collateral ligaments, 431f, 601–602, 601f–602f, 601b–602b, 632f
Collecting system, function of, 518t
Colles' fascia, 452f–453f, 555
Colles' fractures, of radius, 406f, 406b
Colliculus, 249f, 251
Colloid, 341f
Colon, 470f, 472–476, 473f–474f, 475b, 511f
    arterial supply to, 475–476, 476f, 476b
    irritation of, 496b
    lymphatic drainage of, 475–476
    venous drainage of, 475–476
Colorectal cancer, 477b
Comminuted fracture, of bone, 34, 34f
Commissural fibres, 259–260
Common carotid artery, 312f, 319f, 321f
Common fibular nerve, 581f, 593f, 611f, 639f, 640
Common iliac artery, 91f, 477f, 525f
Common palmar digital arteries, 437f
Common peroneal nerve, 612f, 639f, 640
Compact bone, 30f, 32f–33f
Compartments, 325

Compensatory hyperplasia, 481b
Complement proteins, immunity and, 177t
Complement system, 178
Complete facet, on transverse process, 195f
Complete fracture, of bone, 33
Complete heart block, 131–132
Complete transection, in spine, 219
Compliance, breathing and, 102, 103f
Compression fracture, of bone, 34
Conchae, 304, 306f, 315f
Conducting system, 126–127, 126f, 127b
Condyloid joint, of bone, 38
Congestive cardiac failure, 160
Conjoint tendon, 455f–456f, 458f
Conjunctiva, 297, 297f, 302f
Connective tissues, 25–38, 26f, 139f
    blood, 38
    capsule of, 341f
    cells, 25–26
    fibres, 26–27
    ground substance in, 26f, 27
    type of, 27–38
        adipose tissue, 27–28, 28b
        bone, 29–34, 29f, 29b
        cartilage, 28–29, 28b, 31f
Conoid ligament, 387f
Constipation, 495b
Contractile cells, function of, 9t
Contrecoup injuries, 259f, 259b
Conus arteriosus, 121
Conus elasticus, 330f
Conus medullaris, of spinal cord, 208f
Copper, 507
Coracoacromial ligament, 386f, 391f
Coracobrachialis muscle, 394t, 399f, 439f
Coracoclavicular ligament, 391f
Coracohumeral ligament, 391f
Coracoid process, 385f–386f
Cornea, 297, 297f–298f
Corniculate cartilage, 330, 330f
Cornu, 197f
    of coccyx, 197f
    of sacrum, 197f
Corona radiata, 357f
Coronal suture, 235f, 240f
Coronary arteries, 124, 138
Coronary sinus, 120f, 125–126, 125f
Coronoid fossa, 390f

Coronoid process, 282f, 405f

Corpora cavernosa, 540f, 552f

Corpus callosum, 255f, 257f, 260, 267–268, 268b

Corpus cavernosum, 539f

Corpus luteum, 357f, 358

Corpus spongiosum, 539f–540f

Corpus striatum, 260, 260b, 269

Corrugator supercilii, 293f

Cortex, of kidney, 162f, 344f, 512f

Cortical nephron, 513b, 514f

Corticonuclear fibres, 215f

Corticonuclear tract, 216, 216b

Corticopontocerebellar pathway, 216–217

Corticospinal fibres, 215f

Corticospinal tract, 215–216, 216b, 263

Cortisol, 344f
  regulation of, 346, 346f

Costal cartilage, 68, 68f, 72f, 382f

Costal facet, on transverse process, 195f

Costal fibres, 75f

Costal margin, 470f

Costal pleura, 95

Costocervical trunk, 76f, 333f

Costochondral joint, 69f

Costoclavicular ligament, 382f, 384f

Costoclavicular roughened area, 382f

Costodiaphragmatic recess, 95, 97b

Costomediastinal recess, 95

Costosternal joint, 69f

Costotransverse joint, 69f, 73f

Costovertebral joint, 69f, 73f

Cough reflex, 116

Coup injuries, 259f, 259b

Coup-contrecoup injuries, 259f, 259b

Cowper's gland, 535f, 537

Cranial cavity, 234–235, 242–243
  drainage to cavernous sinus in, 308f

Cranial nerve nuclei, 251

Cranial nerves, 270–280

Cretinism, 342

Cribriform plate, 243t

Cricoid cartilage, 329, 329f–330f

Cricothyroid ligament, 329f

Cricothyroid membrane, 330

Crista terminalis, 120f

Crohn disease, 475b, 476f

Crossed dystopia, 510b

Crossed extensor reflex, 218, 218f

CRT. *See* Capillary refill time

Cruciate ligaments, 602–604, 603f–604f, 603b–604b

Crus
  of clitoris, 552f
  of penis, 540f

Crus cerebri, 249f, 254f

C-type lectin, 176

C-type natriuretic peptide, 151

Cubital fossa, 411–412, 411b–412b, 412f–413f

Cubital lymph nodes, 402f

Cuboid bone, 566f, 625f, 628f, 630f

Cuneiform bones, 566f, 625f, 628f

Cuneiform cartilage, 330

Curvatures, 189–190, 189f

Cushing syndrome, 502b

Cushing's disease, 340

Cutaneous nerves, of lumbar plexus, 578f

Cyanosis, 113

Cystic duct, 469f

Cystic fibrosis, 507b

Cystitis, 527b

Cytokines, 178–179, 179t

Cytoplasm, 9f–10f, 12–15
  cytoskeleton, 15, 15f
  endoplasmic reticulum, 12, 13f, 15f–16f
  Golgi apparatus, 10f, 12, 13f
  lysosome, 10f, 12–13, 13f, 13b
  mitochondria, 10f, 14f, 14b
  in myelinated axon, 48f
  peroxisome, 10f, 13–14, 14b
  proteasomes, 14, 14b

Cytoskeleton, 15, 15f

Cytotoxic reactions, 180

Cytotoxic T (CD8) cells, 177

Cytotrophoblast, 362f

Cytotrophoblastic shell, 549f

D

Dartos fascia, 452f–453f

Decidua basalis, 549f

Decidua parietalis, 549f

Decussation, of pyramids, 208f

Deep cardiac plexus, 126

Deep cervical artery, 333f

Deep cervical lymph chain, 319f

Deep cervical lymph nodes, 403f

Deep external pudendal artery, 591f

Deep facial vein, 292f

Deep fascia
  in ankle joint, 623f
  of forearm, 412f

Deep fibular/peroneal nerve, 613, 613b, 614f, 616f, 623f, 629–634, 639f, 640

Deep inguinal nodes, 557f

Deep inguinal ring, 458f

Deep lingual vein, 312f

Deep palmar arch, 437f

Deep part medial (tibial) collateral ligaments, 601f

Deep perineal pouch, 554f

Deep transverse metacarpal ligament, 427f, 431f

Deep transverse metatarsal ligament, 632f

Deep vein thrombosis (DVT), 142

Defaecation, 496, 496f, 496b

Defensins, 178, 179t

Degenerating corpus luteum, 357f

Delayed compensatory effects, 158

Deltoid ligament, 620f

Deltoid muscle, 392f, 394t, 397f, 399f

Deltoid tubercle, 382f

Deltoid tuberosity, 390f

Deltopectoral lymph nodes, 402f

Dendrites, in neuron, 46f, 47

Dens, facet for, 193f

Dense connective tissue, of scalp, 237, 237f

Dense granules, 174t

Denticulate ligament, 208f, 220f

Dentine, 310f

Depressor anguli oris muscle, 293f, 294

Depressor labii inferioris muscle, 293f, 294

Depressors, of vasomotor centre, for hypertension, 149

Dermal papilla, 55f–56f

Dermatomes, of lower limb and foot, 640f

Dermis, 55f–56f, 56–57, 56b

Descending aorta, 87, 87b, 123f, 483f

Descending branch, of lateral circumflex artery, 591f

Descending colon, 473f

Descending genicular artery, 591f

Descending (motor) tracts, of spinal cord, 212f, 214–217, 215f, 215b–216b

Dextrocardia, 118b

Diabetes insipidus, 340
Diabetes mellitus, 349–351, 350t, 484b, 515b
    type I, 349–350, 350t
    type II, 350
Diapedesis, 172–173
Diaphragm, 73–75, 74b, 81f–82f, 85f, 96f, 451f, 454f, 478f, 511f
    inferior aspect of, 75f
    oesophageal opening in, 91f
Diaphragma sellae, 264
Diaphragmatic peritoneum, 92b
Diaphragmatic pleura, 95
Diaphragmatic surface, of heart, 119
Diaphysis, of bone, 30f
Diarrhoea, 494b
Diastole, 127
Diastolic pressure, 147, 148t
Dicoumarol, 176
Diencephalon, 253–256
Dietary fats, 498, 499t
Dietary fibre, 494–495
Differentiation, stages of, 353f
Diffusion, 156, 156f
Digastric muscle, 278f, 281f, 289t–290t, 323f, 324t
    anterior belly of, 318f
    posterior belly of, 318f
Digestion, 485
Digestive gland cells, function of, 9t
Digestive system, 461–464
    development of, 461b, 462f, 463b, 478f
    physiology of, 485–508
        chewing (mastication) and swallowing, 488
        energy storage, 485–488
        mixing and propulsion of food, 488–496
        mixing of food, 489–495, 490f, 490b–493b, 492f–494f
        movement of food through, 495–496
        nutrition, 497–508
        regulation of food intake, 485–488
        secretion, 488–489, 488b
Digestive tract, 463f, 464–485
    layers of, 463f
    movement of food through, 495–496
    structure of, 463–464, 463f, 464b
Digestive vesicle, lysosome enzymes in, 13f

Digital arteries, in foot, 615f
Digital fibrous sheath, 427f
Digital lymphatic vessels, 402f
Digital synovial sheath, 426f
Diploe, 234
Displaced fracture, of bone, 33
Dissecting aneurysms, 142f, 142b
Distal convoluted tubule, 519, 519b
    cellular structure and transport characteristics of, 520f
    function of, 518t
Distal phalanx, 60f, 426f–427f
Distal tubule, 516f–517f
Diuretics
    for hypertension, 148
    urine formation and, 521–522
Diurnal variation, arterial blood pressure and, 148
Dorsal branch of ulnar nerve, 439f
Dorsal calcaneocuboid ligament, 627f
Dorsal column, 213f
Dorsal cutaneous branch of ulnar nerve, 419f
Dorsal digital artery, 426f
Dorsal digital expansion, 434f
Dorsal digital nerve, 426f
Dorsal horn, of spinal cord, 210f
Dorsal interossei muscle, 429t–430t, 433t, 633f, 633t–634t
    4th, 434f
Dorsal lingual vein, 312f
Dorsal metatarsal arteries, in foot, 615f
Dorsal motor nucleus, of vagus, 279
Dorsal nasal artery, 291f, 296f
Dorsal nasal vein, 291f
Dorsal nuclei, 253
Dorsal pancreas, 478f
Dorsal rami, 79f, 222f, 594f
Dorsal respiratory group, 110, 110f
Dorsal root, 220f, 222f
Dorsal root ganglion, 217f, 220f
Dorsal scapular nerve, 401t
Dorsal surface, of hand, 380f
Dorsal talonavicular ligament, 627f
Dorsal tarsometatarsal ligaments, 631f
Dorsal tubercle, 405f
Dorsal venous arch, 437f, 592f
Dorsal venous network, 629–634
Dorsalis pedis artery, 615f, 629, 629b

Dorsum
    of foot, 619f, 629–634
        deep fibular/peroneal nerve in, 629–634
        dorsal venous network in, 629–634
        dorsalis pedis artery in, 629, 629b
        superficial fibular/peroneal nerve in, 629
    of lower limb, 566f
Double gallbladder, 482b
Drooling, 489
Duct of sweat gland, 55f
Duct system, 367f
Ductule, 367f
Ductus arteriosus, 123f
Ductus deferens, 533f, 534–535, 535f, 535b, 575f
Ductus venosus, 123f
Duodenal papilla, 469f
Duodenal ulcer, 467b, 491b
Duodenojejunal junction, 473f
Duodenum, 454f, 468, 468b, 469f, 478f, 483f, 492f, 511f
Dupuytren's contracture, 425f, 425b
Dura mater, 208f, 220f, 264, 265f, 272f, 315f
Dural sac, 220f
Dural sleeve, 220f
Dural venous sinuses, 138
DVT. See Deep vein thrombosis
Dwarfism, 340
Dyspnoea, 111
Dystrophia adiposogenitalis (Frolich's syndrome), 340, 340b

E
Ear, 314–317, 314b
Eccrine sweat glands, 60–61, 61b
ECG. See Electrocardiogram
Ectopic arrhythmias, 131–133
Edinger-Westphal nucleus, 251, 273
EDTA. See Ethylenediaminetetraacetic acid
Efferent arteriole, 516f–517f
Efferent ductules, 533f
Efferent lymphatic vessel, 162f
Efferent pathways, of autonomic nervous system, 224f
Efferent tracts, of spinal cord, 212–217, 212f
Ejaculation, 539–541, 541b

Ejaculatory duct, 535f
Elastic cartilage, 29
Elastic fibres, 26f, 27, 139f
Elasticity, breathing and, 102
Elbow joint, 380f, 407–409, 407f–408f, 407b
  attachments, action and innervation of muscles, 410t
  axis of, 407f
  of upper limb, 442t
Electrocardiogram (ECG), 127–130, 128f–129f
  in bradycardia, 131f
  cardiac cycle and, 129–130, 129f
  recording, 130
  in tachycardia, 131f
Electrolytes, active reabsorption of, diuretics inhibiting, 522
Ellipsoid joint, of bone, 38
Embryo, veins of, 137b
Embryonic ectoderm, 362f
Embryonic endoderm, 362f
Emotions, 287
  arterial blood pressure and, 148
  heart rate and, 135
Emphysema, 114–115, 115f, 115b
Empyema, 97b
Enamel, 310f
Endocardium, 20
Endochondral ossification, of bone, 31
Endocrine cells, 466f
Endocrine glands, 23–25, 24f, 334–370, 334b
  adrenal (suprarenal) glands, 343–347
  gonads, 351–367
  heart, 368–369
  hypothalamus, 369
  Islets of Langerhans, 347–351, 347f
  kidneys, 368
  local hormones, 369–370
  parathyroid glands, 342–343
  pineal gland, 368, 368b
  pituitary gland, 335–340, 338f, 339t
  position of, 337f
  thymus, 369
  thyroid gland, 340–342, 341b
Endocrine hypertension, 149
Endocrine messenger, 336f
Endocrine system, 333–334, 334b
Endocytosis, 11–12, 11f
Endometrial epithelium, 362f
Endometriosis, 547b

Endometrium, 362f, 546, 548f
  arterial supply to, 546f
  changes of, 545f
Endomysium, 40f
Endoneurium, 50, 51f
Endoplasmic reticulum, 12, 13f, 15f–16f
  rough endoplasmic reticulum, 10f, 12, 12b
  smooth endoplasmic reticulum, 10f, 12, 12b
Endosteal cells, 31f
Endosteum, of bone, 30f
Endothelial cell, 155f
Endothelium, 20, 137, 139f, 155f
Enteric nervous system, 464, 464f, 464b
Enterocytes, 469
Eosinopenia, 173
Eosinophils, 172f, 172t, 173
Ependymal cells, 247, 247f
Epicardium, 85
Epicondyles, of humerus, 407b
Epidermis, 55–56, 55f–56f, 55b–56b
Epididymis, 533f, 534, 534b
Epididymitis, 534b
Epiglottis, 311f, 329, 329f–330f
Epimysium, 40f
Epinephrine, 497–498
Epineurium, 50, 51f
Epiphyseal line, 30f, 392f
Epiphysis, of bone, 30f
Epispadias, 539b
Epithalamus, 254f, 255
Epithelial alveolar cell, 367f
Epithelial cells
  function of, 9t
  junctional complexes of, 22f
Epithelium, in tissues, 19–25
  classification of, 20, 21f
  function of, 20–23
    cell apex, 20, 20b
    cell base, 23
    cell-to-cell adhesion, 20–23, 22f
    secretory epithelia and glands, 23–25, 25b
      endocrine glands, 23–25, 24f
      exocrine glands, 23, 24f–25f
Eponychium, 60f
Erection, 539–541, 541b
Erector spinae, 205t–206t
ERV. See Expiratory reserve volume
Erythrocyte sediment rate (ESR), 168

Erythrocytes, 165–172, 167f, 167t, 167b
  destruction of, 168
  function of, 167
  values of, normal, 167t
Erythropoiesis, control of, 167
Erythropoietin, 368, 515, 515b
ESR. See Erythrocyte sediment rate
Essential amino acids, 504
Ethmoid bone, 295f
  orbital plate of, 307f
  perpendicular plate of, 305f
  uncinate process of, 305f
Ethmoid sinus, 306
Ethmoidal bulla, 306f
Ethmoidal cells, 307f
Ethmoidal foramina, 295f
Ethylenediaminetetraacetic acid (EDTA), 176
Eupnoea, 111
Eversion, 626–627, 630f, 630t–631t
Excretory genital ducts, 534–535
Exercise
  arterial blood pressure and, 148
  effect of, in respiratory physiology, 111
  heart rate and, 135
Exocrine glands, 23, 24f–25f
Exocytosis, 11–12
Expiration, 102
Expiratory reserve volume (ERV), 103
Expired air, 105, 105t
Extension
  of metacarpophalangeal joints, 428
  of shoulder joint, 395, 395f
  of wrist, 421–422, 422f
Extensor carpi radialis brevis muscle, 410t, 417f, 419f, 421f, 423t–424t
Extensor carpi radialis longus muscle, 410t, 417f, 419f, 421f, 423t–424t
Extensor carpi radialis muscle, 422f
Extensor carpi ulnaris muscle, 410t, 417f, 419f, 421f–422f, 423t–424t
Extensor digit minimi muscle, 410t, 419f, 421f, 423t–424t, 429t–430t
Extensor digitorum brevis muscle, 619f, 633t–634t
Extensor digitorum longus muscle, 610f, 614f–615f, 619f, 622f, 623f, 630t–631t, 633f
Extensor digitorum muscle, 410t, 417f, 419f, 421f, 423t–424t, 429t–430t
Extensor digitorum tendon, 431f, 434f

Extensor expansion, 426f, 431f
Extensor hallucis brevis muscle, 619f, 633t–634t
Extensor hallucis longus muscle, 614f–615f, 619f, 622t, 623f, 630t–631t
Extensor indicis muscle, 419f, 421f, 423t–424t, 429t–430t
Extensor pollicis brevis muscle, 419f, 421f, 423t–424t, 429t–430t
Extensor pollicis longus muscle, 417f, 419f, 421f, 423t–424t, 429t–430t
Extensor pollicis longus tendon, 431f
Extensor retinaculum, 421f
External anal sphincter, 551f, 555–556, 556f, 556b
External auditory meatus, 315f
External carotid artery, 237f, 266f, 279f–281f, 285f, 291f
External carotid plexus, 90f
External ear, 314
External genitalia
    female, 552–555
    male, 555, 555b
External iliac artery, 524f–525f, 579
External iliac nodes, 557f
External iliac vein, 524f, 575f, 579
External intercostal muscle, 79f
External jugular vein, 237f, 291f, 321f–322f
External nasal artery, 307f, 309f
External nasal nerve, 276f
External nose, 304, 304f, 304b
External oblique muscle, 207f, 452f–453f, 455f–456f, 457t, 458f, 570f
External os, 544f
External respiration, 104–106, 105t, 106f, 106b
External urethral orifice, 540f
Extracardiac pressure, changes in, 136
Extracellular matrix, in connective tissues, 26f
Extra-embryonic endoderm, 362f
Extra-embryonic mesoderm, 362f
Extraglomerular mesangial cells, 517f
Extraocular muscles, 300, 300f, 301t
Extraperitoneal fascia, 452f–453f
Extrapyramidal system, 216, 216b, 263
Extrasystole, 132
Eye
    horizontal section through, 298f
    muscles around, 292–294, 294b

Eyeball, 297–300, 297f, 297b
    arterial supply to, 296f
    horizontal section through, 297f
    inner nervous layer of, 299–300
    middle vascular layer of, 298–299, 299b
    movement of, 300–302
    outer fibrous layer of, 297–298, 298b
    protection of, 300–302
Eyelids, 300, 300b, 302f

F
Face, 287–317
    arterial supply to, 287–288
    blood supply and innervation to, 287–292
    ear, 314–317, 314b
    external nose, 304, 304f, 304b
    innervation of, 292
    lymphatic drainage of, 290
    muscles of, 292–294, 292b, 293f
    nasal cavity, 304–308, 305f, 309f
    oral cavity, 308–314, 310f, 311b
    superficial and deep vasculature of, 291f
    vasculature of, 291f
    venous drainage of, 290b
Facial artery, 291f
Facial nerve, 276–277, 277b, 278f, 316f
    buccal branches, 278f
    cervicofacial branch, 278f
    digastric branch, 278f
    marginal mandibular branches, 278f
    temporal branches, 278f
    temporofacial branch, 278f
    zygomatic branches, 278f
Facial vein, 291f–292f
    drainage to, 308f
Falciform ligament, 478f, 478f
Fallopian tube. See Uterine tube
Fallot's tetralogy, 118b
Falx cerebelli, 264
Falx cerebri, 264, 265f, 271f
Fascia
    compartments of, 325
    prevertebral layer of, 319f
Fascia lata, 452f–453f
Fascial spaces, 325, 326f
Fascicle, in peripheral nerves, 50, 51f
Fasciculus, 40f, 244–245, 245f
Fasciculus uncinatus, 259
Fat cells, function of, 9t

Fat pad, in synovial joints, 37f
Fats, 486f, 498–503
    absorption of, 499–500
    digestion of, 498, 499t
    metabolism of, 501–502, 502f, 502b
        insulin effect on, 348, 348b
        in liver, 508
Fatty liver disease, 480b
Female reproductive system, 541–542
Femoral artery, 524f, 589f, 590, 591f
Femoral branch, of genitofemoral nerve, 578f
Femoral condyles, axes of, 599f
Femoral hernia, 458
Femoral nerve, 578f–579f, 589f, 592–593, 638, 639f
Femoral sheath, 458f, 589f
Femoral triangle, 588–589, 589f, 589b
    lymph nodes of, 589, 590f
    vessels in, 591f
Femoral vein, 524f, 589f, 591–592, 591f, 591b–592b
Femoral vessels, 580f
Femur, 37f, 566f, 582–584, 582b, 583f–584f, 584b
    head of, 583f–584f
    hip joint capsule to, 585f
    patella with, movement of, 608f, 610f
Fenestra, 155f
Fertilisation, 361–363, 361f, 542b
Fetal capillaries, 363f
Fetal circulation, 549f
FEV. See Forced expiratory volume
Fibres connecting sesamoid bone, 431f
Fibrinogen, 165, 504
Fibrinolysis, 175
Fibroblasts, 352f
    in connective tissues, 25, 26f
    function of, 9t
Fibrocartilage, 28
Fibrocartilaginous disc, 570f
Fibroids, 548f, 548b
Fibro-osseous tunnels, 634
Fibroserous sac, 84
Fibrosomes, 10f
Fibrous astrocyte, 246f–247f, 247
Fibrous connective tissue, of scalp, 237
Fibrous flexor sheaths, 427f, 431f
Fibrous joint capsule, 37f, 284, 382
Fibrous joints, of bone, 35, 36f
Fibrous pericardium, 84–85, 85b
Fibrous ring, 119f

Fibrous tissue, 119f
Fibula, 566f, 597f, 598, 598b
  anterior border of, 597f
  anterior surface of, 597f
  head of, 597f
  interosseous border of, 597f
  lateral malleolus of, 597f
  lateral surface of, 597f
  medial crest of, 597f
  neck of, 597f
  shaft of, 597f
  triangular subcutaneous area of, 597f
Fibularis (peroneus) brevis muscle,
    614f, 619f, 622t, 623f, 630t–631t
Fibularis (peroneus) longus muscle,
    610f, 614f, 617f, 619f, 622t, 623f,
    630t–631t
Fibularis (peroneus) tertius muscle,
    619f, 622t, 623f
Fibular/peroneal artery, 614, 618f
Filtration, of substances, 156–157
Filtration membrane, of kidney, 516f
Filum terminale, 208f
Fimbria, 541f
Fingers
  joint, of upper limb, 443, 443t
  movements of, 432f
First metatarsal, of foot, 627f
1st-degree heart block, 131
Flatulence, 496b
Flatus, 496b
Flexion
  axis of, 422f
  of metacarpophalangeal joints, 428
  of shoulder joint, 395, 395f
  of wrist, 421–422, 422f
Flexor accessorius muscle, 633t–634t,
    635f
Flexor carpi radialis muscle, 410t,
    417f, 419f, 421f–422f, 423t–424t,
    426f
Flexor carpi ulnaris muscle, 410t, 417f,
    423t–424t
Flexor digiti minimi brevis muscle,
    429t–430t, 433t, 633t–634t
Flexor digitorum brevis muscle, 633f,
    633t–634t, 635f
Flexor digitorum longus muscle, 614f,
    619f, 622t, 623f, 630t–631t, 633f
Flexor digitorum profundus muscle,
    417f, 419f, 423t–424t, 426f–427f,
    429t–430t, 434f, 439f

Flexor digitorum superficialis muscle,
    410t, 417f, 419f, 423t–424t,
    426f–427f, 429t–430t, 434f, 440f
Flexor hallucis brevis muscle,
    633t–634t
Flexor hallucis longus muscle, 614f,
    619f, 622t, 623f, 630t–631t
Flexor pollicis brevis muscle, 433t
Flexor pollicis longus muscle, 417f,
    419f, 421f, 423t–424t, 426f,
    429t–430t
Flexor reflex, 218, 218f
Flexor retinaculum, 419f, 426f,
    439f–440f, 619f, 623f
Flexor tendons, in fingers, 426f
Fluorine, 507
Foetal adrenal glands, 364
Foetal skull, 236f
Folic acid, 506
  deficiency anaemia, 171
  for red blood cell synthesis, 167
Follicle-stimulating hormone (FSH),
    339t
Follicular cells, 340–341, 341f
Food intake, regulation of, 485–488
  anorexia and, 487
  cachexia and, 487
  factors in, 486–487
  feedback mechanisms in, 486f
  inanition and, 487
  intermediate, 487
  long-term, 487
  neural, 485–486
  obesity and, 487
  short-term, 486–487
  starvation and, 487–488, 488f
Foot, 566f, 624–636, 624b, 625f
  dorsum of, 619f, 629–634
    deep fibular/peroneal nerve in,
      629–634
    dorsal venous network in,
      629–634
    dorsalis pedis artery in, 629, 629b
    superficial fibular/peroneal nerve
      in, 629
  function of, 636, 636b
  interphalangeal joints, 629, 629b, 633f
    movements in, 629
  joints of, 626, 627f
    movements in, 643
  metatarsals, 566f, 625f, 626, 626b,
    632f

Foot (Continued)
  metatarsophalangeal joints,
    627–629, 628b, 632f
    movements in, 628–629, 633f,
      633t–634t
  phalanges, 566f, 625f, 626, 626b
  plantar aspect (sole) of, 634–636
    fibro-osseous tunnels, 634
    lateral plantar artery, 635–636,
      635f, 635b–636b
    lateral plantar nerve, 634–635
    medial plantar artery, 635–636,
      635f, 635b–636b
    medial plantar nerve, 634–635
    plantar aponeurosis, 634–636,
      634b, 635f
  subtalar joint, 626, 628f
    movements in, 626–627, 629f
  tarsus, 625, 625f, 625b
  transverse (mid) tarsal joint,
    626–627, 628f
    movements in, 626–627, 629f
  walking and, 636, 637f
    cycle, 636, 636b, 638f
Foramen caecum, 243t, 308f, 311f
Foramen lacerum, 244t
Foramen magnum, 243f, 244t,
    266f
Foramen of Magendie, 252
Foramen of Monro, 261f
Foramen ovale, 123f, 244t, 276f
Foramen rotundum, 244t, 276f
Foramen spinosum, 244t
Foramen transversarium, 193f
Forced expiratory volume (FEV), 104,
    104f
Forearm, 380f, 404–418
  anterior aspect of, 416f
  attachments, action and innervation
    of muscles, 415t
  axis of, 427f
  compartments of, 414–418
    anterior, 414–418, 417f
    posterior, 418, 418f
  cubital fossa, 411–412, 411b–412b,
    412f–413f
  elbow joint, 407–409, 407f–408f,
    407b
  radioulnar joints, 412, 412b,
    413f–415f
  radius, 404–406, 404b, 405f
  ulna, 406–407, 406b–407b

Foregut
    arterial supply to, 467–468,
        467f–468f, 468b
    lymphatic drainage of, 467–468
    venous drainage of, 467–468
Forehead, muscles of, 292
Foreign bodies, in trachea, 95b
Forward dislocation, 286b
Fossa ovalis, 120, 120f
Fovea capitis, 583f
Fovea centralis, 297f
Frank-Starling mechanism, 133b
FRC. See Functional residual capacity
Free edge, 60f
Free fluid vesicles, 157f
Free nerve endings, 52, 52f, 56f
Frenulum, 310f
Friction, 145
Frontal bone, 234, 234b, 235f–236f,
        240, 240f, 243f, 295f, 305f
Frontal lobe, 257f, 259b, 262f
Frontal nerve, 275f, 296f
Frontal pole, 257f
Frontal sinus, 306, 306f–307f
Functional residual capacity (FRC),
        103
Fundiform ligament, of penis, 540f
Fundus
    of gallbladder, 482b
    of stomach, 465f
    of uterus, 544f
Fusiform aneurysms, 142f, 142b

G
Gait
    cycle of, 636, 638f
    determinates of, 637f
Gallbladder, 469f, 478f, 482, 482b
    emptying, 492f
Gallstones, 493f, 493b
Ganglion, 244–245, 245f
Gartner's duct, 550b
Gas exchange, 104, 104b
Gastric artery, 467f
Gastric atrophy, 491b
Gastric phase, of gastric secretion, 490f
Gastric pit, 466f
Gastric secretion, phases and
        regulation of, 490f
Gastric ulcer, 467b, 491b
Gastric varices, 468f
Gastritis, acute, 491b

Gastrocnemius muscle, 595t–596t,
        610f, 622t
    lateral head of, 599f, 611f, 614f, 617f
    medial head of, 599f, 611f, 614f, 617f
Gastrointestinal capillary membranes,
        154b
Gastrointestinal hormones, 488
Gastrointestinal tract, immunity and,
        177t
Gastro-oesophageal junction, 466b
Gastro-oesophageal reflux disease
        (GORD), 490b
Gastro-oesophageal varices (GOV), 468f
Gastro-omental artery, 467f
Gemelli muscles, 580f, 593f
Gemellus inferior muscle, 575t–577t,
        580f
Gemellus superior muscle, 575t–577t,
        580f
Gender
    arterial blood pressure and, 148
    heart rate and, 135
General resistance, of venous blood
        pressure, 153
General somatic afferent (GSA), 271
General somatic efferent (GSE), 272
General visceral afferent (GVA), 272
General visceral efferent (GVE), 272
Geniculate ganglion, 277
Genioglossus muscle, 313f
Geniohyoid muscle, 289t–290t, 324t
Genital ducts, female, 530f
Genitofemoral nerve, 578f, 639f
Germinal epithelium, 352f
Ghrelin, 485–486, 486f
Gigantism, 339
Glans clitoris, 550b, 552f
Glans penis, 526f, 540f
Glaucoma, 299b
Glenohumeral ligaments, 391f
Glenohumeral thickenings, 392f
Glenoid fossa, 385f
Glenoid labrum, 391f–392f
Glial cells, 247, 247f
Globulins, 146, 165, 504
Globus pallidus, 251
Glomerular capillaries, 154b, 517f
Glomerular filter, 516f
Glomerular filtration rate, diuretics
        inhibiting, 522
Glomerulonephritis, 515b
Glomerulus, 516f

Glossopharyngeal nerve, 248, 248b,
        277–279, 279f, 279b, 312f
Glucagon, 348–349, 497
Glucagon-like peptide, 486–487
Glucocorticoids, 345–347, 345b
Gluconeogenesis, 508, 515
Glucose, 497
Gluteal region, 580–582, 580f
    blood vessels of, 581–582
    intramuscular injection site in, 581f,
        581b
    in lower limb, 566f
    muscles in, 575t–577t
Gluteal tuberosity, 583f
Gluteus maximus muscle, 575t–577t,
        580f, 588b
Gluteus medius muscle, 575t–577t,
        580f
Gluteus minimus muscle, 575t–577t,
        580f
Glycoproteins, 174
Golgi apparatus, 10f, 12, 13f
Golgi tendon organs, location and
        microscopic appearance of, 40–41,
        42f
Golgi vesicle, 10f
Gomphosis, of fibrous joints, 35, 36f
Gonadal arteries, 525f
Gonads, 337f, 351–367
    ovaries, 356–361
    pregnancy, parturition and lactation,
        361–367
    testes, 351–356, 355b
Gonorrhoea, 550
GORD. See Gastro-oesophageal reflux
        disease
GOV. See Gastro-oesophageal varices
Gracile tract, 248
Gracilis muscle, 575t–577t, 580f, 589f,
        595t–596t, 610f–611f
Granulocytes, 172
    progenitor, 31f
Granulosa cell, 360f
Graves disease, 180
Gravity, of venous blood pressure, 153
Great auricular nerve, 239f
Great cardiac vein, 125–126, 125f
Great cerebral vein, 271f
Great saphenous vein, 138
Great vessels, 136–143
Greater auricular nerve, 322f
Greater curvature, of stomach, 465f

Greater occipital nerve, 239f
Greater omentum, 454f, 465, 465f, 465b, 478f
Greater palatine artery, 307f
Greater petrosal nerve, 315f
Greater sac, of peritoneal cavity, 454f
Greater sciatic foramen, 572f
Greater sciatic notch, 568f
Greater splanchnic nerve, 90f–91f, 91–92
Greater trochanter, of femur, 583f
Greater tubercle, 390f
Greater vestibular gland, 550, 552f
Greenstick fracture, 34, 34f, 406f, 406b
Grey matter, 211–212, 217f, 245f
 dorsal horn, 211–212
 lamination of, 211
 lateral horn, 212, 212f
 ventral horn, 212
Grey ramus communicans, 90–91, 90f–91f
Grip, types of, 436f
Groove
 of knee joint, 599f
 on medial condyle, 597f
Ground substance, in connective tissues, 26f, 27
Growth, effect on, 348, 348b
Growth hormone (GH), 337–339, 339t
 regulation of secretion, 338–339
GSA. *See* General somatic afferent
GSE. *See* General somatic efferent
Gums, 309–311
Gut tube, formation of, 462f
GVA. *See* General visceral afferent
GVE. *See* General visceral efferent

H
Haemangiomas, 143, 143b
Haematocrit, 146, 146f
Haematopoiesis, 515
Haematospermia, 537
Haemoglobin
 P50 of, 109
 restoration of, 158
 values of, normal, 167t
Haemolysis, in newborn, 170
Haemolytic anaemia, 169–170, 171t
Haemolytic disease, 169b
Haemophilia, 176b
Haemopoiesis, 166f
Haemorrhage, 157–158

Haemorrhagic anaemia, 169, 171t
Haemorrhoids, 556f, 556b
Haemostasis, 175
Haemothorax, 97b
Hair cells, 316f
Hair follicle, 56f
Hair papilla, 56f
Hairs, 56f, 58–60, 58b, 60b
Hamate bone, 418f–419f
Hamstrings, 580f, 586b
Hand, 380f, 424–435, 425b, 426f
 axis of, 427f
 blood supply and lymphatic drainage, 435, 435b
 carpometacarpal joints, 426–427, 428f
 function of, 432–435
 interphalangeal joints, 430
 metacarpals and phalanges, 425–426, 425b–426b, 427f
 metacarpophalangeal joints, 427–430, 428b, 431f
Hard palate, 310f
Hashimoto thyroiditis, 180
Haversian canal, 32f
Haversian system, 32f
HDLs. *See* High-density lipoproteins
Head, 231–376
 of humerus, 390f–392f
 injury to, 259f, 259b
 of radius, 405f
Hearing, 317, 317b
Heart, 118–127, 119b, 368–369
 apex of, 118
 arterial supply of, 125f
 base of, 118–119
 blood and nerve supply to, 124–127, 124b
 blood flow through, pattern of, 123–124, 123f
 chambers of, 119–121
 clinical physiology of, 126b
 congenital anomalies of, 118b
 coronal section of, 126f
 development of, 117f, 117b
 electrolyte concentrations on, 133
 fibrous framework of, 119f
 valves of, 121–122, 122b
Heart block, 131
Heart failure, 159–160
 compensatory mechanisms of, 159–160
 signs and symptoms of, 160

Heart rate, 134–135, 134f
Heart sounds, 122–123, 123b
Heart valve disorders, 122
Heimler syndrome, 14b
Helfet test, 607f, 607b
Helicobacter pylori, infection of, 467b, 491b
Helix, in ears, 315f
Helper T (CD4) cells, 177
Hemiazygos vein, 77f–78f, 89f
Hemisection, in spine, 219
Heparin, 176, 370
Hepatic artery, 467f, 479f
Hepatic duct, 469f, 478f
Hepatic lobules, 479f
Hepatic portal vein, 479f
Hepatic sinusoid, 479f
Hepatic veins, 524f
Hepatitis, 480b–481b
Hepatocytes, 479f–480f, 480
Hering-Breuer inflation reflex, 110, 110b
Herniae
 abdominal, 458, 458b
 femoral, 458
 inguinal, 458
HEV. *See* High endothelial venule
Hiatus hernia, 74b
High endothelial venule (HEV), 162f
High-density lipoproteins (HDLs), 500
Hilum, 98, 98f, 98b, 162f
Hinge joint, of bone, 38
Hip bone, in synovial joints, 37f
Hip joint, 566f, 584–588, 586b
 anterior relations of, 589f
 capsular attachment of, 585f
 capsular ligaments associated with, 585f, 586b
 movements in, 575t–577t, 586–588, 642
  abduction and adduction, 586, 587f
  flexion and extension, 586, 586b, 587f
  medial and lateral rotation, 586–588, 588f, 588b
 relations of, 580f, 588
Hirschsprung disease, 464b
Hirudin, 176
Histamines, 151, 369
Histotoxic hypoxia, 113
Holocrine secretion, 23, 25f

Homeostasis, 513–515
Hook of hamate, 418f
Horizontal fissure, 99f, 101f
Hormonal regulation, 150
Hormones, 334, 336t
    blood pressure and, 150–151, 151t
Horner syndrome, 248b
Horseshoe kidney, 510b
Human chorionic
    somatomammotropin secretion,
    364
Human spermatozoa, structure of, 354f
Humeral epicondyles, alignment of,
    409f, 409b
Humeral (lateral) lymph nodes,
    402f–403f
Humerus, 380f, 387–391, 387b, 390f,
    391b, 397f, 399f, 403f
    head of, 392f
    long axis of, 407f
    mid-shaft of, 403f
    surgical neck of, 390f
Humoral immunity, development of,
    178
Hunger pangs, 490b
Hyaline cartilage, 28, 28b, 36f, 570f
Hyaloid canal, 297f
Hydrogen ions, 111
Hyoglossus muscle, 279f, 281f,
    312f–313f
Hyoid bone, 318f, 323f, 325, 326f, 329f
Hyperadrenalism (Cushing's
    syndrome), 346–347
Hypercalcaemia, 133
Hypercapnia, 113
Hypereffective heart, 135
Hypergonadism, 356, 361
Hyperkalaemia, 133
Hypermetropia, 297f, 297b
Hyperpnoea, 112
Hypersalivation, 489b
Hypertension, 148
    during pregnancy, 149
    primary, 148
    secondary, 149, 149b
Hyperthyroidism, 342
Hyperventilation, 112
Hypoadrenalism/adrenal insufficiency
    (Addison's disease), 346
Hypocapnia, 113
Hypoeffective heart, 135–136
Hypoglossal canal, 244t

Hypoglossal nerve, 248, 280, 280b,
    281f, 312f
Hypoglossal nucleus, 248b, 280
Hypogonadism, 356, 356b, 361
Hypokalaemia, 133
Hypophysial stalk, 338f
Hypophysis, 255f
Hyposalivation, 489b
Hypospadias, 539b
Hypotension, 149
Hypothalamic-hypophysial portal
    vessels, 338f
Hypothalamic-hypophysial tract, 338f
Hypothalamo-hypophyseal portal
    system, 335–336
Hypothalamus, 248b, 255–256, 255f,
    256b, 337f–338f, 346f, 356f, 360f,
    369, 485–486, 486f
Hypothenar muscles, 419f
    nerve to, 439f
Hypothyroidism, 342
Hypoventilation, 112
Hypovolemic shock, 159
Hypoxia, 112–113
Hypoxic (arterial) hypoxia, 112
Hysterectomy, 548b

I

IBD. *See* Inflammatory bowel disease
IC. *See* Inspiratory capacity
IDDM. *See* Insulin-dependent diabetes
    mellitus
IDL. *See* Intermediate-density
    lipoproteins
IGV. *See* Isolated gastric varices
Ileocaecal fold flaps, 471f
Ileocaecal junction, 471f, 473f
Ileocaecal valve, 495, 495b
    emptying of, 496f
Ileocolic artery, 476f
Ileum, 468–471, 471f, 473f
    arterial supply to, 471f
Iliac crest, 568f
Iliac fossa, 568f
Iliac tuberosity, 568f
Iliacus muscle, 575f, 575t–577t, 579f,
    589f
Iliocostalis cervicis, 204f
Iliocostalis lumborum, 204f
Iliocostalis thoracis, 204f
Iliofemoral ligament, 585f
Iliohypogastric nerve, 511f, 578f, 639f

Ilioinguinal nerve, 511f, 578f, 639f
Iliolumbar ligaments, 572f
Iliopsoas muscle, 580f
Iliopubic eminence, 568f
Iliotibial tract, 599f, 610f
Ilium bone, 567, 568f
Immune deficiency diseases, 179–180
Immunisation, 179
Immunity, 176–180, 177t
Immunoglobulins, 178
Immunological hypersensitivity
    reactions, 180
Impacted fracture, of bone, 34
Implantation, of fertilised egg,
    361–363, 361f
Inanition, 487
Incisor crest, 305f
Incisura angularis, 465f
Incompetence, of heart, 122
Infantile Refsum disease, 14b
Infection, of bronchopulmonary
    segment, 99b
Inferior acromioclavicular ligament,
    386f
Inferior alveolar nerve, 285f
Inferior angle, 385f
Inferior articular facet, of vertebra, 196f
Inferior cerebellar peduncle, 248, 248b,
    252
Inferior cervical ganglion, 335f
Inferior colliculus, 251, 255f
Inferior concha, 306f–307f
Inferior demifacet, 73f
Inferior extensor retinaculum, 615f,
    619f, 623f, 628f
Inferior ganglion, 280f
Inferior gluteal artery, 575f
Inferior gluteal line, 568f
Inferior gluteal nerve, 580f–581f, 638
Inferior gluteal vessels, 580f, 581–582
Inferior horn, 261f
Inferior hypogastric plexus, 91f
Inferior labial artery, 291f
Inferior labial vein, 291f
Inferior lateral angle, of sacrum, 197f
Inferior lateral nasal nerves, nasal
    branch of, 309f
Inferior lobe, of lungs, 99f
Inferior longitudinal bundle, 259
Inferior meati, opening into, 306f
Inferior mesenteric artery, 91f, 476f
Inferior oblique muscle, 301t

Inferior ophthalmic vein, 275f, 296f
Inferior orbital fissure, 240f, 275f, 295f
Inferior parathyroid gland, 332f
Inferior phrenic veins, 524f
Inferior pubic ligament, 551f
Inferior radioulnar joint capsule, 380f, 416f, 419f
Inferior rectal artery, 477f
Inferior rectus muscles, 275f, 301t
Inferior sagittal sinus, 265f, 271f
Inferior salivary nucleus, 277–279
Inferior surface, of cerebral cortex, 269
Inferior thyroid artery, 321f, 332f–333f
Inferior thyroid vein, 332f
Inferior tibiofibular joint, 566f, 612, 613f
Inferior turbinate, 305f
Inferior ulnar collateral artery, 413f
Inferior vena cava, 74, 78f, 86f, 120f, 123f, 125f, 137, 483f, 524f, 589f
Inflammation, of gall bladder, 92b
Inflammatory bowel disease (IBD), 476f
Infraclavicular lymph nodes, 403f
Infraglenoid tubercle, 385f
Infrahyoid muscle, 323f, 324t, 326f
Infraorbital artery, 291f
Infraorbital foramen, 240f, 241t
Infraorbital nerve, 276f
  internal nasal branches of, 309f
Infraorbital vein, 292f, 296f
Infrapatellar branch, of saphenous nerve, 579f
Infrapatellar bursa, 600f
Infrapatellar fat pad, 600f
Infraspinatus muscle, 393f, 394t, 397f, 399f
Infraspinous fossa, 385f
Infratemporal fossa, 276f, 287, 287b
  drainage to pterygoid plexus in, 308f
Infratrochlear nerve, 276f, 296f
Infundibulum, 121, 255f, 262f, 264, 541f
Inguinal canal, 456–458, 457b–458b, 458f
Inguinal hernia, 458
Inguinal ligament, 452f–453f, 455f–456f, 589f
Inhibin, 356f, 360f
Inner ear, 316–317, 316f
Innermost intercostal muscle, 79f

Innervation
  of heart, 126
  of intervertebral disc, 202
  of palate, 314
  of tongue, 312
Innominate bone, 566f, 567–569, 567b, 568f
  ilium, 567, 568f
  ischium, 567, 568f
  pubis, 567–569, 568f, 569b
Inspiration, 75, 101–102
Inspiratory capacity (IC), 103, 103f
Inspiratory reserve volume (IRV), 103
Inspired air, 105, 105t
Insulin, 347–348, 348b, 485–486
Insulin-dependent diabetes mellitus (IDDM), 180, 484b
Insulinoma (hyperinsulinism), 350–351, 351b
Interatrial septum, development of, 117b
Intercalated duct, 483f
Intercarpal joints, 419f
Interchondral joint, 71f
Interclavicular ligament, 382f
Intercondylar eminence, 597f
Intercondylar line, 583f
Intercondylar notch, 583f
Intercostal muscles, 72–73, 73b, 74f
Intercostal nerve, 74f, 79f, 223f
  1st, 79
  2nd, 79
  3rd, 79
  6th, 79
  7th, 79
  11th, 79
Intercostal vessels, 74f
Interferons (IFN), 177t, 178, 179t
Interleukins (IL), 178, 179t
Intermediate cuneiform, 625f
Intermediate filament, 10f, 15, 15f, 15b
Intermediate sacral crest, 197f
Intermediate ventral nucleus, 253
Intermediate-density lipoproteins (IDL), 500
Internal acoustic meatus, 244t
Internal anal sphincter, 556f
Internal capsule, 269
Internal carotid artery, 266–267, 267b, 272f, 281f, 315f
  in carotid canal, 266f
  in cavernous sinus, 266f
  in neck, 266f

Internal carotid plexus, 90f
Internal iliac artery, 477f, 525f, 578–579
Internal iliac vein, 578–579
Internal intercostal muscle, 79f
Internal jugular vein, 237f, 279f–281f, 291f, 312f, 319f, 321f, 334f, 383f
  superior bulb of, 315f
Internal oblique muscle, 207f, 452f–453f, 455f–456f, 457t, 458f
Internal pudendal artery, 477f
Internal pudendal vessels, 582
Internal respiration, 106, 107f
Internal thoracic artery, 76f, 333f
Internal thoracic vein, 77f
Internal vertebral venous plexus, 202
Interneurons, 47b, 218f
Interosseous arteries, 413f
Interosseous ligament, 419f
  attachments of, 613f
Interosseous membrane, 36f, 416f–417f, 612f, 614f
Interosseous recurrent artery, 413f
Interosseous talocalcanean ligament, 627f
Interphalangeal joints, 380f, 430, 434f, 629, 629b, 633f
  movements in, 629
Interphase, 17
Interspinales muscle, 204f, 205t–206t
Interspinous ligament, 201f–202f
Interstitial emphysema, 115, 115b
Interstitial fluid, 157, 157f, 157b
Interstitial space, 107f
Interstitium, 157, 157f, 157b
Intertransversarii muscle, 204f
Intertrochanteric crest, 583f
Intertrochanteric line, 583f
Intertubercular groove, 390f
Interureteric ridge, 526f
Interventricular septum, development of, 117b
Intervertebral disc, 36f, 73f, 194f, 196–198, 196b, 198f
Intervertebral foramen, 201f
Intervertebral joints, 195–200
  between arches, 199–200, 199b–200b, 200f, 200t
  between bodies, 195–199, 198f
Intervillous space, 363f
Intestinal lining cells, function of, 9t
Intestinal phase, of gastric secretion, 490f

Intra-articular disc, 37f, 284, 284f, 382f, 386f
Intra-articular ligament, 71f, 73f
Intracapsular ligament, 37f
Intracranial venous connections, 292f
Intracranial venous sinuses, 270, 270b, 271f
Intraglomerular mesangial cells, 517f
Intrahepatic gallbladder, 482b
Intraligamentary fibroid, 548f
Intramembranous ossification, 31, 234
Intramural fibroid, 548f
Intravillus space, 363f
Intrinsic muscles, of foot, 633t–634t
Inversion, 626–627, 630f, 630t–631t
Investing layer, of fascia, 325, 326f
Iodine, 507
Iris, 297f, 298
Iron, 507
Iron deficiency anaemia, 170, 170b
IRV. See Inspiratory reserve volume
Ischial spine, 568f, 575f
Ischial tuberosity, 551f, 553f, 568f
Ischio-anal fossae, 554f
Ischiocavernosus muscle, 540f, 552f
Ischiofemoral ligament, 585f
Ischiopubic ramus, 551f
  attachment to, 452f–453f
Ischiorectal fossa, infection or tumour in, 555f, 555b
Ischium, 567, 568f
Islets of Langerhans, 347–351, 347f, 483f, 484
  blood glucose regulation, 349–351
  glucagon, 348–349
  insulin, 347–348, 348b
Isolated gastric varices (IGV), 468f
Isthmus, 541f, 544f

J

Jaundice, treatment of, 482b
Jejunum, 468–471
  arterial supply to, 471f
  mucosal wall of, 474f
Joint(s), of thoracic cage, 68–72, 69f
Joint capsule, 194f, 285f, 382f, 387f, 391f–392f, 408f, 431f
  dependent part of, 392f
  of femoral head, 584f
  of knee joint, 600f
  of metatarsophalangeal joints, 632f
  of popliteal fossa, 612f

Joint cavity, in synovial joints, 37f
Joint space, in synovial joints, 37f, 392f
Jugular foramen, 244t
Jugular notch, 68f
Jugular venous pulse
  elevated, 154b
  inspection of, 153b, 154f
Juxtacrine messenger, 336f
Juxtaglomerular apparatus, 515–518, 517f
Juxtaglomerular cells, 517f
Juxtamedullary nephron, 513b, 514f

K

Ketosis, 487–488
Keyhole surgery, 456b
Kidneys, 368, 483f, 509–522, 510b, 512f, 513b, 524f–525f
  blood supply of, 514f
  cells in, function of, 9t
  development of, 509f, 509b
  diseases of, 522
  diuretics and, 521–522
  immediate compensatory effects on, 158
  internal organisation of, 512f
  physiology of, 513–515
    endocrine function, 515
    excretion, 513
    gluconeogenesis, 515
    haematopoiesis, 515, 515b
    homeostasis, 513–515
    regulation, 513
  relations of, 511f
  urine formation in, 515–521
Klinefelter syndrome, 531
Knee joint, 566f, 598–608, 599f–601f, 600b–601b
  movements in, 605–608, 605f, 642–643
    flexion and extension, 606–608, 606f–608f, 607b–608b
    medial and lateral rotation, 608, 609f–610f
Krause end bulbs, 52, 52f
Kupffer cell, 479f, 480
Kussmaul's sign, 154b

L

Labia majora, 555
Labia minora, 552
Labour, stages of, 365–366

Labrum, of femoral head, 584f
Lacerations, to scalp, 238b
Lacrimal apparatus, 302, 302b–303b, 303f
Lacrimal artery, 296f
Lacrimal bone, 295f, 304f–305f
Lacrimal canaliculi, 303f
Lacrimal fossa, 294–295
Lacrimal gland, 226f, 296f, 303f
  orbital part of, 303f
  palpebral part of, 303f
Lacrimal groove, 294–295, 295f
Lacrimal nerve, 275f–276f, 296f, 303f
Lacrimal vessels, 303f
Lactating breast, 367f
Lactation, 366–367
Lactiferous duct, 367f
Lacuna, 32f
Lambdoid suture, 235f
Lamellar bone, 31
Lamina, 191f, 193f, 195f–196f
Lamina terminalis, 255f
Laparoscopic surgery, for abdomen, 456b
Large intestine, 472–476, 473f, 486f
  absorptive and storage functions of, 494, 494f
  arterial supply to, 476f
  movement of, 496, 496b
  wall of, 474f
Larger lymph vessels, 161, 161f
Laryngopharynx, 328
Larynx, 93b, 94, 328–331, 329f
Lateral accessory vein, 592f
Lateral anterior cutaneous nerve, 579f, 639f
Lateral aortic (lumbar) nodes, 557f
Lateral arcuate ligament, 75f
Lateral articular surface, 620f
Lateral cerebral surface, 268f
Lateral circumflex femoral artery, 591f
Lateral collateral ligaments, 599f, 601b, 603f, 613f
Lateral condyle
  of femur, 583f
  of tibia, 597f
Lateral cord, 399f
Lateral cutaneous nerve
  of calf/leg, 611f, 616f, 639f
  of forearm, 412f, 417f, 439f
  of thigh, 578f, 639f

Lateral epicondyle
  of femur, 583f
  of humerus, 390f, 409f
Lateral fornix, 544f
Lateral funiculus, of spinal cord, 210f
Lateral geniculate body, 254f
Lateral horn, of spinal cord, 210f
Lateral inferior genicular artery, 612f,
  618f
Lateral ligament, 285f
Lateral lymph nodes, 399f
Lateral malleolus, 597f, 623f
Lateral marginal vein, 592f
Lateral mass, of vertebra, 197f
Lateral meniscus, 600f, 603f
  flattened area for, of tibia, 597f
Lateral nasal artery, 291f
  alar branch of, 307f
Lateral nasal cartilage, 305f
Lateral nasal vein, 291f
Lateral nuclei, 253
Lateral patellar retinaculum, 599f
Lateral pectoral nerve, 400f, 401t
Lateral perforating cutaneous branch,
  79f
Lateral plantar artery, 635–636, 635f,
  635b–636b
Lateral plantar nerve, 617f, 634–635,
  639f, 640
Lateral pterygoid muscle, 284f–285f,
  289t–290t
Lateral rectus muscle, 275f, 296f, 301t
Lateral reticulospinal tracts, 216, 216b
Lateral sacral crest, 197f
Lateral spinothalamic tract, 214, 214b
Lateral sulcus, 256, 257f
Lateral superior genicular artery, 612f,
  618f
Lateral supracondylar ridge, 390f
Lateral surface, of cerebral cortex, 269
Lateral talocalcanean ligament, 620f,
  627f
Lateral ventricles, 245f
Latissimus dorsi muscle, 394t, 438f,
  440f
LDLs. *See* Low-density lipoproteins
Le Fort fractures, 241f, 241b
Le Fort I fracture, 241f, 241b
Le Fort II fracture, 241f, 241b
Le Fort III fracture, 241f, 241b
Least splanchnic nerve, 90f–91f
Left atrium, 120

Left brachiocephalic vein, 77f, 81,
  81f–82f, 83, 89f
Left bronchomediastinal trunk, 96f
Left common carotid artery, 82f, 83,
  85f, 93f, 266f, 333f
Left coronary artery, 124
Left crus, 75f
Left gastro-omental artery, 467f
Left hilum, 98
Left internal carotid artery, 267f
Left internal iliac artery, 477f
Left jugular trunk, 89
Left lung, 98
  medial and lateral aspects of, 99f
  medial surface of, 98
Left marginal artery, 125f
Left parasternal lymphatic vessel, 96f
Left pericardiacophrenic vessels, 85f
Left phrenic nerve, 82f, 85f, 92, 93f
Left pulmonary artery, 82f, 86f, 93f
Left pulmonary veins, 86f
Left recurrent laryngeal nerve, 70f, 82f,
  84f, 92, 93f
Left subclavian artery, 82f, 83, 93f, 266f
Left superior intercostal vein, 77f–78f
Left vagus nerve, 70f, 81, 82f, 84f, 88f,
  92, 93f
Left ventricle, 93f, 121
Left ventricular failure, 160
Left ventricular impression, 99f
Left ventricular pressure, 153
Left vertebral artery, 266f–267f
Leg, 566f, 594–615
  compartments of, 612–615, 614f
    anterior, 612–614
    lateral, 614, 614f
    muscles, 615
    posterior, 614–615
  fibula, 566f, 597f, 598, 598b
  knee joint, 566f, 598–608, 599f–601f,
    600b–601b
    movements in, 605–608, 605f,
      642–643
  patella, 566f, 598, 598f, 598b
    in knee joint, 601b, 603f
    movement of, with femur and
      tibia, 608f, 610f
  popliteal fossa, 608–611, 609b–610b,
    611f–612f
  tibia, 566f, 596–598, 596b, 597f, 598b
    patella with, movement of, 608f,
      610f

Leg (*Continued*)
  reflections of synovial membrane
    on, 600f
  tibiofibular joints, 611–612, 612f
    inferior, 612, 613f
    superior, 611–612, 613f
Lens, 297f
  biconvex, 299
  suspensory ligament of, 298f
Leptin, 370, 485–486, 486f
Lesser curvature, of stomach, 465f
Lesser occipital nerve, 239f, 322f
Lesser omentum, 454f, 465, 465f
Lesser petrosal nerve, 315f
Lesser sac, of peritoneal cavity, 454f
Lesser sciatic notch, 568f, 572f
Lesser splanchnic nerve, 90f–91f,
  91–92
Lesser trochanter, 583f
Lesser tubercle, of humerus, 390f
Leukocytes, 26, 165, 167t, 172–174,
  172f, 172t, 172b
Leukotrienes, 369
Levator anguli oris muscle, 293f, 294
Levator ani muscle, 459b, 460f, 460t,
  526f, 551f, 554f, 556f, 575f
Levator labii superioris alaeque nasi,
  293f, 294
Levator labii superioris muscle, 293f,
  294
Levator palpebrae superioris muscles,
  275f, 296f, 301t, 302f
  tendon of, 302f–303f
Levator scapulae muscle, 318f–319f,
  320t, 388t–389t, 397f
Levatores costarum muscle, 75
Leydig cells, 352f, 356f
Ligaments
  in cartilaginous joints, 36f
  of larynx, 330, 330b
Ligamentum arteriosum, 70f, 82f, 84f,
  93f, 123f
Ligamentum cervicis, 628f
Ligamentum flavum, 201f–202f
Ligamentum nuchae, 319f
Ligamentum patellae, 599f–600f, 601b,
  608f, 610f
Ligamentum teres, 123f, 584f
Light reflex pathway, 273
Limbic system, 263–264, 263b–264b
Limiting layer, 363f
Line of gravity, 189f

Linea alba, 455f–456f, 458f
Linea aspera, 583f
Lingual artery, 291f, 312f
Lingual nerve, 285f, 312f–313f
Lingula, 282f, 285f
Lipids, formation of, 13f
Lipoproteins, 500
Lipoxin A, 369
Lips, 309
Little finger, 418f
Liver, 123f, 154b, 454f, 470f, 477–482,
    478b, 480f, 480b–482b, 511f
  cancer, 482b
  development of, 477b, 478f
  diaphragmatic and visceral surfaces
    of, 479f
  metabolic functions of, 508, 508b
    carbohydrate metabolism, 508,
      508b
    fat/lipid metabolism, 508
    protein metabolism, 508, 508b
  secretion of, 492f
Liver bud, 478f
Liver disease, 505b
Lobule, 315f
Local hormones, 369–370
  in blood, 370
  in tissues, 369–370
Local regulation, 151
Local vasoconstrictors, 151
Local vasodilators, 151
Long association fibres, 259
Long bone, ossification centres in, 33f
Long buccal nerve, 285f
Long ciliary nerves, 296f
Long curved subcutaneous bone,
    379–381, 382f
Long plantar ligament, 627f
Long posterior sacroiliac ligament,
    572f
Long (great) saphenous vein, 623f
  of calf/leg, 614, 614f
  of thigh, 591f–592f, 592, 592b
Long thoracic nerve, 400f
Long tracts, of spinal cord, 213–217
Longissimus capitis muscle, 204f,
    205t–206t
Longissimus cervicis muscle, 205t–206t
Longissimus thoracis muscle, 204f,
    205t–206t
Longitudinal fissure, 257f, 262f
Longitudinal ligaments, 202f

Longitudinal muscle, 298f
Longus colli, 319f
Loop of Henle, 511–513, 512f, 518t,
    519, 520f
Loose areolar tissue, of scalp, 237
Loose connective tissue, of scalp, 237f
Low-density lipoproteins (LDLs), 500
Lower limb, 563–648, 565b, 566f
  ankle, 615–621, 616b, 619f
    ankle joint, 566f, 616–621, 618b,
      619f–621f, 623f
  calf/leg, 594–615
    compartments of, 612–615, 614f
    fibula, 566f, 597f, 598, 598b
    knee joint, 566f, 598–608,
      599f–601f, 600b–601b
    patella, 566f, 598, 598f, 598b
    popliteal fossa, 608–611,
      609b–610b, 611f–612f
    tibia, 566f, 596–598, 596b, 597f,
      598b
    tibiofibular joints, 611–612, 612f
  dermatomes of, 640f
  development of, 381f
  foot, 566f, 624–636, 624b, 625f
    dorsum of, 619f, 629–634
    function of, 636, 636b
    interphalangeal joints, 629, 629b,
      633f
    joints of, 626, 627f
    metatarsals, 566f, 625f, 626, 626b
    metatarsophalangeal joints,
      627–629, 628b, 632f
    phalanges, 566f, 625f, 626, 626b
    plantar aspect (sole) of, 634–636
    subtalar joint, 626, 628f
    tarsus, 625, 625f, 625b
    transverse (mid) tarsal joint,
      626–627, 628f
    walking and, 636, 637f
  muscles of, 638–643
  nerves of, 638–643
    common fibular nerve, 639f, 640
    common peroneal nerve, 639f,
      640
    femoral nerve, 638, 639f
    inferior gluteal nerve, 638
    obturator nerve, 638, 639f
    sciatic nerve, 638–640
    superior gluteal nerve, 638
    tibial nerve, 640
  pelvic girdle, 567–582

Lower limb (Continued)
    coccyx, 566f, 569–570,
      569b–570b, 571f
    function of, 574, 574b
    gluteal region, 580–582
    innominate, 566f, 567–569, 567b,
      568f
    lumbosacral joint, 573, 573b, 574f
    relations of, 574–580, 575f,
      578f–580f, 579b
    sacrococcygeal joint, 573–574,
      574b
    sacrum, 566f, 569–570,
      569b–570b, 571f
    symphysis pubis, 569, 569b, 570f
  region of, movements in, 642–643
  rotation of, 381f
  thigh, 566f, 582–594, 582b
    compartments of, 589–594
    femoral triangle, 588–589, 589f,
      589b
    femur, 566f, 582–584, 582b,
      583f–584f, 584b
    hip joint, 566f, 584–588, 586b
Lower subscapular nerve, 400f, 401t
Lumbar curve, 189–190
Lumbar enlargement, of spinal cord,
    208f
Lumbar plexus, 223, 223f, 574, 578f
  cutaneous nerves of, 578f
Lumbar region, 189f
  intervertebral disc of, 198f
  zygapophyseal joints of, 200f
Lumbar splanchnic nerves, 90f
Lumbar sympathetic trunk, 91f
Lumbar vertebrae, 194–195, 195b, 196f
Lumbosacral joint, 573, 573b, 574f
Lumbosacral plexus, 223, 223f
Lumbosacral trunk, 578f
Lumbrical muscle, 427f, 429t–430t,
    433t
  3rd, 434f
  in foot, 633f, 633t–634t
Lumen, 543f
Lunate bone, 418f–419f
  articular surface for, 405f
Lung capacity, 103–104
Lungs, 93b, 94f, 97–101, 123f
  air and blood flow in, regulation of,
    109, 109b
  root of, 98, 98f
  surface markings of, 99–100, 100b

Luteal phase, of menstrual cycle, 545f, 546
Luteinising hormone (LH), 339t
Lymph, 160–161
  flow, rate of, 160
  function of, 160
Lymph capillaries, 161
  origin of, 161f
  structure of, 161f
Lymph nodes, 161–162, 400, 400b
  of femoral triangle, 589, 590f
  function of, 162, 162b
  structure of, 162, 162f
Lymph vessels, 163f
  tumours of, 143
Lymphatic drainage
  of chest wall, 78–79, 79b
  of face, 290
  of hand, 435, 435b
  of palate, 313
  right anterior chest wall and breast,
    403f
  of scalp, 238, 238f
  of thyroid gland, 331
  of tongue, 312
  of trachea, bronchi and lungs, 95
Lymphatic duct, right, 403f
Lymphatic plexus, of palm, 402f
Lymphatic system, 157, 160–164
Lymphatic vessel, 107f
Lymphatics
  in femoral canal, 589f
  of heart, 126
Lymphocytes, 164, 172f, 172t, 173
  processing of, 176–179
Lymphocytopenia, 173
Lymphocytosis, 173
Lymphoid tissue (lingual tonsil), 311f
Lysosomes, 10f, 12–13, 13f, 13b

M
Macrocytic anaemia, 506
Macrophages, 108f, 173
  in connective tissues, 25–26, 26f
  function of, 9t
Macula, 299
Macula densa, 515–516, 516f–517f
Magnesium, 507
Main sensory nucleus, 274–275
Main stem villus, 549f
Major alar cartilage, 304f–305f
Male reproductive system, 532–541
  accessory glands of, 535–537, 535f

Malignant hypertension, 148
Malleolus, 612f
MALT. See Mucosa-associated
  lymphoid tissue
Mamillary process, of vertebra, 196f
Mammillary body, 255f, 262, 262f,
  338f
Mandible, 235f, 240f, 278f, 282–287,
  282b, 323f
  body of, 285f
  growth of, 282–283
  head of, 284f
  head of, in synovial joints, 37f
  inferior aspect of, 283f
  lateral aspect of, 283f, 285f
  lateral left aspect of, 288f
  length and height of, 283
  mandibular fossa and, 286f
  medial aspect of, 282f
  movements of, 286–287, 287b,
    289t–290t
Mandibular division, 275, 275b
Mandibular fossa, 37f, 243f, 284f
Mandibular nerve, 276f
Manganese, 507–508
Manubriosternal joint, 69f, 382f
Manubrium, 68, 68f, 382f
Marginal artery, 476f
Marginal sinus, 363f
Masseter muscle, 288f, 289t–290t
Mast cells, in connective tissues, 26,
  26b
Mastication, 292
Mastoid air cells, 315f
Mastoid antrum, 315f
Mastoid nodes, 238f
Mastoid process, 278f, 315f
Maternal circulation, 549f
Maternal vessels, 363f
Matrix
  in bone, 32f
  in skin, 60f
Mature sperm, 353f
Maxilla, 240f, 243f, 295f
  frontal process of, 304f–305f
  palatine process, 305f
Maxillary artery, 285f, 291f
Maxillary division, 275
Maxillary nerve, 276f
Maxillary sinus, 306, 306b, 307f
  opening of, 306f
McBurney's point, 473b

MCHC. See Mean cell haemoglobin
  concentration
Meals, arterial blood pressure after, 148
Mean arterial pressure, 147–148
Mean cell haemoglobin concentration
  (MCHC), 167t
Meckel's diverticulum, 469b
Medial and lateral rotation
  axis of, 395f
  of shoulder joint, 396, 396f
Medial anterior cutaneous nerve, 579f,
  639f
Medial arcuate ligament, 75f
Medial articular surface, 620f
Medial border, 385f
Medial calcaneal branch, of tibial
  nerve, 617f
Medial calcaneal nerve, 617f
Medial cerebral surface, 268f
Medial circumflex femoral artery, 591f
Medial (tibial) collateral ligament, 599f,
  601b, 603f
Medial condyle
  of femur, 583f
  of tibia, 597f
Medial cuneiform, 625f
Medial cutaneous nerve
  of arm, 401f
  of forearm, 400f–401f, 403f, 412f, 417f
Medial epicondyle, 390f, 409f, 439f,
  583f
Medial geniculate body, 254f
Medial head of triceps, 438f
Medial inferior genicular artery, 612f,
  618f
Medial intermuscular septum, 439f
Medial lemniscus, 213f, 248b
Medial longitudinal bundle, 252
Medial malleolus, 597f, 623f
Medial meniscus, 600f, 603f
  anterior part of, 600f
  flattened area for, 597f
  posterior part of, 600f
Medial nuclei, 253
Medial patellar retinaculum, 599f
Medial pectoral nerve, 399f–400f, 401t
Medial plantar artery, 635–636, 635f,
  635b–636b
Medial plantar nerve, 617f, 634–635,
  639f, 640
Medial pterygoid muscle, 285f, 288f,
  289t–290t

Medial rectus muscle, 275f, 296f, 301t
Medial reticulospinal tracts, 216, 216b
Medial superior genicular artery, 612f, 618f
Medial supracondylar ridge, 390f
Medial surface
    of cerebral cortex, 269
    of tibia, 597f
Medial talocalcanean ligament, 628f
Medial umbilical ligament, 123f
Median cubital vein, 402f, 412f, 437f
Median fissure, 262f
Median nerve, 400f–401f, 401t, 403f, 404, 412f, 417f, 419f, 440f
    of forearm, 418
    of upper limb, 438–439, 440f
Median sacral crest, 197f
Median vein, of forearm, 412f
Mediastinal pleura, 95
Mediastinal syndrome, 83b
Mediastinum, 80–93, 80b
    anterior, 83
    divisions of, 83f
    left, 80, 82f
    middle, 83–87
    posterior, 87–93
    right, 80, 81f
    superior, 80–83
Medulla, 162f, 344f
Medulla oblongata, 208f, 213f, 247–248, 248b, 249f, 262f, 269
Medullary cavity, of bone, 30f
Medullary ducts, 519–521, 521f
Medullary sinus, 162f
Meiosis, 19
Meiotic division I, 353f
Meiotic division II, 353f
Meissner plexus. See Submucosal plexus
Meissner's corpuscles, 52, 52f, 55f
Membranes, 330, 330b
Membranous urethra, 526f, 527
Memory B cells, 178
Memory T cells, 177
Menarche, 359–361, 361f
Meninges, 264, 265f
Menisci, 604, 604b, 605f
Meniscofemoral ligament, 603f
Meniscopatellar fibres, 603f
Menopause, 359–361, 361f
Menstrual cycle, 361, 545f, 546–548, 547b
    uterine changes during, 359f

Mental artery, 291f
Mental foramen, 240f, 241t
Mental nerve, 276f
Mentalis, 293f, 294
Merkel's discs, 52, 52f
Merocrine secretion, 23, 25f
Mesangial cells, in renal corpuscle, 517f
Mesencephalic nucleus, 274–275
Mesencephalon, 249f
Mesenchymal stem cells, 26f, 31f
Mesentery, 453f–454f
Mesodermal somites, 381f
Mesonephric system, in embryo, 509f
Mesothelium, 20
Metabolites, accumulation of, 147
Metacarpals, 380f, 418f–419f, 425–426, 425b–426b, 427f, 431f, 434f
Metacarpophalangeal joints, 380f, 427–430, 428b, 431f
    attachments, action and innervation, 429t–430t
    movements of, 432f
Metanephric system, in embryo, 509f
Metaphase, 17
Metaphyseal anastomosis, 203f
Metarterioles, 155f
Metatarsals, 566f, 625f, 626, 626b
Metatarsophalangeal joints, 627–629, 628b, 632f
    movements in, 628–629, 633f, 633t–634t
Metathalamus, 254–255, 254f
Microcirculation, 154–157
Microfilaments, 10f, 15, 15f
Microglial cell, 247, 247f
Microtubules, 10f, 15, 15f, 354f
Microvilli, 472f
Micturition, 528–530, 529f
    abnormalities of, 529–530
    facilitation or inhibition by brain, 529
    voluntary urination and, 529
Midbrain, 250–251, 251b, 254f, 262f, 269
Midcarpal joint, 380f, 419f
Middle cardiac vein, 125–126, 125f
Middle cerebellar peduncle, 252–253, 254f
Middle cerebral artery, 267f–268f, 268, 268b, 272f
Middle cervical ganglion, 335f
Middle collateral artery, 413f

Middle concha, 306f–307f
Middle cranial fossa, 242, 243f, 244t
Middle ear, 314–316, 315f
Middle finger, 418f
Middle genicular artery, 612f
Middle lobe, of lungs, 99f
Middle meati, opening into, 306f
Middle mediastinum, 83–87
Middle scalene muscle, 318f, 321f
Middle thyroid vein, 332f
Middle turbinate, 305f
Midface fractures, 241f, 241b
Midgut, herniation of, 478f
Midline raphe, 540f
Midtarsal joint line, 628f
Milk ejection, 366–367, 367b
Milk lipids, 367f
Milk secretion, 366
Millard-Gubler syndrome, 250b
Mineral metabolism, 506–508
Mineralocorticoids, 344–345
Minimally invasive surgery, for abdomen, 456b
Minor alar cartilage, 305f
Mitochondria
    in cells, 10f, 14f–15f, 14b
    of human spermatozoa, 354f
    in muscle contraction, 43f
Mitosis, 17, 17b
Mitral valve, 119f–120f, 121
Moderator band, 120f, 121
Modiolus, 294
Monocytes, 172f, 172t, 173
    progenitor, 31f
Monocytosis, 173
Monounsaturated fats, 499t
Mons pubis, 553f
Motor area, 269
Motor cranial nerve fibres, 215f
Motor decussation of pyramids, 215f
Motor homunculus, 257, 258f
Motor neuron, 217f–218f
    axon of, in skeletal muscle, 40f
    in muscle contraction, 43f
Motor nucleus, 274–277
Motor speech area, 269
Motor spinal nerve fibres, 215f
Motor system, 263
Mouth, muscles around, 294, 294b
Mucosa, 463f–464f
Mucosa-associated lymphoid tissue (MALT), 164, 464b

Mucosal nerves, 464f
Mucosal villi, 474f
Mucous, 488
Mucous glands, 226f
  cells, function of, 9t
Mucous neck cells, 466f
Multifidus muscle, 204f, 205t–206t
Multipennate muscles, 44, 45f
Multipolar neuron, 46, 46f
Mumps, 489
Mural cells, 155
Muscle, 38–44
  action of, 44, 44b
  attachment of, 44, 44b
  cardiac muscle, 39, 39f, 39b
  cells in, function of, 9t
  contraction, 42–43, 43f, 43b
  fibre
    in muscle contraction, 43f
    organisation, 40, 40f–41f, 40b–41b
  forms of, 43–44, 45f
  sensory receptors in, 40–42
  skeletal muscle, 39–44, 40f
  smooth muscle, 38–39, 38f, 39b
  spindles, 41–42, 42f, 42b
Muscle cell nucleus, in muscle
    contraction, 43f
Muscle stretch reflex, in spine,
    217–218, 217f, 218b
Muscles, 435–444
  of arm, 404
  of calf/leg, 615
  of larynx, 330–331, 330b, 332f
  of lower limb, 638–643
  of pectoral region, 386–387
  of shoulder joint, 397f
  of thigh, 594, 595t–596t
  of thoracic cage, 72–79
Muscular triangle, 318f, 324–325
Muscularis mucosa, 464f
Musculocutaneous nerve, 400f–401f,
    401t, 403–404, 403f, 436, 439f
Musculophrenic artery, 76f
Myasthenia gravis, 180
Myelin sheath
  in muscle contraction, 43f
  in myelinated axon, 47f–48f
Myelination, of axon, 47–48, 47f–48f
Myenteric plexus, 464, 464f
Mylohyoid line, 285f
Mylohyoid muscle, 289t–290t, 323f,
    324t

Myocardium, 118
Myoepithelial cell, 367f
Myofibrils, in muscle contraction,
    43f
Myoglobin, 109, 109b
Myometrium, 544–548, 545b, 549f
  arterial supply to, 546f
Myopia, 297f, 297b
Myxoedema, 342

N
Nail(s), 58, 58b, 60f
Nail bed, 60f
Nail body, 60f
Nail root, 60f
Naris, 304f
Nasal bleeding (epistaxis), 308b
Nasal bone, 235f, 240f, 304f–305f
Nasal cavity, 304–308, 305f, 309f
  paranasal sinuses, 304–308
  venous drainage of, 308f
  walls of, 307f
Nasalis muscle, 293f
Nasociliary nerve, 275f, 296f
Nasolacrimal duct, 303f
  opening of, 306f
Nasolacrimal groove, 304f
Nasopharynx, 327–328
Natural killer cells, 178
Navicular bone, 566f, 625f, 628f, 630f
Navicular fossa, of urethra, 540f
Neck, 317–332
  anterior triangle of, 318f, 320–325
  cervical vertebrae, 317
  compartments of, 325
  of femur, 583f
  of fibula, 597f
  of human spermatozoa, 354f
  hyoid, 325, 326f
  larynx, 328–331, 329f
  nasopharynx, 327–328
  pharynx, 326–328, 326b, 327f
  posterior triangle of, 318f, 319–320,
    320t, 321f–322f
  of radius, 405f
  regions, 317–332, 317b
  root of, 331–332, 333f–334f
  thyroid gland, 331, 331b
  transverse section of, 319f
  triangles of, 318f
Neocerebellum, 252
Neonatal adrenoleukodystrophy, 14b

Nephron, 511–513
  cortical, 513b
  juxtamedullary, 513b
  organisation of, 512f
  tubular system, parts of, 518t
Nerve bundle, in skin, 56f
Nerve endings, 52, 52f
Nerve fibres, types of, activity of, 51,
    51f
Nerve injury, 52–53, 53b
Nerve root sheaths, 220f, 221
Nerve supply, 308, 308b
  to chest wall, 79
  to heart, 124–127, 124b
  to pericardium, 86–87, 87b
  to pleurae, 97b
  to thoracic cage, 75–79
  to trachea and bronchi, 95
Nerves
  of lower limb, 638–643
    common fibular nerve, 639f,
      640
    common peroneal nerve, 639f,
      640
    femoral nerve, 638, 639f
    inferior gluteal nerve, 638
    obturator nerve, 638, 639f
    sciatic nerve, 638–640
    superior gluteal nerve, 638
    tibial nerve, 640
  of neck, 332, 332b, 335f
  of posterior triangle, 320
  summary of, 435–444
Nervous regulation, 149
Nervous system, immediate
    compensatory effects on, 158
Nervous tissue, 44–53, 46b
  action potential in, 50, 50f
  nerve endings, 52, 52f
  nerve injury, 52–53, 53b
  neurons, 46–49
    classes of, 46f
    communication, 48–49
    function of, 9t
  peripheral nervous system, 50–52
Neural canal, 191f, 193f, 195f–196f
Neural tube, 245b
Neurogenic hypertension, 149
Neurogenic shock, 159
Neurogram, of peripheral nerves, 51f
Neurohormone, 336f
Neurolemma, in myelinated axon, 48f

Neurons, 46–49, 245f
  cell body, 46–47, 46f, 245f
  classes of, 46
  communication, 48–49
  function of, 9t
Neuropraxia, 53
Neurotmesis, 53
Neurotransmitter, 336f
Neutral fats, 498
Neutropenia, 172–173
Neutrophilia, 172–173
Neutrophils, 172–173, 172f, 172t
Neutrophils, function of, 9t
Niacin, 506
  deficiency, 506b
Nicotinic acid. *See* Niacin
NIDDM. *See* Non-insulin-dependent
  diabetes mellitus
Nocturnal micturition, 530, 530b
Node of Ranvier, in myelinated axon,
  47f–48f
Non-essential amino acids, 504,
  504b
Non-insulin-dependent diabetes
  mellitus (NIDDM), 484b
Noradrenaline, 150
Normotopic arrhythmias, 130
Nose, 94
  external, 304, 304f, 304b
  muscles around, 294
Nuclear basket, 16f
Nuclear envelope, 16f
Nuclear membrane, 9f, 16–17
Nuclear pores, 16f
Nucleolus, 9f–10f, 16f, 17, 17b
Nucleoplasm, 9f
Nucleus, 245f
  in cells, 9f–10f, 15–17, 16f
    chromatin, 10f, 17
    nuclear membrane, 9f, 16–17
    nucleolus, 9f–10f, 16f, 17, 17b
  in myelinated axon, 48f
Nucleus ambiguus, 277–279
Nucleus cuneatus, 249f
Nucleus gracilis, 249f
Nucleus pulposus, 196, 198f,
  202f–203f
Nucleus tractus solitarius, 276–279
Nutrient foramen, of tibia, 597f
Nutrition, 497–508
Nutrition deficiency anaemias, 170,
  171t

O
Obesity, 487, 503b
Oblique cord, 416f
Oblique fissure, 99f, 101f
Oblique fracture, of bone, 34, 34f
Oblique pericardial sinus, 86f
Oblique popliteal ligament, 599f
Obstructive shock, 159
Obturator artery, 575f
Obturator canal, 575f
Obturator externus muscle, 575t–577t,
  580f
Obturator foramen, 568f, 569, 570f, 572f
Obturator internus muscle, 460f, 554f,
  575t–577t, 580f–581f, 593f
Obturator internus tendon, 580f
Obturator nerve, 638, 639f
  anterior branch of, 579f
  of lumbar plexus, 578f–579f
  of pelvis, 575f
  posterior branch of, 579f
  of thigh, 593
Occipital artery, 281f, 291f, 312f
  sternocleidomastoid branch of, 312f
Occipital bone, 234, 235f–236f, 243f,
  305f
Occipital condyle, 243f
Occipital lobe, 257f, 259b, 262f
Occipital nodes, 238f
Occipital pole, 257f
Occipital vein, 237f, 291f
Occipitofrontalis muscle, 292, 293f
Oculomotor nerve, 251, 255f, 272f,
  273, 273b
  inferior branch of, 296f
  inferior division of, 275f
  superior branch of, 296f
  superior division of, 275f
Odontoid process, of vertebra, 193f
Oesophageal atresia, 87b
Oesophageal constrictions, 87b
Oesophageal impression, 99f
Oesophageal opening, 75f
Oesophageal plexus, 70f, 81f, 88f
Oesophageal varices, 468f
Oesophagus, 74, 81, 81f–82f, 87–88,
  87b, 88f–89f, 319f, 333f–334f,
  383f, 465f
Oestrogens, 351, 358–359, 360f, 368f
Olecranon, 405f, 407b, 409f, 413f
  alignment of, 409f, 409b
  of humerus, 407b

Olecranon fossa, 390f
Olfactory bulb, 262f, 309f
Olfactory nerve, 272, 309f
Olfactory pathway, 272, 272b
Olfactory receptors, reflex and, 116
Olfactory tract, 262f
Oligodendrocytes, 247, 247f
  in myelinated axon, 47f
Oligospermia, 537
Oligozoospermia, 537
Olive, 248, 249f, 262f
Olivospinal tract, 216
Omental bursa
  formation of, 465f
  of peritoneal cavity, 454f
Omental cake, 465b
Omohyoid muscle, 320t, 323f, 324t
  inferior belly of, 318f
  superior belly of, 318f
Omphalocele, 463b
Oophorectomy, 548b
Open fracture, of bone, 33
Ophthalmic artery, 275f, 296f
Ophthalmic division, 275
Ophthalmic nerve, 276f, 296f
Ophthalmic veins, 292f
Opponens digiti minimi muscle, 433t
Opponens pollicis muscle, 433t
Optic axis, 297f
Optic canal, 244t, 295f
Optic chiasm, 255f, 262f, 338f
Optic disc, 297f
Optic nerve, 262f, 272–273, 275f, 297f
Optic tract, 254f, 262f
Oral cavity, 308–314, 310f, 311b
  lips, 309
  oropharyngeal isthmus, 314
  palate, 313–314
  salivary glands, 312–313
  teeth and gums, 309–311
  tongue, 311–312
Orbicularis oculi muscle, 292–293,
  293f, 302f
Orbicularis oris muscle, 293f, 294
Orbit, 276f, 294–302
  arterial supply to, 296f
  bones of, 295f
  fractures, 295b
  nerves of, 296f
  venous drainage of, 296f
  vessels and nerves within, 295–297
Orbital fascia, 295

Orbital periosteum, 295
Orbital septum, 302f–303f
Orchitis, 534b
Organs, 53–61
    golgi tendon, location and
        microscopic appearance of,
        40–41, 42f
    skin, 53–61, 53b–54b
        appendages of, 58–61
        function of, 54
        metabolism of, 54–55
        protection of, 54, 54b
        sensation of, 54, 54b
        sexual signalling of, 55
        structure of, 55–57, 55f, 55b
        thermoregulation of, 54, 54b
        wound repair, 57–58, 58b, 59f
Original position of bones, 387f
Oropharyngeal isthmus, 314
Oropharynx, 328
Orthopnoea, 111
Orthostatic (postural) hypotension,
    149
Osmotic diuretics, 522
Osteoarthritis, 28b, 37b
Osteoblasts, 9t, 30, 31f–33f
Osteoclasts, 30, 31f–33f
Osteocytes, 30, 31f
Osteoprogenitor cells, 30, 31f
Otic ganglion, 225, 226f
Oval window, 315f–316f
Ovarian cycles, 545f
Ovarian cyst, 542b
Ovarian fimbria, 543f
Ovarian tumours, 542b
Ovarian vein, 524f
Ovaries, 337f, 356–361, 541–542, 541f,
    542b, 543f, 548f
    cells in, function of, 9t
    hypergonadism, 361
    hypogonadism, 361
    menstrual cycle, 361
    oestrogens, 358–359
    progesterone, 359, 360f
    puberty, menarche and menopause,
        359–361, 361f
    reproductive hormones, 357–358,
        357f
    round ligament of, 543f
    stages of follicular growth in, 357f
Ovulation, 357f, 358
Ovum, 357f

Oxalate compounds, 176
Oxygen, 105, 108, 108b
Oxygen debt, 111
Oxygen toxicity/poisoning, 113, 113b
Oxygen-haemoglobin dissociation
    curve, 108–109, 109f, 109b
Oxyhaemoglobin, 108b
Oxyntic gland, 466f
Oxytocin, 339t, 365

P

P wave, 127–128
P50, of haemoglobin, 109
Pacinian corpuscles, 52, 52f, 56f
Packed cell volume (PCV), values of,
    normal, 167t
Pain receptors, in foot, 218f
Palate, 313–314
Palatine bone, 243f, 295f
    horizontal plate, 305f
    perpendicular plate of, 305f
Palatine tonsil, 311f, 328, 328b
Palatoglossal arch, 310f–311f
Palatopharyngeal arch, 310f–311f
Paleocerebellum, 252
Palmar aponeurosis, slip from, 431f
Palmar cutaneous branch, of ulnar
    nerves, 419f, 439f
Palmar digital artery, 426f
Palmar digital nerve, 426f
Palmar interossei muscle, 429t–430t,
    433t
    3rd, 434f
Palmar ligament, 431f
Palmar surface, of hand, 380f
Palmaris longus muscle, 410t, 417f,
    419f, 422f, 423t–424t
Palpation
    in lumbar vertebra, 195b
    of sternum, 69–70
Panacinar emphysema, 114, 115f, 115b
Pancreas, 337f, 454f, 482–484,
    482b–484b, 483f, 486f, 492f
    development of, 478f, 482b
    secretions, 491, 492f
Pancreatic bud, 478f
Pancreatic cancer, 483b
Pancreatic duct, 469f
Pancreatitis, 484b, 491b
Paneth cells, 469
Pantothenic acid, 506
Papillary muscle, 120f

Paracentesis, 97b
Paracortex, 162, 162f
Paracrine messenger, 336f
Paralysis
    of buccinator, 294b
    of muscles on one side of face, 294b
    of orbicularis oculi, 294b
    of upper lip muscle, 294b
Paranasal sinuses, 235, 304–308, 307f
Parasternal lymph nodes, 78–79, 96f,
    403f
Parasympathetic nervous system, 225,
    226f–227f
Parasympathetic stimulation, 135, 135b
Parasympathetic vasodilator fibres, 150
Parathyroid glands, 337f, 342–343,
    343b
    adrenal cortex, 343–344, 343b–344b,
        344f
    adrenal medulla, 347
    glucocorticoids, 345–347, 345b
    mineralocorticoids, 344–345
Paraventricular nucleus, 338f
Parietal bone, 235f–236f, 240f, 243f
Parietal cells, 466f
Parietal lobe, 257f, 259b
Parietal peritoneum, 452f–453f
Parietal pleura, 95, 98f
    surface markings of, 99–100, 101f
Parieto-occipital sulcus, 257f
Parotid gland, 226f, 278f, 312–313
Parotid nodes, 238f, 292f
Paroxysmal tachycardia, 132
Pars intermedia, 338f
Partial fracture, of bone, 33
Partial heart block, 131, 132b
Parturition (childbirth), 365–366
    mechanics of, 366
Passive artificial immunisation, 179
Passive immunisation, 179
Passive natural immunisation, 179
Patella, 217f, 566f, 598, 598f, 598b
    in knee joint, 601b, 603f
    movement of, with femur and tibia,
        608f, 610f
Patellar ligament, 217f
Patellar surface
    of femur, 583f
    of knee joint, 599f
Patellar tendon reflex pathway, 217f
Patent ductus arteriosus, 136b
    peripheral pulses in, 153f

PCV. *See* Packed cell volume
Peak expiratory flow rate, 104, 104b
Pectinate line, 556f
Pectineal line, 583f
Pectineus muscle, 575t–577t, 580f, 589f
Pectoral (anterior) axillary lymph
    nodes, 402f
Pectoral girdle, 381f
    bones of, 379
    movements of, 384–386, 388f,
        388t–389t
      elevation and depression, 385
      lateral and medial rotation,
        385–386, 386b
      muscles, 386–387
      protraction and retraction,
        385–386
    of upper limb, 442t–443t
Pectoral lymph nodes, 78, 399f, 403f
Pectoral region
    acromioclavicular joint, 384, 384b,
      386f–387f
    clavicle, 379–381, 379b, 381b, 382f
    movements of pectoral girdle,
      384–386, 388f, 388t–389t
    scapula, 383–384, 383b–384b,
      385f–386f
    sternoclavicular joint, 381–383,
      382f–383f, 382b
    of upper limb, 379–387, 380f
Pectoralis major muscle, 68, 394t, 397f,
    399f
Pectoralis minor muscle, 388t–389t,
    399f
Pedicel, 516f
Pedicle, 191f, 193f, 195f
Pedunculated submucosal fibroid, 548f
Pedunculated subserosal fibroid, 548f
Pellagra, 506b
Pelvic cavity, 451f
Pelvic floor, 458–459, 459b, 460f, 460t
Pelvic girdle, 567–582
    coccyx, 566f, 569–570, 569b–570b,
      571f
    function of, 574, 574b
    gluteal region, 580–582
      blood vessels, 581–582
      intramuscular injection site in,
        581f, 581b
      in lower limb, 566f
      muscles in, 575t–577t
      pelvis and, 580f

Pelvic girdle *(Continued)*
    innominate, 566f, 567–569, 567b,
      568f
      ilium, 567, 568f
      ischium, 567, 568f
      pubis, 567–569, 568f, 569b
    lumbosacral joint, 573, 573b, 574f
    relations of, 574–580, 575f,
      578f–580f, 579b
      external iliac artery, 579
      external iliac vein, 579
      internal iliac artery, 578–579
      internal iliac vein, 578–579
      lumbosacral plexus, 580, 580b,
        581f
    sacrococcygeal joint, 573–574, 574b
    sacrum, 566f, 569–570, 569b–570b,
      571f
    symphysis pubis, 569, 569b, 570f
Pelvic inlet, 451f, 525f
Pelvic splanchnic nerves, 227f
Pelvis, 450–508, 451f, 452f–454f, 453b,
    575f, 580f
Pendular movements, of small
    intestine, 495f
Penis, 452f–453f, 538–541, 539f, 539b
    erectile tissue of, 540f
    major blood vessels of, 539f
Peptic ulcer, 491b
Peptide YY (PYY), 486–487, 486f
Peptone, 176
Perforating cutaneous nerve, 581f, 594,
    594f
Pericardiacophrenic vessels, 85f
Pericardial cavity, 381f
Pericardial pleura, 95
Pericardial sac, 82f
Pericardium, 84–87, 85f
    blood and nerve supply to, 86–87,
      87b
    cut edge of, 86f
Pericranium, 237, 237f
Pericytes, 155, 155f
Perimysium, 40f
Perineal body, 460f, 540f, 551f
Perineal fascia, 555
Perineal membrane
    in females, 551f, 554f
    in males, 528f, 551f
Perineum, 550–557, 551f
    inferior aspect of, 554f
    neurovascular supply of, 556–557

Perineum *(Continued)*
    arteries, 556
    lymphatics, 557, 557f, 557b
    nerves, 556
    veins, 557
    superficial features of, 553f
Perineurium, 50, 51f
Periodic breathing, 112, 112f
Periodontal membrane, 36f, 310f
Periosteal cells, 31f
Periosteum, 302f
    of bone, 30f, 32f
    in fibrous joints, 36f
    of scalp, 237
Peripheral chemoreceptors, 111
Peripheral nerves, structure of, 50–52,
    51f
Peripheral nervous system, 50–52
Peripheral pulses, in patent
    ductus arteriosus and aortic
    regurgitation, 151, 153f
Peripheral resistance, of venous blood
    pressure, 153
Peristalsis, of small intestine, 495, 495f
Peritoneum, arrangement of, 453f
Peritonitis, 453b
Perivascular interstitial space, 107f
Peroneal artery, 612f
Peroxisomes, 10f, 13–14, 14b
Phagocytic cells, immunity and, 177t
Phagocytic vesicle, lysosome enzymes
    in, 13f
Phagocytosis, 11–12
Phalanges, 380f, 418f, 425–426,
    425b–426b, 427f, 434f, 566f, 625f,
    626, 626b
Pharyngeal branch, of
    glossopharyngeal nerve, 279f
Pharyngeal muscles, 326
Pharynx, 94, 326–328, 326b, 327f
Phospholipids, 174, 500
Phosphorus, 507
Phrenic nerve, 92–93, 92b–93b, 93f,
    321f, 334f–335f
    right, 74, 383f
Physical exercise, effect of, in
    respiratory physiology, 111
Physique, arterial blood pressure and,
    148
Pia mater, 208f, 220f, 264, 265f, 315f
Pia sleeve, of nerve root, 220f
Pineal body, 254f–255f, 255

Pineal gland, 337f, 368, 368b
Pinocytosis, 11–12, 157
Pinocytotic vesicle, lysosome enzymes in, 13f
Piriform fossa, 328, 328b
Piriformis muscle, 460f, 575f, 575t–577t, 580f
Pisiform bone, 418f–419f
Pituitary fossa, 243f, 305f
Pituitary gland, 272f, 307f, 335–340, 337f–338f, 339t
    disorders of, 339–340, 339t
    growth hormone, 337–339
    regulation of growth hormone secretion, 338–339
Pivot joint, of bone, 38
Placenta, 363, 364f, 548, 548b, 549f
    organisation of, 363f
Placental septum, 363f, 549f
Plane joint, of bone, 37
Plantar aponeurosis, of foot, 634–636, 634b, 635f
Plantar aspect (sole), of foot, 634–636
    fibro-osseous tunnels, 634
    lateral plantar artery, 635–636, 635f, 635b–636b
    lateral plantar nerve, 634–635
    medial plantar artery, 635–636, 635f, 635b–636b
    medial plantar nerve, 634–635
    plantar aponeurosis, 634–636, 634b, 635f
Plantar calcaneocuboid ligament, 627f
Plantar calcaneonavicular ligament, 620f, 627f–628f
Plantar cuneonavicular ligament, 627f
Plantar digital artery, 635f
Plantar intermetatarsal ligament, 627f
Plantar interossei muscle, 633t–634t
Plantar ligament, of metatarsophalangeal joints, 632f
Plantar surface, of lower limb, 566f
Plantar tarsometatarsal ligaments, 631f
Plantaris muscle, 595t–596t, 599f, 611f, 614f, 622t
Plasma, 165
Plasma cells, 26, 178
Plasma membrane, 10f, 15f
Plasma proteins, 165, 165b, 504, 504f, 504b
    depletion of, 508b
    restoration of, 158

Plasma volume, restoration of, 158
Platelet activating factor, 179, 179t
Platelet cytoplasm, 174, 174t
Platelet disorders, 174
Platelets, 174–176, 174b
    function of, 175
Platysma muscle, 289t–290t, 293f, 319f
Pleasure zone, 263
Pleurae, 95–97, 95b, 97b
    surface markings of, 99–100, 100b
Pleural cavity, 95, 98f
Pleural effusion, 114
Plicae circulares, 469, 472f
Pneumonia, 114
Pneumotaxic centre, 110, 110f, 110b
Pneumothorax, 97b
Podocytes, 515, 516f–517f
Poliomyelitis, 219
Polycystic kidney disease, 513b
Polycythaemia, 146, 172
Polymorphonuclear leukocytes, 172, 172f
Polypnoea, 111
Polyps, 477b
Polyunsaturated fats, 499t
Pons, 208f, 213f, 249–250, 249f, 250b, 254f–255f, 262f, 269
Pontine branches, of basilar artery, 267f
Popliteal artery, 611f–612f, 618f
Popliteal fossa, 608–611, 609b–610b, 611f–612f
Popliteal nodes, 590f
Popliteal surface, of femur, 583f, 611f
Popliteal vein, 592f, 611f
Popliteus muscle, 595t–596t, 599f, 603f, 612f–613f
Pores, 154
Portal systems, 138, 141f
Portal vein, 123f
Postaxial border of limb, 381f
Post-central anastomosis, 203f
Postcentral gyrus, 257f
Postcentral sulcus, 257f
Posterior arch, of vertebra, 193f
Posterior auricular artery, 237f, 291f
Posterior auricular nerve, 278f
Posterior auricular vein, 237f, 291f, 322f
Posterior border, of fibula, 597f
Posterior cerebellar artery, 267f
Posterior cerebral artery, 266f, 268f, 269, 269b

Posterior chamber, 298f
Posterior circumflex humeral artery, 386f, 397f
Posterior commissure, 553f
Posterior communicating artery, 266f–267f, 272f
Posterior condylar canal, 244t
Posterior cord, 399f
    of brachial plexus, 438f
Posterior cranial fossa, 243, 243f, 244t
Posterior cruciate ligament, 600f, 603f–604f
Posterior cutaneous nerve, 417f, 580f–581f, 594f, 639f
Posterior ethmoidal artery, 296f, 307f
    septal branch of, 307f
Posterior ethmoidal nerve, 296f
Posterior fontanelle, 236f
Posterior funiculus, of spinal cord, 210f
Posterior glandular branch, of superior thyroid artery, 332f
Posterior gluteal line, 568f
Posterior head cap, 354f
Posterior horn, 261f, 603f
Posterior inferior cerebellar artery, 267f
Posterior inferior iliac spine, 568f
Posterior intercostal arteries, 75–76, 76f, 87, 386f
    collateral branch of, 76f
Posterior intercostal veins, 77, 77f–78f
Posterior intermediate sulcus, of spinal cord, 208f, 210f
Posterior intermuscular septum, 614f
Posterior internal plexus, 203f
Posterior interosseous arteries, 417f
Posterior interosseous nerve, 412f, 417f, 418
Posterior interventricular artery, 125f
Posterior lateral sulcus, of spinal cord, 208f, 210f
Posterior ligament, 613f
Posterior longitudinal ligament, 199, 199f, 201f, 203f
Posterior median sulcus, of spinal cord, 208f, 210f
Posterior mediastinum, 87–93
Posterior nuclei, 253–254
Posterior pituitary, 338f
Posterior pulmonary plexus, 70f
Posterior sacral foramen, 197f
Posterior scalene muscle, 318f
Posterior spinal arteries, 209f

Posterior spinocerebellar tract, 214, 214b
Posterior subcostal artery, 87
Posterior superior iliac spine, 568f
Posterior superior pancreaticoduodenal artery, 467f
Posterior talocalcanean ligament, 620f
Posterior talofibular ligament, 613f, 620f
Posterior tibial artery, 614f, 615, 618f, 623f
Posterior tibiofibular ligament, 613f
Posterior tibiotalar ligament, 620f
Posterior triangle, of neck, 318f
Posterior tubercle, of vertebra, 193f
Posterior vagal trunk, 88f
Posterior ventral nucleus, 253
Posterolateral ventral nucleus, 253
Posteromedial ventral nucleus, 253
Postganglionic axons, 223–224
Postganglionic fibres, 90, 91f
Post-ileal appendix, 473f
Postjunctional membrane, in muscle contraction, 43f
Posture
    heart rate and, 135
    of venous blood pressure, 153
Potassium, 507
Potassium ions, on heart, 133
Power grips, of hand, 435
P-R interval, 128
Preantral follicle, 357f
Pre-aortic nodes, 557f
Pre-auricular nodes, 238f, 292f
Preaxial border of limb, 381f
Precapillary sphincters, 155f
Precentral gyrus, 256–257, 257f
Precentral sulcus, 257f
Preganglionic axons, 223–224
Preganglionic neurons, 90, 91f
Pregnancy, 361–365, 365b, 547f, 547b
    fertilisation, cleavage and implantation, 361–363, 361f–362f
    hormonal factors during, 363–364
    hypertension during, 149
    maternal responses to, 364–365
    placenta, 363, 364f
Pre-ileal appendix, 473f
Prejunctional membrane, in muscle contraction, 43f

Preovulatory (mature) follicle, 357f
Prepatellar bursa, 600f
Pressure gradients, 145, 146t
Pressure pulse, in ascending aorta, 152f
Pretracheal fascia, 319f, 325, 326f
Pretracheal space, 325, 326f
Prevertebral layer, 326f
    of fascia, 325
    fascial space within, 325, 326f
Primary capillary plexus, 338f
Primary cartilaginous joint, of bone, 35, 36f
Primary hypotension, 149
Primary lymphoid follicle, 162f
Primary spermatocyte, 352f–353f
Primary synaptic cleft, in muscle contraction, 43f
Primordial follicle, 357f
Primordial germ cell, stages of, 353f
Princeps pollicis artery, 437f
Procerus muscle, 293f
Processus vaginalis, 533f
Procoagulants, 176
Profunda brachii artery, 386f, 397f, 403f, 404, 413f, 437f
Profunda femoris artery, 590, 590b, 591f
Profundus muscle, 434f
Progesterone, 359, 360f, 364, 365f, 368f
Progestins, 360f
Projection fibres, 260
Prolactin (PRL), 339t, 366, 368f
Proliferative phase, of menstrual cycle, 545f, 546
Pronator quadratus muscle, 415t
Pronator teres muscle, 410t, 412f, 415t, 417f, 440f
    humeral head, 417f
    ulnar head, 417f
Pronephric system, in embryo, 509f
Proper palmar digital arteries, 437f
Prophase, 17
Prostacyclin, 369
Prostaglandins, 151, 368, 518
    related hormones and, 369
Prostate, 526f, 535–537, 535f–536f, 536b–537b
Prostate cancer, 537b
Prostate-specific antigen (PSA), 535, 536b
Prostatic urethra, 526f, 527
Proteasomes, 14, 14b

Protein deficiency anaemia, 170
Protein fibres, in connective tissues, 26f
Proteins, 503–505
    absorption of, 503, 503b
    digestion of, 503, 503t
    formation of, 13f
    metabolism of, 504–505, 504b–505b, 505f
        insulin effect on, 348, 348b
        in liver, 508
        plasma, 504, 504f, 504b
Proteinuria, 515b
Proteoglycan filament, 157f
Prothrombin, 165
Protoplasmic astrocyte, 246f–247f, 247
Protraction, 286
Proximal convoluted tubule, 516f, 518–519, 518t, 519f, 519b
Proximal nail fold, 60f
Proximal phalanx, 426f, 431f
    base of, 431f
    of metatarsophalangeal joints, 632f
PSA. See Prostate-specific antigen
Pseudostratified epithelium, 20
Psoas bursa, site of, 585f
Psoas major muscle, 207f, 575t–577t, 589f
Psoas muscle, 511f
Pteroylglutamic acid. See Folic acid
Pterygoid plexus, of veins, 292f, 296f
Pterygoid venous plexus, 271f
Pterygomandibular raphe, 313f
Pterygopalatine fossa, 276f
Pterygopalatine ganglion, 225, 226f
Ptosis, 300b
Ptyalism, 489
Puberty, 359–361, 361f
Pubic symphysis, 451f, 551f, 553f, 575f, 589f
Pubic tubercle, 568f
Pubis, 567–569, 568f, 569b, 570f
Pubofemoral ligament, 585f
Pudendal artery, 575f
Pudendal nerve, 575f, 580f–581f
Pudendal vessels, 580f
Pulmonary circulation, 106, 106b, 136
Pulmonary oedema, 114
Pulmonary trunk, 84f, 123f, 137
Pulmonary valve, 119f–121f, 121–122
Pulmonary veins, 93f, 99f
Pulp cavity, 310f
Pulse pressure, 147

Pulse wave, formation and transmission of, 151
Pulsus alternans, 152b
Pulsus deficit, 152b
Pulsus paradoxus, 152b
Puncta, 303f
Pupil, 297f, 299
Purpura, 176b
Pyelonephritis, 513b
Pyloric sphincter, 465–466, 465f
Pylorus, 465f
Pyramid
    of brainstem, 249f, 262f
    of kidney, 512f
    of spinal cord, 208f
Pyramidal decussation, 249f
Pyramidal system, 215, 263
Pyramidal tract, lesions of, 248b
Pyramidalis muscle, 454b, 570f
Pyridoxine (vitamin B$_6$), 506

Q

QRS complex, 128
Q-T interval, 128
Quadrangular membrane, 330, 330f
Quadrangular space, 397f
Quadrate ligament, 413f
Quadrate tubercle, of femur, 583f
Quadratus femoris muscle, 575t–577t, 580f–581f, 593f
Quadratus lumborum muscle, 204f, 205t–206t, 207f, 511f, 578f
Quadratus plantae muscle, 633t–634t
Quadriceps tendon, 600f, 601b

R

Radial artery, 413f, 416, 416b, 417f, 419f, 421f, 437f
Radial collateral artery, 413f
Radial collateral ligament, 408f
Radial fossa, 390f
Radial nerve, 397f, 400f–401f, 401t, 403f, 404, 412f, 436, 438f
Radial nerve palsy, 398f
Radial notch, 413f, 415f
Radial recurrent artery, 413f
Radial styloid process, 405f
Radial tuberosity, 405f
Radialis indicis artery, 437f
Radiocarpal joints, 380f, 419f, 422f
Radioulnar joints, 412, 412b, 413f–415f, 443, 443t

Radius, 404–406, 404b, 405f, 413f, 417f, 419f
    head of, 413f, 415f
Ramus, 282, 282f
Raphe, 553f
Rectal artery, 477f
Rectum, 473f, 476–477, 478f, 526f, 556f
    arterial supply to, 477f, 477b
Rectus abdominis muscle, 454b, 455f–456f, 457t, 570f
Rectus femoris muscle, 575t–577t, 580f, 585f, 589f, 595t–596t, 610f
Rectus sheath, formation of, 455f–456f
Recurrent laryngeal nerve, 319f
    left, 332f
    right, 332f
Red blood cell, count, restoration of, 158
Red marrow cavities, of bone, 30f, 30b
Red nucleus, 251
Red pulp, of spleen, 163f
Refracting media, 299, 299b
Regurgitation, 122
Renal artery, 91f, 511f, 525f
Renal calculi. See Urinary tract stones
Renal cell carcinomas, 521b
Renal column, 512f
Renal corpuscle, 511–513, 515, 515b, 516f–517f
Renal hypertension, 149
Renal papillae, 511
Renal pelvis, 512f
Renal regulation, 150
Renal vein, 511f, 524f
Renin, 368
Renin secretion, immediate compensatory effects on, 158
Renin-angiotensin system, 516–518, 517f
Repetitive strain injury, 616b
Reproductive hormones, 357–358, 357f
Reproductive system, 530–550
    development of, 530f, 530b
    female, 541–542
    male, 532–541
    sex determination, 531–532
RER. See Rough endoplasmic reticulum
Resident cells, in connective tissues, 26f
Residual body, lysosome enzymes in, 13f
Residual volume (RV), 103, 103f

Respiration
    chemical control of, 111
    disturbances of, 111
    immediate compensatory effects on, 158
    mechanics of, 101
    thoracic cage during, 101f
Respiratory bronchiole, 107, 107f, 115f
Respiratory centre, 110, 110f
Respiratory control, 109–110
Respiratory diverticulum, development of, stages in, 94f
Respiratory excursions, 103f
Respiratory physiology, 102–116, 102b
Respiratory protective reflexes, 116
Respiratory sinus rhythm, 130
Respiratory system, 93–116, 93b–94b, 177t
Respiratory unit, 107–109, 107f
Rete testis, 533f
Reticular fibres, in connective tissues, 26f, 27
Retina, 297, 297f, 299
    blood supply to, 299–300, 300b
    cellular organisation of, 299f
Retinitis pigmentosa, 113b
Retinol, 505
Retraction, 286, 287f, 387f
Retrocaecal appendix, 473f
Retromandibular vein, 290, 322f
Retroperitoneal rectum, 476
Retropharyngeal space, 325, 326f
Rhesus system, 168, 169b
Rhomboid major muscle, 388t–389t, 397f
Rhomboid minor muscle, 388t–389t, 397f
Rib cage, 470f
Riboflavin (vitamin B$_2$), 506
Ribosome, 15f
Ribs, 68, 70–71, 71f, 73f, 102, 102f, 333f
    1st, 71, 74f, 82f, 382f, 384f
    10th, 71
    11th, 71
    12th, 71, 578f
Right aortic arch, 136b
Right ascending lumbar vein, 78f
Right atrial impression, 99f
Right atrial pressure, 153
Right atrium, 93f, 119, 120f
Right brachiocephalic vein, 77f, 81, 81f, 83

Right bronchomediastinal trunk, 96f
Right common carotid artery, 89f, 383f
Right common iliac artery, 575f
Right coronary artery, 124, 125f
Right crus, 75f
Right hilum, 98
Right internal carotid artery, 267f
Right lung, 98, 99f
    medial surface of, 97–98
Right lymph trunk, 90
Right marginal artery, 125f
Right parasternal lymphatic vessel, 96f
Right pericardiacophrenic vessels, 85f
Right phrenic nerve, 81, 81f, 85f, 92,
    93f
Right pulmonary arteries, 86f, 93f
Right pulmonary veins, 86f
Right subclavian artery
    abnormal origin of, 136b
    impression, 99f
Right subcostal vein, 78f
Right superior intercostal vein, 77f–78f
Right surface, of heart, 119
Right vagus nerve, 70f, 81f, 84f, 88f,
    92, 93f
Right ventricle, 93f, 121
Right vertebral artery, 266f
Rima glottidis, 329f
Ring finger, 418f
Risorius muscle, 294
Robot-assisted surgery, for abdomen,
    456b
Root canal, 310f
Rotatores muscles, 204f, 205t–206t
Rouget cells, 155
Rough endoplasmic reticulum (RER),
    10f, 12, 12b
Roughage, 494–495
Round window, 315f–316f
R-R interval, 129, 129f
Rubrospinal tract, 216
Ruffini corpuscles, 52, 52f
RV. See Residual volume

S
Saccular aneurysms, 142f, 142b
Saccule, 316f
Sacral body, 197f
Sacral canal, 197f
Sacral cornu, 197f
Sacral curvature, 190
Sacral ganglia, 90f

Sacral hiatus, 197f
Sacral plexus, 223, 223f
Sacral promontory, 197f
Sacral region, 189f
Sacrococcygeal joint, 573–574, 574b
Sacroiliac joint, 566f, 570–573, 571b,
    572f, 573b
    movements in, 573, 573f
Sacrospinous ligament, 554f, 572f
Sacrotuberous ligament, 551f, 554f, 572f
Sacrum, 195, 195b, 197f, 460f, 566f,
    569–570, 569b–570b, 571f
Saddle joint, of bone, 37–38
Sagittal suture, 235f
Saliva, 488–489, 489b
Salivary gland duct cells, function of, 9t
Salivary glands, 312–313
Salpingo-oophorectomy, 548b
Saphenous nerve, 579f, 593, 614, 614f,
    623f, 639f
Sarcolemma, 40f
Sarcoplasm, 43f
Sartorius muscle, 575t–577t, 580f, 589f,
    595f–596f, 610f
Saturated fats, 499t
Scala tympani, 316f
Scala vestibuli, 316f
Scalene muscles, 383f
Scalene tubercle, 74f
Scalenus anterior muscle, 319f, 320t
Scalenus medius muscle, 319f, 320t
Scalenus posterior muscle, 320t
Scalp, 236–239
    blood supply to, 237–238, 237f
    lacerations to, 238b
    layers of, 237f
Scaphoid, 405f, 418f–419f
Scapula, 380f, 383–384, 383b–384b,
    385f–386f, 395f, 399f
Scarpa's fascia, 451, 452f–453f
Schwann cells
    in muscle contraction, 43f
    in unmyelinated axon, 47–48, 48f
Sciatic nerve, 580f–581f, 593–594, 593f,
    594b, 638–640
Sclera, 297, 297f, 300
Scoliosis, 190, 190f, 190b
Scrotal varicoceles, 143b
Scrotum, 452f–453f, 553f
Scurvy, 506, 506b
Sebaceous gland, 56f, 60, 60b
    of eyelash, 302f

Secondary cartilaginous joint, of bone,
    35, 36f
Secondary hypotension, 149
Secondary peritonitis, 453b
Secondary spermatocytes, 352f–353f
Secondary synaptic cleft, in muscle
    contraction, 43f
Secretin, 492f
Secretion, control of, 348–349
Secretory lobules, 367f
Secretory vesicle, 10f, 13f
Segmental fracture, of bone, 34, 34f
Segmentation contractions, of small
    intestine, 495, 495f
Selective lesions, of spinal cord,
    219–220
Semen, 537
    anomalies of, 537
Semicircular canals, 316f
Semicircular ducts, 316f, 317b
Semilunar hiatus, 306f
Semimembranosus muscle, 575t–577t,
    593f, 595t–596t, 599f, 610f–611f
Seminal vesicle, 535, 535f
Seminiferous tubules, 352f, 533f
Semispinalis capitis muscle, 204f,
    205t–206t, 319f, 320t
Semispinalis cervicis muscle, 204f,
    205t–206t
Semispinalis thoracis muscle, 204f,
    205t–206t
Semitendinosus muscle, 575t–577t,
    593f, 595t–596t, 610f–611f
Sensory area, 134–135, 269
Sensory cells, function of, 9t
Sensory innervation, of scalp, 238–239,
    239f
Sensory neuron, 217f–218f
Sensory system, 263
Septal cartilage, 305f
    lateral process of, 304f
    superior margin of, 304f
Septal defects, 118b
Septic shock, 159
SER. See Smooth endoplasmic
    reticulum
Serosa, 464f
    of digestive tract, 463, 463f
    of large intestine, 474f
Serotonin (5-hydroxytryptamine), 369
Serous acinus, in pancreas, 483–484,
    483f

Serous pericardium, 85–86, 86b
Serous visceral pericardium, 126
Serratus anterior muscle, 388t–389t
Serratus posterior inferior, 207f
Sertoli cells, 351, 352f, 356f, 534
Sesamoid bones, 431f, 625f
Sex, determination of, 531–532
Shaft
   of femur, 583f
   of fibula, 597f
   of tibia, 597f
Sheehan's syndrome, 340b
Shock, 158–159
Short association fibres, 259
Short ciliary nerves, 296f
Short gastric arteries, 467f
Short posterior ciliary artery, 296f
Short posterior sacroiliac ligament,
   572f
Short (small) saphenous vein, 592f,
   614f, 615, 623f
Shoulder joint, 380f, 391–398,
   392f–393f, 393b
   attachments, action and innervation
      of, 394t
   movements of, 393–396, 393b, 395f,
      395b
   muscles of, 397f
   relations of, 396–398, 398b
   of upper limb, 442t–443t
Sickle cell anaemia, 170
Sigmoid arteries, 476f
Sigmoid colon, 473f
Sigmoid sinus, 271f
Simmonds' disease/syndrome, 340
Sinoatrial block, 131
Sinuatrial node, 120f, 126f
Sinus arrhythmia, 130
Sinus bradycardia, 130
Sinus tachycardia, 130
Sinuses, 338f
Sjögren syndrome, 489
Skeletal muscle, 39–44, 40f
Skin, 53–61, 53b–54b
   allergies, 173
   in ankle joint, 623f
   appendages of, 58–61
      glands, 60–61
      hair, 56f, 58–60, 58b, 60b
      nails, 58, 58b, 60f
   in calf/leg, 614f
   function of, 54

Skin (Continued)
   immediate compensatory effects on,
      158
   immunity and, 177t
   metabolism of, 54–55
   protection of, 54, 54b
   of scalp, 237, 237f
   sensation of, 54, 54b
   sexual signalling of, 55
   structure of, 55–57, 55f, 55b
      dermis, 55f–56f, 56–57, 56b
      epidermis, 55–56, 55f–56f,
         55b–56b
      subcutaneous connective tissue
         layer, 56f, 57, 57b
   thermoregulation of, 54, 54b
   wound repair, 57–58, 58b, 59f
Skull, 234–243, 234b–235b
   adult, 235f
   anterior aspect of, 240, 240f, 241t,
      241b
   base of, 242, 243f
   external features of, 236–242
   foetal, 236f
   growth of, 235–236, 235b–236b
   lateral aspect of, 239–240, 240b, 285f
   lateral left aspect of, 288f
   posterior aspect of, 239
   vault, 236–239, 236b
Sleep, arterial blood pressure during,
   148
Slow/delayed hypersensitivity, 180
Small cardiac vein, 125–126, 125f
Small intestine, 454f, 468–471, 471b,
   486f, 511f
   within the abdominopelvic cavity,
      470f
   arterial supply of, 471–472, 472f,
      472b
   layers of, 472f
   lymphatic drainage of, 471–472,
      472b
   movements of, 495, 495f, 495b
   secretions from, 493–494
   venous drainage of, 471–472, 472b
Smith's fractures, of radius, 406f, 406b
Smooth endoplasmic reticulum (SER),
   10f, 12, 12b
Smooth muscle, 38–39, 38f, 39b, 107f,
   139f
   fibre, 155f
Sneezing reflex, 116

Sodium, 507
Sodium ions, on heart, 133
Soft palate, 310f
Soleal line, of tibia, 597f
Soleus muscle, 610f, 614f, 622t
Somatic nerves, of perineum, 556
Somatic nervous system and, 221–223,
   222f–223f
Somatostatin, 349, 349b
Special somatic afferent (SSA), 272
Special visceral afferent (SVA), 272
Special visceral efferent (SVE), 272
Sperm, 537, 538f
   anomalies of, 537
Spermatic cord, 458f
Spermatids, 352f–353f
Spermatogenesis, 351–354, 352b, 354b,
   356f
Spermatogonia, 351, 352f–353f
Spermatozoa, 352f
Sphenoid bone, 240, 243f
   greater wing of, 240f, 294–295, 295f
   lesser wing of, 240f, 295f
   medial pterygoid plate of, 305f
   spine of, 285f
Sphenoid sinus, 306–308, 307f
Sphenoidal recess, opening into, 306f
Sphenoidal sinus, 272f, 305f
Sphenomandibular ligament, 285f
Spheno-occipital synchondrosis, 235b
Sphenopalatine artery, 307f
   posterior lateral nasal branches of,
      307f
   posterior septal branch of, 307f
Sphenopalatine foramen, 309f
Sphenoparietal sinus, 271f
Sphincter of Oddi, 492f
Sphincter pupillae, 226f, 273
Sphincter vagina, 460f
Spinal cord, 204–227, 208f, 248f
   autonomic nervous system and,
      223–227, 224f
   dural sac of, 265f
   internal structure and organisation
      of, 210–220, 210f, 211t
      afferent and efferent tracts,
         212–217, 212f
      grey matter, 211–212
      white matter, 212
   lesions of, 219–220
   meninges of, 206–210, 207b, 208f
      blood supply, 207–210, 209f, 210b

Spinal cord *(Continued)*
  epidural space, 207, 207b
  short tracts of, 212–213
  somatic nervous system and, 221–223, 222f–223f
  spinal nerves in, 220–221, 220f, 220b–221b, 222f
  ventral aspect of, 208f
Spinal nerve, 213f, 220–221, 220f, 221b, 222f, 319f
Spinal nucleus, 274–275
Spinal reflex, 217–218
  flexor reflex and crossed extensor reflex in, 218, 218f
  muscle stretch reflex in, 217–218, 217f, 218b
Spinalis capitis, 205t–206t
Spinalis cervicis, 205t–206t
Spinalis thoracis, 204f, 205t–206t
Spine, 385f
Spinocerebellar tract, 248b
Spinoglenoid notch, 385f
Spinothalamic pathway, to brain, 218f
Spinothalamic tract, 213f, 248b
Spinous process, of vertebra, 191f, 193f, 196f
Spinous tubercles, on median sacral crest, 197f
Spiral artery, 546, 546f, 549f
Spiral fractures, of bone, 34
Spiral groove, 390f, 438f
Splanchnic nerves, 91f
Spleen, 162–163, 470f, 483f, 484–485, 485b, 511f
  development of, 484b
  function of, 163, 163b
  rupture of, 485b
  structure of, 163, 163f
Splenic artery, 163f, 467f
Splenius capitis muscle, 318f–319f, 320t
Splenomegaly, 163b
Spongy urethra, 526f, 527
Spontaneous bacterial peritonitis, 453b
SSA. *See* Special somatic afferent
S-T segment, 128–129
Stable fracture, of bone, 33
Stagnant (hypokinetic) hypoxia, 113
Stapedius muscle, 316b
  nerve to, 315f
Starvation, 487–488, 488f
Steatohepatitis, 480b
Steatorrhea, 492b

Stellate ganglion, 90f
Stem cells, 17–19, 18f
  in meiosis, 19
Stenosis, 122
Sternal angle, 68f, 68b, 69, 70f
Sternal fibres, 75f
Sternebrae, 68
Sternoclavicular joint, 380f, 381–383, 382f–383f, 382b
Sternocleidomastoid muscle, 281f, 318f, 321f–322f
Sternocostal joints, 71f
Sternocostal surface, 119
Sternocostalis muscle, 75
Sternohyoid muscle, 319f, 323f, 324t, 383f
Sternomastoid muscle, 317b, 319f, 320t, 383f, 397f
Sternothyroid muscle, 319f, 323f, 324t, 383f
Sternum, 68–70, 68f–69f, 68b–69b, 383f–384f, 451f
  articular facet for, 382f
Sternum, manubrium of, 326f
Stimulatory reactions, 180
Stokes-Adams syndrome, 132b
Stomach, 88f, 454f, 465–468, 465b–467b, 470f, 478f, 486f, 492f, 511f
  anterior aspect of, 465f
  cancer, 468b
  development of, 465f, 465b
  gastric pit and gland in, 466f
  innervation of, 467, 467f, 467b
  rotation of, 465f
Straight sinus, 270, 271f
Straight tubule, 533f
Stratum basale, 55f
Stratum corneum, 55f
Stratum granulosum, 55f
Stratum lucidum, 55f
Stratum spinosum, 55f
Stratum spongiosum, 363f
Stress (hairline) fracture, of bone, 34
Stress incontinence, 459b
Stretch receptor, 217f
Stroke volume, 133–134
Stroma, 546f
Stylohyoid muscle, 281f, 318f, 323f, 324t
Styloid process, 243f, 284f–285f, 315f
Stylomandibular ligament, 285f

Stylopharyngeus muscle, 279f
Subacromial bursa, 392f
Subacute combined degeneration, 219–220
Subarachnoid space, 220f, 265f
Subcaecal appendix, 473f
Subcapsular sinus, 162f
Subclavian artery, 74f, 76f, 335f, 437f
  1st part of, 321f
  3rd part of, 321f
  left, 332f–333f, 386f
  right, 333f
Subclavian groove, 382f
Subclavian lymphatic duct, 403f
Subclavian vein, 74f, 321f, 334f–335f, 383f
Subclavius muscle, 388t–389t, 399f
  nerve to, 400f
Subcostal artery, 77
Subcostal groove, 72f
Subcostal nerves, 79, 511f
Subcostalis muscle, 75
Subcutaneous connective tissue layer, 56f, 57, 57b
Subcutaneous fat, in calf/leg, 614f
Subcutaneous papilla, 56f
Subdiaphragmatic lymphatics, 403f
Sublingual fold, 310f
Sublingual gland, 226f, 313, 313f
Submandibular duct, 310f, 313f
Submandibular ganglion, 225, 226f
Submandibular gland, 226f, 313, 313f
Submandibular nodes, 238f, 292f
Submandibular triangle, 321
Submental nodes, 238f, 292f
Submental triangle, 318f, 321
Submucosa, 463f–464f
Submucosal fibroid, 548f
Submucosal plexus, 464, 464f
Subscapular fossa, 385f
Subscapular (posterior) lymph nodes, 402f–403f
Subscapularis muscle, 393f, 394t, 399f
Subserosal fibroid, 548f
Substance P, 370
Substantia nigra, 250
Subtalar joint, 626, 628f
  movements in, 626–627, 629f
Subthalamus, 256
Sulcus terminalis, 311f
Superficial cardiac plexus, 84f, 126
Superficial circumflex iliac artery, 591f

Superficial circumflex iliac vein, 592f
Superficial dorsal artery, of penis, 539f
Superficial epigastric artery, 591f
Superficial epigastric vein, 592f
Superficial external pudendal artery, 591f
Superficial external pudendal vein, 592f
Superficial fascia, 451, 455f–456f, 539f, 555, 555b
  arrangement of, 452f–453f
  investing layer of, 319f
  membranous layer of, 528f
Superficial fibular/peroneal nerve, 623f, 639f, 640
  in calf/leg, 614, 614f, 616f
  in foot, 629
Superficial inguinal lymph nodes, 557f, 590f
Superficial inguinal ring, 458f
Superficial palmar arch, 435b, 437f
Superficial radial nerve, 412f, 417f, 419f
Superficial temporal artery, 237f, 285f, 291f
Superficial temporal vein, 237f, 291f
Superficial terminal branch, of ulnar nerve, 439f
Superficial thrombophlebitis, 142
Superficial transverse perineal muscle, 540f, 552f
Superior alveolar nerve, anterior, nasal branch of, 309f
Superior angle, 385f
Superior articular facet, 193f, 195f–196f
Superior articular processes, of vertebra, 197f
Superior border, 385f
Superior cerebellar artery, 267f
Superior cerebellar peduncle, 250, 253, 254f
Superior cerebral veins, 271f
Superior cervical ganglion, 335f
Superior colliculus, 251, 255f
Superior concha, 306f–307f
Superior conjunctival fornix, 302f
Superior constrictor muscle, 313f
Superior costotransverse ligament, 73f
Superior demifacet, 73f
Superior epigastric artery, 76f
Superior extensor retinaculum, 615f, 619f

Superior fibular retinaculum, 623f
Superior gluteal artery, 575f
Superior gluteal nerve, 580f–581f, 638
Superior gluteal vessels, 580f, 581–582
Superior hypogastric plexus, 91f
Superior labial artery, 291f
  septal branch from nasal artery from, 307f
Superior labial vein, 291f
Superior ligament, of symphysis pubis, 570f
Superior lobe, of lungs, 99f
Superior longitudinal bundle, 259
Superior meatus, 306f
Superior mediastinum, 80–83
Superior mesenteric artery, 91f, 476f
Superior oblique muscle, 275f, 296f, 301t
Superior ophthalmic vein, 296f
Superior orbital fissure, 240f, 244t, 275f–276f, 295f
Superior parathyroid gland, 332f
Superior petrosal sinus, 271f
Superior radioulnar joint, 380f, 413f
Superior rectal artery, 476f–477f
Superior rectus muscle, 275f, 296f, 301t
Superior sagittal sinus, 265f, 270, 271f
Superior salivary nucleus, 276–277
Superior surface
  of 1st left rib, 74f
  of diaphragm, 74
Superior tarsal muscle, 302f
Superior thyroid artery, 332f
Superior thyroid vein, 332f
Superior tibiofibular joint, 566f, 611–612, 613f
Superior turbinate, 305f
Superior ulnar collateral artery, 403f, 413f
Superior vena cava, 81, 81f, 83, 83b, 84f–86f, 89f, 120f, 123f, 125f, 137
Superior vesical artery, 123f
Supinator crest, 405f
Supinator muscle, 415t, 417f
Suppressor T cells, 177
Supraclavicular lymph nodes, 403f
Supracondylar fractures, 407b
Supracondylar lines, of femur, 583f
Suprahyoid muscle, 323f, 324t
Supraoptic nucleus, 338f
Supraorbital artery, 237f, 291f, 296f
Supraorbital foramen, 241t

Supraorbital nerve, 239f, 276f, 296f
Supraorbital notch, 240f
Supraorbital veins, 237f, 291f, 296f
Suprapatellar bursa, 600f, 608f
Suprapleural membrane, 80b
Suprascapular artery, 321f, 333f, 386f
Suprascapular nerve, 401t
Suprascapular notch, 385f
Suprascapular vein, 322f
Supraspinatus muscle, 392f–393f, 394t, 397f
Supraspinous fossa, 385f
Supraspinous ligament, 201f–202f
Supratrochlear artery, 237f, 291f, 296f
Supratrochlear nerve, 239f, 276f, 296f
Supratrochlear vein, 237f, 291f
Supravaginal cervix, 543f
Supreme intercostal artery, 76f, 333f
Sural nerve, 611f, 614f, 615, 617f, 623f, 639f
Surface membrane, 354f
Surface mucous cells, 466f
Suspensory ligament
  of axilla, 399f
  of clitoris, 552f
  of penis, 540f
Sutural ligament, in fibrous joints, 36f
Sutures, of fibrous joints, 35, 35b, 36f
SVA. See Special visceral afferent
SVE. See Special visceral efferent
Swallowing, 328, 328b
  reflex, 116
Sweat glands, 56f, 60–61
Sympathetic chain, 90–92, 90f, 90b, 332
Sympathetic nerves, 91f
Sympathetic nervous system, 225–227
Sympathetic plexus, 315f
Sympathetic stimulation, 135, 147
Sympathetic trunk, 70f, 335f
Sympathetic vasodilator fibres, 150
Sympatheticomimetic drugs, 159
Symphysis menti, 282
Symphysis pubis, 458f, 460f, 569, 569b, 570f
Synapse, in neuron, 48–49, 49f, 49b, 217f, 245f
Syncytiotrophoblast, 362f
Syndesmosis, 35, 36f
Syndrome of inappropriate hypersecretion of antidiuretic hormone, 340
Synovial condyloid joint, 283–284

Synovial joints, 36–38, 36b, 37f, 68
Synovial membrane, 37f, 392f, 600f, 608f
  protrusion of, 408f
Synovial sheath, 392f, 419f, 427f
Syringomyelia, 219
Systemic circulation, 136
Systole, 127
Systolic pressure, 147, 148t

T
T lymphocytes, 176–177
T wave, 127–128
Tabes dorsalis, 219
Tachycardia, electrocardiogram in, 131f
Tachypnoea, 111
Tactile corpuscle, 56f
Taeniae coli, 473f
Talus, 566f, 623f, 625f, 628f, 630f
Target tissues, 360f
Tarsal gland, 302f
Tarsal plates, 300
Tarsometatarsal joints, 627, 631f
  movements in, 627, 627b, 632f
Tarsus, 300, 302f, 625, 625f, 625b
Taste (gustatory) pathway, 279
Tectorial membrane, 316f
Tectospinal tract, 216, 216b
Tectum, 251
Teeth, 36f, 309–311, 310f
Tegmental syndrome, 251b
Tegmentum, 250
Tela choroidea, 260
Telophase, 17
Temporal bone, 235f–236f, 240, 243f, 315f
Temporal lobe, 257f, 259b, 262f
Temporal pole, 257f
Temporalis muscle, 288f, 289t–290t
Temporomandibular joint, 283–287
  lateral, 285f
  movements of, 286–287, 287b
  sagittal, 284f
Tendocalcaneus, 617f, 623f
Tendon, 44b, 217f
  of biceps femoris, 613f
  of fibularis (peroneus) longus, 627f
  of popliteus, 600f, 613f
  of rectus femoris, 599f
  of tibialis anterior, 627f
  of tibialis posterior, 627f

Tennis elbow, 409b
Tension, 145
Tension pneumothorax, 97b
Tensor fascia lata, 575t–577t, 580f, 595t–596t
Tensor tympani, 315f, 316b
Tentorium cerebelli, 264, 271f
Teratozoospermia, 537
Teres major muscle, 394t, 397f, 399f
Teres minor muscle, 393f, 394t, 397f, 399f
Testes, 337f, 351–356, 355b–356b, 356f, 532–534, 533f, 533b–534b
  cells in, function of, 9t
  coverings of, 532f
  development of, 532f, 532b
  hypergonadism, 356
  hypogonadism, 356, 356b
  spermatogenesis, 351–354, 352b, 354b
  testosterone, 354–356, 354b
Testicular torsion, 534b
Testicular vein, 524f
Testosterone, 354–356, 354b, 356f
  functions of, 355–356, 355f–356f, 355b
Thalamus, 245f, 253–256, 254f–255f, 257f, 269
  blood supply to, 254b
  function of, 254
Thalassaemia, 170
Theca cell, 360f
Thenar muscles, 419f
Thiamine (vitamin B₁), 505–506
Thiamine deficiency, 505–506
Thiazide diuretics, 519b
Thigh, 566f, 582–594, 582b
  compartments of, 589–594
    anterior, 590–593
    medial, 593
    muscles, 594, 595t–596t
    posterior, 593–594
  femoral triangle, 588–589, 589f, 589b
    lymph nodes of, 589, 590f
    vessels in, 591f
  femur, 566f, 582–584, 582b, 583f–584f, 584b
    hip joint capsule to, 585f
    patella with, movement of, 608f, 610f
  hip joint, 566f, 584–588, 586b

Thigh (Continued)
  anterior relations of, 589f
  capsular attachment of, 585f
  capsular ligaments associated with, 585f, 586b
  movements in, 575t–577t, 586–588, 642
  relations of, 580f, 588
Third occipital nerve, 239f
Thoracic aorta, 82f, 86f
Thoracic cage, 66–80, 68b, 201
  anterior aspect of, 67f
  lateral aspect of, during respiration, 101f
  muscles attached to, 75–79
Thoracic cavity, 80–180
Thoracic curve, 189
Thoracic duct, 88–90, 89f, 96f, 334f, 383f
Thoracic inlet, 67f, 79–80, 81f–82f, 97
Thoracic outlet, 80
Thoracic outlet syndrome, 387b
Thoracic region, 189f
  intervertebral disc of, 198f
  zygapophyseal joints of, 200f
Thoracic splanchnic nerves, 90f
Thoracic sympathetic chain, 91
Thoracic vertebrae, 72, 194, 194b, 195f
Thoracoacromial trunk, 399f
Thoracodorsal nerve, 400f, 401t
Thoracolumbar fascia, 207f, 451
Thorax (chest), 65–186
  anterior aspect of, 120f, 455f–456f
  thoracic cage, 66–80, 67f–68f, 68b
  thoracic cavity, 80–180
Thready (weak) pulse, 152b
Thrombocytes, 165, 174–176, 174b
Thrombocythaemia, 174
Thrombocytopenia, 174
Thrombocytosis, 174
Thrombopoietin, 368
Thrombosis, 139, 176, 176b
Thromboxane A₂, 369
Thrombus, 142
Thumb, 418f
  joint, of upper limb, 443–444, 443t
  movements of, 432f
Thymus gland, 163–164, 164b, 337f, 369
Thyrocervical trunk, 321f, 332f–333f
Thyrohyoid membrane, 324t, 329f, 330
Thyrohyoid muscle, 332f

Thyroid cartilage, 266f, 329, 329f
Thyroid follicles, 340–341, 341f
Thyroid gland, 319f, 331, 331b, 340–342, 341f, 341b
   function of thyroid hormones, 341–342, 341b
   regulation of secretion of, 341
Thyroid hormones, function of, 341–342, 341b
Thyroid-stimulating hormone (TSH), 339t
Thyroxine, 150–151
Tibia, 566f, 596–598, 596b, 597f, 598b
   patella with, movement of, 608f, 610f
   reflections of synovial membrane on, 600f
Tibial nerve, 581f, 593f, 611f, 614f, 615, 617f, 623f, 640
Tibial plateau, 603f
Tibial surface, 599f
Tibial tuberosity, 597f
Tibialis anterior muscle, 610f, 614f, 619f, 622t, 623f
Tibialis posterior muscle, 614f, 619f, 622t, 623f
Tibiocalcaneal ligament, 620f
Tibiofibular joints, 611–612, 612f
   inferior, 612, 613f
   superior, 611–612, 613f
Tibionavicular ligament, 620f
Tidal volume (TV), 103
Tinel's test (Hoffmann-Tinel sign), 421b
Tissue fluid, immediate compensatory effects on, 158
Tissues, 19–53
   connective, 25–38, 26f
     blood, 38
     cells, 25–26
     fibres, 26–27
     ground substance in, 26f, 27
     type of, 27–38
   epithelium in, 19–25
     classification of, 20, 21f
     function of, 20–23
     secretory epithelia and glands, 23–25, 25b
   muscle, 38–44
     action of, 44, 44b
     attachment of, 44, 44b
     cardiac muscle, 39, 39f, 39b
     cells in, function of, 9t

Tissues (Continued)
     contraction, 42–43, 43f, 43b
     forms of, 43–44, 45f
     sensory receptors in, 40–42
     skeletal muscle, 39–44, 40f
     smooth muscle, 38–39, 38f, 39b
     spindles, 41–42, 42f, 42b
   nervous, 44–53, 46b
     action potential in, 50, 50f
     nerve endings, 52, 52f
     nerve injury, 52–53, 53b
     neurons, 46–49
     peripheral nervous system, 50–52
TLC. See Total lung capacity
TNF. See Tumour necrosis factors
Tongue, 311–312
   dorsum of, 310f–311f
Total lung capacity (TLC), 103f
Trabeculae, 162, 162f–163f, 192
Trabeculae carneae, 121
Trachea, 81f, 85f, 93b, 94–95, 94f, 95b, 319f, 329f, 333f–334f, 383f
   anterolateral aspect of, 96f
   blood and nerve supply to, 95
Tracheobronchial lymph nodes, 95, 96f
Tragus, 315f
Trans fats, 499t
Transitional epithelium (urothelium), 20
Transpyloric plane, 69–70
Transversalis fascia, 452f–453f, 455f–456f, 458f
Transverse band, 408f
Transverse cervical artery, 321f, 333f
   deep branch of, 386f
Transverse cervical nerve, 322f
Transverse cervical vein, 322f
Transverse colon, 454f
Transverse facial artery, 291f
Transverse facial vein, 291f
Transverse fracture, of bone, 34f
Transverse humeral ligament, 391f
Transverse intermuscular septum, 614f
Transverse ligament, 600f, 603f
Transverse mesocolon, 454f
Transverse process, of vertebra, 73f, 191f, 193f–194f, 196f
Transverse ridges, 197f
Transverse sinus, 85–86, 86f, 271f
Transverse talofibular ligament, 620f
Transverse (mid) tarsal joint, 626–627, 628f
   movements in, 626–627, 629f

Transversus abdominis, 207f, 457t, 458f, 511f
Trapezius muscle, 281f, 318f–319f, 320t, 321f–322f, 388t–389t, 390b, 397f, 399f, 418f–419f
Trapezoid bone, 418f–419f
Trapezoid ligament, 387f
Trapezoid line, 382f
Triangular interval, 397f, 438f
Triangular space, 397f
Triangular subcutaneous area, 597f
Triceps, 403f
   lateral head, 397f
   long head of, 438f–440f
Triceps brachii muscle, 394t, 410t
Trichomoniasis, 550
Tricuspid valve, 119f–120f, 121
Trigeminal ganglion, 213f, 276f
Trigeminal nerve, 213f, 274–275, 276f
   cutaneous distribution of, 293f
Trigeminal sensory nucleus, 277–279
Triglycerides. See Neutral fats
Trigone, 526f
Triple X (trisomy X) syndrome, 531
Triquetral bone, 418f–419f
Trochanteric fossa, 583f
Trochlea, 390f, 411f
Trochlear nerve, 249f, 251, 273–274, 274b, 275f, 296f
Trochlear notch, 405f, 413f
Trochlear surface, 620f
Trophoblast, 363f
True capillary, 155f
Tubal ligation, 542b
Tubal pregnancy, 542b
Tubercle of crest, 568f
Tubular pole, 516f
Tumour necrosis factors (TNF), 178, 179t
Tunica adventitia, 137–138, 140t–141t
Tunica albuginea, 533, 533f, 539f
Tunica externa, 139f
Tunica intima, 137, 139f, 140t–141t
Tunica media, 137–138, 139f, 140t–141t
Tunica vaginalis, 533, 533f
Turner's syndrome, 531–532
TV. See Tidal volume
Tympanic membrane, 315f
Typical ribs, 70–71, 72f

U

U wave, 129
Ulcerative colitis, 475b, 476f, 496b
Ulna, 406–407, 406b–407b, 417f, 419f
  abduction of, 415f
  articular surface for, 405f
  extension of, 415f
  head of, 413f
  long axis of, 407f
  movements of, 408–409, 408f–409f, 408b–409b, 411f
Ulnar artery, 412f–413f, 416, 416b, 417f, 419f, 437f
Ulnar collateral ligament, 407b, 408f
Ulnar groove, 390f
Ulnar nerve, 400f–401f, 401t, 403f, 404, 417f, 418, 419f, 439f
  compression of, 412b
  deep branch of, 439f
  deformity, 420f, 420b
  of upper limb, 436–438, 439f
Ulnar notch, 413f
Ulnar recurrent arteries, 413f
Ulnar styloid process, 405f
Umbilical arteries, 363f, 549f, 575f
Umbilical cord, 363f, 381f
Umbilical vein, 123f, 363f, 549f
Uncovertebral joint, 194f
Uncus, 262f
Uninhibited neurogenic bladder, 530
Unipennate muscles, 44, 45f
Unipolar neuron, 46, 46f
Unmyelinated axons, 47–48, 48f
Unsaturated fats, 498
Upper body surface, raised lip of, of vertebra, 193f
Upper lateral cutaneous nerve, of arm, 438f
Upper limb, 377–448, 379b
  anterior surface of, 402f
  arm, 387–404
  cutaneous innervation of, 401f
  deep fascia of, 379
  development of, 379b, 381f
  forearm, 404–418
  hand, 424–435, 425b, 426f
  major nerves of, 435–439
  movements in each region of, 442–444
  pectoral region, 379–387, 380f
  rotation of, 381f

Upper limb (Continued)
  summary of nerves and muscles, 435–444
  wrist, 418–424, 418b, 419f, 420b, 421f
Upper molars, posterior, roots of, 307f
Upper subscapular nerve, 400f, 401t
Ureter, 483f, 511f–512f, 523, 523b, 535f, 541f, 543f, 575f
  arterial supply to, 525f
  course and relationships of, 524f
  development of, 523b
Ureteropelvic junction, 525f
Urethra, 460f, 526f, 527–528, 527b, 535f, 539f
Urethral sphincters, nerve supply to, 528, 528b
Urethritis, 527b
Urinary bladder, development of, 509f
Urinary system, 508–530
Urinary tract stones, 521b
Urine, diluted or concentrated, 521
Urogenital hiatus, 460f
Urogenital system, immunity and, 177t
Urogenital triangle, 550–555, 550b, 551f, 553f
Uterine artery, 541f, 543f, 546f
Uterine cavity, 543f–544f
Uterine gland, 546f
Uterine involution, 366
Uterine tube, 541f, 542, 542b, 543f–544f, 548f
Uterus, 526f, 541f, 543–550, 543b–544b, 544f
  blood supply to, 543f, 544
  layers of, 544
  during pregnancy, 547f, 547b
  wall, 548f
Utricle, 316f, 535f
Uvea, 298
Uvula, 310f

V

'v' wave, 154
Vacuole
  in cells, 10f
  in spermatozoa, 354f
Vagal stimulation, 492f
Vagina, 460f, 526f, 543f–544f, 549–550, 550b
  conditions of, 550
Vaginal cervix, 543f

Vaginismus, 550
Vaginitis, 550
Vagotomy, 467f, 467b
Vagus nerve, 74, 92, 92b, 248, 248b, 279–280, 280f, 280b, 319f, 321f, 332, 486f
  left, 332f, 335f
  parasympathetic innervation from, 88
  right, 332f
Valgus (knock knee) malalignment, 601f
Valveless diploic veins, 234b
Varicose veins, 142
Varus (bowleg) malalignment, 601f
Vas deferens. See Ductus deferens
Vasa recta, 471f
Vasa vasorum, 139f
Vascular endothelial growth factor, 137–138
Vasculogenesis, 137–138
Vasectomy, 535b
Vasoactive intestinal polypeptide, 151
Vasoconstrictor area, 134
Vasoconstrictor fibres, 150
Vasoconstrictors, local, 151
Vasodilator area, 134
Vasodilator fibres, 150
Vasodilators, for hypertension, 149
Vasogenic shock, 159
Vasomotion, 155
Vasomotor centre, 149
Vasopressin, 151
Vastus intermedius muscle, 595t–596t
Vastus lateralis muscle, 589f, 595t–596t, 599f, 610f–611f
Vastus medialis muscle, 589f, 595t–596t, 599f, 610f
VC. See Vital capacity
Veins, 107f
  development of, 137b
  function of, 143
  of lymph nodes, 162f
  of posterior triangle, 320
  structure of, 139f
Vena caval opening, 75f
Vena comitans, 403f
Venae cordis minimae, 125–126
Venous blood, volume of, 153
Venous blood pressure, 153
  pathological variation in, 153
  physiological variation in, 153
  regulation of, 153

Venous drainage
  of brain, 269–270
  of chest wall, 77–78, 77f
  of face, 290, 290b
  of hand, 435, 437f
  of orbit, 296f
  of palate, 313
  of scalp, 237–238
  of thyroid gland, 331
  of tongue, 312, 312f
Venous lakes, 546f
Venous pulse, 153–154, 153b
Venous return, 134
Venous return curves, 136, 136f
Venous thrombosis, 142–143, 143b
Venous valve, 139f
Ventilation-perfusion ratio, 109, 109b
Ventral horn, of spinal cord, 210f
Ventral pancreas, 478f
Ventral posterior nucleus of thalamus, 213f
Ventral rami, of spinal nerves, 91b, 222f
Ventral respiratory group, 110, 110f
Ventral root, of nerve, 220f, 222f
Ventral tegmental decussation, 250
Ventricular contraction, 122, 130
Ventricular fibrillation, 132–133
Ventricular pressure, 130
Ventricular relaxation, 130
Ventricular system, of brain, 260–262
Venules, 143, 155f
Vertebra prominens, 193f, 194, 194b
Vertebrae, 188, 191–195, 191f–192f, 191b
  cervical, 193–194, 193f–194f, 193b
  internal architecture of, 192, 192f, 192b
  lumbar, 194–195, 195b, 196f
  thoracic, 194, 194b, 195f
Vertebral arch, 191, 191f
Vertebral artery, 266, 268f, 319f, 333f
Vertebral body, 36f, 73f, 191f, 193f–196f
Vertebral canal, 197f
Vertebral column, 188–204, 189f
  blood supply of, 201–202, 202b, 203f
  bones of, 191–195
  intervertebral joints of, 195–200
  movements of, 200, 200t, 201f

Vertebral column (Continued)
  muscles of trunk in, 202–204, 204f, 205t–206t, 207f
  nerve supply of, 201–202, 202b
  stability of, 200–201, 202f
Vertex, 239f
Vertical line, of tibia, 597f
Very-low-density lipoproteins (VLDL), 500
Vessel diameter, 146
Vessels, of neck, 331–332
Vestibular fold, 329f
Vestibular ligament, 330f
Vestibular nerve, 316f
Vestibule, of mouth, 310f
Vestibulocochlear nerve, 277
Vestibulospinal tract, 216, 216b
Villus, 363f, 469, 472f
Visceral peritoneum, 453f
Visceral (pulmonary) pleura, 95, 98f, 101f
Viscosity, of blood, 146
Visual area, 269
Visual axis, 297f
Visual pathway, 272–273, 273b, 274f
Vital capacity (VC), 103, 103b
Vitamin(s), 505–506
Vitamin A, 505
Vitamin B$_1$ (thiamine), 505–506
Vitamin B$_2$ (riboflavin), 506
Vitamin B$_6$ (pyridoxine), 506
Vitamin B$_{12}$, 506
  deficiency anaemia, 170
  for red blood cell synthesis, 167
Vitamin C (ascorbic acid), 506
Vitamin D, 506
Vitamin E, 506
Vitamin K, 506, 506b
Vitreous chamber, 297f
VLDL. See Very-low-density lipoproteins
Vocal fold, 329f
Vocal ligament, 330f
Volkmann canals, in compact bone, 32f
Vomer, 305f
von Willebrand disease, 176b

W
Walking, 636, 637f
  cycle, 636, 636b, 638f
Warfarin, 176

Weber paralysis, 251b
White adipose tissue, 502
White matter, 210f, 212, 245f
White pulp, of spleen, 163f
White ramus communicans, 90, 91f
Whole-body protein deficiency, 504b
Wilson disease, 481b
Woven bone, 31
Wrist, 418–424, 418f, 419f, 420b, 421f
  attachments, action and innervation of muscles, 423t–424t
  carpus, 420, 420f, 420b
  drop, 398f
  joint, 420–424
    movements, 420–424, 420b–421b
    of upper limb, 443, 443t

X
'x' wave, 154
'x$_1$' wave, 154
Xerostomia, 489
Xiphisternal junction, 69, 69f
Xiphoid process, 68f, 69
XYY syndrome, 532

Y
'y' wave, 154
Yellow marrow, of bone, 30f
Yolk sac cavity, 362f

Z
Zellweger syndrome, 14b
Zinc, 507
Zollinger-Ellison syndrome, 491b
Zona fasciculata, 343, 344f
Zona glomerulosa, 343, 344f
Zona orbicularis, 584f–585f
Zona pellucida, 357f
Zona reticularis, 343–344, 344f
Zygomatic arch, 235f, 285f
Zygomatic bone, 235f, 240f, 243f, 295f
Zygomaticofacial artery, 291f
Zygomaticofacial nerve, 276f
Zygomaticofacial vein, 291f
Zygomaticotemporal artery, 291f
Zygomaticotemporal nerve, 239f, 276f
Zygomaticotemporal vein, 291f
Zygomaticus major, 293f, 294
Zygomaticus minor, 293f, 294
Zymogen granules, 483f